ANTIEPILEPTIC DRUGS TO TREAT PSYCHIATRIC DISORDERS

MEDICAL PSYCHIATRY

ANTIEPILEPTIC DRUGS TO TREAT PSYCHIATRIC DISORDERS

Edited by

Susan L. McElroy
Lindner Center of HOPE
Mason, Ohio, USA
University of Cincinnati College of Medicine
Cincinnati, Ohio, USA

Paul E. Keck, Jr.
Lindner Center of HOPE
Mason, Ohio, USA
University of Cincinnati College of Medicine
Cincinnati, Ohio, USA

Robert M. Post
Bipolar Collaborative Network
Bethesda, Maryland, USA

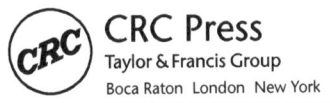

CRC Press
Taylor & Francis Group
Boca Raton London New York

CRC Press is an imprint of the
Taylor & Francis Group, an **informa** business

First published 2008 by Informa Healthcare USA, Inc.

Published 2021 by CRC Press
Taylor & Francis Group
6000 Broken Sound Parkway NW, Suite 300
Boca Raton, FL 33487-2742

© 2008 by Taylor & Francis Group, LLC
CRC Press is an imprint of Taylor & Francis Group, an Informa business

No claim to original U.S. Government works

ISBN 13: 978-0-8493-8259-8 (hbk)

Library of Congress Cataloging-in-Publication Data

Antiepileptic drugs to treat psychiatric disorders / edited by Susan L. McElroy, Paul E. Keck Jr., Robert M. Post.
      p. ; cm. — (Medical psychiatry ; 39)
   Includes bibliographical references and index.
   ISBN-13: 978-0-8493-8259-8 (hardcover : alk. paper)
   ISBN-10: 0-8493-8259-9 (hardcover : alk. paper) 1. Anticonvulsants—
   Therapeutic use. 2. Mental illness—Chemotherapy. 3. Psychopharmacology. I. McElroy, Susan L. II. Keck, Paul E. III. Post, Robert M. IV. Series.
      [DNLM: 1. Anticonvulsants—pharmacology. 2. Anticonvulsants—
   therapeutic use. 3. Epilepsy—drug therapy. 4. Mental Disorders—drug
   therapy. W1 ME421SM v.39 2008 / QV 85 A6296 2008]
      RC483.5.A56A62 2008
      616.8'53061—dc22
                                                                    2008013317

Visit the Taylor & Francis Web site at
http://www.taylorandfrancis.com

and the CRC Press Web site at
http://www.crcpress.com

Preface

Antiepileptic drugs (AEDs) are increasingly being used in conditions other than epilepsy. Their most common area of "off label" use is in psychiatric and neuropsychiatric disorders. Indeed, several AEDs, namely, divalproex sodium, lamotrigine, and carbamazepine, have United States Food and Drug Administration indications for treating various phases of bipolar disorder. These drugs are now viewed as major treatments for bipolar disorder, with new AEDs often evaluated as potential mood-stabilizing agents.

However, it has become evident that anticonvulsant properties do not automatically predict antimanic or mood-stabilizing effects and that many AEDs have beneficial psychotropic properties, whether or not they have efficacy in bipolar disorder. Thus, while some anticonvulsants may have antimanic or mood-stabilizing effects, others may have anxiolytic, anticraving, or weight-loss properties. Controlled trials that have been conducted suggest that divalproex sodium, lamotrigine, and topiramate may have beneficial effects when used adjunctively with antipsychotics in schizophrenia; that pregabalin may reduce anxiety in generalized anxiety disorder; that topiramate may reduce alcohol and cocaine craving and use in substance use disorders; and that topiramate and zonisamide may have therapeutic effects on eating pathology and weight in eating disorders. These properties need to be properly "profiled" so that they can be used to benefit patients and further advance neuropsychopharmacology research.

Despite the increased clinical use and research with these compounds, the diverse therapeutic effects of AEDs in psychiatric and neuropsychiatric conditions has not been gathered and scrutinized in one source for many years. This book provides an accessible and expert summary of currently available AEDs and their use in these disorders for the mental health professional. The first part of the book (chaps. 1–6) reviews available AEDs, their putative mechanisms of action in epilepsy and other neurological conditions in which they are commonly used (e.g., neuropathic pain and migraine), their use in epilepsy and neuropsychiatric disorders often accompanied by seizures and psychopathology (e.g., traumatic brain injury, autism, and intellectual disability), and their side effects and drug-drug interactions. The second part of the book (chaps. 7–20) is devoted to providing a state-of-the-art update on the use of AEDs in a broad range of psychiatric disorders and disorders with psychiatric features. Specifically, AEDs in the treatment of bipolar and major depressive disorder, schizophrenia, anxiety disorders, substance use disorders, eating and weight disorders, impulse control disorders, personality disorders, sleep disorders, and fibromyalgia are reviewed and summarized. The third part of the book (chap. 21) discusses the mechanisms of action of currently available AEDs potentially underlying their therapeutic properties in psychiatric conditions, with a focus on mood disorders.

Altogether, this book provides a resource for clinicians who treat patients with psychiatric and neuropsychiatric conditions and for researchers studying the expanding role of AEDs in neuropsychopharmacology.

Susan L. McElroy
Paul E. Keck, Jr.
Robert M. Post

Contents

III. Potential Psychotropic Mechanisms of Action of AEDs

Contributors

Robert M. Anthenelli Tri-State Tobacco and Alcohol Research Center, Department of Psychiatry, University of Cincinnati College of Medicine and Cincinnati Veterans Affairs Medical Center, Cincinnati, Ohio, U.S.A.

Lesley M. Arnold Department of Psychiatry, University of Cincinnati College of Medicine, Cincinnati, Ohio, U.S.A.

Heather A. Berlin Department of Psychiatry, Mount Sinai School of Medicine, New York, New York, U.S.A.

Charles L. Bowden Department of Psychiatry, University of Texas Health Science Center at San Antonio, San Antonio, Texas, U.S.A.

Jan Lewis Brandes Department of Neurology, Vanderbilt University School of Medicine and Nashville Neuroscience Group, Nashville, Tennessee, U.S.A.

Joseph R. Calabrese Bipolar Disorders Center for Intervention and Services Research, Case Western Reserve University, Cleveland, Ohio, U.S.A.

Doo-Sup Choi Departments of Psychiatry and Psychology and Molecular Pharmacology, Mayo Clinic, Rochester, Minnesota, U.S.A.

Leslie Citrome New York University School of Medicine, New York, New York, and Clinical Research and Evaluation Facility, Nathan S. Kline Institute for Psychiatric Research, Orangeburg, New York, U.S.A.

Mark A. Frye Department of Psychiatry and Psychology, Mayo Clinic, Rochester, Minnesota, U.S.A.

Keming Gao Bipolar Disorders Center for Intervention and Services Research, Case Western Reserve University, Cleveland, Ohio, U.S.A.

Aaron P. Gibson College of Pharmacy, University of New Mexico, Albuquerque, New Mexico, U.S.A.

David R. P. Guay Department of Experimental and Clinical Pharmacology, College of Pharmacy, University of Minnesota and Consultant, Division of Geriatrics, HealthPartners, Inc., Minneapolis, Minnesota, U.S.A.

Anna I. Guerdjikova Lindner Center of HOPE, Mason, and Department of Psychiatry, University of Cincinnati College of Medicine, Cincinnati, Ohio, U.S.A.

Daniel Hall-Flavin   Department of Psychiatry and Psychology, Mayo Clinic, Rochester, Minnesota, U.S.A.

Benjamin L. Handen   Western Psychiatric Institute and Clinic, University of Pittsburgh School of Medicine, Pittsburgh, Pennsylvania, U.S.A.

Jaimee L. Heffner   Tri-State Tobacco and Alcohol Research Center, Department of Psychiatry, University of Cincinnati College of Medicine, Cincinnati, Ohio, U.S.A.

Eric Hollander   Department of Psychiatry, Mount Sinai School of Medicine, New York, New York, U.S.A.

James I. Hudson   Department of Psychiatry, Harvard Medical School, Boston, and McLean Hospital, Belmont, Massachusetts, U.S.A.

Candace S. Johnson   Tri-State Tobacco and Alcohol Research Center, Department of Psychiatry, University of Cincinnati College of Medicine, Cincinnati, Ohio, U.S.A.

Kyle M. Kampman   University of Pennsylvania School of Medicine, Philadelphia, Pennsylvania, U.S.A.

Victor M. Karpyak   Department of Psychiatry and Psychology, Mayo Clinic, Rochester, Minnesota, U.S.A.

Paul E. Keck, Jr.   Lindner Center of HOPE, Mason, and Department of Psychiatry, University of Cincinnati College of Medicine, Cincinnati, Ohio, U.S.A.

David E. Kemp   Bipolar Disorders Center for Intervention and Services Research, Case Western Reserve University, Cleveland, Ohio, U.S.A.

Hochang Lee   Department of Psychiatry, Johns Hopkins School of Medicine, Baltimore, Maryland, U.S.A.

Catherine Mancini   Department of Psychiatry and Behavioural Neurosciences, McMaster University and Anxiety Disorders Clinic, McMaster University Medical Centre—HHS, Hamilton, Ontario, Canada

Maria McCarthy   Western Psychiatric Institute and Clinic, University of Pittsburgh School of Medicine, Pittsburgh, Pennsylvania, U.S.A.

Susan L. McElroy   Lindner Center of HOPE, Mason, and Department of Psychiatry, University of Cincinnati College of Medicine, Cincinnati, Ohio, U.S.A.

Andrew McKeon   Department of Neurology, Mayo Clinic, Rochester, Minnesota, U.S.A.

David J. Muzina   Cleveland Clinic Psychiatry and Psychology, Cleveland, Ohio, U.S.A.

Erik Nelson   Department of Psychiatry, University of Cincinnati Medical Center, Cincinnati, Ohio, U.S.A.

Nick C. Patel   College of Pharmacy, University of Georgia, Department of Psychiatry & Health Behavior, Medical College of Georgia, Augusta, Georgia, U.S.A.

Beth Patterson   Anxiety Disorders Clinic, McMaster University Medical Centre—HHS, Hamilton, Ontario, Canada

David T. Plante   Department of Psychiatry, Massachusetts General Hospital and McLean Hospital, Harvard Medical School, Boston, Massachusetts, U.S.A.

Harrison G. Pope, Jr.   Department of Psychiatry, Harvard Medical School, Boston, and McLean Hospital, Belmont, Massachusetts, U.S.A.

Robert M. Post   Head, Bipolar Collaborative Network, Bethesda, Maryland, U.S.A.

Vani Rao   Department of Psychiatry, Johns Hopkins School of Medicine, Baltimore, Maryland, U.S.A.

Patricia Roy   Department of Psychiatry, Johns Hopkins School of Medicine, Baltimore, Maryland, U.S.A.

Ihsan M. Salloum   Department of Psychiatry, University of Miami, Miller School of Medicine, Miami, Florida, U.S.A.

Vivek Singh   Department of Psychiatry, University of Texas Health Science Center at San Antonio, San Antonio, Texas, U.S.A.

Sharon B. Stanford   Department of Psychiatry, University of Cincinnati College of Medicine, Cincinnati, Ohio, U.S.A.

Jeffrey R. Strawn   Lindner Center of HOPE, Mason, and Department of Psychiatry, University of Cincinnati College of Medicine, Cincinnati, Ohio, U.S.A.

Torbjörn Tomson   Department of Clinical Neuroscience, Karolinska Institutet, Stockholm, Sweden

Christine Truong   Anxiety Disorders Clinic, McMaster University Medical Centre—HHS, Hamilton, Ontario, Canada

Michael Van Ameringen   Department of Psychiatry and Behavioural Neurosciences, McMaster University and Anxiety Disorders Clinic, McMaster University Medical Centre—HHS, Hamilton, Ontario, Canada

K. M. A. Welch   Rosalind Franklin University of Medicine and Science and Department of Neurology, Chicago Medical School, Chicago, Illinois, U.S.A.

John W. Winkelman   Divisions of Sleep Medicine and Psychiatry, Brigham & Women's Hospital, Harvard Medical School, Boston, and the Sleep Health Center®, affiliated with Brigham & Women's Hospital, Brighton, Massachusetts, U.S.A.

Mary C. Zanarini   Laboratory for the Study of Adult Development, McLean Hospital, Belmont and the Department of Psychiatry, Harvard Medical School, Boston, Massachusetts, U.S.A.

Mechanisms of Action of Antiepileptic Drugs

Aaron P. Gibson
College of Pharmacy, University of New Mexico, Albuquerque, New Mexico, U.S.A.

Nick C. Patel
College of Pharmacy, University of Georgia, Department of Psychiatry & Health Behavior, Medical College of Georgia, Augusta, Georgia, U.S.A.

INTRODUCTION

Antiepileptic drugs (AEDs) have been utilized in the treatment of various psychiatric disorders for several decades. As early as the 1960s, it was recognized that AEDs had remedial effects on mood and behavior (1–4). Over time and with an accumulating body of evidence, the psychiatric application of AEDs has grown significantly, with a number of these agents being approved for specific disorders and considered mainstays of treatment. The precise mechanisms of action by which AEDs are useful in patients with epilepsy remain largely unknown. Elucidation of AED mechanisms of action in the context of epilepsy has been challenging because agents may have multiple mechanisms of action and there may be differential interaction at the same molecular target between agents. However, a common link among proposed AED mechanisms of action involves the modulation of excitatory and inhibitory neurotransmission via effects on ion channels and certain neurotransmitters. Although an assumption that the putative mechanisms of action of AEDs are similar for both epilepsy and psychiatric disorders may be premature (5), a clearer understanding of the mechanisms of action of AEDs is necessary and may lead to improved predictions about an agent's clinical efficacy and safety profiles across the spectrum of psychiatric disorders. Ultimately, this information may contribute toward targeted treatment interventions with a higher likelihood of response and a subsequent improvement in patient psychosocial functioning.

In this chapter, we summarize the concepts of ion channel and neurotransmitter modulation and review the proposed mechanisms of action of AEDs currently available, as well as those in the development pipeline.

TARGETS FOR ANTIEPILEPTIC DRUGS

Ion Channels

Voltage-dependent sodium (Na^+) and calcium (Ca^{2+}) channels are the primary ion channels associated with the mechanisms of action of a large number of available AEDs. Both ion channels are involved in the regulation of the flow of cations from the extracellular space into the neuron (6) (Fig. 1).

Voltage-dependent Na^+ channels control the intrinsic excitatory activity of the nervous system. At resting membrane potential, Na^+ channels are closed, or inactive. During depolarization, these channels are opened, or activated, and allow for the influx of Na^+ ions. Spontaneous closure of Na^+ channels, termed "inactivation," follows, and it is during this period of time that Na^+ channels cannot be reactivated to evoke another action potential. Repolarization of the membrane potential results in the recovery of Na^+ channels to a resting state (7,8). The duration of

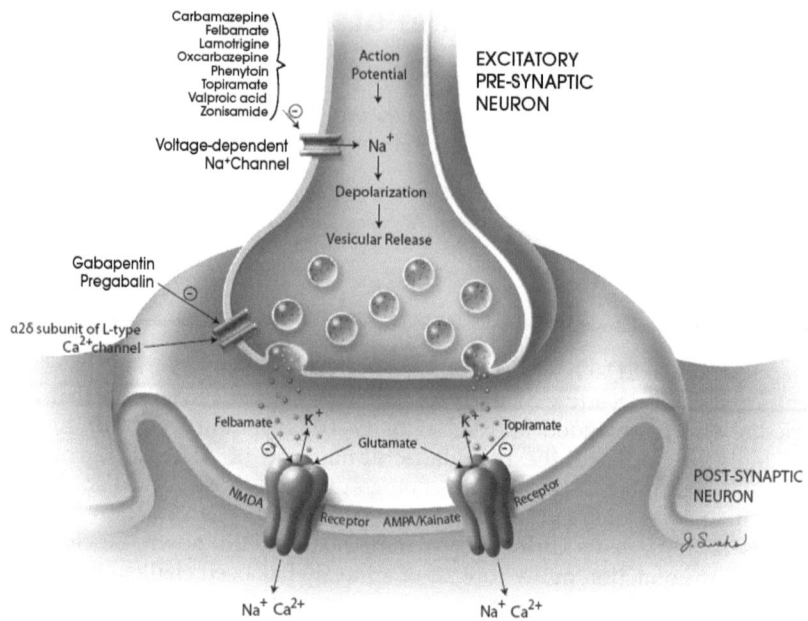

FIGURE 1 Putative mechanisms of action of AEDs at an excitatory synapse in the central nervous system. *Abbreviations*: AEDs, antiepileptic drugs; Na⁺, sodium; Ca²⁺, calcium; K⁺, potassium; NMDA, N-methyl-ᴅ-aspartate; AMPA, α-amino-3-hydroxy-5-methyl-isoxazole-4-propionic acid. *Source*: Illustrations courtesy of Jennifer A. Suehs, Biomedical Illustration, Austin, Texas, U.S.A.

Na^+ channel inactivation is brief, permitting sustained high-frequency repetitive firing. Prolongation of the inactive state of these Na^+ channels limits neuronal excitability and confers protection against partial and generalized tonic-clonic seizures (7,8).

Voltage-dependent Ca^{2+} channels are also involved in the excitatory activity of neurons and have been implicated in epileptogenic discharge. Ca^{2+} channels are classified on the basis of the membrane potential at which they are activated: low- and high-threshold (9). Low-threshold T-type Ca^{2+} channels are expressed in thalamic relay neurons, whereas high-threshold Ca^{2+} channels are distributed throughout the nervous system (10). T-type Ca^{2+} channels play a role in the regulation of the T current, which amplifies thalamic oscillations including the characteristic three-per-second spike and wave pattern of absence seizures (11). Some AEDs reduce the flow of Ca^{2+} through T-type channels, thereby reducing the T current (10,11). High-threshold Ca^{2+} channels may also be potential drug targets as these channels have been reported to be associated with neuronal processes important in epileptogenesis. Specifically, the L-type Ca^{2+} channels may modulate the slow after hyperpolarization and the release of neurotransmitters (12,13).

Voltage-dependent potassium (K^+) channels are involved in the repolarization of the membrane potential. Activators of the K^+ channel limit neurons from rapidly firing and may have antiepileptic effects (14).

GABA-Mediated Inhibition

Gamma-aminobutyric acid (GABA) is one of the main inhibitory neurotransmitters and is widely distributed throughout the central nervous system (15). Enhanced GABAergic tone has a broad antiepileptic effect (16) and has served as a principal target for a number of AEDs. Mechanisms by which GABA-mediated inhibition occurs include augmentation of GABA-activated currents and increased GABA supply (Fig. 2).

GABA acts upon three receptor classes: $GABA_A$, $GABA_B$, and $GABA_C$ (17,18). $GABA_A$ receptors are ligand-operated ion channels that increase the influx of chloride anions (Cl⁻) following postsynaptic GABA binding. This, in turn, results in hyperpolarization of the neuron. The role of ionotropic $GABA_A$ receptors in the context of AED mechanisms of action is well established, specifically allosteric modulation related to benzodiazepines and barbiturates. $GABA_B$ receptors are G-protein coupled metabotropic receptors that, when activated, lead to increased K^+ conductance, decreased Ca^{2+} entry, and suppression of the release of other neurotransmitters (15,19). It has been suggested that GABA binding to the $GABA_B$ receptor may result in activation of K^+ channels through a second messenger pathway involving arachidonic acid (20). Although the role of $GABA_B$ receptors is currently limited to potential treatments for absence seizures, enhanced GABA binding or allosteric receptor facilitation at these receptors may indeed have anti-epileptic effects in other types of seizure activity (18). The significance of $GABA_C$ receptors, which are also ligand-operated ion channels, in the brain is unclear (17).

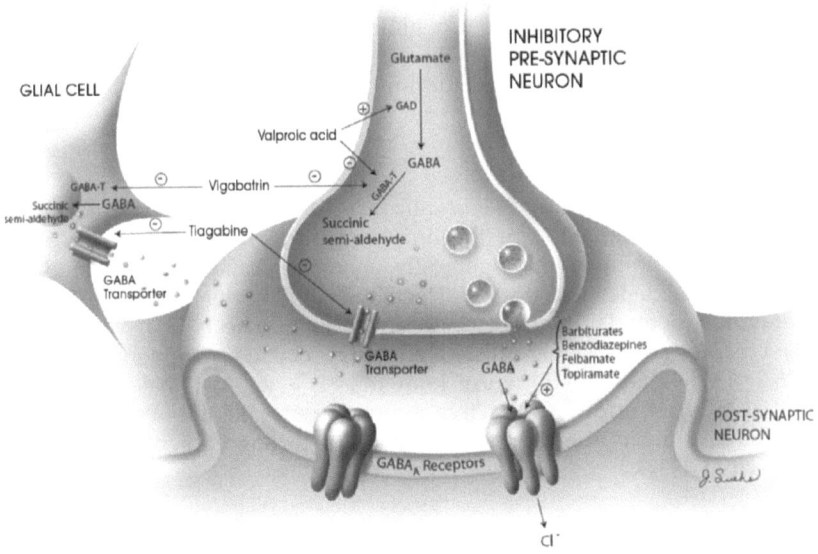

FIGURE 2 Putative mechanisms of action of AEDs at an inhibitory synapse in the central nervous system. *Abbreviations*: AEDs, antiepileptic drugs; Cl⁻, chloride; GABA, γ-aminobutyric acid; GAD, glutamic acid decarboxylase, GABA-T, GABA transaminase. *Source*: Illustrations courtesy of Jennifer A. Suehs, Biomedical Illustration, Austin, Texas, U.S.A.

In inhibitory presynaptic terminals, synthesis of GABA from glutamic acid is dependent on glutamic acid decarboxylase (GAD). Following vesicular release and subsequent receptor activation, GABA is removed from the synaptic cleft by GABA reuptake transporters into presynaptic terminals and glial cells. Thereafter, GABA is recycled for release from presynaptic terminals or metabolized into succinic acid semialdehyde by GABA transaminase (GABA-T) (21,22). Increased availability of GABA resulting from increased GABA production by GAD, inhibition of reuptake transporters, or inhibition of GABA-T forms the basis of antiseizure actions of some newer AEDs.

Glutamate-Mediated Excitation

In contrast to GABA, glutamate is the major excitatory neurotransmitter in the brain (21), and decreased glutamatergic tone may have antiepileptic effects. Glutamate has activity at the following ionotropic glutamate receptors: N-methyl-D-aspartate (NMDA), α-amino-3-hydroxy-5-methyl-isoxazole-4-propionic acid (AMPA), and kainate (Fig. 1). These ligand-operated ion channels allow for the flow of Na^+ and Ca^{2+}. The NMDA receptor subtype is associated with slower kinetics compared with the AMPA/kainate receptor subtypes. Antagonism at NMDA and AMPA receptors are targets for AEDs, although few available AEDs act via these particular mechanisms (23).

Glutamate also has activity at metabotropic glutamate (mGlu) receptors, which have effects on neuronal excitability through G-protein-linked modifications of enzymes and ion channels. The mGlu receptors are predominantly presynaptic and have been classified into three groups (I, II, and III). Furthermore, these receptors have been shown to modify glutamatergic and GABAergic neuro-transmission. Antagonists of group I mGlu receptors and agonists of groups II and III mGlu receptors may confer anticonvulsant properties (23,24).

Serotonergic Neurotransmission

Recent developments suggest that serotonin may have a role in epileptogenesis. Specifically, serotonin depletion in the brain may lower the seizure threshold, increasing the susceptibility to audiogenically, chemically, and electrically induced seizures. Current evidence indicates that activation of the serotonin-2C (5-HT$_{2C}$) receptor may be a potential mechanism for antiepileptic effects (25). Mutations of the 5-HT$_{2C}$ receptor genes have been shown to be associated with increased risk of seizure (26,27), while administration of known 5-HT$_{2C}$ agonists has reduced sei-zure activity (28,29). In addition, selective serotonin reuptake inhibitors have been reported to have anticonvulsant properties, perhaps through potentiation of sero-tonergic activity (30,31).

MECHANISMS OF ACTION OF ANTIEPILEPTIC DRUGS

The mechanisms of action of AEDs are diverse, affecting one or more of the potential targets detailed above. In this section, we review the proposed mecha-nisms of action of first- and second-generation AEDs, as well as those related to compounds in development. Table 1 summarizes the mechanisms of action of available AEDs.

TABLE 1 Summary of Principal Mechanisms of Action of First- and Second-Generation Antiepileptic Drugs

AED	Na$^+$ channel blockade	Ca^{2+} channel blockade	K$^+$ channel activation	Enhanced GABA-mediated inhibition	Reduced glutamate-mediated excitation	Other
First-Generation						
Carbamazepine	+	+	+			
Valproate	+			+		
Phenytoin	+					
Benzodiazepines				+		
Barbiturates				+		
Ethosuximide		+				
Acetazolamide						+
Second-Generation						
Felbamate	+	+		+	+	
Topiramate	+	+		+	+	
Gabapentin		+		+		
Zonisamide	+	+				
Lamotrigine	+	+				
Levetiracetam						+
Oxcarbazepine	+	+	+			
Pregabalin		+				
Tiagabine				+		
Vigabatrin				+		

Abbreviations: AED, antiepileptic drug; Ca^{2+}, calcium; GABA, γ-aminobutyric acid; K$^+$, potassium; Na$^+$, sodium.

First-Generation Antiepileptic Drugs
First-generation AEDs include carbamazepine, valproate, phenytoin, benzodiazepines, barbiturates, ethosuximide, and acetazolamide.

Carbamazepine
Carbamazepine (CBZ) limits the sustained, high-frequency repetitive firing of neurons through the stabilization of inactivated Na$^+$ channels in a voltage-, frequency-, and time-dependent fashion (32). The effectiveness of CBZ in extending the inactive phase of Na$^+$ channels and inhibiting action potentials may be higher during periods of neuronal excitability as Na$^+$ channels may be more susceptible to blockade. It has also been reported that CBZ may have activity at K$^+$ channels, thereby increasing K$^+$ conductance (33), and may inhibit L-type Ca^{2+} channels (34). The CBZ metabolite 10,11-epoxycarbamazepine also contributes to CBZ's overall antiepileptic effects by limiting repetitive neuronal firing (35). Given these pharmacological properties, CBZ is widely used for the treatment of partial seizures and primary generalized tonic-clonic seizures.

CBZ has also been shown to have effects on GABA$_A$ (36) and GABA$_B$ (37,38) receptors, inhibits the increase in intracellular free Ca^{2+} induced by NMDA and glycine (39), and inhibits glutamate release (40). Furthermore, it has been reported that CBZ may act as an antagonist of adenosine A$_1$ receptors (41) and "peripheral-type" benzodiazepine receptors (42), attenuate cAMP production (43), induce the release of serotonin (40,44,45), and decrease the release of the excitatory amino acid aspartate (42). It is unclear whether these additional pharmacological effects of CBZ contribute to its antiepileptic profile.

Valproate

Much of the attention regarding the broad antiepileptic effects of valproate (VPA) has focused on its mechanisms of action on the GABAergic system. Specifically, VPA has been shown to elevate whole-brain GABA levels and potentiate response by inhibiting GABA-T and activating GAD (16). VPA may enhance GABA release via activity at presynaptic $GABA_B$ receptors, and may block GABA reuptake (46). The GABAergic effects of VPA may indeed be specific to certain regions of the brain (16).

At therapeutically relevant concentrations, VPA has been reported to suppress sustained, high-frequency repetitive neuronal firing through blockade of voltage-dependent Na^+ channels (35). VPA may reduce peak conductance and slow the recovery of Na^+ channels from fast inactivation, although these proposed actions remain controversial (47–49). VPA may also reduce T-type Ca^{2+} channel currents, although this effect is considered modest (50). Other potential mechanisms involved in the antiepileptic effects of VPA are the inhibition of NMDA-evoked depolarizations (51,52) and decreased release of aspartate (53).

Phenytoin

Similar to CBZ, phenytoin (PHT) is effective for partial and generalized seizures as it limits the repetitive firing of action potentials mediated through Na^+ channel blockade (54). This action is both voltage- and frequency-dependent; PHT binds with greater affinity to channels in the inactive state, and reductions in neuronal firing are increased after depolarization and decreased after hyperpolarization (54,55). PHT may also modulate postsynaptic, high voltage-activated Ca^{2+} currents (56), possibly contributing to its antiseizure activity. Other effects of PHT include potentiation of GABA at the $GABA_A$ receptor (36), attenuation of glutamatergic neurotransmission (57,58), and inhibition of Ca^{2+}/calmodulin-regulated protein phosphorylation and neurotransmitter release (59).

Benzodiazepines

Benzodiazepines (BZDs) have broad-spectrum AED activity, with demonstrated efficacy in partial and generalized tonic-clonic seizures, as well as status epilepticus. Clonzepam, diazepam, and lorazepam are among the most commonly used BZDs for seizure treatment. The antiseizure properties of BZDs result primarily from their positive allosteric activation of postsynaptic $GABA_A$ receptors and subsequent increase in the frequency of Cl^- channel opening and augmentation of GABA-activated currents. BDZs do not affect the mean open time or conductance of the Cl^- channel (60). In the absence of GABA, however, BZDs are unable to directly activate $GABA_A$ receptors (61). In addition to their established effects on the GABAergic system, there is evidence suggesting that high concentrations of BZDs inhibit currents carried by Na^+ and Ca^{2+} channels (62,63). This action indicates that BZDs, like CBZ, VPA, and PHT, can reduce sustained, high-frequency repetitive neuronal firing.

Barbiturates

The principal molecular target of barbiturates, including phenobarbital (PB) and pentobarbital (PTB), is the $GABA_A$ receptor. These agents are similar to BZDs in that the antiepileptic effects result from enhanced effects of GABA-evoked Cl^- currents. In contrast to BZDs, PB and PTB increase the mean open time of Cl^- channels, but do not affect the frequency of Cl^- channel openings or conductance of these channels (60,64). Furthermore, PB and PTB can directly activate $GABA_A$ receptors without the presence of GABA (61). Secondary mechanisms by which PB and PTB may exert antiseizure activity include blockade of voltage-dependent Na^+ channels at high concentrations (62), blockade of high-voltage-activated Ca^{2+} channels (65), and inhibition of the AMPA/kainate glutamate receptor subtype (66).

Ethosuximide
Ethosuximide (ESM) is protective against absence seizures because it reduces T-type Ca^{2+} currents in thalamic relay neurons (11). ESM has also been reported to have effects on Na^+ and K^+ currents (67,68), and $GABA_A$ receptors (69). However, it is unclear whether these secondary mechanisms are associated with ESM's antiepileptic properties.

Acetazolamide
While acetazolamide (AZM) has been used as an adjunct for the treatment of partial and generalized seizures for several decades, its precise mechanism of action related to antiepileptic effects remains unclear. Because AZM is a potent carbonic anhydrase inhibitor (70), it has been postulated that an increase in carbon dioxide concentrations in neurons and an increase in pH and a decrease in bicarbonate concentrations in neuroglia may confer its antiseizure activity (71). As a result of these ionic and acid-base changes, extracellular K^+ concentrations decrease, leading to reduced neuronal excitability (72). Extracellular pH levels also decrease, leading to NMDA receptor blockade (73) and enhanced $GABA_A$ receptor response (74).

Second-Generation Antiepileptic Drugs
Second-generation AEDs include felbamate, topiramate, gabapentin, zonisamide, lamotrigine, levetiracetam, oxcarbazepine, pregabalin, tiagabine, and vigabatrin.

Felbamate
Felbamate (FBM) possesses clinical efficacy across a wide spectrum of seizure types, which is attributed to its multiple mechanisms of action (75). FBM is unique in that it is the first to have direct action on the NMDA glutamate receptor subtype. Clinically relevant concentrations of FBM have been shown to inhibit NMDA/glycine-stimulated increases in intracellular Ca^{2+} (76) and block NMDA receptor–mediated excitatory postsynaptic potentials (77). Although some studies suggest that FBM block of NMDA receptors occurs at the glycine recognition site (78,79), other studies indicate that this may not be the site at which FBM interacts (80,81). FBM may also inhibit AMPA/kainate receptors (82).

In addition to its glutamatergic effects, FBM potentiates GABA responses via barbiturate-type action on $GABA_A$ receptors (80,83). FBM may stabilize the inactive state of voltage-dependent Na^+ channels, reducing sustained, high-frequency repetitive firing of neurons (84). Furthermore, FBM may reduce high-voltage-activated Ca^{2+} channels (85).

The clinical use of FBM has been limited due to postmarketing surveillance reports of fatal aplastic anemia and hepatoxicity (75).

Topiramate

Topiramate (TPM) has multiple mechanisms of action and is protective against partial and generalized tonic-clonic seizures (86). TPM reduces Na^+ and Ca^{2+} currents through prolongation of the inactivation of Na^+ channels (87) and inhibition of L-type Ca^{2+} channels (88), respectively. These effects are believed to be associated with TPM's ability to reduce sustained repetitive firing and spontaneous bursting (89).

TPM interacts with both the GABA and glutamate neurotransmitter systems. TPM potentiates GABA response by acting at a site on the $GABA_A$ receptor to enhance Cl^- influx and increase Cl^- currents (90). The $GABA_A$ receptor site at which TPM acts is different from that at which BZDs act because flumazenil, a BZD antagonist, does not reverse the effects of TPM (91). TPM also blocks the AMPA/ kainate glutamate receptor subtype (92).

Interestingly, TPM is a weak inhibitor of carbonic anhydrase (93). It is unlikely that this property contributes much to TPM's antiepileptic profile as it does for AZM, a potent carbonic anhydrase inhibitor.

Gabapentin

Gabapentin (GBP) is a synthetic GABA analogue that is recommended as adjunct treatment of partial seizures with or without secondary generalization (94). GBP does not act at $GABA_A$ or $GABA_B$ receptors despite its structural similarities with GABA (95), nor does it affect GABA reuptake or synthesis (61). GBP has been shown to promote GABA release (96), although the precise mechanism of this is unknown. It has been reported that GBP enhances nipecotic acid–promoted nonvesicular release of GABA (97).

GBP has not been found to have direct actions on voltage-dependent Na^+ channels. However, GBP may modulate Ca^{2+} currents through high-affinity binding at the $\alpha_2\delta$-subunit of the L-type voltage-dependent Ca^{2+} channels (98). The relevance of this pharmacological property in the context of GBP's antiepileptic effects remains unclear.

Zonisamide

Zonisamide (ZNS) is a broad-spectrum AED that is effective against localization-related and generalized epilepsies, and appears to be potent in progressive myoclonic epilepsy syndromes (99). Effects on ion channels are believed to be the principal mechanisms involved in ZNS's antiseizure activity; specifically, ZNS inhibits voltage-dependent Na^+ channels and T-type Ca^{2+} channels (100,101).

Other potential pharmacological actions of ZNS possibly conferring antiepileptic properties include weak inhibition of carbonic anhydrase (102), inhibition of monoamine release and metabolism (103,104), inhibition of K^+-evoked glutamate release (105), and free radical scavenging (106).

Lamotrigine

Lamotrigine (LTG) was initially developed as a folate antagonist on the basis of the presumed correlation between antifolate and antiepileptic properties (107).

However, LTG shares a pharmacological profile similar to that of CBZ and PHT and possesses a broad spectrum of clinical efficacy for generalized tonic-clonic, partial, and absence seizures. LTG inhibits sustained repetitive neuronal firing by prolonging the inactivated state of Na^+ channels in a voltage-, use-, and frequency-dependent manner (108,109). LTG may exhibit selectivity for neurons that synthesize glutamate and aspartate (110). In addition to its effects on Na^+ channels, LTG reduces Ca^{2+} currents through a voltage-dependent block of Ca^{2+} channels (111,112).

Levetiracetam

Levetiracetam (LEV) is a recent AED effective against partial seizures with or without secondary generalization (113). The mechanism of action of LEV is unknown, as this agent does not interact with either Na^+, Ca^{2+}, or K^+ channels or the GABAergic or glutamatergic systems. It is believed that LEV does interact with a specific synaptic membrane-binding site because LEV is displaced from this site by ESM, pentylenetetrazol, and bemegride (114). Recently, the binding site of LEV was identified as SV2A, a synaptic vesicle protein. Although the molecular action of SVA2 is unclear, there is a strong correlation between the affinities of agents that act at SVA2 and antiseizure potency (115).

Oxcarbazepine

Oxcarbazepine (OXC) is effective against partial and generalized tonic-clonic seizures (61). Structurally related to CBZ, OXC displays similar mechanisms of action, including inhibition of voltage-dependent Na^+ and Ca^{2+} channels (116,117) and increased K^+ conductance (116). The block of high-threshold Ca^{2+} currents by OXC may reduce presynaptic glutamate release (117,118). OXC does have an active monohydroxy metabolite, known as licarbazepine, which may contribute to its antiepileptic properties.

Pregabalin

Similar to GBP, pregabalin (PGL) is a GABA analogue and is effective against partial seizures (119). The putative mechanism of action of PGL is the binding to voltage-dependent Ca^{2+} channels at the $\alpha_2\delta$-subunit and modulation of Ca^{2+} influx. PGL also reduces the synaptic release of several neurotransmitters, including noradrenaline and glutamate, possibly accounting for its ability to reduce neuronal excitability (120).

Tiagabine

Tiagabine (TGB) is an analogue of nipecotic acid, a GABA uptake antagonist. TGB exhibits potent inhibition of neuronal and glial GABA uptake transporters, specifically the GABA transporter-1 (121). This pharmacological action results in higher GABA levels in the synaptic cleft and possibly, a subsequent prolongation of the duration of the peak inhibitory postsynaptic current (122). TGB is effective as an adjunct for partial seizures with or without secondary generalization (123).

Vigabatrin

Vigabatrin (VGB) is a structural analogue of GABA that demonstrates protection against partial seizures with or without secondary generalization (124). VGB is an irreversible inhibitor of GABA-T, particularly in neurons (125). Inhibition of GABA-T leads to elevated brain GABA levels and enhancement of inhibitory neurotransmission. VGB may also block glial cell uptake of GABA (126).

Future Antiepileptic Drugs

Some compounds in the AED pipeline have been based on the structures of existing AEDs and target conventional molecular targets. These include: CBZ analogues racemic licarbazepine and (S)-licarbazepine acetate; VPA-like agents valrocemide, valnoctamide, propylisopropyl acetamide, and isovaleramide; selective partial BZD receptor agonists such as TPA023 and ELB139; FBM analogue flurofelbamate and another carbamate, RWJ-333369; and, LEV analogues brivaracetam and seletracetam (127).

Other compounds in the pipeline capitalize on novel mechanisms of action potentially conferring antiepileptic effects. Lacosamide is a functional amino acid that may allosterically inhibit NMDA receptors. Talampanel is a 2,3-benzodiazepine selective noncompetitive AMPA receptor antagonist, while NS1209 is a water-soluble, competitive AMPA receptor antagonist. Retigabine and ICA-27243 are KCNQ K^+ channel openers with and without $GABA_A$ receptor modulation, respectively. Finally, ganaxolone is a neuroactive steroid that modulates $GABA_A$ receptors, and rufinamide is a triazole that is believed to have Na^+ channel–blocking activity (127).

CONCLUSION

Available and future AEDs exhibit a variety of mechanisms of action that may be attributed to antiseizure activity. Oftentimes, multiple pharmacological actions have been suggested for one agent. In the treatment of epilepsy, an AED's pharmacological profile may reliably predict its spectrum of clinical efficacy, as well as certain side effects. It is unknown whether an AED's mechanisms of action relevant to epilepsy are indeed relevant to its psychotropic effects. As AEDs have and will continue to be valuable in the treatment armamentarium of psychiatric disorders, a better understanding of their pharmacology may help guide the field to determine which psychiatric disorders or symptoms where particular agents could be of benefit.

REFERENCES

1. Dalby MA. Antiepileptic and psychotropic effect of carbamazepine (Tegretol) in the treatment of psychomotor epilepsy. Epilepsia 1971; 12(4):325–334.
2. Lambert PA, Carraz G, Borselli S, et al. Neuropsychotropic action of a new anti-epileptic agent: depamide. Ann Med Psychol (Paris) 1966; 124(5):707–710.
3. Okuma T, Kishimoto A, Inoue K, et al. Anti-manic and prophylactic effects of carbamazepine (Tegretol) on manic depressive psychosis. A preliminary report. Folia Psychiatr Neurol Jpn 1973; 27(4):283–297.
4. Okuma T, Kishimoto A. A history of investigation on the mood stabilizing effect of carbamazepine in Japan. Psychiatry Clin Neurosci 1998; 52(1):3–12.
5. Ovsiew F. Antiepileptic drugs in psychiatry. J Neurol Neurosurg Psychiatry 2004; 75 (12):1655–1658.
6. Barchi RL. Ion channel mutations affecting muscle and brain. Curr Opin Neurol 1998; 11(5):461–468.
7. Errington AC, Stohr T, Lees G. Voltage gated ion channels: targets for anticonvulsant drugs. Curr Top Med Chem 2005; 5(1):15–30.

8. Ragsdale DS, Avoli M. Sodium channels as molecular targets for antiepileptic drugs. Brain Res Brain Res Rev 1998; 26(1):16–28.
9. Hoffman F, Biel M, Flockerzi V. Molecular basis for Ca2+ channel diversity. Annu Rev Neurosci 1994; 17:399–418.
10. Stefani A, Spadoni F, Bernardi G. Voltage-activated calcium channels: targets of antiepileptic drug therapy? Epilepsia 1997; 38(9):959–965.
11. Coulter DA, Huguenard JR, Prince DA. Characterization of ethosuximide reduction of low-threshold calcium current in thalamic neurons. Ann Neurol 1989; 25(6):582–593.
12. Blalock EM, Chen KC, Vanaman TC, et al. Epilepsy-induced decrease of L-type Ca2+ channel activity and coordinate regulation of subunit mRNA in single neurons of rat hippocampal 'zipper' slices. Epilepsy Res 2001; 43(3):211–226.
13. Otoom S, Hasan Z. Nifedipine inhibits picrotoxin-induced seizure activity: further evidence on the involvement of L-type calcium channel blockers in epilepsy. Fundam Clin Pharmacol 2006; 20(2):115–119.
14. Porter RJ, Rogawski MA. New antiepileptic drugs: from serendipity to rational discovery. Epilepsia 1992; 33(suppl 1):S1–S6.
15. Olsen RW, Avoli M. GABA and epileptogenesis. Epilepsia 1997; 38(4):399–407.
16. Loscher W. Valproate: a reappraisal of its pharmacodynamic properties and mechanisms of action. Prog Neurobiol 1999; 58(1):31–59.
17. Chebib M. GABAC receptor ion channels. Clin Exp Pharmacol Physiol 2004; 31(11): 800–804.
18. Sperk G, Furtinger S, Schwarzer C, et al. GABA and its receptors in epilepsy. Adv Exp Med Biol 2004; 548:92–103.
19. Gage PW. Activation and modulation of neuronal K+ channels by GABA. Trends Neurosci 1992; 15(2):46–51.
20. Misgeld U, Bijak M, Jarolimek W. A physiological role for GABAB receptors and the effects of baclofen in the mammalian central nervous system. Prog Neurobiol 1995; 46(4):423–462.
21. Meldrum BS. Update on the mechanism of action of antiepileptic drugs. Epilepsia 1996; 37(suppl 6):S4–S11.
22. Tillakaratne NJ, Medina-Kauwe L, Gibson KM. Gamma-Aminobutyric acid (GABA) metabolism in mammalian neural and nonneural tissues. Comp Biochem Physiol A Physiol 1995; 112(2):247–263.
23. Meldrum BS. Glutamate as a neurotransmitter in the brain: review of physiology and pathology. J Nutr 2000; 130(suppl 4S):S1007–S1015.
24. Moldrich RX, Chapman AG, De Sarro G, et al. Glutamate metabotropic receptors as targets for drug therapy in epilepsy. Eur J Pharmacol 2003; 476(1–2):3–16.
25. Isaac M. Serotonergic 5-HT2C receptors as a potential therapeutic target for the design antiepileptic drugs. Curr Top Med Chem 2005; 5(1):59–67.
26. Applegate CD, Tecott LH. Global increases in seizure susceptibility in mice lacking 5-HT2C receptors: a behavioral analysis. Exp Neurol 1998; 154(2):522–530.
27. Heisler LK, Chu HM, Tecott LH. Epilepsy and obesity in serotonin 5-HT2C receptor mutant mice. Ann N Y Acad Sci 1998; 861:74–78.
28. Gobert A, Rivet JM, Lejeune F, et al. Serotonin (2C) receptors tonically suppress the activity of mesocortical dopaminergic and adrenergic, but not serotonergic, pathways: a combined dialysis and electrophysiological analysis in the rat. Synapse 2000; 36(3):205–221.
29. Hutson PH, Barton CL, Jay M, et al. Activation of mesolimbic dopamine function by phencyclidine is enhanced by 5-HT (2C/2B) receptor antagonists: neurochemical and behavioral studies. Neuropharmacology 2000; 39(12):2318–2328.
30. Pasini A, Tortorella A, Gale K. The anticonvulsant action of fluoxetine in substantia nigra is dependent upon endogenous serotonin. Brain Res 1996; 724(1):84–88.
31. Favale E, Audenino D, Cocito L, et al. The antcionvulsant effect of citalopram as an indirect evidence of serotonergic impairment in human epileptogenesis. Seizure 2003; 12(5):316–318.
32. Macdonald RL. Antiepileptic drug actions. Epilepsia 1989; 30(suppl 1):S19–S28 (discussion S64–S18).
33. Zona C, Tancredi V, Palma E, et al. Potassium currents in rat cortical neurons in culture are enhanced by the antiepileptic drug carbamazepine. Can J Physiol Pharmacol 1990; 68(4):545–547.

34. Ambrosio AF, Silva AP, Malva JO, et al. Carbamazepine inhibits L-type Ca2+ channels in cultured rat hippocampal neurons stimulated with glutamate receptor agonists. Neuropharmacology 1999; 38(9):1349–1359.
35. McLean MJ, Macdonald RL. Carbamazepine and 10,11-epoxycarbamazepine produce use- and voltage-dependent limitation of rapidly firing action potentials of mouse central neurons in cell culture. J Pharmacol Exp Ther 1986; 238(2):727–738.
36. Granger P, Biton B, Faure C, et al. Modulation of the gamma-aminobutyric acid type A receptor by the antiepileptic drugs carbamazepine and phenytoin. Mol Pharmacol 1995; 47(6):1189–1196.
37. Motohashi N, Ikawa K, Kariya T. GABAB receptors are up-regulated by chronic treatment with lithium or carbamazepine. GABA hypothesis of affective disorders? Eur J Pharmacol 1989; 166(1):95–99.
38. Zhang JD, Saito K. Carbamazepine facilitates effects of GABA on rat hippocampus slices. Zhongguo Yao Li Xue Bao 1997; 18(3):230–233.
39. Hough CJ, Irwin RP, Gao XM, et al. Carbamazepine inhibition of N-methyl-D-aspartate-evoked calcium influx in rat cerebellar granule cells. J Pharmacol Exp Ther 1996; 276(1): 143–149.
40. Waldmeier PC, Baumann PA, Wicki P, et al. Similar potency of carbamazepine, oxcarbazepine, and lamotrigine in inhibiting the release of glutamate and other neurotransmitters. Neurology 1995; 45(10):1907–1913.
41. Biber K, Walden J, Gebicke-Harter P, et al. Carbamazepine inhibits the potentiation by adenosine analogues of agonist induced inositolphosphate formation in hippocampal astrocyte cultures. Biol Psychiatry 1996; 40(7):563–567.
42. Post RM, Weiss SR, Chuang DM. Mechanisms of action of anticonvulsants in affective disorders: comparisons with lithium. J Clin Psychopharmacol 1992; 12(1 suppl):S23–S35.
43. Chen G, Pan B, Hawver DB, et al. Attenuation of cyclic AMP production by carbamazepine. J Neurochem 1996; 67(5):2079–2086.
44. Dailey JW, Reith ME, Yan QS, et al. Carbamazepine increases extracellular serotonin concentration: lack of antagonism by tetrodotoxin or zero Ca2+. Eur J Pharmacol 1997; 328(2-3):153–162.
45. Dailey JW, Reith ME, Yan QS, et al. Anticonvulsant doses of carbamazepine increase hippocampal extracellular serotonin in genetically epilepsy-prone rats: dose response relationships. Neurosci Lett 1997; 227(1):13–16.
46. Fraser CM, Sills GJ, Butler E, et al. Effects of valproate, vigabatrin and tiagabine on GABA uptake into human astrocytes cultured from fetal and adult brain tissue. Epileptic Disord 1999; 1(3):153–157.
47. Albus H, Williamson R. Electrophysiologic analysis of the actions of valproate on pyramidal neurons in the rat hippocampal slice. Epilepsia 1998; 39(2):124–139.
48. Remy S, Urban BW, Elger CE, et al. Anticonvulsant pharmacology of voltage-gated Na+ channels in hippocampal neurons of control and chronically epileptic rats. Eur J Pharmacol 2003; 17(12):2648–2658.
49. Vreugdenhil M, van Veelan CW, van Rijen PC, et al. Effect of valproic acid on sodium currents in cortical neurons from patients with pharmaco-resistant temporal lobe epilepsy. Epilepsy Res 1998; 32(1–2):309–320.
50. Kelly KM, Gross RA, Macdonald RL. Valproic acid selectively reduces the low-threshold (T) calcium current in rat nodose neurons. Neurosci Lett 1990; 116(1-2):233–238.
51. Gean PW, Huang CC, Hung CR, et al. Valproic acid suppresses the synaptic response mediated by the NMDA receptors in rat amygdalar slices. Brain Res Bull 1994; 33(3): 333–336.
52. Zeise ML, Kasparow S, Zieglgansberger W. Valproate suppresses N-methyl-D-aspartate-evoked, transient depolarizations in the rat neocortex in vitro. Brain Res 1991; 544(2): 345–348.
53. Chapman AG, Croucher MJ, Meldrum BS. Anticonvulsant activity of intracerebroventricularly administered valproate and valproate analogues. A dose-dependent correlation with changes in brain aspartate and GABA levels in DBA/2 mice. Biochem Pharmacol 1984; 33(9):1459–1463.
54. McLean MJ, Macdonald RL. Multiple actions of phenytoin on mouse spinal cord neurons in cell culture. J Pharmacol Exp Ther 1983; 227(3):779–789.

55. Schwarz JR, Grigat G. Phenytoin and carbamazepine: potential- and frequency-dependent block of Na currents in mammalian myelinated nerve fibers. Epilepsia 1989; 30(3):286–294.
56. Schumacher TB, Beck H, Steinhauser C, et al. Effects of phenytoin, carbamazepine, and gabapentin on calcium channels in hippocampal granule cells from patients with temporal lobe epilepsy. Epilepsia 1998; 39(4):355–363.
57. Tunnicliff G. Basis of antiseizure action of phenytoin. Gen Pharmacol 1996; 27(7):1091–1097.
58. Wamil AW, McLean MJ. Phenytoin blocks N-methyl-D-aspartate responses of mouse central neurons. J Pharmacol Exp Ther 1993; 267(1):218–227.
59. DeLorenzo RJ. Calmodulin systems in neuronal excitability: a molecular approach to epilepsy. Ann Neurol 1984; 16(suppl): S104–S114.
60. Twyman RE, Rogers CJ, Macdonald RL. Differential regulation of gamma-aminobutyric acid receptor channels by diazepam and phenobarbital. Ann Neurol 1989; 25(3):213–220.
61. White HS. Comparative anticonvulsant and mechanistic profile of the established and newer epileptic drugs. Epilepsia 1999; 40(suppl 5):S2–S10.
62. McLean MJ, Macdonald RL. Benzodiazepines, but not beta carbolines, limit high frequency repetitive firing of action potentials of spinal cord neurons in cell culture. J Pharmacol Exp Ther 1988; 244(2): 789–795.
63. Skerritt JH, Werz MA, McLean MJ, et al. Diazepam and its anomalous p-chloro-derivative Ro 5-4864: comparative effects on mouse neurons in cell culture. Brain Res 1984; 310(1): 99–105.
64. Macdonald RL, Rogers CJ, Twyman RE. Barbiturate regulation of kinetic properties of the GABAA receptor channel of mouse spinal neurones in culture. J Physiol 1989; 417: 483–500.
65. Rogawski MA, Porter RJ. Antiepileptic drugs: pharmacological mechanisms and clinical efficacy with consideration of promising developmental stage compounds. Pharmacol Rev 1990; 42(3):223–286.
66. Marszalec W, Narahashi T. Use-dependent pentobarbital block of kainate and quisqualate currents. Brain Res 1993; 608(1):7–15.
67. Crunelli V, Leresche N. Block of thalamic T-type Ca(2+) channels by ehtosuximide is not the whole story. Epilepsy Curr 2002; 2(2):53–56.
68. Leresche N, Parri HR, Erdemli G, et al. On the action of the anti-absence drug ethosuximide in the rat and cat thalamus. J Neurosci 1998; 18(13):4842–4853.
69. Kaminski RM, Tochman AM, Dekundy A, et al. Ethosuximide and valproate display high efficacy against lindane-induced seizures in mice. Toxicol Lett 2004; 154(1–2):55–60.
70. Reiss WG, Oles KS. Acetazolamide in the treatment of seizures. Ann Pharmacother 1996; 30(5):514–519.
71. Woodbury DM, Engstrom FL, White HS, et al. Ionic and acid-base regulation of neurons and glia during seizures. Ann Neurol 1984; 16(suppl): S135–S144.
72. Schwartzkroin PA. Cellular electrophysiology of human epilepsy. Epilepsy Res 1994; 17 (3):185–192.
73. Traynelis SF, Cull-Candy SG. Proton inhibition of N-methyl-D-aspartate receptors in cerebellar neurons. J Physiol 1990; 345(6273):347–350.
74. Krishek BJ, Amato A, Connolly CN, et al. Proton sensitivity of the GABA (A) receptor is associated with the receptor subunit composition. J Physiol 1996; 492(pt 2):431–443.
75. Pellock JM. Felbamate. Epilepsia 1999; 40(suppl 5):S57–S62.
76. Taylor LA, McQuade RD, Tice MA. Felbamate, a novel antiepileptic drug, reverses N-methyl-D-aspartate/glycine-stimulated increases in intracellular Ca2+ concentration. Eur J Pharmacol 1995; 289(2):229–233.
77. Corradetti R, Pugliese AM. Electrophysiological effects of felbamate. Life Sci 1998; 63 (13):1075–1088.
78. McCabe RT, Wasterlain CG, Kucharczyk N, et al. Evidence for anticonvulsant and neuroprotectant action of felbamate mediated by strychnine-insensitive glycine receptors. J Pharmacol Exp Ther 1993; 264(3):1248–1252.
79. White HS, Harmsworth WL, Sofia RD, et al. Felbamate modulates the strychnine-insensitive glycine receptor. Epilepsy Res 1995; 20(1):41–48.
80. Rho JM, Donevan SD, Rogawski MA. Mechanism of action of the anticonvulsant felbamate: opposing effects on N-methyl-D-aspartate and gamma-aminobutyric acid A receptors. Ann Neurol 1994; 35(2):229–234.

81. Subramaniam S, Rho JM, Penix L, et al. Felbamate block of the N-methyl-D-aspartate receptor. J Pharmacol Exp Ther 1995; 273(2):878–886.
82. De Sarro G, Ongini E, Bertorelli R, et al. Excitatory amino acid neurotransmission through both NMDA and non-NMDA receptors is involved in the anticonvulsant activity of felbamate in DBA/2 mice. Eur J Pharmacol 1994; 262(1–2):11–19.
83. Rho JM, Donevan SD, Rogawski MA. Barbiturate-like actions of the propanediol dicarbamates felbamate and meprobamate. J Pharmacol Exp Ther 1997; 280(3):1383–1391.
84. Taglialatela M, Ongini E, Brown AM, et al. Felbamate inhibits cloned voltage-dependent Na+ channels from human and rat brain. Eur J Pharmacol 1996; 316(2–3):373–377.
85. Stefani A, Calabresi P, Pisani A, et al. Felbamate inhibits dihydropyridine-sensitive calcium channels in central neurons. J Pharmacol Exp Ther 1996; 277(1):121–127.
86. Privitera MD. Topiramate: a new antiepileptic drug. Ann Pharmacother 1997; 31(10):1164–1173.
87. Zona C, Ciotti MT, Avoli M. Topiramate attenuates voltage-gated sodium currents in rat cerebellar granule cells. Neurosci Lett 1997; 231(3):123–126.
88. Zhang X, Velumian AA, Jones OT, et al. Modulation of high-voltage-activated calcium channels in dentate granule cells by topiramate. Epilepsia 2000; 41(suppl 1):S52–S60.
89. DeLorenzo RJ, Sombati S, Coulter DA. Effects of topiramate on sustained repetitive firing and spontaneous recurrent seizure discharges in cultured hippocampal neurons. Epilepsia 2000; 41(suppl 1): S40–S44.
90. White HS, Brown SD, Woodhead JH, et al. Topiramate enhances GABA-mediated chloride flux and GABA-evoked chloride currents in murine brain neurons and increases seizure threshold. Epilepsy Res 1997; 28(3):167–179.
91. White HS, Brown SD, Woodhead JH, et al. Topiramate modulates GABA-evoked currents in murine cortical neurons by a nonbenzodiazepine mechanism. Epilepsia 2000; 41(suppl 1): S17–S20.
92. Gibbs JW, Sombati S, DeLorenzo RJ, et al. Cellular actions of topiramate: blockade of kainate-evoked inward currents in cultured hippocampal neurons. Epilepsia 2000; 41(suppl 1):S10–S16.
93. Shank RP, Gardocki JF, Vaught JL, et al. Topiramate: preclinical evaluation of structurally novel anticonvulsant. Epilepsia 1994; 35(2):450–460.
94. Morris GL. Gabapentin. Epilepsia 1999; 40(suppl 5):S63–S70.
95. Taylor CP, Gee NS, Su TZ, et al. A summary of mechanistic hypotheses of gabapentin pharmacology. Epilepsy Res 1998; 29(3):233–249.
96. Honmou O, Oyelese AA, Kocsis JD. The anticonvulsant gabapentin enhances promoted release of GABA in hippocampus: a field potential analysis. Brain Res 1995; 692(1-2):273–277.
97. Honmou O, Kocsis JD, Richerson GB. Gabapentin potentiates the conductance increase induced by nipecotic acid in CA1 pyramidal neurons in vitro. Epilepsy Res 1995; 20(3):193–202.
98. Gee NS, Brown JP, Dissanayake VU, et al. The novel anticonvulsant drug, gabapentin (Neurontin): binds to the alpha2delta subunit of a calcium channel. J Biol Chem 1996; 271(10):5768–5776.
99. Sobieszek G, Borowicz KK, Kimber-Trojnar Z, et al. Zonisamide: a new antiepileptic drug. Pol J Pharmacol 2003; 55(5):683–689.
100. Schauf CL. Zonisamide enhances slow sodium inactivation in Myxicola. Brain Res 1987; 413(1):185–188.
101. Suzuki S, Kawakami K, Nishimura S, et al. Zonisamide blocks T-type calcium channel in cultured neurons of rat cerebral cortex. Epilepsy Res 1992; 12(1):21–27.
102. Masuda Y, Karasawa T. Inhibitory effect of zonisamide on human carbonic anhydrase in vitro. Arzneimittelforschung 1993; 43(4):416–418.
103. Kawata Y, Okada M, Murakami T, et al. Effects of zonisamide on K+ and Ca2+ evoked release of monamine as well as K+ evoked intracellular Ca2+ mobilization in rat hippocampus. Epilepsy Res 1999; 35(3):173–182.
104. Okada M, Kaneko S, Hirano T, et al. Effects of zonisamide on dopaminergic system. Epilepsy Res 1995; 22(3):193–205.

105. Okada M, Kawata Y, Mizuno K, et al. Interaction between Ca2+, K+, carbamazepine and zonisamide on hippocampal extracellular glutamate monitored with a microdialysis electrode. Br J Pharmacol 1998; 124(6):1277–1285.
106. Mori A, Noda Y, Packer L. The anticonvulsant zonisamide scavenges free radicals. Epilepsy Res 1998; 30(2):153–158.
107. Reynolds EH, Chanarin I, Milner G, et al. Anticonvulsant therapy, folic acid and vitamin B12 metabolism and mental symptoms. Epilepsia 1966; 7(4):261–270.
108. Cheung H, Kamp D, Harris E. An in vitro investigation of the action of lamotrigine on neuronal voltage-activated sodium channels. Epilepsy Res 1992; 13(2):107–112.
109. Zona C, Avoli M. Lamotrigine reduces voltage-gated sodium currents in rat central neurons in culture. Epilepsia 1997; 38(5):522–525.
110. Leach MJ, Marden CM, Miller AA. Pharmacological studies on lamotrigine, a novel potential antiepileptic drug: II. Neurochemical studies on the mechanism of action. Epilepsia 1986; 27(5):490–497.
111. Stefani A, Spadoni F, Siniscalchi A, et al. Lamotrigine inhibits Ca2+ currents in cortical neurons: functional implications. Eur J Pharmacol 1996; 307(1):113–116.
112. Wang SJ, Huang CC, Hsu KS, et al. Inhibition of N-type calcium currents by lamotrigine in rat amygdalar neurones. Neuroreport 1996; 7(18):3037–3040.
113. Hovinga CA. Levetiracetam: a novel antiepileptic drug. Pharmacotherapy 2001; 21 (11):1375–1388.
114. Noyer M, Gillard M, Matagne A, et al. The novel antiepileptic drug levetiracetam (ucb L059) appears to act via a specific binding site in CNS membranes. Eur J Pharmacol 1995; 286(2):137–146.
115. Lynch BA, Lambeng N, Nocka K, et al. The synaptic vesicle protein SV2A is the binding site for the antiepileptic drug levetiracetam. Proc Natl Acad Sci U S A 2004; 101 (26):9861–9866.
116. McLean MJ, Schmutz M, Wamil AW, et al. Oxcarbazepine: mechanisms of action. Epilepsia 1994; 35(suppl 3):S5–S9.
117. Stefani A, Pisani A, De Murtas M, et al. Action of GP 47779, the active metabolite of oxcarbazepine, on the corticostriatal system. II. Modulation of high-voltage-activated calcium currents. Epilepsia 1995; 36(10):997–1002.
118. Calabresi P, de Murtas M, Stefani A, et al. Action of GP 47779, the active metabolite of oxcarbazepine, on the cotricostriatal system. I. Modulation of corticostraital synaptic transmission. Epilepsia 1995; 36(10):990–996.
119. Warner G, Figgitt DP. Pregabalin: as adjunctive treatment of partial seizures. CNS Drugs 2005; 19(3):265–272 (discussion 273–274).
120. Taylor CP, Angelotti T, Fauman E. Pharmacology and mechanism of action of pregabalin: the calcium channel alpha2-delta (alpha2-delta) subunit as a target for antiepileptic drug discovery. Epilepsy Res 2007; 73(2):137–150.
121. Borden LA, Murali Dhar TG, Smith KE, et al. Tiagabine, SK&F 89976-A, CI-966, and NNC-711 are selective for the cloned GABA transporter GAT-1. Eur J Pharmacol 1994; 269(2):219–224.
122. Roepstorff A, Lambert JD. Comparison of the effect of the GABA uptake blockers, tiagabine and nipecotic acid, on inhibitory synaptic efficacy in hippocampal CA1 neurones. Neurosci Lett 1992; 146(2):131–134.
123. Leach JP, Brodie MJ. Tiagabine. Lancet 1998; 351(9097):203–207.
124. Mumford JP, Cannon DJ. Vigabatrin. Epilepsia 1994; 35(suppl 5):S25–S28.
125. Lippert B, Metcalf BW, Jung MJ, et al. 4-amino-hex-5-enoic acid, a selective catalytic inhibitor of 4-aminobutyric-acid aminotransferase in mammalian brain. Eur J Pharmacol 1977; 74(3):441–445.
126. Leach JP, Sills GJ, Majid A, et al. Effects of tiagabine and vigabatrin on GABA uptake into primary cultures of rat cortical astrocytes. Seizure 1996; 5(3):229–234.
127. Rogawski MA. Diverse mechanisms of antiepileptic drugs in the development pipeline. Epilepsy Res 2006; 69(3):273–294.

2 Antiepileptics in the Treatment of Epilepsy

Torbjörn Tomson
Department of Clinical Neuroscience, Karolinska Institutet, Stockholm, Sweden

INTRODUCTION

Effective antiepileptic drugs (AEDs) have been available for the treatment of epilepsy since bromides were introduced in 1857 (1). The introduction of phenobarbital in 1912 marked the next important step in the development of the therapeutic armamentarium (2), and phenobarbital is still a first-line AED in many parts of the world (3). A slow development followed and only a few major new AEDs—phenytoin, carbamazepine, and valproate—were introduced during the following close to eight decades. However, the situation has now changed dramatically with more than 10 new AEDs licensed since 1990. This has provided epileptologists and their patients with more treatment options, but at the same time the much more challenging task of being rational in drug selection.

From early on, AEDs have been tried successfully for conditions other than epilepsy and had their indications extended to pain syndromes, to migraine, and, in more recent years, to psychiatric conditions (4). While such exploration of new potential indications in the early years was mainly based on case series and small uncontrolled studies, randomized controlled trials in pain and psychiatric disorders are now frequently included in the original development program for a new potential AED. Nevertheless, much of the vast experience of the use of AEDs in the treatment of epilepsy should be of some relevance for their use in psychiatric patients. The objective of this chapter is, therefore, to provide an overview of the use of AEDs in the treatment of epilepsy. Specifically, general principles of the pharmacological treatment of epilepsy will be discussed, including drug selection and treatment strategies.

OBJECTIVES OF TREATMENT

Although the term "antiepileptic drug," or AED, is well established and widely accepted, it is a misnomer or at least somewhat misleading in that AEDs do not cure epilepsy. In fact clinical evidence for a modifying effect of AEDs on the natural course of the epileptic disorder is lacking. Antiseizure drugs might be a more appropriate designation, since these drugs are used to reduce the likelihood or risk of seizures in patients with "a disorder of the brain characterized by an enduring predisposition to generate epileptic seizures," the most recent definition of epilepsy suggested by the International League Against Epilepsy (ILAE) (5).

The general objective of treatment is to ensure the best possible quality of life according to the patient's individual circumstances. This is best achieved if the patient can be rendered free from seizures by the prophylactic use of AEDs. The primary objective of treatment is therefore to obtain complete seizure freedom with no or minimal adverse effects from AEDs. This is often, but far from always, a realistic goal. Dose-related adverse effects often limit the use of AEDs and a compromise may be necessary between the wish to control seizures completely and the risk of significant adverse effects. A common modified treatment goal is therefore a reduction in seizure frequency and severity without embarrassing or intolerable side effects. Initiation of treatment with AEDs should therefore always be preceded by an individual careful evaluation of the risks and benefits of the treatment under consideration.

AVAILABLE ANTIEPILEPTIC DRUGS

The discovery and development of AEDs that are available today have been based on different approaches. Phenytoin is the first example of an AED that was identified and characterized in animal experiments (6). Some major AEDs, e.g., valproate, were discovered by serendipity. Others were developed through structure modifications of well-known AEDs, e.g., oxcarbazepine and pregabalin. Many of the newer-generation AEDs have been developed through the National Institutes of Neurological Disorders and Stroke Antiepileptic Drug Screening and Development Program (7). However, very few AEDs have been designed to interact with specific neuronal mechanisms thought to be of importance for seizure occurrence, and these drugs, e.g., vigabatrin and tiagabine, have for different reasons been less successful.

Hence, in most cases, AEDs have not been developed to work through predefined mechanisms. As a result, our understanding of their mode of action is far from complete. Four different major targets can, however, be identified: (1) blockade of voltage-sensitive sodium channels; (2) enhanced gamma-aminobutyric acid (GABA)-mediated inhibition, either by raising GABA levels or by potentiating GABA responses; (3) blockade of voltage-sensitive calcium channels; and (4) decreased glutamate-mediated excitation (8). Many AEDs have multiple modes of action as well as mechanisms other than those mentioned. AEDs and their postulated modes of action are listed in Table 1.

TABLE 1 Proposed Mechanisms of Action of Older- and Newer-Generation AEDs

	Sodium channel blocker	Calcium channel blocker	GABA$_A$ receptor modulator	Inhibitor of GABA reuptake or metabolism	NMDA/AMPA/ Kainate receptor antagonist	Others
Older-generation AEDs						
Benzodiazepines			+			
Carbamazepine	+					
Ethosuximide		+				
Phenobarbital			+		+	
Phenytoin	+					
Valproate	+	+				
Newer-generation AEDs						
Felbamate	+	+	+		+	
Gabapentin		+				
Lamotrigine	+	+				
Levetiracetam		+				+
Oxcarbazepine	+					
Pregabalin		+				
Tiagabine				+		
Topiramate	+	+	+		+	
Vigabatrin				+		
Zonisamide	+	+	+			

Abbreviation: AEDs, antiepileptic drugs.
Source: Based on Ref. 8.

Partly because of these deficiencies in our understanding, AEDs are normally not classified by their mode of action, but usually by the time when they were introduced, as older-generation AEDs (phenobarbital, phenytoin, primidone, ethosuximide, carbamazepine, valproate and bensodiazepines) or newer-generation AEDs (drugs introduced from 1990 on).

PRINCIPLES FOR DRUG SELECTION

General Principles

Epilepsy is a very heterogeneous condition encompassing different disorders with varying manifestations, etiologies, and prognosies. On the basis of the recommendations of the ILAE (9), seizures are classified into two broad categories, partial (focal) or generalized, depending on whether seizure onset is in a limited part of the brain (focal onset) or whether both hemispheres are symmetrically engaged at onset (generalized onset) (Table 2). Additionally, taking into account etiology, age of onset, and typical combinations of seizures, the ILAE has suggested a classification of the epileptic syndrome of which seizures are the most obvious expression (10). However, because of limited available information, it is frequently difficult to classify the epileptic syndrome of patients with newly diagnosed epilepsy (11).

The seizure and epilepsy classifications are the basis for drug selection, because AEDs vary with respect to efficacy in different seizure types. The spectrum of efficacy by seizure types is summarized in Table 3 and is partly related to the mechanisms of AED action. However, since our knowledge of the pathophysiology underlying the different types of seizures and epilepsies is poor and our understanding of the modes of action of AEDs incomplete, the selection of a drug for an individual epilepsy patient is not mechanistically based. Rather, the choice depends on the clinical efficacy and effectiveness of a drug for the type of seizure or syndrome. The best evidence for efficacy and effectiveness comes from randomized clinical trials (RCTs), but a number of other variables need to be taken into account in selecting an AED for a patient. Examples of such drug properties that rarely lend themselves to an evidence-based analysis are idiosyncratic reactions, chronic toxicity, teratogenicity, pharmacokinetics including interaction potential, and drug formulations. Patient-specific variables of importance may be age, gender, genetic background, comorbidities, and comedication. In addition,

---

TABLE 2 International Classification of Epileptic Seizures

Partial seizures (seizures beginning locally)
   Simple partial seizures (consciousness not impaired)
   Complex partial seizures (with impairment of consciousness)
   Partial seizures secondarily generalized
Generalized seizures (bilaterally symmetrical and without local onset)
   Absence seizures
   Myoclonic seizures
   Clonic seizures
   Tonic seizures
   Tonic-clonic seizures
   Atonic seizures
Unclassified epileptic seizures (inadequate or incomplete data)

Source: Simplified after Ref. 9.

TABLE 3 Efficacy Spectrum of Different Antiepileptic Drugs for Some Common Seizure Types

	Partial seizures	Generalized tonicclonic seizures	Absence seizures	Myoclonic seizures
Older-generation AEDs				
Benzodiazepines	a	a		a
Carbamazepine	a	a	b	b
Ethosuximide			+	
Phenobarbital	a	a	b	
Phenytoin	a	a	b	b
Valproate	a	a	a	a
Newer-generation AEDs				
Felbamate	a	a		
Gabapentin	a	a		b
Lamotrigine	a	a	a	ab
Levetiracetam	a	a		a
Oxcarbazepine	a	a	b	b
Pregabalin	a	a		
Tiagabine	a	a	b	b
Topiramate	a	a		a
Vigabatrin	a	a	b	b
Zonisamide	a	a		a

[a]Indicates efficacy based on randomized controlled trials as well as other types of studies.
[b]Indicates that the drug may aggravate or precipitate the seizure type on the basis of uncontrolled studies or case reports.
Source: From Ref. 12.

drug cost and insurance coverage may be important (12). Recommendations from evidence-based treatment guidelines therefore need to be put into context.

Evidence-Based Treatment Guidelines

A number of organizations have published treatment guidelines on AED selection for new-onset or newly diagnosed epilepsy (12–14). While all have applied an evidence-based strategy, their methodologies vary and it is not surprising that their recommendations differ somewhat. The American Academy of Neurology and American Epilepsy Society restricted their analysis to the newer-generation AEDs (14). On the basis of the available randomized controlled trials, they concluded that there is evidence that gabapentin, lamotrigine, topiramate, and oxcarbazepine have efficacy as monotherapy in newly diagnosed adolescents and adults with either partial or mixed seizure disorders. They also concluded that there was evidence for the effectiveness of lamotrigine for newly diagnosed absence seizures in children, but that evidence for the effectiveness of the newer AEDs in other newly diagnosed generalized epilepsy syndromes was lacking. Unfortunately, since the standard older-generation AEDs were not included in this analysis, the question whether newer AEDs should replace these traditional agents was left unanswered.

The ILAE guidelines differ from those of the American Academy of Neurology and American Epilepsy Society in that all AEDs were included (12). Furthermore, these guidelines set up criteria for what was considered to be a clinically relevant study design, incorporating outcome measures, duration of trial, blinding, the use of acceptable comparators, and an acceptable statistical power to detect meaningful differences between treatment arms. The evidence was analyzed for different seizure types; for children, adults, and elderly, separately; and for two epilepsy syndromes. Overall, very few trials met the criteria for class I evidence. Out of 50 RCTs evaluated by meta-analyses, only four had class I evidence and two fulfilled criteria for class II evidence. There was an especially alarming lack of well-designed, properly conducted RCTs for patients with generalized seizures/epilepsies and for children in general (12).

On the basis of these guidelines, level A recommendations (highest level) were made for carbamazepine and phenytoin in adults with partial onset seizures. For children with partial onset seizures, oxcarbazepine received a level A recommendation, and for elderly patients with the same seizure type, gabapentin and lamotrigine were awarded a level A recommendation. The evidence was insufficient to make level A or B recommendations for several important seizure types and epilepsy syndromes, including generalized onset tonic-clonic seizures, absence seizures, and juvenile myoclonic epilepsy. Of note, the ILAE guidelines are probably the strictest and most demanding with respect to assessment of the available evidence and, as a result, leave the practitioner with little guidance in many instances.

The National Institute of Clinical Excellence (NICE) in the United Kingdom has also issued evidence-based guidelines, specifically assessing the role of the newer-generation AEDs (13). They conclude that evidence does not suggest differences in effectiveness in seizure control between newer and older AEDs in monotherapy. Furthermore, they conclude that evidence is inadequate to support the conclusion that newer AEDs are generally associated with improved quality of life. On the basis of these considerations, and given the higher cost of newer AEDs, the NICE guidelines conclude that first-line monotherapy should be an older AED, such as carbamazepine or valproate, unless these are unsuitable because of contraindications (13).

Although treatment guidelines are useful in that they provide an objective assessment on the basis of scientifically sound criteria, they are often of limited value for the practitioners in their choice of treatment for an individual patient. First, while guidelines may reveal differences in the level of evidence for efficacy between two AEDs, this is not equivalent to evidence of a difference in efficacy. Second, guidelines are outdated as soon as new RCTs are published. Although the ILAE guidelines were published in 2006, important RCTs have been published since. As an example, an RCT compared levetiracetam and carbamazepine in newly diagnosed patients with partial or generalized tonic-clonic seizures (15). This study, showing equivalent seizure freedom rates for the two treatment arms, would meet the class I criteria and qualify levetiracetam for a level A recommendation. Furthermore, the largest ever RCTs of AEDs in epilepsy, SANAD, have also been published after the treatment guidelines (16). In part A of this unblinded RCT, carbamazepine was compared with gabapentin, lamotrigine, oxcarbazepine, and topiramate in patients for whom carbamazepine was deemed to be standard treatment (16). On the basis of retention on the drug patients were randomized to, Marson et al. concluded that lamotrigine is clinically better than carbamazepine, the standard drug treatment for patients diagnosed with partial onset epilepsy (16). The apparent better outcome with lamotrigine was due to fewer withdrawals for adverse events, whereas there was no indication of lamotrigine being superior to carbamazepine in terms of seizure control. The conclusion that lamotrigine is clinically better than carbamazepine has been questioned, however, in part because some patients randomized to carbamazepine used a suboptimal drug formulation (immediate release rather than controlled release) with lower tolerability. Additionally, as SANAD was on open study, the reliability of assessments of tolerability could be biased, and this RCT would be downgraded to evidence level III in the ILAE system (12). With an identical open design, SANAD B assessed the effectiveness of valproate, lamotrigine, and topiramate for newly diagnosed generalized and unclassifiable epilepsy patients, for whom recruiting clinicians regarded valproate as standard treatment (16). Valproate was better tolerated than topiramate and more efficacious than lamotrigine. It was thus concluded that valproate should remain the first-line treatment for most patients with an idiopathic generalized epilepsy or seizures that are difficult to classify (16).

Finally, recommendations from treatment guidelines should not be over-interpreted since only some of the many variables of importance for drug selection can be assessed in an evidence-based analysis based on RCTs. Most would agree that in general carbamazepine is a drug of first choice for partial-onset seizures, while valproate has a role as a first-line AED for most forms of generalized-onset seizures. However, due to individual factors, there are special situations and populations where other priorities would seem more rational. Evidence-based analyses thus need to be put into clinical context, and it must ultimately remain for the individual physician to use his or her judgement and expertise when deciding on the most appropriate AED for a specific epilepsy patient (12).

Drug Selection in Special Populations

Some individual patient factors with bearing on AED selection are related to special situations such as specific stages in life, the occurrence of comorbidity, or concomitant medications. Several special populations requiring particular considerations in AED selection are briefly discussed below.

Women of Childbearing Potential

The treatment of women with epilepsy who are of childbearing potential needs special consideration because of the adverse fetal effects of AEDs. Older-generation AEDs have been associated with a two- to threefold increased risk for major congenital malformations in the offspring exposed to these agents in utero (17,18). Such risks, however, have to be balanced against the fetal and maternal risks associated with uncontrolled epileptic seizures during pregnancy (17). The strategy has been to use the appropriate AED for the patient's type of epilepsy in monotherapy at the lowest effective dosage to maintain seizure control throughout pregnancy. With this strategy, the vast majority of women with epilepsy will have uncomplicated pregnancies and give birth to normal children.

However, recent data indicate that there may be differences among AEDs with respect to teratogenic potential and this may affect drug selection for this special population. Independent prospective and retrospective pregnancy registries have reported particularly high risks with exposure to valproate, with malformation rates ranging from approximately 6% to 10% in monotherapy (19–22). This has been two to three times greater than with carbamazepine. The risk with valproate appears to be dose dependent, being significantly higher at daily doses above 800 to 1000 mg (23–25). Little is known of the teratogenic risks associated with the newer generation AEDs, with the exception of lamotrigine, a drug quite frequently used during pregnancy. The malformation rate with lamotrigine in monotherapy was initially reported to be 2.9% to 3.2% (22,26), similar to the risk associated with carbamazepine (22). However, one study found a dose-effect relationship also for lamotrigine teratogenicity, so that at lamotrigine dosages greater than 200 mg/day, the malformation rate was similar to that associated with exposure to valproate 600 to 1000 mg/day (22). In addition, the North American epilepsy and pregnancy registry recently reported a significantly increased risk for nonsyndromic cleft palate among infants exposed to lamotrigine during pregnancy (27).

Adding to the complexity of this issue, a retrospective study suggested that compared with carbamazepine and phenytoin, exposure to valproate in utero was associated with lower verbal IQ in the offspring. This association remained after adjustment for several potential confounding factors, including maternal IQ. It also seemed to be dose-dependent, appearing at dosages above 600 mg/day (28,29).

Although further studies are needed, a conservative approach to the use of valproate is recommended in women of childbearing potential, whereby alternative AEDs should be proposed to those planning pregnancies, so that satisfactory seizure control can be maintained. However, in the treatment of epilepsy during pregnancy, the importance of seizure control should not be neglected. Preliminary data suggest that this may be more difficult with lamotrigine and oxcarbazepine (30,31). The reason for this could be that the disposition of these two AEDs is markedly affected by pregnancy, with pronounced decreases in plasma concentrations as a consequence (32).

Prepregnancy counselling is essential, as any attempt for a major change in therapy (e.g., a switch from valproate to another AED) should ideally be accomplished before conception. Such counselling should include information on teratogenic risks, the importance of seizure control, possibilities and limitations with prenatal screening, drug-level monitoring, and breast-feeding.

The Elderly

Epilepsy is common among the elderly. In fact, the highest risk in life of acquiring epilepsy is after the age of 70 years (11). For many reasons, special considerations are justified in the management of epilepsy in older age. This may be due to differences in the spectrum of seizure types, etiological factors, comorbidities, and age-related pharmacokinetic and pharmacodynamic alterations (33). The latter contributes to an increased sensitivity to the effects of AEDs, and lower target dosages are generally appropriate. Drug selection may also be affected by age. The vast majority of people with epilepsy onset at high age have partial onset seizures, and broad-spectrum AEDs are thus not necessary. The increased sensitivity to adverse drug effects is also reflected in comparatively high dropout rates for tolerability problems among elderly in clinical trials (34). Unlike the situation in other age groups, RCTs in elderly with newly diagnosed epilepsy have reported better effectiveness (encompassing both efficacy and tolerability and reflected by greater retention on the treatment that the patient was allocated to) with some of the newer-generation AEDs (35,36). A 24-week double-blind study comparing lamotrigine and carbamazepine reported higher retention on lamotrigine, 71% versus 42% on carbamazepine (35). In this RCT, rated by the ILAE guidelines as class II evidence because of the short duration, the difference in retention was explained by more frequent dropouts for adverse events in the carbamazepine arm, as there were no apparent differences in efficacy. A larger and more recent class I study compared lamotrigine and gabapentin with carbamazepine in 593 elderly epilepsy patients (36). More patients allocated to lamotrigine (66%) and gabapentin (51%) remained on their treatment at 12 months compared with those allocated to carbamazepine (36%). Again, differences in retention were explained by withdrawals due to adverse effects. The unfavorable outcome for carbamazepine might, however, be explained by use of a suboptimal drug formulation since immediate-release carbamazepine tablets were used. A subsequent RCT compared lamotrigine and sustained-release carbamazepine in newly diagnosed epilepsy in elderly (37) and found no difference in effectiveness between the two. Retention on carbamazepine using the sustained-release formulation in this study was much higher (67%) than with immediate-release carbamazepine in the study by Rowan et al. (36). These data illustrate that AED tolerability is a major issue among the elderly and that special attention must be paid not only in the selection of the pharmacological substance but also in choosing the most appropriate drug formulation.

Comorbidities and Concomitant Medication

Comorbidity is another issue of major relevance for drug selection in epilepsy. A substantial proportion of patients with epilepsy at all ages have other conditions that may be of relevance in this respect. Some AEDs may have beneficial effects on that other condition that could be exploited. Psychiatric disorders, the topic of this book, is one example. Pain syndromes are another example where drugs such as carbamazepine (trigeminal neuralgia) or gabapentin or pregabalin (neuropathic pain) have documented efficacy (4). Selection of an AED with multiple therapeutic effects might be considered in epilepsy patients with coexisting psychiatric or medical syndromes. On the other hand, some adverse effects of AEDs may be particularly relevant in patients with specific comorbidities and should be used with caution or be avoided under certain circumstances. Use of vigabatrin and topiramate has been associated with an increased incidence of psychosis and depression (38). For similar reasons, levetiracetam should be used with caution in patients predisposed to mood disorders (39). Weight gain is a common side effect of valproate and pregabalin, which should be taken into account in the selection of treatment of epilepsy in obese persons. Because of its potential hepatotoxic effects, valproate should be used cautiously or avoided in patients with hepatic disease, while carbamazepine should not be used in patients with preexisting dysfunction of the cardiac conduction system or cardiomyopathies (40).

Many AEDs (phenobarbital, primidone, phenytoin, carbamazepine, and to a lesser extent oxcarbazepine) are potent enzyme inducers, whereas others inhibit drug-metabolizing enzymes (e.g., valproate). Hence, AEDs are frequently involved in pharmacokinetic drug-drug interactions (41,42). In addition to changing the disposition of other drugs that patients may use, AEDs can be the substrate for interactions caused by other pharmaceutical agents. It is beyond the scope of this chapter to discuss this in detail. The reader is referred to comprehensive reviews on the subject (41,42). Suffice it to say that many of these interactions can be managed by dose adjustments guided by drug-level monitoring, but some are so complicated, and with potentially serious consequences, that the combinations are best avoided. In such situations, preference might be given to an AED devoid of interaction potential.

TREATMENT STRATEGIES

Initiation of Treatment

Treatment with AEDs is generally considered indicated after recurrent (two or more) unprovoked seizures. It is seldom initiated after a first seizure, because only about half of those patients will have a recurrence (43). The likelihood of further seizures, however, is considerably higher after two seizures. Long-term prophylactic use of AEDs is also not indicated after provoked seizures, but there are situations where treatment might be started after a first attack. This could be considered when the likelihood of further seizures is high and the consequences of such seizures can be expected to be particularly serious, e.g., in a fragile elderly patient with seizure onset after a stroke. On the other hand, some patients with very short and mild seizures with long intervals might prefer to stay off treatment.

The present strategy is based on the assumption that treatment with AEDs is purely symptomatic and does not affect the natural course of epilepsy. However, it has been debated for more than a century whether early aggressive treatment could modify the long-term prognosis and possibly prevent the development of chronic refractory epilepsy (44) or, if used prophylactically after an insult (e.g., traumatic brain injury) but before seizure onset, might modify the risk of developing epilepsy. Randomized placebo-controlled studies have failed to show any effect of AEDs on the development of epilepsy after such insults (45). The effects of immediate versus deferred AED treatment after onset of unprovoked seizures have also recently been assessed in RCTs (46,47). These studies indicate that while early treatment after seizure onset may have an effect on seizure control in the short term, it does not affect long-term remission (46,47).

Monotherapy or Polytherapy

Monotherapy with the appropriate AED according to the type of seizure or epilepsy syndrome and taking other patient-specific factors into account has been the prevailing treatment strategy in epilepsy since the 1970s (48). Monotherapy is preferred to combination treatment in newly diagnosed epilepsy since (1) it is effective in the majority of patients, (2) drug-drug interactions are avoided, (3) polytherapy makes it difficult to evaluate the contribution of individual AEDs, (4) polytherapy may increase the risk of chronic toxicity, and (5) the risk of paradoxical seizure aggravation is probably higher with polytherapy. Some 50% to 60% of patients with newly diagnosed epilepsy can expect to achieve a satisfactory seizure control with an appropriate AED as monotherapy (48,49). Whether to change to another monotherapy or to add another AED if the first monotherapy trial fails is more controversial (50). A randomized open trial compared the two strategies, alternative monotherapy versus adjunctive therapy, in patients who failed a single AED and found no difference between the groups (51). In clinical practice, the strategy after first monotherapy failure will depend on the reason for failure. Patients with idiosyncratic adverse effects will, for obvious reasons, change to an alternative AED, but this will also be the choice in patients who fail because of other adverse effects. On the other hand, patients who experience some, but insufficient, benefit from their first AED will more often be prescribed a drug to combine with their original medication (50).

Changing from one AED to another can be a fairly complicated procedure. It is done gradually over weeks to months.

Individualization of Dosage

AED dosage needs to be tailored to the needs of the individual patient. The general strategy is to use the lowest effective dosage aiming at complete seizure control without embarrassing or intolerable adverse effects. There is a marked inter-individual variability in the dosage that provides the optimal balance between efficacy and tolerability, and this has to be achieved in each patient in a systematic manner. To improve tolerability, AEDs generally need to be introduced with slow titration before reaching the first-target maintenance dosage. The necessary dosage titration time varies among AEDs from a few days for drugs such as gabapentin, levetiracetam, phenytoin, and valproate to several weeks for carbamazepine, lamotrigine, and topiramate (52). The initial target maintenance dosage is selected on the basis of the known dose-response profile of the AED as well as on patient characteristics (e.g., seizure type, epilepsy severity, and patient preference) (52). If seizures continue, the dosage is gradually increased until seizures are controlled or until intolerable adverse effects occur. This is a time-consuming process, which, depending on the seizure frequency, could take months up to a few years. In this dose escalation procedure, it is important to be aware that some AEDs may have paradoxical effects at higher dosages. This possibility should be considered with the occurrence of new types of seizures or deterioration in seizure control following a dose increase (53).

Treatment Monitoring

For several reasons, it may be difficult to find the individual optimal dosage of an AED in the treatment of a patient with epilepsy with clinical monitoring alone. This is partly related to the nature of epilepsy: seizures may be infrequent and occur irregularly. Symptoms and signs of AED toxicity may be subtle and sometimes difficult to distinguish from manifestations of the condition under treatment. In addition, the pharmacokinetics of many AEDs vary considerably between patients, making it further difficult to predict clinical effects. For these reasons, therapeutic drug monitoring has been frequently used to guide the pharmacological treatment of epilepsy. By measuring AED plasma concentrations, the clinician can control for the pharmacokinetic contribution to the variability in drug response. The concept rests on the assumption that drug concentrations correlate better with clinical effects than with dose, which is reasonable for most AEDs, but less so for drugs with irreversible actions (vigabatrin) or for which tolerance is likely to develop (benzodiazepines).

Therapeutic ranges have been proposed for AEDs in the effort to assist in dosage individualization. These are plasma concentrations associated with high likelihood of seizure control and minimal risk of dose-related adverse effects (Table 4). Traditionally, the AED dosage has often been adjusted in the individual patient to reach a plasma concentration within this range. However, the documentation underlying the therapeutic ranges is scarce and the optimal plasma concentration will vary considerably, depending on individual factors such as seizure type and the severity of epilepsy. Thus, it has become apparent that a large proportion of patients with easy-to-treat new-onset epilepsy will respond at levels below the lower limit of many ranges (54,55). On the basis of this finding, it has been recommended that the therapeutic ranges of AEDs be redefined by omitting the lower limit.

TABLE 4 Often-Quoted Tentative Therapeutic Ranges for Antiepileptic Drugs

Drug	Time to steady state (days)	Tentative therapeutic range (μg/mL)
Carbamazepine	2–7	(4)–11
Ethosuximide	4–10	(40)–100
Phenobarbital	8–30	(10)–40
Phenytoin	3–15	(10)–20
Valproate	2–4	(50)–100
Felbamate	3–5	(30)–60
Gabapentin	2	(12)–20
Lamotrigine	3–15	(2.5)–15
Levetiracetam	2	(8)–26
Oxcarbazepine	2–3	(12)–35[a]
Pregabalin	2	(2.8)–8.2
Tiagabine	2	(20)–100[b]
Topiramate	4–6	(5)–20
Vigabatrin	1–2	NA
Zonisamide	5–12	(10)–38

Note: The documentation of the ranges is particularly scarce for the newer-generation drugs. The lower limit of the therapeutic range is of limited value, because many patients do well at serum concentrations below this limit. It is, therefore, indicated in parenthesis.
[a]Monohydroxy derivative, the active component of oxcarbazepine.
[b]ng/mL.
Abbreviation: NA, not applicable.

It has even become customary to move away from the concept of general therapeutic ranges and instead establish and utilize the "individualized reference concentration." This is defined as the concentration that has been measured in an individual patient after that individual had been stabilized on a dosage that produced the best response (56). Knowledge of the serum concentration at which the individual patient has shown a good response provides a useful reference in understanding the causes of potential future treatment failures. It has therefore become common to measure the plasma concentration when the patient has been stabilized on a maintenance dosage that seems to provide a good response. However, the dosage will not necessarily be adjusted if the drug level was found to be below the traditional therapeutic range. Should breakthrough seizures occur in the future, a new plasma concentration will reveal if this was associated with a decline from the individual reference concentration, and appropriate measures could be made to restore the optimal plasma concentration. An advantage of the individualized reference concentration approach is that it does not rely on fixed therapeutic ranges and can be applied to any AED, including newer-generation AEDs for which the very existence of a therapeutic range has been questioned (56,57).

Duration of Treatment and Withdrawal

Treatment of epilepsy is generally maintained for years and is sometimes life long. However, some patients will remit and can successfully withdraw their AEDs after years of seizure control. In a population-based study, Annegers and collaborators found that 20 years after diagnosis, 70% of patients had entered remission lasting five years or more and almost 50% were seizure free without medication (58).

Withdrawal of AEDs may thus be an option for many patients after some years of seizure freedom. This option is often considered after three to five years in adults and perhaps after two years in children. The likelihood of a successful AED withdrawal depends on a number of individual factors. Some epilepsy syndromes, e.g., juvenile myoclonic epilepsy, are associated with a very high relapse rate. An underlying neurological disorder or brain lesion is another factor associated with high relapse risks, while childhood onset of epilepsy suggests a low risk (59). Although there are methods to estimate the risk of recurrence on drug withdrawal, the outcome can never be predicted with certainty. A British study randomized patients who had been seizure free for at least two years to slow AED withdrawal or continued medication. Two years after randomization, 78% of those in whom treatment continued and 59% of those in whom it was withdrawn remained seizure free (60). It is ultimately for the patient to decide on the basis of the best possible information whether to take this risk of relapse. If a withdrawal is attempted, it should be performed gradually, probably over months.

CONCLUSIONS

AEDs are the mainstay of epilepsy treatment. The treatment is prophylactic aiming at seizure control without embarrassing adverse effects. There are as yet no clinical data indicating that AEDs modify the natural course of epilepsy; AED treatment of epilepsy should therefore be considered symptomatic. Treatment is normally initiated after two or more unprovoked seizures. Individualization has been a key concept in the pharmacological treatment of epilepsy, with respect to choice of AEDs as well as drug dosage. A number of new drugs have been introduced during the last 15 years, but some older-generation AEDs are still considered first-line therapies. The selection of an AED is based on the drugs' efficacy and effectiveness for the specific type of seizures and epilepsy syndrome of the individual patient, but other clinical factors are also taken into account. Treatment is started with the appropriate AED as monotherapy generally in a low first-target maintenance dose. The dosage is adjusted on the basis of the clinical response aiming at the lowest effective dosage. The prognosis is favorable for patients with newly diagnosed epilepsy, the majority achieving remission on treatment. Many of those can also successfully withdraw their treatment after some years of seizure freedom. For others, however, treatment may be lifelong.

REFERENCES

1. Locock C. Discussion of paper by EH Sieveking: analysis of fifty-two cases of epilepsy observed by the author. Lancet 1857; i:527.
2. Hauptman A. Luminal bei epilepsie. MMW Munch Med Wochenschr 1912; 59:1907–1909.
3. Kale R, Perucca E. Revisiting phenobarbital for epilepsy. BMJ 2004 Nov 20; 329 (7476):1199–1200.
4. Spina E, Perugi G. Antiepileptic drugs: indications other than epilepsy. Epileptic Disord 2004; 6(2):57–75.
5. Fisher RS, van Emde Boas W, Blume W, et al. Epileptic seizures and epilepsy: definitions proposed by the International League Against Epilepsy (ILAE) and the International Bureau for Epilepsy (IBE). Epilepsia 2005; 46(4):470–472.
6. Merritt HH, Putnam TJ. A new series of anticonvulsant drugs tested by experiments on animals. Arch Neurol Psychiatry 1938; 39:1003–1015.

7. Smith M, Wolcox KS, White HS. Discovery of antiepileptic drugs. Neurotherapeutics 2007; 4(1):12–17.
8. White HS, Smith MD, Wilcox KS. Mechanisms of action of antiepileptic drugs. Int Rev Neurobiol 2007; 81:85–110.
9. Commission on Classification and Terminology of the International League Against Epilepsy. Proposal for revised clinical and electroencephalographic classification of epileptic seizures. Epilepsia 1981; 22:489–501.
10. Commission on Classification and Terminology of the International League Against Epilepsy. Proposal for revised classification of epilepsies and epileptic syndromes. Epilepsia 1989; 30(4):389–399.
11. Olafsson E, Ludvigsson P, Gudmundsson G, et al. Incidence of unprovoked seizures and epilepsy in Iceland and assessment of the epilepsy syndrome classification: a prospective study. Lancet Neurol 2005; 4(10):627–634.
12. Glauser T, Ben-Menachem E, Bourgeois B, et al. ILAE treatment guidelines: evidence-based analysis of antiepileptic drug efficacy and effectiveness as initial monotherapy for epileptic seizures and syndromes. Epilepsia 2006; 47:1094–1120.
13. Stokes T, Juarez-Garcia A, Camosso-Stefinovic J, et al. Clinical Guidelines and Evidence Review for the Epilepsies: Diagnosis and Management in Adults and Children in Primary and Secondary Care. London, UK: Royal College of General Practitioners, 2004.
14. French JA, Kanner AM, Bautista J, et al. Efficacy and tolerability of the new antiepileptic drugs, I: treatment of new-onset epilepsy: report of the TTA and QSS Subcommittees of the American Academy of Neurology and the American Epilepsy Society. Epilepsia 2004; 45:401–409.
15. Brodie MJ, Perucca E, Ryvlin P, et al. for the Levetiractem Monotherapy Study Group. Comparison of levetiracetam and controlled-release carbamazepine in newly diagnosed epilepsy. Neurology 2007; 68(6):402–408.
16. Marson AG, Al-Kharusi AM, Alwaidh M, et al. for the SANAD Study Group. The SANAD study of effectiveness of carbamazepine, gabapentin, lamotrigine, oxcarbazepine, or topiramate for treatment of partial epilepsy: an unblinded randomized comparison. Lancet 2007; 369:1000–1026.
17. Tomson T, Perucca E, Battino D. Navigating toward foetal and maternal health: the challenge of treating epilepsy in pregnancy. Epilepsia 2004; 45:1171–1175.
18. Perucca E. Birth defects after prenatal exposure to antiepileptic drugs. Lancet Neurol 2005; 4:781–786.
19. Wide K, Winbladh B, Kallen B. Major malformations in infants exposed to antiepileptic drugs in utero, with emphasis on carbamazepine and valproic acid: a nation-wide, population-based register study. Acta Paediatr 2004; 93:174–176.
20. Artama M, Auvinen A, Raudaskoski T, et al. Antiepileptic drug use of women with epilepsy and congenital malformations in offspring. Neurology 2005; 64:1874–1878.
21. Wyszynski DF, Nambisan M, Surve T, et al. Increased rate of major malformations in offspring exposed to valproate during pregnancy. Neurology 2005; 64:961–965.
22. Morrow J, Russell A, Guthrie E, et al. Malformation risks of antiepileptic drugs in pregnancy: a prospective study from the UK Epilepsy and Pregnancy Register. J Neurol Neurosurg Psychiatry 2006; 77:193–198.
23. Samren EB, van Duijn CM, Christiaens GC, et al. Antiepileptic drug regimens and major congenital abnormalities in the offspring. Ann Neurol 1999; 46:739–746.
24. Kaneko S, Battino D, Andermann E, et al. Congenital malformations due to antiepileptic drugs. Epilepsy Res 1999; 33:145–158.
25. Vajda FJ, Eadie MJ. Maternal valproate dosage and foetal malformations. Acta Neurol Scand 2005; 112(3):137–143.
26. Cunnington M, Tennis P, and The International Lamotrigine Pregnancy Registry Scientific Advisory Committee. Lamotrigine and the risk of malformations in pregnancy. Neurology 2005; 64:955–960.
27. Holmes LB, Wyszynski DF, Baldwin EJ, et al. Increased risk for non-syndromic cleft palate among infants exposed to lamotrigine during pregnancy. Birth Def Res (Part A): Clin Mol Teratol 2006; 76:318.

28. Adab N, Kini U, Vinten J, et al. The longer term outcome of children born to mothers with epilepsy. J Neurol Neurosurg Psychiatry 2004; 75:1575–1583.
29. Vinten J, Adab N, Kini U, et al. Neuropsychological effects of exposure to anti-convulsant medication in utero. Neurology 2005; 64:949–954.
30. The EURAP Study Group. Seizure control and treatment in pregnancy. Observations from the EURAP Epilepsy Pregnancy Registry. Neurology 2006; 66:354–360.
31. Vajda FJ, Hitchcock A, Graham J, et al. Foetal malformations and seizure control: 52 months data of the Australian Pregnancy Registry. Eur J Neurol 2006; 13(6):645–654.
32. Tomson T, Battino D. Pharmacokinetics and therapeutic drug monitoring of newer antiepileptic drugs during pregnancy and the puerperium. Clin Pharmacokinet 2007; 46:209–219.
33. Perucca E, Berlowitz D, Birnbaum A, et al. Pharmacological and clinical aspects of antiepileptic drug use in the elderly. Epilepsy Res 2006; 68 (suppl 1):S49–S63.
34. Ramsay RE, Rowan AJ, Slater JD, et al. The VA cooperative study group. Effect of age on epilepsy and its treatment: results from the VA cooperative study. Epilepsia 1994; 35 (suppl 8):91 (abstr).
35. Brodie MJ, Overstall PW, Giorgi L. for the UK Lamotrigine Elderly Study Group. Multicentre, double-blind, randomised comaprison between lamotrigine and carbama-zepine in elderly patients with newly diagnosed epilepsy. Epilepsy Res 1999; 37:81–87.
36. Rowan AJ, Ramsay RE, Collins JF, et al. VA cooperative study 428 group. New onset geriatric epilepsy: a randomised study of gabapentin, lamotrigine, and carbamazepine. Neurology 2005; 64:1868–1873.
37. Saetre E, Perucca E, Isojärvi J, et al. for the LAM 40089 Study Group. An international multicenter randomized double-blind controlled trial of lamotrigine and sustained-release carbamazepine in the treatment of newly diagnosed epilepsy in the elderly. Epilepsia 2007; 48(7):1292–1302.
38. Ben-Menachem E, Schmitz B, Tomson T, et al. Role of valproate across the ages. Treatment of epilepsy in adults. Acta Neurol Scand Suppl 2006; 184:14–27.
39. Mula M, Trimble MR, Yuen A, et al. Psychiatric adverse events during levetiracetam therapy. Neurology 2003; 61(5):704–706.
40. Perucca E, Beghi E, Dulac O, et al. Assessing risk to benefit ratio in antiepileptic drug therapy. Epilepsy Res 2000; 41(2):107–139.
41. Patsalos PN, Perucca E. Clinically important drug interactions in epilepsy: interactions between antiepileptic drugs and other drugs. Lancet Neurol 2003; 2(8):473–481.
42. Patsalos PN, Perucca E. Clinically important drug interactions in epilepsy: general features and interactions between antiepileptic drugs. Lancet Neurol 2003; 2(6):347–356.
43. Berg AT, Shinnar S. The risk of seizure recurrence following a first unprovoked seizure: a quantitative review. Neurology 1991; 41:965–972.
44. Reynolds EH, Elwes RDC, Shorvon S. Why does epilepsy become intractable? Preven-tion of chronic epilepsy. Lancet 1983; 356:952–954.
45. Temkin NR. Antiepileptogenesis and seizure prevention trials with antiepileptic drugs: meta-analysis of controlled trials. Epilepsia 2001; 42(4):515–524.
46. Marson A, Jacoby A, Johnson A, et al. for the Medical Research Council MESS Study Group. Immediate versus deferred antiepileptic drug treatment for early epilepsy and single seizures: a randomised controlled trial. Lancet 2005; 365:2007–2013.
47. Leone MA, Solari A, Beghi E, FIRST Group. Treatment of the first tonic-clonic seizure does not affect long-term remission of epilepsy. Neurology 2006; 67(12):2227–2229.
48. Reynolds EH, Shorvon SD. Monotherapy or polytherapy for epilepsy? Epilepsia 1981; 22:1–10.
49. Mattson RH, Cramer JA, Collins JF, et al. Comparison of carbamazepine, phenobarbital, phenytoin, and primidone in partial and secondarily generalized tonic-clonic seizures. N Engl J Med 1985; 313:145–151.
50. Brodie MJ. Medical therapy of epilepsy: when to initiate treatment and when to com-bine? J Neurol 2005; 252(2):125–130.
51. Beghi E, Gatti G, Tonini C, et al. BASE study group. Adjunctive therapy versus alter-native monotherapy in patients with partial epilepsy failing on a single drug: a multi-centre, randomised, pragmatic controlled trial. Epilepsy Res 2003; 57(1):1–13.

52. Perucca E, Dulac O, Shorvon S, et al. Harnessing the clinical potential of antiepileptic drug therapy: dosage optimisation. CNS Drugs 2001; 15(8):609–621.
53. Perucca E. Overtreatment in epilepsy: adverse consequences and mechanisms. Epilepsy Res 2002; 52(1):25–33.
54. Shorvon SD, Chadwick D, Galbraith AW, et al. One drug for epilepsy. Br Med J 1978; 25(1): 474–476.
55. Shorvon SD, Galbraith AW, Laundy M, et al. Monotherapy for epilepsy. In: Johannessen SI, Morselli PL, Pippenger CE, et al. eds. Antiepileptic Therapy: Advances in Drug Monitoring. New York, NY: Raven Press, 1980:213–219.
56. Perucca E. Is there a role for therapeutic drug monitoring of new anticonvulsants? Clin Pharmacokin 2000; 38:191–204.
57. Johannessen SI, Tomson T. Pharmacokinetic variability of newer antiepileptic drugs: when is monitoring needed? Clin Pharmacokin 2006; 45:1061–1075.
58. Annegers JF, Hauser WA, Elveback LR. Remission of seizures and relapse in patients with epilepsy. Epilepsia 1979; 20(6):729–737.
59. Specchio LM, Beghi E. Should antiepileptic drugs be withdrawn in seizure-free patients? CNS Drugs 2004; 18(4):201–212.
60. Medical Research Council Antiepileptic Drug Withdrawal Study Group. Randomized study of antiepileptic drug withdrawal in patients in remission. Lancet 1991; 337:1175–1180.

3   Antiepileptic Drugs in the Treatment of Neuropathic Pain

David R. P. Guay
Department of Experimental and Clinical Pharmacology, College of Pharmacy,
University of Minnesota and Consultant, Division of Geriatrics, HealthPartners, Inc.,
Minneapolis, Minnesota, U.S.A.

INTRODUCTION

Chronic neuropathic pain syndromes are common, especially in older individuals. Examples include painful diabetic peripheral neuropathy, postherpetic neuralgia, phantom limb pain, central poststroke pain, and trigeminal neuralgia. Tricyclic antidepressants have been extensively used in the treatment of chronic neuropathic pain for many years (1). However, tricyclic antidepressants can be difficult to use due to their side-effect profile (1). Antiepileptic drugs (AEDs) such as phenytoin and clonazepam do not appear to be particularly effective in chronic neuropathic pain (see below). However, the same cannot be said for other AEDs, including the older agents carbamazepine and valproate and the newer agents gabapentin, lamotrigine, levetiracetam, oxcarbazepine, pregabalin, and topiramate. AEDs are an advance in the management of chronic neuropathic pain based upon their equivalent or superior clinical efficacy and superior tolerability compared with other pharmacologic modalities. This chapter will review the role of older and newer AEDs in the management of neuropathic pain, with an emphasis on data published from the year 2000 to the present.

ANALGESIC MECHANISMS OF ACTION

The analgesic mechanisms of action of the AEDs are not well understood but are presumed to be related to their antiepileptic mechanisms of action. For example, the hypothesized analgesic mechanisms of action of gabapentin include increase in concentration and rate of synthesis of gamma-aminobutyric acid (GABA) in the brain, modulation of specific types of calcium currents, reduction in the release of several monoamine neurotransmitters, inhibition of voltage-activated sodium channels, increase in serotonin (5-HT) concentrations, and inhibition of glutamate synthesis by branched-chain amino acid aminotransferase (2). More recent data speculate roles for 5-HT$_3$ receptors in spinal neuronal responses, the nitric oxide–cyclic guanosine monophosphate (cGMP) protein kinase G-potassium channel in the spinal cord, and spinal release of glutamate/aspartate in the dorsal horn in the analgesia induced by gabapentin (3–5).

PHARMACODYNAMICS

AEDs are active in a wide variety of laboratory (animal) models of neuropathic pain as illustrated in Table 1 (6–31). In addition, levetiracetam has recently been evaluated in a human experimental pain model in 16 healthy volunteers. Using a randomized, double-blind, placebo-controlled, crossover format, the effect of a

TABLE 1 Activities of AEDs in Laboratory Models of Neuropathic Pain

Model	Drug	Effect	References
Partial ligation of sciatic or saphenous nerve	Carbamazepine	PO has minimal effect on mechanical hyperalgesia in rats. IP dose-dependently ↓ mechanical hyperalgesia in rats.	10,12
		PO has no effect on tactile hyperalgesia in rats.	10
		PO dose-dependently ↓ mechanical hyperalgesia in guinea pigs.	10
	Ethosuximide	IP dose-dependently ↓ tactile hypersensitivity and thermal hyperalgesia in rats.	7
	Felbamate	IP dose-dependently ↓ thermal hyperalgesia, mechanical allodynia, and mechanical hyperalgesia in rats.	6
	Gabapentin	IP dose-dependently ↓ mechanical hypersensitivity and allodynia but not mechanical hyperalgesia in rats.	17,27
		IP dose-dependently ↓ cold and mechanical allodynia and mechanical and thermal allodynia/hyperalgesia in mice.	29,30
	Lamotrigine	Dose-dependently ↓ mechanical hyperalgesia (PO/IP); has no effect on tactile or cold allodynia (PO/IP); and has either no effect or ↓ mechanical allodynia in a dose-independent fashion in rats (PO/IP).	10,16,25
		PO lamotrigine dose-dependently ↓ mechanical hyperalgesia in guinea pigs.	10
	Levetiracetam	IP levetiracetam has only a marginal effect on mechanical hyperalgesia in rats.	12
	MHD[a] Oxcarbazepine	PO MHD and oxcarbazepine have no effect on mechanical hyperalgesia, and PO oxcarbazepine has no effect on tactile allodynia in rats.	10
		PO MHD and oxcarbazepine dose-dependently ↓ mechanical hyperalgesia in guinea pigs (MHD is slightly less potent than parent compound).	10
		IP oxcarbazepine dose-dependently ↓ mechanical and cold allodynia in rats.	15
	Topiramate	IP topiramate ↓ mechanical allodynia in rats.	21
		IP topiramate ↓ mechanical hyperalgesia and cold allodynia but has no effect on mechanical allodynia in rats after chronic constriction injury (sciatic nerve). IP topiramate ↓ cold allodynia and thermal hyperalgesia but has no effect on mechanical allodynia in rats after crush injury (sciatic nerve).	9
	Valproic acid	IP valproic acid dose-dependently ↓ tactile allodynia in rats.[b]	14
		IP valproic acid dose-dependently ↓ tactile allodynia in rats.[c]	23
	Vigabatrin	PO vigabatrin dose-dependently ↓ thermal allodynia in rats.	20
	Zonisamide	SC, ICV, IT zonisamide dose-dependently ↓ thermal hyperalgesia and tactile allodynia in rats.	8
		IP zonisamide dose-dependently ↓ thermal hyperalgesia but has minimal effect on mechanical allodynia in rats.	13

TABLE 1 (*Continued*)

Model	Drug	Effect	References
Sciatic transection and dorsal cervical rhizotomy (models of deafferentation pain)	Phenobarbital	IM phenobarbital dose-dependently delays the onset and reduces the magnitude of pain.	11
Streptozotocin (model of diabetic neuropathy)	Carbamazepine	IP carbamazepine dose-dependently ↓ mechanical hyperalgesia in rats.	12
	Lamotrigine	IV lamotrigine has no effect on thermal allodynia or mechanical hyperalgesia in rats.	31
	Levetiracetam Pregabalin	IV levetiracetam and pregabalin ↓ thermal allodynia and mechanical hyperalgesia in rats.	31
	Levetiracetam	IV levetiracetam dose-dependently ↓ mechanical hyperalgesia in rats.	12
Photochemical-induced nerve injury	Lamotrigine	IP lamotrigine has no effect on mechanical or cold allodynia in rats.	16
Toxin-induced models			
Capsaicin	Ethosuximide Trimethadione	IP ethosuximide dose-dependently ↓ mechanical allodynia in rats while IP trimethadione only marginally ↓ mechanical allodynia.	18
Dynorphin	Tiagabine	IP tiagabine dose-dependently ↓ chronic allodynia in mice while IT tiagabine has no such effect.	22
Late phase Postformalin	Ethosuximide Trimethadione	IP ethosuximide dose-dependently ↓ formalin-induced behaviors in rats while IP trimethadione only marginally ↓ such behaviors.	18
	Tiagabine	IT tiagabine only marginally reduces formalin-induced behaviors in mice.	22
Paclitaxel	Ethosuximide	IP ethosuximide dose-dependently ↓ mechanical and cold allodynia in rats.	19
	Gabapentin	IP gabapentin dose-dependently ↓ mechanical allodynia and thermal hyperalgesia in mice.	28
Resinoferatoxin	Gabapentin	IP and IT gabapentin dose-dependently ↓ tactile allodynia in rats.	26
Vincristine	Lamotrigine Ethosuximide	PO lamotrigine and IP ethosuximide dose-dependently ↓ mechanical allodynia in rats.	22,24

[a]Monohydroxy metabolite of oxcarbazepine.
[b]Valpromide, valnoctamide, and diisopropylacetamide are more potent than valproic acid itself.
[c]The tetramethylcyclopropyl analogues are much more potent than valproic acid itself.
Abbreviations: IP, intraperitoneal; PO, oral; SC, subcutaneous; ICV, intracerebroventricular; IT, intrathecal; IM, intramuscular; IV, intravenous; ↓, decrease.

single 1500 mg oral dose on pain detection and tolerance to single electrical stimuli and temporal pain summation threshold to repetitive electrical stimuli of the sural nerve was evaluated. Measurements were performed before drug administration and at 2, 4, 6, 8, and 24 hours after administration. Levetiracetam significantly increased pain tolerance thresholds ($p = 0.04$) and trended towards increasing pain detection thresholds ($p = 0.06$) to single stimuli. It had no effect on pain summation thresholds ($p = 0.30$). There was a significant correlation of two-hour postdose drug concentrations with placebo-corrected effects on pain tolerance ($r = 0.67, p < 0.01$). The delay in the peak pain tolerance threshold effect until six to eight hours postdosing, while peak plasma drug concentrations occurred at two hours postdosing, was consistent with an effect in a deep central nervous system (CNS) compartment or delayed blood-brain barrier transfer of the drug into the CNS. No significant drug effect was noted on auditory reaction time. Slight or moderate sedation and/or dizziness occurred during the first four to six hours after administration of levetiracetam and placebo in eight and three subjects, respectively (32).

Gabapentin and gabapentin plus morphine do not alter the circadian variation in the neuropathic pain characteristic of painful diabetic peripheral neuropathy and postherpetic neuralgia (33).

A few studies have been performed to assess whether or not there are therapeutic plasma drug concentration ranges for analgesia as there are for antiepileptic activity. In an open trial in sciatica, lamotrigine plasma concentrations correlated with weekly pain diary scores (using a numerical pain scale) ($r^2 = 0.945$, $p = 0.001$), mean pain intensity scores (by visual analogue scale) ($r^2 = 0.94$, $p = 0.001$), mean straight leg raise improvement (in degrees) ($r^2 = 0.919$, $p = 0.003$), and mean bending towards the affected side (in degrees) ($r^2 = 0.816$, $p = 0.014$). However, correlations with McGill Pain questionnaire scores or forward bending improvement (in degrees) were not significant. Despite these results, a therapeutic plasma lamotrigine concentration range could not be derived (34).

One study conducted with carbamazepine in intractable neuropathic pain (4 patients with trigeminal neuralgia, 12 patients with peripheral nerve injury) found no significant correlation of individual pain score or decrease in score from baseline with plasma carbamazepine concentration in the five "responders." When data from all seven patients completing all three dose levels (which included the 5 "responders") were evaluated, a significant correlation was only noted between individual sedation scores and drug concentration ($r = 0.65$, $p < 0.005$) (35). In another trial utilizing seven patients with trigeminal neuralgia exposed to three dose levels, a carbamazepine plasma concentration–effect relationship was seen in six of seven (86%), with the best effect noted between 5.7 and 10.1 mg/L. In one patient studied on two occasions, the relationship differed each time (36). Finally, in a trial examining carbamazepine in a variety of neuropathic pain states (10 cases of trigeminal neuralgia, 4 of postherpetic neuralgia, 4 of phantom limb pain, and 13 of reflex sympathetic dystrophy), logistic regression analysis found significant plasma concentration–effect relationships for carbamazepine and, in selected cases, its active epoxide metabolite. The pain parameter evaluated was pain reduction by 25%, 30%, and 75% from baseline. The carbamazepine plasma concentrations having the highest probability of response in 50% of patients (C_{50}) were 5.1 mg/L (for a 50% pain reduction) and 7 mg/L (for a 75% pain reduction). When drug plasma concentrations associated with 25% to 75% pain reduction were compared with C_{50} data, a therapeutic plasma concentration range for analgesia of 2 to 7 mg/L was derived (37). It thus appears that for carbamazepine, the antiepileptic and analgesic plasma concentration ranges overlap considerably.

CLINICAL PHARMACOLOGY

As an aid in rational prescribing of AEDs for the treatment of neuropathic pain, the clinical pharmacology of selected agents will be reviewed: valproate, gabapentin, pregabalin, lamotrigine, carbamazepine, oxcarbazepine, topiramate, zonisamide, and levetiracetam. Table 2 illustrates the major pharmacokinetic properties of these nine agents (38–48).

TABLE 2 Pharmacokinetic Parameters of Selected AEDs

Drug	F (%)	T_{max} (hr)	PPB (%)	V_d/F (L/kg)	$t_{\varnothing}$ (hr)	CL/F (mL/min)
Valproate	90[a]	3–5[a]	90→82[b]	11[c]	9–16	0.56[d]
Gabapentin	60→27[e]	1.5–4	<3	58[f]	5–7	190
Pregabalin	≥90	1.5	0	0.5	6	—
Lamotrigine	98	1.5–5	55	0.9–1.3	25–33	0.44–0.58[g]
Carbamazepine	—	4–5	76	0.8–2	25–65→12–17[h]	25→80[h]
Oxcarbazepine[i]	—	4–6	37–43	0.7–0.8	9	0.85[g]
Topiramate	81–95	1–4	9–17	0.6–0.8	20–30 8–15[j]	20–30 40–60[j]
Zonisamide	≥50	2–5	40–50	1.5	56[k] 63–69[l] 105[m] 25–35[j]	17–24 30–50[j]
Levetiracetam	>95	1	<10	0.5–0.7	6–8 5–8[j]	0.96[g]

[a]Divalproex delayed-release tablets/capsules.
[b]PPB falls as concentration increases (e.g., 90% at 40 μg/mL down to 82% at 130 μg/mL).
[c]L/1.73 m^2.
[d]L/hr/1.73 m^2.
[e]Bioavailability falls as the dose is increased (e.g., 60% with 300 mg thrice daily down to 27% with 1600 mg thrice daily).
[f]L.
[g]mL/min/kg.
[h]Autoinduction of metabolism causes $t_{\varnothing}$ to fall and CL/F to increase with time (complete after 3–5 wk on a fixed dose).
[i]Data refer to the active 10-monohydroxy metabolite.
[j]Recipients of enzyme-inducing AEDs.
[k]Single dose.
[l]Multiple dose to steady state.
[m]Red blood cells.
Abbreviations: F, oral bioavailability; T_{max}, time to peak plasma concentration; PPB, plasma protein binding; V_d/F, apparent volume of distribution; $t_{\varnothing}$, terminal disposition half-life; CL/F, apparent total body clearance.
Source: From Refs. 38–48.

Valproate

Pharmacokinetics

The term valproate refers to valproic acid, sodium valproate, and divalproex sodium (the latter being a stable coordination compound containing equal proportions of valproic acid and sodium valproate). After oral administration, divalproex is rapidly converted to valproic acid in the gastrointestinal tract. Food does not affect the absorption of valproic acid to a clinically relevant degree. Divalproex in the form of delayed-release tablets is over 90% bioavailable while divalproex in the extended-release tablet formulation is 10% to 20% less bioavailable than the delayed-release tablets. Thus, interconversion of these two formulations requires adjustment for this difference in bioavailability (dose conversion chart is available in the Depakote ER® product information) (49).

Mean volume of distribution of total/unbound valproic acid is 11/92 L/1.73 m^2. The plasma protein binding of the drug is concentration-dependent (90% at 40 μg/mL to 82% at 130 μg/mL) and can be reduced in the elderly, in those with chronic liver or renal disease, and in the presence of other highly bound drugs. Valproic acid can also displace other drugs from their plasma protein–binding sites (46).

Elimination occurs principally via metabolism (30–50% via glucuronidation, >40% via β-oxidation, <15–20% via other forms of oxidation), with renal excretion of parent drug being less than 3%. Mean terminal disposition half-life ranges from 9 to 16 hours, while mean systemic clearance of total/unbound drug is 0.56/ 4.6 L/hr/1.73 m² in healthy volunteers. Advancing age is associated with decreased plasma protein–binding (mean decrease of 44%) and decreased plasma systemic clearance (mean decrease of 39%). In the presence of cirrhosis and acute viral hepatitis, mean systemic clearance of unbound drug falls by 50% and 16%, respectively. In liver disease, the unbound fraction is increased by 2- to 2.6-fold. In severe renal impairment [creatinine clearance (CrCl) < 10 mL/min], mean systemic clearance of unbound drug falls by 27%. Hemodialysis reduces serum drug concentrations by approximately 20% (46).

Drug Interactions

Serum concentrations of valproic acid can be elevated by concomitant chlorpromazine (mean 15%), felbamate (mean 35%), sertraline, and cimetidine therapies. The converse can occur during concurrent bile acid–binding resin, rifampin (mean 40%), carbamazepine, ethosuximide, lamotrigine, and phenytoin therapies. Valproic acid can raise the serum concentrations of amitriptyline/nortriptyline (mean 21%/34%), carbamazepine-10,11-epoxide (mean 45%), diazepam (mean 25%), lamotrigine (mean 165%), barbiturates (mean 30%), phenytoin (mean 25%), and zidovudine (mean 38%) (49,50).

Adverse Effects

On the basis of epilepsy trials conducted with divalproex delayed-release tablets, the most common adverse effects are asthenia and somnolence (27% each), dizziness and tremor (25% each), headache (31%), nausea (48%), vomiting (27%), abdominal pain (23%), diplopia (16%), and blurred vision (12%) (49). Pancreatitis is a rare but potentially serious adverse effect, occurring once every 522 patient-years of exposure. Thrombocytopenia appears to be dose- or concentration-dependent, the probability increasing significantly at serum concentrations exceeding 110 µg/mL (females) or 135 µg/mL (males). It is reversible upon drug discontinuation. Hepatotoxicity is very uncommon in the adult patient population, even during concurrent use of hepatic enzyme–inducing drugs.

Dosing

Valproate is available as valproic acid 250 mg capsules and 50 mg/mL oral liquid; divalproex delayed-release (enteric-coated) 125, 250, and 500 mg tablets and 125 mg sprinkle capsules; and divalproex extended-release 250 and 500 mg tablets. Therapy should be initiated at 10 to 15 mg/kg/day, followed by titration in increments of 5 to 10 mg/kg/day at weekly intervals based on response. The usual maximum recommended dose is 60 mg/kg/day (49). Valproic acid, divalproex delayed-release, and divalproex extended-release should be administered in three or four, two, and one dose(s) per day, respectively.

However, many older patients cannot tolerate the rapidity of this dosage escalation scheme and require a more conservative approach. A suggested regimen is 125 mg twice daily to start, followed by titration in increments of 125 to 250 mg/day at weekly intervals, based upon response, to the lesser of the dose attaining therapeutic goal, 60 mg/kg/day, or the maximum tolerated dose. Serum concentration monitoring plays a limited role in optimizing valproate therapy of neuropathic pain. It may be useful in suspected cases of nonadherence, malabsorption, and drug-drug interactions and in establishing a maximum dosage beyond which risk potential exceeds that of benefit (i.e., once a plasma concentration of 120 to 150 µg/mL is reached, further dose escalation is not recommended).

Gabapentin
Pharmacokinetics
Gabapentin bioavailability falls as dose increases. At daily doses of 900, 1200, 2400, 3600, and 4800 mg (in 3 divided doses), the mean bioavailability is approximately 60%, 47%, 34%, 33%, and 27%, respectively. Peak plasma concentrations are achieved from 1.5 to 4 hours following dose administration. Food exerts no clinically significant effect on bioavailability. Gabapentin undergoes virtually no metabolism. Elimination occurs almost exclusively via renal excretion of parent drug. In subjects with normal renal function, the mean terminal disposition half-life ranges from five to seven hours (51).

As might be expected for a drug virtually 100% dependent on intact renal function for its elimination, renal impairment exerts profound effects on gabapentin pharmacokinetics. From subjects with "normal" renal function (CrCl $\geq$ 60 mL/min) to those with severe renal impairment (CrCl 0–29 mL/min) with or without hemodialysis support, the mean terminal disposition half-life ranges from 6.5 to 52 hours, mean renal clearance from 90 to 10 mL/min, and mean systemic clearance from 190 to 20 mL/min. Hemodialysis efficiently removes gabapentin as noted by comparing mean interdialytic and intradialytic terminal disposition half-lives (132 vs. 3.8 hours, respectively). The significant effect of advancing age on drug pharmacokinetics can be explained solely by the age-associated reduction in CrCl (51).

Drug Interactions
The only drug-drug interaction of documented clinical relevance with gabapentin occurs with aluminum-based antacids. Coadministration of the two agents produces a mean reduction in bioavailability of 20%. If gabapentin administration occurs two hours after that of antacid, the mean reduction in bioavailability is only 5%. Administration of 60 mg morphine two hours prior to 600 mg of gabapentin results in a mean reduction in gabapentin bioavailability of 44%. The mechanism and magnitude of this interaction at other doses is unknown, as is its clinical relevance (51).

Adverse Effects
Examining clinical trial data in postherpetic neuralgia/epilepsy, the most common adverse effects of gabapentin are dizziness (28/19%), somnolence (21/19%), ataxia (3/13%), tremor (−/7%), peripheral edema (8/2%), and blurred vision (3/4%) (51). A withdrawal reaction consisting of anxiety, diaphoresis, palpitations, musculoskeletal complaints, somatic chest pain, and, if severe, seizures has also been described after abrupt discontinuation or overly rapid dosage tapering in nonepileptic subjects. Symptoms emerge the day after discontinuation/excessive taper and peaks over the next one or two days. Reintroduction of gabapentin or restoration of the previous dosage regimen lead to normalization within one or two

days (52,53). Exaggerated effects such as profound somnolence, severe asterixis, myoclonus (new onset or worsened preexisting), dyskinesias, severe arthralgias, and painful gynecomastia have been reported (54–60). Severe renal impairment was reported to be the precipitating factor in two cases (54,60). Rare adverse events such as neutropenia, visual impairment (concentric visual field constriction), and exacerbation of muscle weakness in myasthenia gravis have also been recently reported (61–63). Of interest, the related GABAergic drug, vigabatrin, produces a similar form of visual impairment but does so much more commonly (in up to 40%), and this is one of the reasons that it failed to be approved for use in the United States.

Dosing

Gabapentin is available as 100, 300, and 400 mg capsules, 600 and 800 mg tablets, and a 50 mg/mL oral liquid. For postherpetic neuralgia, the recommended initiation schedule is 300 mg on day 1, 300 mg twice daily on day 2, and 300 mg thrice daily on day 3. Subsequent titration to 1800 mg daily (in 3 divided doses) can be performed on the basis of response. Further dose escalation to 3600 mg daily (in 3 divided doses) may be worthwhile in selected patients (64). As expected, on the basis of its elimination pathways, the presence of renal impairment mandates dosage adjustment. Although there are specific dosage regimens recommended to mimic 900, 1200, 1800, 2400, and 3600 mg daily regimens in subjects with "normal" renal function (i.e., CrCl $\geq$ 60 mL/min) for CrCl ranges of 31 to 59, 16 to 30, and 0 to 15 mL/min, these are only useful in subjects who develop renal impairment acutely (51). In subjects with chronic renal impairment, it is prudent to reduce the initial, incremental, and maintenance doses and prolong the time interval between dosage adjustments, but precise recommendations are not available. An initial dose of 100 to 300 mg once daily, titrated to three or four times daily with intervals of 7 to 10 days between dose adjustments, is reasonable. Response (therapeutic and toxic) is the ultimate guide to gabapentin dosage regimen adjustment in the presence of renal impairment. The ceiling (maximum) dosage may be as high as 4800 mg/day. Post hemodialysis supplementation with single doses of 125 to 350 mg is also recommended to compensate for intradialytic losses. A frequent reason for "therapeutic failure" with gabapentin is the decision not to exceed some arbitrary daily maximum dose, for example 900 mg/day, in the absence of dose-limiting side effects. Some studies suggest that the analgesic effects of the drug may not begin until a daily dose of 900 mg is achieved.

Pregabalin

Pharmacokinetics

Pregabalin is a close structural analogue of gabapentin. Unlike gabapentin, it is well absorbed after oral administration ($\geq$90%) and peak plasma concentrations and areas under the plasma concentration–time curve rise in proportion to dose (linear pharmacokinetics). Peak plasma concentration occurs approximately 1.5 hours after dosing. Pregabalin undergoes virtually no metabolism. At least 90% of the radiolabel is recovered in the urine as parent compound, with approximately 1% appearing as the N-methylated derivative, the major metabolite. Elimination occurs via renal excretion of unchanged drug, with a mean terminal disposition half-life of approximately six hours in subjects with normal renal function. Renal clearance ranges from 67 to 81 mL/min in young healthy volunteers. Renal elimination involves both glomerular filtratrion and tubular secretion (47,65).

Since pregabalin systemic and renal clearances are correlated with CrCl, a significant alteration in drug kinetics is expected in patients with renal impairment. Mean systemic clearance falls from 56.5 mL/min in subjects with CrCl exceeding 60 mL/min to 30.6 mL/min (CrCl 30–60 mL/min), 16.7 mL/min (CrCl 15–29 mL/min), and 8.30 mL/min (CrCl < 15 mL/min). Corresponding mean terminal disposition half-lives are 9.11, 16.7, 25.0, and 48.7 hours. In addition, pregabalin is efficiently removed during hemodialysis (a 4-hour session reduces plasma concentrations by 50%) (66). Hepatic dysfunction would be expected to exert little influence on pregabalin kinetics due to the limited role of metabolism in elimination of the compound. Oral clearance falls with increasing age in elderly subjects, likely due to the age-associated reduction in CrCl (47,65).

Drug Interactions

Pharmacokinetic interactions have not been identified involving pregabalin. Pharmacodynamic interactions involving additive CNS depressant effects have been noted with opioids, benzodiazepines, and ethanol (65).

Adverse Effects

On the basis of the results of double-blind neuropathic pain and epilepsy trials, the most common adverse effects of pregabalin include dizziness (9–37%), somnolence (6–25%), difficulty with concentration/attention (0–6%), peripheral edema, blurred vision (1–9%), dry mouth (2–15%), and weight gain (2–7%) (65). The majority of these effects appear to be dose-dependent, occurring at higher frequencies as the dose increases. Severe asterixis, which compromised mobility and standing, leading to multiple falls, has been reported (67). As with gabapentin, a withdrawal reaction can be precipitated by abrupt drug discontinuation or an overly rapid dose-tapering schedule.

Dosing

Pregabalin is available as 25, 50, 75, 100, 150, 200, 225, and 300 mg oral capsules. In diabetic peripheral neuropathic pain, dosing should be initiated at 50 mg thrice daily and, if necessary and tolerated, increased to 100 mg thrice daily after one week. The maximum recommended dose is 300 mg per day. In postherpetic neuralgia, dosing should be initiated at 75 mg twice or 50 mg thrice daily and, if necessary and tolerated, increased to 300 mg daily after one week. Depending on response, the dose can be escalated to a maximum of 600 mg per day (as 300 mg twice or 200 mg thrice daily) (65).

Dosage regimen adjustment is necessary in the presence of renal impairment (CrCl < 60 mL/min). To mimic 150, 300, and 600 mg/day regimens in the presence of normal renal function, patients with moderate renal impairment (CrCl 30–59 mL/min) should receive total daily doses of 75, 150, and 300 mg, respectively (in 2 or 3 divided doses). Patients with severe renal impairment (CrCl 15–29 mL/min and <15 mL/min) should receive total daily doses of 25 to 50, 75, and 150 mg (in single or 2 divided doses) and 25, 25 to 50, and 75 mg (in single daily doses), respectively. In patients undergoing hemodialysis, a single supplemental dose is necessary after the dialysis session is completed to compensate for dialytic loss.

Patients on 25, 25 to 50, and 75 mg once-daily regimens should receive single supplemental doses of 25 to 50, 50 to 75, and 100 to 150 mg, respectively (65).

Lamotrigine
Pharmacokinetics
Lamotrigine is rapidly and completely absorbed after oral administration with mean time to peak plasma concentration ranging from 1.5 to 5 hours after dosing. The chewable/dispersible tablets are bioequivalent to the compressed tablet formulation, whether swallowed whole, chewed and then swallowed, or dispersed in water and then swallowed (68).

The volume of distribution is dose-independent and similar in patients and healthy volunteers. Lamotrigine is 55 % plasma protein bound (68).

Metabolism occurs primarily via glucuronidation, the major metabolite being an inactive 2-*N*-glucuronide conjugate. After administration of radiolabeled drug to healthy volunteers, 94% and 2% were recovered in the urine and feces, respectively. The radioactivity in the urine consisted of parent compound (10%), the 2-*N*-glucuronide (76%), the 5-*N*-glucuronide (10%), a 2-*N*-methyl metabolite (0.14%), and other unidentified minor metabolites (4%). Although there is evidence of autoinduction in healthy volunteers (i.e., the drug stimulates its own metabolism, causing mean terminal disposition half-life to fall by 25% and mean systemic clearance to increase by 37%), this does not appear to occur in patients concurrently receiving enzyme-inducing AEDs (68).

Advancing age does not appear to alter lamotrigine pharmacokinetics. Severe renal impairment (CrCl < 30 mL/min) is associated with a mean 1.6-fold increase in terminal disposition half-life while in patients undergoing hemodialysis, the inter-dialytic terminal disposition half-life is increased a mean 2.2-fold compared with that in healthy volunteers. A four-hour hemodialysis session removes approximately 20% of the body burden. Moderate and severe hepatic impairment (Child-Pugh grades B and C, respectively) prolong the mean terminal disposition half-life by 1.9- and 3.4-fold, respectively, and reduce the mean systemic clearance by 29% and 71%, respectively, compared with healthy volunteers (68).

Drug Interactions
Carbamazepine, phenobarbital, primidone, phenytoin, and rifampin (via enzyme induction) and oral contraceptive/hormone replacement therapy (due to the estrogen component) can reduce serum lamotrigine concentrations substantially (mean 40%). Valproate coadministration can increase serum lamotrigine concentrations by more than twofold. Lamotrigine coadministration can reduce serum valproate concentrations (mean 25%) (68).

Adverse Effects
Monotherapy with lamotrigine is most frequently associated with dizziness (50%), diplopia (33%), ataxia (24%), blurred vision (23%), and somnolence (14%) (68). Skin rash is the most frequent cause of therapy withdrawal with lamotrigine ($\simeq$4% in clinical trials). It is typically maculopapular or erythematous and displays characteristics of a delayed type hypersensitivity reaction, appearing within the first month of therapy and resolving rapidly on treatment withdrawal. In rare cases (0.3%), it may progress to potentially fatal forms such as erythema multiforme,

Stevens-Johnson syndrome, and toxic epidermal necrolysis. The latter finding mandates that the drug be stopped at the first sign of rash and not restarted. The risk of rash appears to be enhanced significantly when lamotrigine is started in a valproate recipient and also when dose escalation is performed rapidly. In contrast, the risk is significantly reduced when dose escalation is performed slowly (68).

Dosing
Lamotrigine is available as 25, 100, 150, and 200 mg tablets and 2, 5, and 25 mg chewable/dispersible tablets. Patients receiving concurrent therapy with enzyme-inducing drugs and valproate should receive 25 mg every other day for 14 days followed by 25 mg once daily for 14 days followed by dose escalation in 25 to 50 mg/day increments every one to two weeks to the maintenance dose. Patients receiving concurrent therapy with enzyme-inducing drugs but no valproate should receive 50 mg once daily for 14 days followed by dose escalation in 100 mg/day increments every one to two weeks to the maintenance dose. A regimen intermediate to these two would appear to be appropriate for those individuals receiving neither enzyme-inducing drugs nor valproate. No specific dosing recommendations are available for patients with severe renal impairment with or without hemodialysis support. In patients with moderate or severe hepatic impairment, initial, incremental, and maintenance doses should be reduced by 50% and 75%, respectively (68).

Carbamazepine
Pharmacokinetics
The conventional and extended-release tablet and oral suspension formulations are bioequivalent. Mean times to peak plasma concentrations are 1.5 hours (oral suspension), 4 to 5 hours (conventional tablets), and 3 to 12 hours (extended-release tablets) (45,69). Carbamazepine is approximately 76% plasma protein bound with a mean volume of distribution ranging from 0.8 to 2 L/kg. Carbamazepine is primarily eliminated via metabolism followed by renal excretion of hydroxylated and conjugated metabolites. Cytochrome P450 isozyme 3A4 is responsible for generation of the major metabolite, carbamazepine-10,11-epoxide, which is active as well. Clearance increases over the initial few weeks at a fixed-dose level (known as autoinduction). Thus, terminal disposition half-life falls from mean initial values of 25 to 65 hours to 12 to 17 hours after steady state is achieved after three to five weeks on a fixed regimen. After oral administration of radiolabeled carbamazepine, a mean of 72% of radioactivity is found in the urine and 28% in the feces. Urinary radioactivity is principally composed of metabolites, with only a mean of 3% being parent compound (45,69).

Drug Interactions
Cytochrome P-450 isozyme 3A4 inhibitors can increase plasma carbamazepine concentrations (e.g., cimetidine, diltiazem, macrolide antimicrobials, fluoxetine, fluvoxemine, nefazodone, isoniazid, propoxyphene, systemic azole antifungals, metronidazole, verapamil, risperidone, grapefruit juice, and protease inhibitors) (45,50,69). Valproate, felbamate, and quetiapine can increase plasma concentrations of the active 10,11-epoxide metabolite (45,50,69). Cytochrome P-450 isozyme 3A4 inducers can reduce plasma carbamazepine concentrations (e.g., cisplatin,

doxorubicin, rifampin, barbiturates, phenytoin, and primidone) (45,50,69). Carbamazepine can increase plasma concentrations of phenytoin and primidone and decrease those of dihydropyridine calcium channel blockers, cyclosporine, corticosteroids, selected benzodiazepines, selected traditional and atypical neuroleptics, itraconazole, lamotrigine, methadone, oral contraceptives/hormone replacement therapy, phenytoin, protease inhibitors, tiagabine, topiramate, tricyclic antidepressants, valproate, and warfarin (45,50,69).

Adverse Effects

The major adverse effects of carbamazepine involve the CNS and gastrointestinal tract and include drowsiness, dizziness, confusion, headache, fatigue, nystagmus, incoordination, nausea, and vomiting. In addition, rare cases of bone marrow depression of one to all cell lines, hepatotoxicity, and dermatologic reactions have been reported. Carbamazepine is one of the most frequent causes of drug-induced syndrome of inappropriate antidiuretic hormone (SIADH) secretion. Occasional monitoring of serum sodium concentration, complete blood count with differential, and liver function tests are appropriate (69).

Dosing

Carbamazepine is available as chewable 100 mg tablets, conventional 200 mg tablets, 20 mg/mL oral suspension, and 100, 200, and 400 mg extended-release tablets. The recommended initial dose is 200 mg twice daily (tablets) or 100 mg four times daily (oral suspension), with subsequent titration in 200 mg/day increments at weekly intervals, to a maximum of 1200 (rarely, 1600) mg/day. In older individuals, a lower initial dose of 100 mg twice daily (tablets) or 50 mg four times daily (oral suspension) is prudent, with titration occurring at 7 to 14 day intervals. For the role of serum drug concentration monitoring, see "Dosing" under the heading "Valproate."

Oxcarbazepine

Pharmacokinetics

Oxcarbazepine is a keto analogue of carbamazepine (its chemical formula being 10,11-dihydro-10-oxo-carbamazepine). Oxcarbazepine may be considered a prodrug for the active moiety 10,11-dihydro-10-hydroxy-5H-dibenzo(b,f)azepine-5-carboxamide (MHD). After absorption of oxcarbazepine (essentially 100%), conversion to MHD occurs almost immediately by reduction of the keto group by cytosol arylketone reductase. Food exerts no clinically significant effect on oxcarbazepine absorption. The pharmacokinetics of MHD are linear (i.e., peak plasma concentrations and areas under the plasma concentration–time curve rise in proportion to increasing doses). Plasma protein binding of oxcarbazepine and MHD are not altered in patients with trigeminal neuralgia (70) The metabolite MHD is, in turn, glucuronidated or converted to the dihydroxy or transdiol derivative, 10,11-dihydro-10,11-trans-hydroxycarbamazepine (DHD), this reaction being catalyzed by cytochrome P450. In contrast to carbamazepine, oxcarbazepine/MHD do not undergo autoinduction (i.e., stimulate their own metabolism). Ninety-six percent of the oxcarbazepine dose is excreted in the urine (83% as MHD or MHD glucuronide, ≤3% as oxcarbazepine, 4–7% as DHD).

On the basis of single- and multiple-dose studies, MHD peak plasma concentration and area under the plasma concentration–time curve are 30% to 60%

higher in elderly (60–82 years old) as compared with young volunteers (18–32 years old). Age-related reduction in CrCl accounts for these differences (71). Mild to moderate (Child-Pugh classes A and B, respectively) hepatic impairment does not significantly alter the pharmacokinetics of oxcarbazepine or MHD. Data are not available regarding the effect of severe (Child-Pugh class C) hepatic impairment (71). A linear correlation exists between CrCl and renal MHD clearance. When CrCl is less than 30 mL/min, the mean MHD terminal disposition half-life is prolonged to 19 hours and mean area under the plasma concentration–time curve is increased twofold (71).

Drug Interactions
In contrast to carbamazepine, oxcarbazepine/MHD are not generalized hepatic enzyme inducers. Oxcarbazepine/MHD selectively induce cytochrome P450 isozyme 3A4/3A5, enhancing the metabolism of estrogen (mean area under the curve decrease of 48%), progestogen (mean area under the curve decrease of 32%), felodipine (mean peak concentration decrease of 34%, mean area under the curve decrease of 28%), and carbamazepine. In addition, induction of UDP-glucuronyl transferase activity occurs, leading to enhanced glucuronidation and elimination of lamotrigine (mean peak concentration decrease of 29%). Furthermore, inhibition of cytochrome P450 isozyme 2C19 by oxcarbazepine/MHD can produce increases in phenytoin and phenobarbital concentrations of up to 40% and 14%, respectively. Hepatic enzyme inducers such as carbamazepine, phenobarbital, and phenytoin enhance MHD systemic clearance by 25% to 40%. Verapamil and valproate may also reduce MHD plasma concentrations by unknown mechanisms (38,41–43,50).

Adverse Effects
On the basis of the results of double-blind epilepsy trials, the most common adverse effects of oxcarbazepine include sedation, headache, dizziness, rash, vertigo, ataxia, nausea, and diplopia. These effects appear to be dose-dependent, occurring at higher frequencies as the dose increases (71,72). Behavioral effects such as depression and mania occur rarely (73). Rash occurs less frequently with oxcarbazepine compared with carbamazepine and the rate of cross-reactivity is approximately 30%. In contrast to carbamazepine, no hepatic or hematologic toxicities have occurred with oxcarbazepine. Although hyponatremia is felt to occur more frequently in oxcarbazepine as compared with carbamazepine recipients, at least some of the frequency difference may be accounted for by enhanced monitoring in the oxcarbazepine recipients as mandated by study protocols. The frequency of hyponatremia due to oxcarbazepine ranges from 22% to 73%. Most cases are asymptomatic, but occasionally severe cases can be seen. Most cases arise in the first three months of therapy and risk factors include old age, menstruating females, much increased fluid intake (e.g., psychogenic polydipsia), renal impairment, postoperative period, and concurrent use of other drugs that can also reduce serum sodium. Concurrent use of natriuretic drugs may increase the risk of hyponatremia due to oxcarbazepine (74,75). The mechanism of this effect is unclear but presumed complex, including changes in osmoreceptor sensitivity, release of antidiuretic hormone (ADH), sensitivity of kidney ADH receptors, direct effects on renal tubular cells, and/or suppression of ADH breakdown. Serum ADH can be normal, increased, or decreased in a given case. Frequent electrolyte monitoring, especially during the first three months of therapy, is recommended.

The safety/tolerability of oxcarbazepine has been compared between patients with epilepsy 65 years of age and older ($N = 52$) and 18 to 64 years old ($N = 1574$). The premature discontinuation rates (due to adverse events) and adverse event profiles were similar in the two populations. The most common adverse events in the older group were vomiting (19%), dizziness (17%), nausea (17%), and somnolence (15%). Asymptomatic hyponatremia occurred in three older patients (74).

Dosing
Oxcarbazepine is available as 150, 300, and 600 mg oral tablets and 60 mg/mL oral suspension. On the basis of epilepsy data, the recommended adult starting dose of oxcarbazepine is 300 to 600 mg/day with slow dose titration at weekly intervals based on response to a usual maintenance dose of 600 to 1200 mg/day. The drug should be given two or three times daily. Oxcarbazepine can also replace carbamazepine at a dose 1.5-fold (1.2-fold in elders) that of carbamazepine. When this is done, deinduction will occur with the removal of carbamazepine. As a result, the metabolism of oxcarbazepine (and other agents) will slow over a period of several weeks, necessitating dose reductions in some cases. When CrCl is less than 30 mL/min, the initial starting dose should be halved, followed by dose titration to desired response (38,41,44,71).

Topiramate
Pharmacokinetics
First evaluated as an oral hypoglycemic, topiramate is a sulfamate-substituted monosaccharide derived from D-fructose (39). Food has no clinically significant effect on oral bioavailability. Despite its low-capacity, saturable binding to the carbonic anhydrase of red blood cells (RBCs), topiramate exhibits linear pharmacokinetics. Topiramate is principally eliminated by the renal route (55–66% of dose as parent drug). Although metabolism (via oxidation, glucuronidation) is usually of minor importance, this becomes a more important process in patients receiving hepatic enzyme inducer(s).

Healthy volunteer studies have suggested that the pharmacokinetics of topiramate are not altered by advancing age (76). However, in patients with epilepsy, topiramate systemic clearance is negatively correlated with advancing age (77). This may be explained, at least in part, by the effect of age-related reduction in renal function. In studies utilizing subjects with varying degrees of renal impairment, moderate (CrCl 30–69 mL/min) and severe (CrCl < 30 mL/min) renal impairment reduced mean systemic clearance by 42% and 54%, respectively, compared with subjects with CrCl greater than 70 mL/min. Hemodialysis clearance of topiramate was substantial (mean 120 mL/min) and may necessitate dosage supplementation at the end of the procedure (76).

Drug Interactions
The enzyme inducers carbamazepine and phenytoin enhance topiramate systemic clearance by 40% to 50%. Primidone, phenobarbital, and oxcarbazepine also enhance topiramate systemic clearance. Valproate, by an as-yet-undetermined mechanism, reduces topiramate plasma concentrations by a mean of 15%. Gabapentin and lamotrigine have no effect on topiramate systemic clearance. Topiramate reduces phenytoin systemic clearance by up to 25% in selected patients.

This effect, which is due to cytochrome P450 isozyme 2C19 inhibition, is inconsistent, occurring principally in patients at or near the saturation point of phenytoin metabolism. Topiramate reduces ethinyl estradiol plasma concentrations by a mean of 30% (possibly mediated by induction of cytochrome P450 isozyme 3A4) and digoxin peak plasma concentration and area under the plasma concentration–time curve by means of 16% and 12%, respectively (mediated by a nonrenal effect). By an as-yet-unknown mechanism, topiramate may enhance the hypoglycemic effect of metformin (39,41–43,50,76).

Adverse Effects

The commonest adverse effects of topiramate, as identified in double-blind epilepsy trials, are referable to the central nervous system (ataxia, impaired concentration, confusion, dizziness, fatigue, digital and perioral paresthesias, somnolence, abnormal thinking, speech disturbances, and language problems). These effects are increased in frequency and severity with increasing doses, increased speed of dose escalation, and when topiramate is used as a component of combination therapy (as compared with topiramate monotherapy) (39,41,72,76). Topiramate has negative effects on cognitive function in patients with epilepsy, with significant declines occurring in fluency, attention/concentration, processing speed, language skills, perception, and working memory (but not retention) (78). Behavioral events such as aggression/agitation, emotional lability, euphoria, psychosis, and depression are seen uncommonly (73). Nephrolithiasis (mainly with calcium phosphate stones) is seen in about 1.5% of topiramate recipients, most stones being very small and eliminated by spontaneous passage. This is probably mediated by a combination of hypocitraturia, increased calcium phosphate saturation in the urine, and increased urine pH due to carbonic anhydrase inhibition (79–82).

Two non-CNS adverse effects are of special interest. Topiramate may cause acute myopia and secondary angle-closure glaucoma, presumably mediated by carbonic anhydrase inhibition. This almost always occurs in the first month of therapy and is manifested bilaterally by severe ocular pain and ocular hyperemia. This almost always remits within 24 hours of drug withdrawal (83–87). Weight loss occurs in most topiramate recipients. It is manifest within the first three months and peaks by 12 to 18 months of therapy. It appears to be dose-related, with a 2% weight loss at doses below 200 mg/day and 7% at doses above 1000 mg/day. Anorexia is a major contributor to this effect, at least initially. Obese patients experience greater weight loss than nonobese patients. Beneficial effects on plasma glucose and lipids have been noted concurrent with the weight loss (88).

The toxicity risk of combination topiramate-zonisamide therapy, especially with respect to nephrolithiasis and weight loss, is unclear at present.

Dosing

Topiramate is available as 25, 100, and 200 mg oral tablets and 15 and 25 mg sprinkle capsules. On the basis of epilepsy data, the recommended starting dose in adults is 25 to 50 mg/day, followed by dose titration in increments of 25 to 50 mg/day every one to two weeks based on response to a usual maintenance dose of 200 to 400 mg/day (maximum 600 mg/day). Doses should be given twice daily. The sprinkle capsules may be swallowed whole or the contents can be sprinkled on a small amount of soft food. This sprinkle/food mixture should not be chewed. When CrCl is below 70 mL/min, the initial dose should be halved, followed by dose titration at a longer interval than that described above (longer terminal disposition half-life prolongs time to steady state). No specific postdialysis dose supplementation recommendations are available (39,76).

Zonisamide

Zonisamide is 1,2-benzisoxazole-3-methanesulfonamide. Use of this agent in patients with sulfonamide allergies is contraindicated. Such use has resulted in several deaths secondary to complications of severe rashes (including toxic epidermal necrolysis and Stevens-Johnson syndrome), leukopenia, and aplastic anemia.

Pharmacokinetics

Food has no clinically significant effect on oral bioavailability. The pharmacokinetics of this agent are nonlinear (i.e., peak concentration and area under the concentration-time curve do not increase in proportion to increasing dose). This is secondary to the extensive and saturable binding of zonisamide to the carbonic anhydrase of RBCs (RBC: plasma concentration $\simeq 8:1$) (89).

Although the drug's terminal disposition half-life is sufficiently long to allow once-daily dosing, twice-daily dosing is recommended in order to reduce the percentage fluctuation around the steady-state plasma concentration (from 27% with once-daily to 14% with twice-daily dosing). Zonisamide is eliminated via both hepatic metabolism and renal and fecal excretion. Metabolism involves acetylation, reduction, and glucuronidation. The reduction reaction converting zonisamide to 2-(sulfamoylacetyl)-phenol (SMAP) is mediated by cytochrome P450 isozyme 3A. In urine, 35% of the dose appears as parent drug, 15% as N-acetylzonisamide, and 50% as SMAP glucuronide (89).

The pharmacokinetics of zonisamide are not significantly altered by advancing age (89). No data are available regarding the effect of hepatic impairment on drug pharmacokinetics. Renal drug clearance falls as CrCl falls so that when CrCl is less than 20 mL/min, mean zonisamide area under the plasma concentration–time curve is increased by 35% (89).

Drug Interactions

Concurrent use of hepatic enzyme inducers such as phenobarbital, carbamazepine, and phenytoin enhances zonisamide systemic clearance by 30% to 50%. In contrast, valproate and lamotrigine may increase zonisamide plasma concentrations. Zonisamide added to phenytoin therapy produces a modest increase in phenytoin plasma concentrations (mean 16%), probably via a weak inhibitory effect on cytochrome P450 isozyme 2C19. The effect of zonisamide on carbamazepine pharmacokinetics is controversial, although most data support metabolic inhibition (i.e., plasma concentrations of carbamazepine rise and those of its epoxide metabolite fall) (40,42–44,50).

Adverse Effects

The most common adverse effects of zonisamide, as identified in double-blind epilepsy trials, are somnolence, ataxia, anorexia, confusion, abnormal thinking, nervousness, fatigue, and dizziness (40,89). Paresthesias, seen with other carbonic anhydrase inhibitors, are infrequently seen with zonisamide. Behavioral effects such as psychosis, mania, depression, agitation, and irritability are uncommonly seen (73).

Although less problematic than that seen with topiramate (vide supra), significant weight loss may be seen with zonisamide. Nephrolithiasis is a unique adverse effect that led to suspension of U.S./European trials of the drug in the 1980s. Rare in Japan (incidence < 0.2%), 2% to 4% of U.S./European patients develop stones of varied composition (urate, calcium oxalate, calcium phosphate). The majority are small, and no treatment is needed. Urine pH alteration (alkalinization) due to carbonic anhydrase inhibition is the probable mechanism of this effect. Adequate hydration is necessary in order to use this agent safely (40). Again, an unresolved issue concerns the potential for additive toxicity when zonisamide and topiramate are used together, as both have similar biochemical effects (especially nephrolithiasis and weight loss).

Dosing
Zonisamide is available as 100 mg oral capsules. On the basis of epilepsy data, the recommended starting dose in adults is 100 to 200 mg/day, followed by dose titration every two weeks based on response to a usual maintenance dose of 400 to 600 mg/day. Doses should be given twice daily. No specific recommendations are available for dosing zonisamide in patients with hepatic or renal impairment (40,44,89).

Levetiracetam
Pharmacokinetics
Levetiracetam is the S-enantiomer of a racemic (R,S) pyrrolidine acetamide (43). Food has no clinically significant effect on oral bioavailability. Pharmacokinetics of levetiracetam are linear. Metabolism and renal excretion both contribute to drug elimination. Metabolism occurs principally by hydrolysis of the acetamide group, a reaction that is not cytochrome P450–dependent, to the main metabolite UCB-LO57 (accounts for 24% of the dose). Two other minor metabolites are produced, both accounting for less than 3% of the dose. Renal elimination of parent compound and metabolites account for 66% and 27% of the dose, respectively.

Mean systemic clearance is reduced by 38% and mean terminal disposition half-life is prolonged by 2.5 hours in the elderly (61–88 years old) as compared with young volunteers. These differences can be explained by the age-related reduction in CrCl (90,91). Levetiracetam pharmacokinetics are not significantly altered in mild or moderate hepatic impairment but mean systemic clearance is reduced by 50% in severe hepatic impairment (majority of reduction is accounted for by reduction in renal clearance) (90,91). Levetiracetam systemic clearance correlates with CrCl, such that clearance is reduced by means of 40%, 50%, 60%, and 70% in mild (CrCl 50–80 mL/min), moderate (CrCl 30–50 mL/min), severe (CrCl < 30 mL/min) and end-stage (anuric) renal disease, respectively. A four-hour hemodialysis session removes approximately 50% of the levetiracetam body pool (90,91).

Drug Interactions
No clinically significant pharmacokinetic interactions have been identified to date (41,43,50).

Adverse Effects
On the basis of results of double-blind epilepsy trials, the most frequent adverse effects of levetiracetam include dizziness, headache, fatigue, somnolence, and

asthenia (91). Behavioral effects such as psychosis, depression, emotional lability, hostility, and nervousness are uncommonly seen, although their risk is increased in the developmentally disabled and those with a history of psychiatric disorders (41,73).

Dosing

Levetiracetam is available as 250, 500, and 750 mg oral tablets. On the basis of epilepsy data, the recommended adult starting dose is 500 to 1000 mg/day, followed by dose titration every two weeks based on response to a usual maintenance dose of 1000 to 3000 mg/day. The drug should be dosed twice daily. Assuming a target dose of 500 to 1500 mg twice daily when CrCl is normal (>80 mL/min), the respective target doses in mild, moderate, severe, and end-stage renal disease (as defined earlier in this section) are as follows: 500 to 1000 mg twice daily, 250 to 750 mg twice daily, 250 to 500 mg twice daily, and 500 to 1000 mg once daily, with a 250 to 500 mg supplemental dose after each hemodialysis session (41,91).

CLINICAL EFFICACY

Table 3 illustrates case report data for AEDs in neuropathic pain from the year 2000 to the present (92–107), while Table 4 presents clinical trial data over the same time period (34,98,108–154). A major deficiency of virtually all clinical trials of AEDs in neuropathic pain is the lack of "head-to-head" trials where one AED is compared

TABLE 3 Case Reports of AEDs in Neuropathic Pain Since 2000

Reference (year)	Type of neuropathic pain	No. of patients	Maximum dosage (mg/day)
Carbamazepine			
92 (2007)	"First bite" syndrome	1	800 mg/day
Felbamate			
93 (2003)	Trigeminal neuralgia	3	2400, 1200, 1200 mg/day
Gabapentin			
94 (2005)	Chronic cortical limb ischemia and rest pain	1	3600 mg/day
95 (2004)	"Painful legs and moving toes" syndrome	1	900 mg/day
96 (2004)	Cancer-related (Ewing's sarcoma)	1	900 mg/day
97 (2003)	Orbital pain	1	900 mg/day
98 (2003)	Traumatic central cervical cord lesion	1	600 mg/day
99 (2002)	SUNCT	1	900 mg/day
100 (2002)	SUNCT	1	1200 mg/day
101 (2002)	Central poststroke pain	1	900 mg/day
102 (2001)	Genitofemoral neuralgia	1	1200 mg/day
	Ilioinguinal neuralgia	1	1200 mg/day
Lamotrigine			
103 (2003)	SUNCT	1	300 mg/day
Oxcarbazepine			
104 (2005)	Complex regional pain syndrome, type 1	1	300 mg/day
105 (2004)	Postherpetic neuralgia	2	900, 900 mg/day
Topiramate			
106 (2003)	Diabetic neuropathy	1	200 mg/day
107 (2003)	Spinal cord injury–associated pain	2	200, 200 mg/day

Abbreviations: SUNCT, short-lasting, unilateral neuralgiform headache attacks with conjunctival injection and tearing.

(*text continues on page 76*)

TABLE 4 Clinical Trials of AEDs in Neuropathic Pain Since 2000

Reference (year)	Study design	Pain type	Number enrolled	Drug dosing regimen	Clinical results	Adverse events
Carbamazepine						
108 (2005)	R/DB/PC/CO trial	Guillain-Barre syndrome with neuritic pains (ICU)	12	CBZ 100 mg thrice daily for 3 days PLAC for 3 days 1-day washout period between treatment phases	In pts. receiving PLAC first, sign. ↓ in pain and sedation scores were noted on days 6 + 7 as well as a ↓ in the need for meperidine (all $p < 0.05$). In pts. receiving CBZ first, the need for meperidine ↓ sign. on days 1–3 and the washout day, sedation scores ↓ sign. on day 3 and the washout day, and the pain scores ↓ sign. on days 2–5 (all $p < 0.05$). Need for meperidine and pain scores gradually ↑ during PLAC period. Pooling CBZ and PLAC days together (36 of each), mean pain score was sign. ↓ on CBZ days (1.7) vs. PLAC days (3.1) ($p < 0.001$). Meperidine dose on PLAC days (mean 3.7 mg/kg/day) was sign. ↑ compared with that on CBZ days (1.1 mg/kg/day, $p < 0.001$). Mean sedation score on PLAC days (4.2) was sign. ↑ compared with that on CBZ days (2.3, $p < 0.001$)	No sign. AEs were noted
109 (2002)	CR	Neuropathic pain in feet (mountain climbers)	2	CBZ 200 mg thrice daily (regimen of other patient NS)	Marked improvement was seen in symptoms after initiation but even in untreated pts., pain resolves in 4–8 wk	No mention was made of any AEs

(Continued)

TABLE 4 Clinical Trials of AEDs in Neuropathic Pain Since 2000 (*Continued*)

Reference (year)	Study design	Pain type	Number enrolled	Drug dosing regimen	Clinical results	Adverse events
110 (2000)	DB/R/PC trial	Guillain-Barre with neuritic pains (ICU)	36	CBZ 100 mg thrice daily ×7 days ($N = 12$) GBP 300 mg thrice daily ×7 days ($N = 12$) PLAC ×7 days ($N = 12$)	Median pain rating scores favored GBP over PLAC and CBZ ($p < 0.05$ for both). ↓ in pain scores was sign. for all 7 days for GBP vs. PLAC ($p < 0.05$ for all 7 days) but only for days 4–7 for CBZ vs. PLAC ($p < 0.05$ for all 4). GBP effect was sign. greater than CBZ effect on all 7 study days ($p < 0.05$ for all 7). Median Ramsey sedation scores were sign. ↓ on all 7 study days vs. PLAC for both GBP and CBZ ($p < 0.05$ for all 14). GBP scores were sign. less than those of CBZ on all 7 study days ($p < 0.05$ for all 7). Mean consumption of rescue medication (fentanyl IV) was sign. ↓ in both active groups vs. PLAC group on all 7 study days ($p < 0.05$ for all 14) and that with GBP was less than that with CBZ on all 7 study days ($p < 0.05$ for all 7)	No AEs were reported
Clonazepam						
111 (2003)	O, NC trial	Cancer-related neuropathic pain	10	CLON 0.5 mg/day ×1 day → ↑ to 1 mg/day ×3 days → ↑ to 2 mg/day and titrated on the basis of response	Day 5 doses ranged from 0.5 to 2 mg/day (3 received 1 mg/day). Only 5 pts. were evaluable. 3 pts. D/C early due to escalating opioid doses during concurrent CLON dose titration. Pain scores fell in all 5 evaluable subjects from day 1 to day 5 (on a scale of 0–3, 3 pts. fell 1 point, 1 pt. fell 2 points, and 1 pt. fell 3 points)	2 D/C early due to sedation on day 2 (moderate in 1 pt., severe in 1 pt.)

Gabapentin						
112 (2006)	DB/R/PC trial	PHN	76	GBP 300 mg thrice daily → 600 mg thrice daily → 900 mg thrice daily ($N = 34$) NT 25 mg twice daily → 50 mg twice daily ($N = 36$) 2-wk interval between dose changes 8-wk trial duration	6 pts. did not complete the trial (5 lost to follow-up, 1 D/C without giving a reason). Data from 70 pts. were available for analysis. Intergroup differences were NS for pain scales (Likert scale, VAS, SF-MPQ), sleep assessment scale, percentages with at least a 50% improvement in pain, pt. GIC and disability ratings	47 AEs occurred in 58.3% of NT recipients and 9 AEs in GBP recipients (number of GBP pts. NS). 1 pt. D/C early due to severe urinary retention and 1 due to lack of efficacy (both in NT group). Frequencies of xerostomia (50% vs. 0, $p < 0.001$), constipation (22% vs. 0, $p = 0.003$), and orthostatic hypotension (33.3% vs. 0, $p < 0.001$) were sign. higher in NT compared with GBP recipients, respectively
113 (2006)	DB/R/PC trial	Postamputation pain (lower limbs)	46	GBP 300 mg/day on day 1; 900 mg/day on days 2–4; 1200 mg/day on days 5 + 6; 1500 mg/day on days 7 + 8; 1800 mg/day on days 9 + 10; 2100 mg/day on days 11 + 12; and 2400 mg/day on days 13–30 (with CrCl 30–60 mL/min, maximum daily dose = 1200 mg) ($N = 21$) PLAC ×30 days ($N = 20$) Therapy started on the first postoperative day	15 GBP and 18 PLAC recipients completed 6 mo follow-up. Intergroup differences were NS for risk of developing phantom pain; median intensity of phantom and stump pain; median rank scores of frequency, duration, and intensity by pts. of phantom pain; description of pain (McGill Pain Questionnaire); and opioid consumption (at 7, 14, 21, 30 days and 3, 6 mo). Only sign. intergroup difference was in duration of epidural analgesia postoperatively for stump pain (GBP 72.8 hr, PLAC 94.5 hr; $p = 0.01$)	2 pts. in each group D/C early due to AEs. AEs were reported in 9 GBP and 8 PLAC pts. (nausea, stomachache, fatigue, confusion, nightmares, itching, and ataxia were reported but these were not attributed to a specific treatment)

(Continued)

TABLE 4 Clinical Trials of AEDs in Neuropathic Pain Since 2000 (*Continued*)

Reference (year)	Study design	Pain type	Number enrolled	Drug dosing regimen	Clinical results	Adverse events
114 (2005)	O, NC trial	Cancer-related neuropathic pain	62[a]	GBP 300 mg/day → titrated to 1800 mg/day over 15 days (N = 41)	21 pts. (34%) did not complete the trial (protocol violation in 1, lost to follow-up in 3, pt. request in 1, medical deterioration in 10, AEs in 6). At the last timepoint, GBP produced, compared with baseline, sign. ↓ in mean worst pain, average pain, and pain "right now" and ↑ in percentage pain relief, activity, mood, walking, working, relationships, sleep, and enjoyment (p value range p < 0.0001 to p = 0.003). Only least pain was NS affected. 45.2% had a pain score reduction of at least 1/3 (NNT = 2.2). Pain scores on day 8 vs. day 15 were NS. Post hoc analysis suggested that GBP might only be beneficial in females (univariate p = 0.032)	AEs producing early study D/C were drowsiness in 3 and unsteady gait/ headaches, tremor, and nausea in 1 each. Overall AEs were blurred vision and drowsiness (in 5 each), headache and dizziness (in 3 each), unsteady gait (in 2), and heartburn, hallucinations, tremor, and nausea (in 1 each). 15 pts. (24%) had ≥1 AE thought to be due to GBP
115 (2005)	R/DB/PC/CO trial	SCI neuropathic pain	14	GBP 300 mg/day ×2 days → 600 mg/day ×5 days → 900 mg/day ×7 days → 1200 mg/ day ×7 days → 1800 mg/day to complete 4 wk PLAC ×4 wk 2-wk washout period between treatment phases	7 pts. withdrew early from the trial (lack of adherence in 4, AE in 1, and other reasons in 2). Only sign intergroup difference was a ↓ in "unpleasant feeling" by wk 4 with GBP vs. PLAC (p = 0.028). Pain intensity and other pain descriptors were NS different	No AEs were mentioned
116 (2005)	O, R trial	PHN (to establish initial dose to use)	61	GBP 100 mg twice daily (N = NA), GBP 100 mg 4 times daily (N = NA), GBP 200 mg thrice daily (N = NA); each treatment given for 3 days	Mean ± SD pain intensity was sign. ↓ by GBP (pooled VAS: day 1 = 6.5 ± 1.6 vs. day 3 = 4.5 ± 2.1, p < 0.05). Intergroup differences were NS.	AE demographics were NS different between the groups.

| 117 (2005) | O, NC trial | Pain of late stage Lyme disease[b] | 10 | GBP 300 mg/day → titrated over 4–12 wk on the basis of response to effective or maximum tolerated dose. Remained on therapy until pain ceased then gradually ↓ over wk. If relapsed, GBP restarted or dose was ↑. 1–2 yr follow-up | Dosage range of 500 to 1200 mg/day. Improvement occurred in "crawling" and "burning" sensations, and neck and radiating lumbar pain in 90%. Positive effect on mood, general feeling of health, and sleep quality in 50%. "Clearcut" pain ↓ at a mean dose of 700 mg/day | No AEs were mentioned |
| 118 (2004) | DB/R/PC trial | Cancer-related neuropathic pain (adding GBP to opioids) | 121 | GBP titrated from 600 to 1200 to 1800 mg/day (N = 58) PLAC (N = 31) 10-day trial duration. Opioid dose remained the same throughout study period | 21 GBP and 10 PLAC recipients did not complete the study (6 GBP and 3 PLAC pts. because of AEs, 11 GBP and 6 PLAC pts. needed prohibited therapy, 3 GBP pts. withdrew consent, and 1 GBP pt. had a protocol violation). Maximum daily GBP doses were 600, 1200, and 1800 mg in 7.5%, 22.7%, and 69.6% of pts., respectively. Mean follow-up global pain intensity and dysesthesia scores sign. favored GBP over PLAC (4.6 vs. 5.4, p = 0.025 and 4.28 vs. 5.24, p = 0.0077, respectively). GBP also was sign. better than PLAC in ↓ time needed to reach a pain intensity difference ≥33% (p = 0.048). Mean % of follow-up days with a pain intensity difference ≥33% were 51.6% (GBP) and 37.8% (PLAC) (p = 0.039). Only 15% of GBP vs. 40% of PLAC pts. never reached a pain-intensity difference ≥33% (p value NS). However, shooting or burning pain, number of episodes of lancinating pain, allodynia, use of additional analgesic doses, and use of "as needed" opioid doses were NS affected by GBP therapy | AEs included somnolence (23% vs. 0%), dizziness (9% vs. 0%), and nausea/vomiting (6% vs. 0%) in GBP and PLAC recipients, respectively (no statistical results available). |

(*Continued*)

TABLE 4 Clinical Trials of AEDs in Neuropathic Pain Since 2000 (*Continued*)

Reference (year)	Study design	Pain type	Number enrolled	Drug dosing regimen	Clinical results	Adverse events
119 (2004)	R/DB/PC trial	Painful HIV sensory neuropathy	26	GBP 400 mg/day → titrated over 2 wk to 1200 mg/day (given thrice daily) → titrated over 2 wk to 2400 mg/day (titration in 400 mg/day increments every 4 days) ($N = 14$ at wk 4, 13 at wk 6) PLAC ($N = 10$ at wk 4, 8 at wk 6) 4 wk DB phase followed by a 2 wk open phase where pts. could choose to initiate GBP (titrated to 1200 mg/day), maintain GBP at 1200 or 2400 mg/day or ↑ GBP to 3600 mg/day	2 pts. D/C from the study during the DB phase (1 GBP pt. due to AEs, 1 PLAC pt. for personal reasons). 3 more pts. D/C from the study during the open phase (1 GBP pt. due to lack of efficacy and 2 PLAC pts. for personal reasons). At the end of the DB phase, 4 and 10 GBP recipients were receiving 1200 and 2400 mg/day, respectively. At the end of the open phase, 2, 5, and 6 GBP recipients were receiving 1200, 2400, and 3600 mg/day, respectively. All 8 PLAC recipients had switched over to GBP 1200 mg/day. At the end of the DB phase, GBP had sign. ↓ median pain and sleep interference scores by 44.1% and 48.9%, respectively, from baseline. The effect of PLAC on these 2 parameters was NS	During the DB phase, somnolence occurred in 80% vs. 18.2% of GBP and PLAC pts., respectively ($p < 0.05$), and it was more severe in the GBP pts. The rates of dizziness, ataxia, nausea, vomiting, and headache were NS different
120 (2004)	O^e trial	PDN	6	GBP 300 mg thrice daily → 600 mg thrice daily → 900 mg thrice daily → 1200 mg thrice daily ($N = 3$) GBP (as above) + Vit. B1 100 mg/Vit. B12 0.2 mg per 300 mg GBP ($N = 3$) Doses were titrated at 7-day intervals	GBP alone: A trend to dose-dependent improvement in pain scores occurred with 600- and 900-mg doses (not 300 mg). At the end of wk 3, pooled pain scores were 60.5% of baseline. A similar pattern was noted with ADL interference scores (at the end of wk 3, pooled ADL interference scores were 55.1% of baseline) GBP + Vits: A dose-dependent ↓ in pain scores was seen at all 3 dose levels, and at the end of wk 3, pooled pain scores were 35.1% of baseline. A similar pattern was seen with ADL interference scores, wherein at the end of wk 3, pooled ADL interference scores were 36.1% of baseline	During wk 1 + 2, in the GBP group, dizziness, nausea, somnolence, and blurred vision occurred in 2, 1, 3, and 1 pt., respectively. Over the same time period, there were no AEs in the GBP + Vits. group. During wk 3, dizziness occurred in 1 GBP pt. and nausea and vomiting in 1 GBP + Vits. pt. (results suggest that Vit. B1/B12 ameliorate or delay the emergence of AEs to GBP)

| 98 (2004) | DB/R/PC/CO trial | Traumatic SCI neuropathic pain | 20 | GBP 300 mg thrice daily by the end of wk 1 → 600 mg thrice daily by the end of wk 2 → 800 mg thrice daily by the end of wk 3 → 1200 mg thrice daily by the end of wk 4
PLAC ×4 wk
2 wk washout period between treatment phases | Mean ± SD daily dose of GBP (without AEs) = 2235 ± 501 mg (range 900–2700). Mean ± SD maximum tolerated daily dose of GBP = 2850 ± 751 mg (range 1200–3600). All pts. completed trial participation. At all times, GBP was sign. superior to PLAC in ↓ pain scores from baseline ($p < 0.001$). Similar findings were noted for pain episode frequency, sleep interference scores, and disability due to pain. There were sign. differences between groups favoring GBP, for sharp, hot, unpleasant, deep, and surface pain types but not dull, cold, sensitive, or itchy pain types (% relief values: GBP 53–62%, PLAC 8–13%) | Only AE demographic parameter that was sign. different between treatments was the overall frequency (AEs in 65% of GBP treatments vs. 25% of PLAC treatments, $p < 0.05$) |
| 121 (2003) | O, NC trial | Cauda aquina or SCI neuropathic pain (efficacy as a function of disease duration) | 31 | GBP 300 mg/day → titrated every 3 days to 600, 900, 1200, 1500, 1800 mg/day (total = 18 days) → 5-wk maintenance phase (could ↑ to 2400 or 3600 mg/day, if necessary) Group 1: pain <6 mo in duration (13 pts, 9 with sleep interference; 11 pts. completed the trial). Group 2: pain >6 mo in duration (18 pts., 13 with sleep interference; 14 pts. completed the trial) | 25 (81%) completed the trial. 6 D/C early (3 with difficulty making visits, 2 disliked chronic meds., 1 had AE). Pain and sleep interference scores ↓ sign. from baseline in both groups ($p < 0.05$) and at all assessment time points (2, 4, 6, 8 wk). ↓ in both scores was sign. greater for group 1 than group 2 from wk 2–8 (all $p < 0.05$). ↓ in pain score ≥2 points occurred in 100% group 1 and 71% group 2 pts. (results of statistical analyses NA). ↓ in sleep interference score ≥2 points in 89% group 1 and 62% group 2 pts. (results of statistical analyses NA) | Somnolence occurred in 32% (dose dependent but data not shown). Edema, dizziness, headache, perioral numbness, and worsened preexisting renal insufficiency occurred in 3% each. 9 pts. had somnolence alone while 1 had somnolence with all other listed AEs |

(Continued)

TABLE 4 Clinical Trials of AEDs in Neuropathic Pain Since 2000 (*Continued*)

Reference (year)	Study design	Pain type	Number enrolled	Drug dosing regimen	Clinical results	Adverse events
122 (2003)	Retrospective chart review[d]	PHN (change in opioid dosing after starting GBP)	45	35 pts. (78%) received $\geq$2 prescriptions for GBP	Overall proportion receiving opioids fell from 88.9% pretreatment to 71.1% at follow-up ($p = 0.03$). Proportion receiving short-acting agents fell from 86.7% to 62.2% ($p = 0.01$) while proportion receiving long-acting agents was NS changed. Overall number of opioid prescriptions/pt. fell sign. (3.9 → 3.0, $p = 0.03$), especially short-acting agents (3.3 → 2.4, $p = 0.04$). Number of opioid prescriptions fell only in recipients of $\geq$2 GBP prescriptions (overall, 4.3 → 3.1, $p = 0.02$; short-acting agents, 3.6 → 2.4, $p = 0.03$). No effect was seen in recipients of only 1 GBP prescription	No AEs were reported
123 (2003)	O, NC trial	Fabry disease	6	GBP (no details were provided regarding the initial regimen or titration scheme)	Mean daily dose = 917 mg (range 100–1200 mg). Although pain scores fell over 4 wks from baseline (mean average pain score: 5.0 → 3.7 and mean pain "at its worst": 6.8 → 4.8), these changes were NS. No pt. became pain free	Vertigo and blurred speech occurred in 1 pt. (disappeared after dose reduction)
124 (2002)	O, NC trial	Cancer-related neuropathic pain	23	GBP 100 mg thrice daily on day 1 → 200 mg thrice daily on day 2 → 300 mg thrice daily on day 3 → titrated per pt. response 4-wk trial duration	15 (65%) completed the trial. 5 (22%) D/C treatment early on day 15 due to treatment failure. Pain intensity was ↓ by > 50% in 11 (48%) at wk 4. Mean pain relief increased from 8.33% at baseline to 66.58% at wk 4 ($p < 0.01$; where 0% = none → 100% = complete). Mean pain intensity fell from 60.93 → 30.20 mm ($p < 0.01$) or 2.60 → 1.27 ($p < 0.01$). Mean pain quality (from the sensory sets of the SF-MPQ) fell from 13.20 → 3.00 ($p < 0.01$) while the effect on daily life fell from 63.60 → 24.67 ($p < 0.01$)	3 (13%) D/C treatment early (on day 8) due to AEs. Somnolence and mental clouding occurred in 14 (61%) and 13 (57%) pts., respectively. Headache, confusion, dizziness, disequilibrium, and LOC occurred in 5, 4, 3, 1, and 3 pts., respectively. Hyperglycemia occurred in 1 pt

| 125 (2002) | O, NC trial | SCI neuropathic pain | 38 | GBP 300 mg thrice daily → titration based on response [median maintenance dose = 2400 mg/day (range 900–4800 mg/day) (N = 29)] | 9 pts. D/C early (5 due to lack of efficacy). 76% of pts. reported a ↓ in pain. 11 pts. had complete data (0, 1, 3, 6 mo): mean pain scores of 8.86 → 5.23 → 4.59 → 4.13, respectively (p < 0.001 for trend). By verbal descriptions, there was a trend for improvement from "unbearable" pretreatment to "livable" during treatment | 4 pts. D/C early due to AEs. AEs occurred in 8 pts. (primarily drowsiness, dizziness, somnolence) |
| 126 (2002) | DB/R/PC trial | Multiple neuropathic pain syndromes | 305 | GBP titrated to 900 mg/day over 3 days → 1800 mg/day after 2 wk → 2400 mg/day after another 2 wk (N = 121) PLAC (N = 111) 5-wk titration phase → 3-wk maintenance phase | 32 GBP pts. D/C early (AEs in 24, lack of efficacy in 1, other reasons in 7) and 41 PLAC pts. D/C early (nonadherence in 2, AEs in 25, lack of efficacy in 5, other reasons in 9). At end of titration phase, 101 were taking 2400 mg/day, 19 were taking 1800 mg/day, and 27 were taking 900 mg/day. Mean diary-pain scores improved by 21% (GBP) and 14% (PLAC) (p = 0.048). Intergroup differences were sign. at wk 1, 3, 4, 5, 6. In wk 7 and 8, scores stayed constant in the GBP group and fell in the PLAC group; thus differences became NS. Pt. GIC of "very much" or "much improved" was noted in 34% (GBP) and 16% (PLAC) (p = 0.03) while investigator GIC rates were 38% and 18%, respectively (p = 0.01). In the SF-MPQ instrument, GBP vs. PLAC was sign. only for the sensory and total scores (favored GBP). GBP was sign. superior to PLAC in the SF-36 QOL instrument domains of bodily pain, social functioning, and emotional role (all p < 0.05). Response rates (>50% ↓ in mean pain score from baseline to wk 8) were 21% (GBP) and 14% (PLAC) (p = NS). Only sign. intergroup differences in pain types occurred with burning pain (wk 1, 3) and hyperalgesia (wk 3–6), all favoring GBP | Overall AE rates (probably or possibly trial-related) were 58% (GBP) vs. 37% (PLAC). The rates of individual AEs (GBP/PLAC) were: dizziness (24/8%), somnolence (14/5%), headache (9/14%), nausea (9/9%), and abdominal pain (7/4%) (no statistical results were available) |

(Continued)

TABLE 4 Clinical Trials of AEDs in Neuropathic Pain Since 2000 (*Continued*)

Reference (year)	Study design	Pain type	Number enrolled	Drug dosing regimen	Clinical results	Adverse events
127 (2002)	DB/R/PC/CO trial	Guillain-Barre syndrome (ICU)	18	GBP 5 mg/kg thrice daily ×7 days PLAC ×7 days 2-day washout period between phases	In GBP phase, mean pain score ↓ from baseline 7.22 → 2.33 on day 2 → 2.06 on day 7 (sign. different from PLAC on all study days; $p < 0.001$ for all). Sign. ↓ in opioid utilization as well (mean for PLAC of 319 μg on day 1 → 317 μg on day 7. Mean for GBP 211 μg on day 1 → 65 μg on day 7. Intergroup differences were sign. on all study days; $p < 0.001$ for all). Ramsey Sedation Scores were sign. ↑ in GBP compared with PLAC recipients on all 7 days ($p < 0.001$ for all)	During the GBP phase, there was 1 case of nausea while, in the PLAC phase, there were 2 cases of nausea and 3 of constipation. This finding was probably a consequence of increased opioid use in the PLAC recipients
128 (2001)	DB/R/PC trial	PHN	334	GBP 1800 mg/day via forced titration schedule (N = 93) GBP 2400 mg/day via forced titration schedule (N = 85) PLAC (N = 94) 7-wk trial duration (titration schedule: 300 mg on day 1, 600 mg on day 2, 900 mg on day 3, 1200 mg on days 4–7, 1500 mg on day 8, 1800 mg on days 9–14, 2100 mg on day 15, 2400 mg on days 16-end)	18.6% (62 pts.) D/C early. At end of trial, mean pain scores had been reduced, compared with baseline, by 34.5% with GBP 1800 mg/day and 34.4% with GBP 2400 mg/day vs. 15.7% with PLAC ($p < 0.01$ for both). Percentages of responders (defined as ≥50% ↓ in pain scores) were 32% (GBP 1800 mg/day), 34% (GBP 2400 mg/day), and 14% (PLAC) ($p = 0.001$ for both). Sign. intergroup differences occurred from wk 1 onward. Sleep interference score results paralleled those of pain scores. In terms of the components of the SF-MPQ instrument, GBP was sign. superior to PLAC for sensory scores (both doses), total scores (both doses), and VAS of pain scores during the previous week (GBP 2400 mg/day only) (all $p < 0.05$). For the pt. GIC "much" or "very much improved" was noted by 41% of GBP 1800 mg/day ($p = 0.003$) and 43% of GBP 2400 mg/day ($p = 0.005$) recipients vs. 23% of PLAC recipients.	Early D/C was primarily due to AEs (PLAC = 6.3%, GBP 1800 mg/day = 13%, GBP 2400 mg/day = 17.6%). 38% of early D/C due to AEs occurred within the first week and 76% within the first 3 wk. Overall AE rates (possibly/probably trial related) for PLAC/ 1800 mg/GBP 2400 mg were 28/57/60%. AEs with rates ≥5% included dizziness (10/31/33%), somnolence (6/17/ 20%), peripheral edema (0/5/11%), and asthenia (4/6/6%), and

Ref (year)	Design	Condition	N	Treatment	Results	Adverse events
					For the clinician GIC, "much" or "very much improved" was noted in 44% of 1800 mg/day ($p = 0.002$) and 2400 mg/day ($p = 0.001$) recipients vs. 19% of PLAC recipients. For the SF-36 QOL instrument, GBP produced sign. improvements in the bodily pain (1800 mg/day only, $p < 0.01$), vitality (both doses, both $p < 0.05$), and mental health (1800 mg/day only, $p < 0.05$) domains vs. PLAC	diarrhea and xerostomia (1/6/5%, each). Results of statistical analyses were not available
129 (2001)	O, NC trial	Painful HIV neuropathy (drug- or disease-related)	19	GBP 300 mg/day to start → ↑ by 300 mg/day every 2 days to adequate relief or maximum tolerated dose (maximum allowed dose = 3600 mg/day)	Mean ± SD GBP daily dose = 1480 ± 646 mg/day. No effect was noted by 1 pt. (5%). Improvement of pain began after a mean of 6 days and maximal relief was achieved after a mean of 12 days. After 4 mo, mean ± SD pain score had fallen from 55.7 ± 19.1 mm at baseline to 14.7 ± 18.6 mm ($p = 0.0001$). A parallel finding was noted for sleep interference scores (60.4 ± 31.9 mm → 15.5 ± 27.7 mm, $p = 0.0001$). 15 pts. (79%) remained on GBP after 1 to 11 mo follow-up while 4 pts. (21%) stopped GBP after 1 to 3 mo as they had achieved complete/near complete pain relief. No relapse was noted at 1 mo after D/C	Only 1 AE was reported (left leg edema). In 12 pts. where electrophysiologic studies of nerve conduction were performed, the effect of GBP was NS
Lamotrigine 34 (2003)	O, NC trial	Sciatica	14	LTG titrated from 25 to 400 mg/day on weekly basis over 6-wk. Maintenance phase of 4-wk duration	8 pts. (57%) completed the titration period and 7/14 (50%) completed the entire trial (4 left early for personal reasons and 1 due to lack of efficacy). Spontaneous pain, pain intensity, and SF-MPQ scores only sign. improved from baseline with 400 mg dose ($p < 0.05$ for all). Similar findings were noted with leg and LS movement testing ($p < 0.05$ for all). For the 8 completing the titration phase, 2 (25%) had no improvement in pain scores (<1 point) while 6 (75%) had substantial ↓ in scores [from mean of 6.7 (baseline) to 4.7 at wk 6 and 4.0 at wk 10] (statistical results NA). Rescue analgesia use fell from mean of 3.5 pills (baseline) to 2.2 pills (wk 10) (statistical results NA)	2 pts. left study early because of AEs (diarrhea and dizziness in 1 each). AEs in 4/14 (29%) (diarrhea in 1, dizziness in 3)

(Continued)

TABLE 4 Clinical Trials of AEDs in Neuropathic Pain Since 2000 (*Continued*)

Reference (year)	Study design	Pain type	Number enrolled	Drug dosing regimen	Clinical results	Adverse events
130 (2002)	CS	Neuralgia postnerve sectioning	6	LTG 25 mg/day → ↑ in 25 mg/day increments every 6 days to 100 mg/day → ↑ in 50 mg increments, every 6 days, to maximum of 300 mg/day. Trial duration of 1–23 mo, with 4–29 mo follow-up	Maximum LTG dose ranged from 25 to 300 mg/day. Burning/shooting pain intensity ↓ 33–100% and attack frequency fell 80–100% (statistical analyses were not performed)	No mention was made of AEs
Levetiracetam						
131 (2005)	CS	Neoplastic plexopathies (brachial and lumbosacral)	7	Initial LEV regimen was 500–1000 mg/day. Titrated over several days to 2 wk to effective or maximum tolerated dose (details NA)	Maximum LEV dose ranged from 1000–3000 mg/day (twice daily). 7/7 had improved pain control (VAS 8–9 → 0–3 within 2–14 days of initiating LEV). Mean ↓ in opioid use of 70%	No drug-related AEs were mentioned
132 (2004)	CS	Bilateral lower extremity peripheral neuropathy	3	Details of initial LEV regimen and titration schedule NA	Maximum LEV dose ranged from 500 to 3000 mg/day (once or twice daily). 2/3 (67%) had a complete remission and 1/3 (33%) had a 60% remission of pain	No mention was made of AEs
133 (2003)	O, NC trial	PHN	10	LEV 500 mg/day → ↑ by 500 mg/day each week to maximum of 3000 mg/day (twice daily). 12-wk trial duration	Maximum LEV doses ranged from 1500 to 3000 mg/day (mean 2200 mg/day). 3/10 (30%) were "responders" (67–75% improvement in pain, improved sleep, 61–64% ↓ in allodynia, 40–80% ↓ in area of pain/allodynia. Pt. GIC ratings of "much" or "very much improved"). 3/10 (30%) were partial responders (11–50% improvement in pain, improved sleep, 1 pt. had ↓ allodynia severity but no change in area of pain/allodynia while 2 pts. had slight ↑ in allodynia but 50% ↓ in area of pain/allodynia. Pt. GIC rating as "improved"). 4/10 (40%) were clinical failures and left study early	Mild-moderate drowsiness and lack of energy were commonest AEs (no details provided). 1 pt. D/C LEV early (hypertensive urgency on day 27)

Oxcarbazepine

Ref (year)	Study	Pain type	N	Dosing	Results	Adverse events
134 (2006)	O, NC trial	PDN	43	OXCARB 150 mg/day → titrated up to 1200 mg/day at rate allowed by tolerance of pt. 6-mo trial duration	38 (88%) completed trial participation (none left due to AEs). Mean ± SD maximum OXCARB daily dose = 1089.5 ± 146.6 mg (median = 1200 mg). Sign. ↓ occurred in mean worst pain intensity (7.6 → 4.2), least pain intensity (6.3 → 3.2), pain intensity "right now" (5.7 → 2.8), and average pain intensity (6.3 → 3.2), at 6 mo vs. baseline (all p < 0.001). 59% had ≥50% ↓ in pain intensity scores (≥50% ↓ in worst pain, least pain, pain "right now," and average pain in 52.7%, 63.1%, 55.3%, and 63.2%, respectively). Social interference scores improved ≥50% in 62% (≥50% improvement in general activities, mood, walking, working, relationships, and sleep/life enjoyment scores in 60.6%, 63.2%, 52.6%, 60.5%, 68.4%, and 63.2%, respectively)	No hyponatremia was noted. 12 pts. (28%) had AEs (dizziness in 7, nausea in 5, profound sleepiness in 1)
135 (2005)	O, NC trial	PHN[e]	24	150 mg/day to start → ↑ by 150 mg/day every 2 days → maximum 900 mg/day 8-wk trial duration	19 (79%) completed trial participation (3 D/C early due to lack of efficacy). Sign. pain reduction occurred at 8 wk compared with baseline (p < 0.001). Sign. reduction occurred by the end of wk 1. Investigators felt that there was a clinically-sign. ↓ in allodynia (no quantitative data or statistics were provided). Responder rates (>50% ↓ in pain scores) were 4.8%, 36.8%, 52.6%, 84.2%, and 84.2% at wk 2, 3, 4, 6, and 8, respectively. OXCARB was judged as "very good," "good," and "not satisfactory" by 50%, 29%, and 13% of pts., respectively	2 D/C early due to AEs (mild-moderate dizziness, nausea, and sedation). No AEs were reported by the other 22 pts
136 (2005)	O, NC trials (pooled analysis of 7 trials)	Variety of neuropathic pain types	136	OXCARB 150 mg/day → ↑ by 150 mg/day every 2–3 days over 4 wk → 1800 mg/day or maximum tolerated dose 8-wk trial duration	Mean pain score fell 50.2% (77.13 → 38.41). Response rate (≥50% ↓ in pain score) was 49.2%	Most common AEs were vertigo, tremors, somnolence, hypotension, and nausea

(Continued)

TABLE 4 Clinical Trials of AEDs in Neuropathic Pain Since 2000 (*Continued*)

Reference (year)	Study design	Pain type	Number enrolled	Drug dosing regimen	Clinical results	Adverse events
137 (2005)	DB/R/PC trial	PDN	146	OXCARB 300 mg/day → 600 mg/day on day 3 → ↑ by 300 mg/day every 5 days to maximum tolerated dose or 1800 mg/day by wk 4 (N = 44) PLAC (N = 62) 16 wk trial duration (treatments given twice daily)	6 and 9 pts. D/C therapy early in the OXCARB and PLAC groups, respectively, for reasons other than AEs. Mean ± SD maintenance phase dose = 1445 ± 389 mg/day. 55% of OXCARB pts. were maintained on 1800 mg/day. Mean ↓ in pain score (baseline → wk 16) was −24.3 (OXCARB) and −14.7 (PLAC) ($p = 0.0108$). Sign. intergroup differences in pain ↓ occurred in wk 2 [−8.0 (OXCARB) vs. −4.7 (PLAC), $p < 0.05$]. Response rates (> 50% ↓ in pain scores) were 35.2% (OXCARB) and 18.4% (PLAC) ($p = 0.0156$). Response rates (>30% ↓ in pain scores) were 45.6% (OXCARB) and 28.9% (PLAC) ($p = 0.0288$). NNT = 6.0 (at both response thresholds). Pt. GIC of "much" or "very much improved" by treatment occurred in 48% (OXCARB) and 22% (PLAC) pts. ($p = 0.0025$). NNT = 3.9. A "therapeutic effect" (2 consecutive days with ≥20 unit ↓ in pain score from baseline) occurred in 56.5% of OXCARB and 46.8% of PLAC pts. ($p = 0.0209$). The improvement from baseline in pain scores favored OXCARB over PLAC in wk 2, 4–8, 10–16 ($p ≤ 0.05$ in all). The mean proportion of days awakened from sleep by pain was sign. lower for OXCARB pts. (31%) vs. PLAC pts. (49%) ($p = 0.02$). The only sign. intergroup difference in the SF-36 QOL instrument occurred in the aggregate mental health score ($p = 0.03$). In the Profile of Mood States instrument, most intergroup comparisons were NS. PLAC was favored over OXCARB for the confusion-bewilderment scale (3.8 vs. 5.1, respectively; $p = 0.003$) and the vigor-activity scale (8.6 vs. 7.8, respectively; $p = 0.006$)	AEs led to premature study D/C in 19 (28%) of OXCARB and 6 (8%) of PLAC recipients. During the titration phase, the frequencies of AEs to OXCARB/PLAC were as follows: Dizziness 45/8% Headache 25/8% Nausea 23/9% Somnolence 12/3% Fatigue 12/7% Vomiting 9/4% These frequencies dropped during the maintenance phase (due to D/C from the study or the development of tolerance). A clinically-relevant decline in serum sodium to below 125 mEq/L occurred in 3 OXCARB recipients (4.3%). Dose reduction normalized the serum sodium in 2 pts. and the other pt. was D/C early from the study

			N			
138 (2004)	O, NC trial	PDN	30	OXCARB 150 mg/day → daily dose doubled every wk and titrated per tolerability over 4 wk to maximum tolerated dose or 1200 mg/day 8-wk trial duration	20 (67%) completed the trial (5 were D/C due to non-AE-related issues). Mean OXCARB dose during the maintenance phase was 814 mg/day. Maintenance phase dose distribution: 150 mg/day in 1, 300 mg/day in 2, 450 mg/day in 1, 600 mg/day in 10, 900 mg/day in 4, and 1200 mg/day in 10. Mean pain scores ↓ from 66.3 → 34.3 ($p = 0.0001$) (mean ↓ 48.3%). Similar sign. findings were also found with use of the SF-MPQ and PPI pain instruments. 47% were responders (≥50% ↓ pain scores). In the SF-36 QOL instrument, the only sign. difference from baseline was in the domain of bodily pain ($p = 0.0115$). In the Profile of Mood States instrument, no sign. effect was seen with any of the 6 mood items	5 were D/C due to AEs (panic attack, stroke, and pregnancy in 1 each and mild dizziness + diarrhea in 2 each). AEs occurring in ≥10% of pts. included drowsiness (43%), dizziness (37%), headache (30%), nausea/vomiting (23%), and diarrhea (10%). Mild asymptomatic hyponatremia occurred in 1 pt. (no details provided)
Phenytoin 139 (2001)	CS	TN (acute crisis)	3	Fosphenytoin IV (total doses of 11, 14, and 18 mg/kg given in single or multiple fractions)	PO intake compromised by acute TN crises. In all cases, complete pain relief lasted for 2 days, allowing preparation for surgery or modification of baseline PO therapy	No mention was made of AEs
Pregabalin 140 (2006)	DB/R/PC trial	PHN	370	PGB 600 mg/day (N = 60) PGB 300 mg/day (N = 62) PGB 150 mg/day (N = 61) PLAC (N = 59) All treatments given twice daily 13-wk trial duration	34% D/C early (16% due to AEs, 16% due to lack of efficacy, 1% due to lack of adherence, 6% for other reasons). Dose-dependent ↓ in pain scores vs. baseline compared with PLAC (for PGB 150, 300, and 600 mg/day, differences $=-0.88$, -1.07, and -1.79, respectively; $p = 0.0077, 0.0016$, and 0.0003, respectively). Sign. differences emerged as early as wk 1. PGB produced ↓ sleep interference vs. PLAC ($p < 0.001$), beginning in wk 1 ($p < 0.01$). Pts. receiving 150 mg/day and 600 mg/day reported more global improvement than did PLAC pts. ($p = 0.02$ and 0.003, respectively)	Most AEs were mild-moderate in severity. 13.5% of PGB recipients prematurely D/C study participation due to AEs [most commonly due to dizziness (5.8%), somnolence (2.9%), and ataxia (2.5%)]

(Continued)

TABLE 4 Clinical Trials of AEDs in Neuropathic Pain Since 2000 (*Continued*)

Reference (year)	Study design	Pain type	Number enrolled	Drug dosing regimen	Clinical results	Adverse events
141 (2006)	DB/R/PC trial	SCI neuropathic pain	137	PGB flexible dose (150–600 mg/day) (N = 49) (initiated at 150 mg/day × 7 days → 300 mg/day × 7 days → 600 mg/day. Dose could be reduced, if not tolerated.) PLAC (N = 37) Treatments were given twice daily 12-wk trial duration	Withdrawal rates were 30% (PGB) and 45% (PLAC), due to lack of efficacy in 7% and 30%, respectively. Mean PGB dose after 3-wk stabilization phase was 460 mg/day. PGB reduced mean pain score (6.54 → 4.62) sign. more than did PLAC (6.73 → 6.27) ($p <$ 0.001). Sign. PGB effect was noted after 1 wk of therapy. Responder rates were sign. ↑ with PGB vs. PLAC ($\geq$30% ↓ in pain score: 42% vs. 16%, $p = 0.001$; $\geq$50% ↓ in pain score: 22% vs. 8%, $p < 0.05$). PGB sign. improved disturbed sleep (intergroup difference of 1.37, $p < 0.001$) and anxiety (intergroup difference of 1.1, $p = 0.043$) compared with PLAC. Pt. GIC favored PGB over PLAC ($p < 0.001$). PGB produced sign. greater improvement on the total score, affective score, sensory score, VAS score, and present pain intensity index components of the SF-MPQ ($p \leq 0.002$ for all)	Withdrawal rates due to AEs were 21% (PGB, included somnolence, edema, asthenia, amnesia, blurred vision, urinary incontinence) and 13% (PLAC, included edema, blurred vision, myasthenia, abnormal thinking, and paresthesia). Treatment-emergent AEs occurred in 75% of PLAC and 96% of PGB patients. Major AEs included somnolence (41.4% vs. 9%, PGB vs. PLAC), dizziness (24.3% vs. 9%), edema (20% vs. 6%), asthenia (15.7% vs. 6%), and dry mouth (15.7% vs. 3%). Results of statistical analyses were NA

142 (2005) DB/R/PC trial	PDN PHN	338	PGB fixed-dose: 300 mg/day × 1 wk → 600 mg/day × 11 wk ($N = 82$) PGB flexible-dose: 150 mg/day × 1 wk → 300 mg/day × 1 wk → 450 mg/day × 1 wk → 600 mg/day (dose ↓ due to intolerance was allowed) to complete 12 wk ($N = 92$) PLAC × 12 wk ($N = 35$)	Withdrawal rates were 35% (flexible-dose PGB), 38% (fixed-dose PGB), and 46% (PLAC). Both flexible- and fixed-dose PGB regimens sign. ↓ mean end point pain scores vs. PLAC [for flexible-dose: sign. at wk 2 ($p = 0.021$) and wk 3–12 (all $p < 0.013$); for fixed-dose, sign. at wk 1 ($p = 0.007$) and wk 2–12, (all $p < 0.001$)]. Both were also sign. superior to PLAC in improving pain-related sleep interference (for both, $p ≤ 0.01$ for wk 1–5 and $p ≤ 0.05$ for wk 9-end point). Responder rates were sign. ↑ for PGB vs. PLAC recipients (for ≥30% ↓ in pain scores, 59/66/37% of flexible-dose PGB/fixed-dose PGB/PLAC, $p = 0.003$ for flexible-dose and $p < 0.001$ for fixed-dose; for ≥50% ↓, 48/52/24% of flexible-dose PGB/fixed-dose PGB/PLAC, both $p < 0.001$). Patient GIC favored both PGB regimens over PLAC (both $p < 0.01$)	Withdrawal due to AEs occurred in 17%, 25%, and 8% of flexible-dose PGB, fixed-dose PGB, and PLAC recipients, respectively. Most frequent AEs due to PGB flexible-dose/ PGB fixed-dose/ PLAC were dizziness (2/8/2%), peripheral edema (2/1/0%), wt. gain (1/1/0%), and somnolence (0/4/0%). Results of statistical analyses were NA
143 (2005) R/DB/PC trial	PDN	246	PGB 150 mg/day ($N = 75$) PGB 600 mg/day ($N = 72$) PLAC ($N = 72$) 6-wk trial duration	Withdrawal rates were 5%, 12%, and 15% in PGB 150 mg/day, PGB 600 mg/day, and PLAC pts., respectively. PGB 600 mg/day ↓ mean pain score sign. more than did PLAC (to 4.3 vs. 5.6, $p = 0.0002$). Sign. intergroup differences in pain scores occurred from wk 2 to end point. Proportion of responders (≥50% ↓ from baseline pain) was sign. greater for PGB 600 mg/day recipients (39%) than PLAC recipients (15%, $p = 0.002$). PGB 600 mg/day also sign. ↓, compared with PLAC, sleep interference scores (all $p < 0.05$, wk 1 to end point), SF-MPQ present pain intensity scores ($p = 0.002$), SF-MPQ sensory pain scores ($p = 0.002$), SF-MPQ affective pain scores ($p = 0.0028$), SF-MPQ total pain scores ($p = 0.0002$), and SF-MPQ VAS scores ($p = 0.0002$). Investigators rated	Withdrawal due to AEs occurred in 3%, 9%, and 5% of PGB 150 mg/day, PGB 600 mg/day, and PLAC recipients, respectively. The most common AEs with PGB 150 mg/ day/PGB 600 mg/day/ PLAC were dizziness (10/38/2%), somnolence (5/22/4%), edema (4/17/5%), headache (8/16/11%), and asthenia (4/12/ 4%). Results of

(Continued)

TABLE 4 Clinical Trials of AEDs in Neuropathic Pain Since 2000 (*Continued*)

Reference (year)	Study design	Pain type	Number enrolled	Drug dosing regimen	Clinical results	Adverse events
					more PGB 600 mg/day than PLAC recipients as improved (73% vs. 45%, respectively, $p = 0.002$), while patient GIC favored PGB 600 mg/day over PLAC (85% vs. 47% were improved, respectively, $p = 0.002$). PGB 150 mg/day was essentially no different from PLAC	statistical analyses were NA
144 (2004)	R/DB/PC trial	PDN	146	PGB 300 mg/day ($N = 65$) PLAC ($N = 62$) Doses were administered twice daily 8-wk trial duration	Withdrawal rates were 15% (PGB) and 11% (PLAC). PGB produced sign. improvements vs. PLAC in mean pain scores (intergroup difference -1.47, $p = 0.0001$), sleep interference scores (-1.54, $p = 0.0001$), SF-36 bodily pain domain ($+6.87$, $p = 0.0294$), SF-MPQ total scores (-4.41, $p = 0.0033$), SF-MPQ VAS scores (-16.19, $p = 0.0002$), SF-MPQ PPI scores (-0.37, $p = 0.0364$), patient GIC ($p = 0.001$), POMS Total Mood Disturbance component (-9.95, $p = 0.0234$), and POMS Tension-Anxiety component (-2.10, $p = 0.0264$). Sign. pain relief and sleep improvement began during wk 1 of therapy with PGB. Investigator and patient GIC favored PGB over PLAC ($p = 0.004$ and $p = 0.001$, respectively)	Withdrawal due to AEs occurred in 3% of PLAC and 11% of PGB recipients. The most common AEs (PGB/PLAC) were dizziness (36/11%), somnolence (20/3%), edema (11/1%), and blurred vision (5/1%). Results of statistical analyses were NA
145 (2004)	R/DB/PC trial	PHN (failed $\geq$ 1200 mg/day GBP)	238	PGB 150 mg/day ($N = 71$) PGB 300 mg/day ($N = 60$) PLAC ($N = 61$) 8-wk trial duration	Withdrawal occurred in 12% of PGB 150 mg/day, 21% of PGB 300 mg/day, and 25% of PLAC pts. End point mean pain scores were ↓ sign. more by PGB 150 mg/day (-1.20) and 300 mg/day (-1.57) than by PLAC ($p = 0.0002$ and $p = 0.0001$, respectively). SF-MPQ VAS scores were ↓ sign. more by PGB 150 mg/day (-10.02, $p = 0.006$) and 300 mg/day (-13.64,	Withdrawal due to AEs occurred in 10% of PLAC, 11% of PGB 150 mg/day, and 16% of PGB 300 mg/day recipients. The most common AEs (PGB 150 mg/PGB 300 mg/

						Results	Adverse events
						$p = 0.0003$) than by PLAC. Response rates (≥50% ↓ in mean pain scores) were 26%, 28%, and 10% with PGB 150 mg/day, PGB 300 mg/day, and PLAC, respectively ($p = 0.006$ and $p = 0.003$, respectively). PGB 150 mg/day and 300 mg/day also ↓ mean sleep interference scores more than did PLAC (-1.11 and -1.43, respectively; $p = 0.0003$ and $p = 0.0001$, respectively). Patient GIC favored only PGB 300 mg/day over PLAC ($p = 0.002$). PGB 150 mg/day sign. improved SF-36 mental health domain scores ($p = 0.043$), while 300 mg/day did so for mental health ($p = 0.043$), bodily pain ($p = 0.005$), and vitality ($p = 0.044$) domains	PLAC) were dizziness (12/28/15%), somnolence (15/24/8%), edema (3/13/0%), headache (11/11/4%), and dry mouth 11/7/4%). Results of statistical analyses were NA
146 (2004)	R/DB/PC trial	PDN	338	PGB 75 mg/day ($N = 67$) PGB 300 mg/day ($N = 76$) PGB 600 mg/day (titrated to target dose over 6 days) ($N = 70$) PLAC ($N = 89$) 5-wk trial duration		PGB 300 mg/day and 600 mg/day sign. ↓ mean end point pain scores compared to PLAC (differences of -1.26 and -1.45, respectively; both $p = 0.0001$). Corresponding values for differences in end point sleep interference scores were -1.3 and -1.6 (both $p = 0.0001$). Corresponding values for differences in SF-MPQ total scores were -4.89 and -5.18 (both $p = 0.0001$). Similar findings were noted in SF-MPQ VAS and PPI scores (all $p = 0.0001$). Both investigator and patient GIC evaluations favored PGB 300 and 600 mg/day over PLAC (both $p = 0.001$). Sign. intergroup differences began as early as the wk 1 evaluation. Response rates (≥50% ↓ in pain) were 46, 48, and 18% for PGB 300 mg/day, 600 mg/day, and PLAC, respectively (both $p = 0.0001$)	Withdrawal due to AEs occurred in 3.1%, 2.6%, 3.7%, and 12.2% of PLAC, PGB 75 mg/day, 300 mg/day, and 600 mg/day recipients, respectively. The most frequent AEs were dizziness (39/27/8/5% for PGB 600 mg daily/300 mg daily/75 mg daily/PLAC), somnolence (27/24/4/4%), and edema (13/7/4/2%)

(Continued)

TABLE 4 Clinical Trials of AEDs in Neuropathic Pain Since 2000 (*Continued*)

Reference (year)	Study design	Pain type	Number enrolled	Drug dosing regimen	Clinical results	Adverse events
147 (2003)	R/DB/PC trial	PHN	173	PGB 600 mg/day (CrCl > 60 min/mL) or 300 mg/day (CrCl 30–60 mL/min) (N = 58) PLAC (N = 74) 8-wk trial duration All PGB pts. received 150 mg/day ×3 days → 300 mg/day	34.8% of PGB recipients withdrew early while 11.9% of PLAC recipients did so (7.1% of latter due to lack of efficacy). Intergroup mean differences sign. favored PGB over PLAC for end point mean pain scores (−1.69, $p = 0.0001$), SF-MPQ sensory scores (−3.75, $p = 0.0002$), SF-MPQ affective scores (−1.07, $p = 0.0047$), SF-MPQ total scores (−4.87, $p = 0.0002$), SF-MPQ VAS scores (−17.62, $p = 0.0001$), SF-MPQ PPI scores (−0.40, $p = 0.0127$), end point mean sleep interference scores (−1.58, $p = 0.0001$), MOS Sleep Scale sleep problem index scores (−9.80, $p = 0.0001$), SF-36 bodily pain domain (9.00, $p = 0.0021$), and SF-36 general health perception domain (4.21, $p = 0.0488$). Sign. analgesic effects of PGB were apparent as early as day 2 of therapy. Most end points were sign. different at the wk 1 evaluation. Patient GIC sign. favored PGB over PLAC ($p = 0.001$)	31.5% of PGB and 4.8% of PLAC recipients withdrew early due to AEs. The most common AEs (PGB/PLAC) were dizziness (28/12%), somnolence (25/7%), edema (19/2%), blurred vision (11/1%), and dry mouth (11/2%). Results of statistical analyses were NA
Tiagabine						
148 (2001)	O, NC trial	Chronic neuropathy of feet (not PDN)	17	TIA 4 mg/day × 1 wk → 8 mg/day × 1 wk → 12 mg/day × 1 wk → 16 mg/day × 1 wk 4-wk trial duration	9 (53%) completed trial participation. 4/8 mg doses sign. ↓ surface pain (mean 21/38%), skin sensitivity (NS/33%), burning (32/39%), cold (22/25%), pain sharpness (29/17%), and unpleasant feeling + deep pain intensity (17/13%) ($p < 0.03$ for 4 mg, $p < 0.02$ for 8 mg). 12/16-mg doses not evaluated statistically as AEs → discomfort (confounder), and overall, pain did not appear to be improved. 4 (29%) had improved sleep patterns and skin temperatures	Premature D/C due to AEs occurred in 7 pts. (41%) and 1 pt. D/C for another reason (5 at 4-mg level, 2 at 8-mg level, 1 at 12-mg level). AE severity ↑ with ↑ dose and overall frequency was higher in those completing the trial (mean 2.5 vs. 1.1 events/pt., $p < 0.02$). Dizziness, nausea, and impaired concentration were the most common AEs

Topiramate
149 (2004) DB/R/PC trial PDN

317

TOP 25 mg/day → ↑ by 25 mg/day in wk 2, 3, 4 → ↑ by 50 mg/day in wk 5, 6 → ↑ by 100 mg/day in wk 8–12 (maximum dose = 400 mg/day) ($N = 115$) PLAC ($N = 80$) 12-wk trial duration

Mean TOP doses were 161 mg/day (over entire study) and 320 mg/day (wk 9–12). 52.3% (TOP) and 73.4% (PLAC) pts. completed the trial. ↓ in mean pain scores (baseline to wk 12) was sign. greater with TOP (68.0 → 46.2) than PLAC (69.1 → 54.0) ($p = 0.038$) (sign. intergroup differences began at wk 8). TOP sign. ↓ worst-pain scores over previous wk compared to PLAC at wk 8 ($p = 0.03$) and 12 ($p = 0.003$). Responder rates (>30% ↓ in pain scores) were 50% (TOP) and 34% (PLAC) ($p = 0.004$) and for >50% ↓ were 36% (TOP) and 21% (PLAC) ($p = 0.005$). TOP also sign. ↓ mean worst-pain intensity scores ($p = 0.003$), sleep disruption ($p = 0.020$), and improved the mental component summary term of the SF-36 QOL instrument ($p = 0.023$) compared with PLAC. TOP was superior to PLAC in pt. GIC ($p = 0.002$)

24.3% and 8.3% left study early because of AEs to TOP and PLAC, respectively (primarily nausea, somnolence, dizziness, paresthesias, and cognitive dysfunction). TOP ↓ body wt. sign. (mean −2.6 kg vs. PLAC + 0.2 kg, $p < 0.001$). Wt. loss occurred in 76.2% (TOP) and 43.1% (PLAC) pts. ($p < 0.001$). Wt. gain occurred in 16.5% (TOP) and 55% (PLAC) pts. ($p < 0.001$). The most-frequent AEs to TOP were dizziness (11.4%), anorexia (10.9%), somnolence (10%), nausea (9.5%), paresthesias (8.5%), dizziness and fatigue (7.1% each), taste alteration (6.6%), and difficulty concentrating (5.2%)

(Continued)

TABLE 4 Clinical Trials of AEDs in Neuropathic Pain Since 2000 (*Continued*)

Reference (year)	Study design	Pain type	Number enrolled	Drug dosing regimen	Clinical results	Adverse events
150 (2004)	DB/R/PC trial (pooled analysis of 3 trials)	PDN	253 (TOP 100 mg) 372 (TOP 200 mg) 260 (TOP 400 mg) 384 (PLAC)	TOP 25 mg/day × 1 wk → ↑ in 25 mg/day increments every 7 days to 100 mg/day → ↑ in 50 mg/day increments every 7 days to target dose or maximum tolerated dose Completers 134 (TOP 100 mg) 172 (TOP 200 mg) 108 (TOP 400 mg) 225 (PLAC) Study 1: TOP 100 mg/day vs. TOP 200 mg/day vs. TOP 400 mg/day vs. PLAC Study 2: TOP 200 mg/day vs. TOP 400 mg/day vs. PLAC Study 3: TOP 100 mg/day vs. TOP 200 mg/day vs. PLAC Trial durations of 18 wk (N = 1) or 22 wk (N = 2)	D/C due to lack of efficacy occurred in 12–17% of TOP and 20–24% of PLAC pts. In all 3 trials, differences between TOP and PLAC groups in pain scores were NS. TOP and PLAC NS different in Categorical Pain and Sleep Disruption Scale results *except p = 0.02* favoring PLAC over TOP 100 mg/day in Sleep Disruption Scale results in 1 trial. In 1 trial, TOP produced sign. improvements vs. PLAC in bodily pain (100 and 200 mg/day) and physical functioning (100 mg/day) subscales of the SF-36 QOL instrument (in the other 2 trials, these results were NS different). Rescue meds. were needed by 53% PLAC, 47% TOP 100 mg/day, 53% TOP 200 mg/day, and 55% TOP 400 mg/day recipients	D/C due to AEs occurred in 16–31% of TOP and 8% of PLAC pts. D/C rate ↑ with ↑ dose. AEs with frequencies in TOP recipients ≥5% greater than PLAC recipients included fatigue, nausea, paresthesias, somnolence, anorexia, wt. loss, taste perversion, memory difficulty, and confusion. The most common treatment-limiting AEs were (TOP/PLAC): nausea (4/1%), fatigue (4/0%), dizziness (3/2%), difficulty in concentration/attention (3/2%), somnolence (3/1%), and anorexia (3/0%). D/C due to nephrolithiasis occurred in 3 TOP and 1 PLAC pt. Serious AEs occurred in 7% of TOP and 8% of PLAC pts. 19–38% of TOP pts. had

clinically-sign. wt. loss vs. 7% of PLAC pts. (defined as ≥5% of baseline body wt.). Glucose control was sign. better in TOP pts. than in PLAC pts. (≥5% ↓ in HgbA1c in 55% TOP 100 mg/day, 60% of TOP 200 mg/day, 62% of TOP 400 mg/day, and 29% of PLAC pts.). No correlation was noted between ↓ in HgbA1c and ↓ in wt. Results of statistical analyses were not available except for HgbA1c results

Valproate

151 (2005)　DB/R/PC trial　PHN　45

VA titrated to 1000 mg/day (N = 22) PLAC (N = 18) 8-wk study duration

40 pts. (89%) completed the trial. The difference in pain response (baseline → wk 8) was sign. and in favor of VA over PLAC for the SF-MPQ (−4.21), PPI (−1.27), VAS (−23.67), and 11-PLS (−1.7) pain instruments (all $p < 0.0001$). Pt. GIC was "much" or "moderate improvement" in 58.2% (VA) and 14.8% (PLAC) pts. (statistical results NA). NNT for at least 50% pain relief compared to PLAC (by VAS) = 2

1 pt. developed severe vertigo after 10 days therapy with VA → D/C. 3 pts. c/o nausea, vomiting, dizziness, drowsiness, and mild appetite change which gradually ↓ over 3–5 days and did not mandate D/C

(Continued)

TABLE 4 Clinical Trials of AEDs in Neuropathic Pain Since 2000 (*Continued*)

Reference (year)	Study design	Pain type	Number enrolled	Drug dosing regimen	Clinical results	Adverse events
152 (2004)	DB/R/PC/CO trial	Painful polyneuropathy	34	VA titrated over 5 days to 1500 mg/day ×4 wk. PLAC ×4 wk No washout period between treatment phases	Data from 31 pts. could be analyzed (3 pts. had inconsistent VA serum conc.). NS differences between treatments in total and individual pain ratings, in subgroups, and in response rates. No relationship was found between degrees of pain relief and serum drug conc. (responders and nonresponders had similar serum drug conc.)	During the placebo phase, 1 pt. reported headache and during the VA phase, 1 pt. each had headache + nausea and skin rash/flu-like signs/ symptoms
153 (2002)	R/DB/PC trial	PDN	52	VA 200 mg thrice daily for 1 wk. 400 mg thrice daily × 3 wk (N = 28). PLAC (N = 24) 4-wk trial duration	After 1 wk, intergroup differences in pain scores were NS. At 4 wk, they favored VA (3.41 vs. 4.6, p = 0.028). Motor and sensory electrophysiology studies revealed no drug effect	1 VA recipient was D/C early due to ↑ LFTs
154 (2001)	O, NC trial	Cancer-related neuropathic pain	25	VA 200 mg twice daily →↑ by 400 mg/day every 2–3 days to a maximum of 1200 mg/day 15-day study duration	19 (76%) completed the trial. 5 D/C early (4 due to progressive disease and 1 due to lack of efficacy). Median doses on day 8 and day 15 were 800 and 1200 mg/day, respectively (range on both days of 200–1200 mg/day). Response rate was 39–56% (based on ↓ in pain category), 33.3–66.7% (based on ↓ in absolute score), and 22.2–27.8% (based on >50% ↓ in pain score). Pain relief occurred in 56.3–62.5%. Reductions in interference in ADLs were as follows:	1 pt. D/C due to AEs (tremors). Most frequent AEs were drowsiness, unsteadiness, nausea, and anorexia (no quantitative data were presented)

General activities = 23.5%
Mood = 17.7%
Walking = 35.3%
Working = 23.5%
Relationships = 23.5%
Sleep = 12.5%
Enjoyment = 23.5%
Total activity = 58.8%

[a]25 were treatment related, 37 were tumor related.
[b]After IV ceftriaxone therapy had been completed.
[c]Method of treatment assignment NS. No statistical analyses were performed because of small number of subjects in each group.
[d]Of health insurance claims database.
[e]Nonresponse to CBZ/GBP and local anesthetic blockade.

Abbreviations: R, randomized; DB, double-blind; PC, placebo-controlled; CO, crossover; ICU, intensive care unit; CBZ, carbamazepine; PLAC, placebo, ↓, reduction; sign., significantly; AE, adverse event; O, open; NC, non-controlled; GBP, gabapentin; CLON, clonazepam; D/C, discontinued; PHN, postherpetic neuralgia; NT, nortriptyline; NS, not statistically significant; VAS, visual analogue scale; SF-MPQ, Short Form-McGill Pain Questionnaire; GIC, global impression of change; CrCl, creatinine clearance; pts., patients; NNT, number needed to treat (to produce 1 pt. having the outcome-of-interest), SCI, spinal cord injury; PDN, painful diabetic neuropathy; ADL, activities of daily living; LOC, loss of consciousness; QOL, quality of life; HIV, human immunodeficiency virus; NA, not available; LTG, lamotrigine; LEV, levetiracetam; CS, case series; OXCARB, oxcarbazepine; TN, trigeminal neuralgia; PO, oral; PGB, pregabalin; wt., weight; TIA, tiagabine; TOP, topiramate; HgbA1c, hemoglobin A1c; VA, valproate; PPI, present pain intensity score; MOS, Medical Outcomes Study; 11-PLS, 11-point Likert scale; LFT, liver function test.

to another with or without placebo. Such trials would certainly provide data on relative efficacy/tolerability that could help to establish preferred agents. However, as long as large clinical trials in this area are funded principally by the pharmaceutical industry, there will be no head-to-head trials for corporate competitive reasons.

Other areas in which study methodology needs to be improved in order to better distinguish between AEDs in neuropathic pain include quality-of-life and cost-effectiveness assessments. A recent example of utilizing quality-of-life assessments in distinguishing between treatments for neuropathic pain can be found in a secondary analysis of a monotherapy versus combination therapy trial with gabapentin, morphine, and gabapentin plus morphine in the treatment of painful diabetic peripheral neuropathy and postherpetic neuralgia (155). Authors sought to assess the impact of pain reduction on quality of life (using the SF-36 instrument) and mood (using the Profile of Mood States [POMS] instrument). Pain reduction with all three treatments significantly correlated with improved quality of life (for gabapentin, in the domains of role physical, bodily pain, vitality, role emotional, and mental health; for morphine, in the domains of bodily pain, vitality, and social functioning; and for the combination, in the domains of bodily pain, vitality, social functioning, and mental health). In terms of mood, pain reduction with all three treatments significantly correlated with improved mood (for gabapentin, in the domains of tension-anxiety, depression-dejection, and anger-hostility; for morphine, in the domains of depression-dejection, anger-hostility, fatigue-inertia, and vigor-activity; for the combination, in the domain of anger-hostility). The severity of adverse events (sedation, constipation, dry mouth) did not significantly correlate with any quality-of-life or mood parameters, probably since the study was not adequately powered to examine these outcomes. An important result of this analysis is that with increasing analgesia, more substantial improvements in quality of life and mood can be expected (155). However, more work is needed in the area of adverse effects and their relationship to quality of life (156).

In terms of cost-effectiveness evaluation, the recent development of a stochastic simulation model of treatment outcomes of peripheral neuropathic pain is a significant advance upon the usual pharmacoeconomic evaluations. Although treatment and health-state utilities costs need to be added to this model, the importance of clinically relevant outcome data generated by this model should not be understated. The model was developed using data from a 12-week trial of pregabalin in painful diabetic peripheral neuropathy and postherpetic neuralgia (142). Model-projected treatment effects over 12 weeks included the following: 26 ± 0.4 additional days (vs. no treatment) with no/mild pain, 33 ± 0.5 days with a 30% or greater reduction in pain intensity, 28 ± 0.4 days with a 50% or greater reduction in pain intensity, 34 ± 0.5 days with a 2 point or greater fall in pain intensity, and 30 ± 0.5 days with a 3 point or greater fall in pain intensity. Quality-of-life and mood states data would be valuable additions to the model (157).

Selection of Antiepileptic Therapy

Virtually no head-to-head trial data are available upon which to make evidence-based decisions between antiepileptic agents for chronic neuropathic pain in general or specific types of neuropathic pain. Thus, clinicians must use the next best alternative, systematic reviews/meta-analyses, to make therapeutic decisions.

In this section, systematic reviews/meta-analyses and clinical guidelines will be reviewed as an aid to the reader in making appropriate drug choices.

The most recently published systematic review/meta-analysis of pharmacotherapy of neuropathic pain occurred in November 2006, with the promulgation of the EFNS (European Federation of Neurological Societies) treatment guidelines. Only class I and II controlled trials (using the EFNS evidence classification scheme) were assessed, unless top-level trials were unavailable in specific pain types. Higher quality evidence was available for the efficacy of tricyclic antidepressants, opioids, gabapentin, and pregabalin followed by topical lidocaine (in postherpetic neuralgia), the dual serotonin-norepinephrine reuptake inhibitors venlafaxine and duloxetine (in painful diabetic peripheral neuropathy), lamotrigine, and tramadol. In painful polyneuropathy, tricyclic antidepressants and gabapentin/pregabalin are recommended first-line agents. Venlafaxine/duloxetine are considered second-line agents while second-/third-line agents include the opioids and lamotrigine. Oxcarbazepine, topiramate, carbamazepine, and valproate are generally not recommended because of efficacy and/or safety concerns. In postherpetic neuralgia, tricyclic antidepressants, gabapentin/pregabalin, and topical lidocaine are recommended first-line agents. However, topical lidocaine is best suited to older individuals, especially those with allodynia and small pain areas. "Strong" opioids are considered to be second-line agents with topical capsaicin, tramadol and valproate being second-/third-line agents. The main peripheral pain states are felt to respond similarly well to tricyclic antidepressants, gabapentin, and pregabalin. In trigeminal neuralgia, carbamazepine and oxcarbazepine are recommended first-line agents. Baclofen or lamotrigine are proposed as add-on agents in patients refractory to the first-line agents. On the basis of very limited data, in central pain states, amitriptyline and gabapentin/pregabalin are recommended first-line agents while cannabinoids, lamotrigine, and opioids are second-/third-line agents. Data were insufficient to make any conclusions regarding combination therapy and head-to-head comparisons (158).

Comorbidities may impact upon drug selection as well. For example, tricyclic antidepressants should be used cautiously in older individuals, especially those with cardiac risk factors. Opioids have been relegated to second-/third-line status in chronic neuropathic noncancer pain because of potential safety concerns, especially with long-term use. In the context of cancer-associated neuropathic pain, available efficacy data probably justify a first-line status for the opioids. Venlafaxine and duloxetine have been relegated to second-line status because of comparatively lower efficacy, but may be justifiably elevated to first-line status when tricyclic antidepressants are contraindicated or cardiac risk factors are present. The first-line status (although limited) of topical lidocaine is justified, in large part, by its excellent tolerability. Lamotrigine has been relegated to second-/third-line status because of safety concerns (severe dermatologic reactions). Oxcarbazepine is preferred in trigeminal neuralgia over carbamazepine due to lesser safety concerns with the former. Lastly, gabapentin/pregabalin or duloxetine may be preferable in patients where pain exerts a severe impact on quality of life or comorbidities as only these three agents have been adequately studied, having positive effects on quality of life (158).

The most recently updated systematic review/meta-analysis of pharmacologic treatments for neuropathic pain by Finnerup and colleagues appeared in late 2005. Treatments were compared using NNT (number needed to treat, defined by ≥ 50% pain relief from baseline) and NNH (number needed to harm, defined by trial withdrawal due to adverse effects) data in different pain syndromes. One hundred and five controlled trials were evaluated. In peripheral neuropathic pain, the lowest NNT values (i.e., greatest efficacy) were seen with tricyclic antidepressants (range 2–3) followed by opioids (morphine 2.5, oxycodone 2.6) followed by pregabalin (range 3.4–5.4) and then by gabapentin (range 4.1–6.8). In terms of NNH values (where larger values are indicative of greater safety), tricyclic antidepressants had a pooled NNH value of 14.7 (95% CI of 10–25), opioids of 17.1 (10–66), gabapentin of 26.1 (14–170) and pregabalin of 11.7 (8–20). When the authors evaluated treatments using several criteria beyond absolute pain relief (e.g., persistence of analgesia, frequency and severity of adverse effects, effect on quality of life, cost), an algorithm for the treatment of peripheral neuropathic pain emerged as follows: If the condition was postherpetic neuralgia or another focal neuropathy, topical lidocaine was the initial recommended treatment. If such condition failed topical therapy or another condition was present, the additional/initial choices recommended were gabapentin/pregabalin or a tricyclic antidepressant. If a tricyclic antidepressant was desired but contraindicated, the initial choice became a dual selective serotonin-norepinephrine reuptake inhibitor. Gabapentin/pregabalin failures were followed by addition/substitution of a tricyclic antidepressant/dual selective serotonin-norepinephrine reuptake inhibitor and vice versa. The final choice recommended was addition of either oxycodone or tramadol. Available data were insufficient to generate a treatment algorithm for central neuropathic pain (159).

In mid-2005, results of a systematic review/meta-analysis of pharmacologic treatments of postherpetic neuralgia pain were published. Thirty-one trials were suitable for meta-analysis, from which it was possible to extract dichotomous efficacy outcome data (i.e., $\geq$ 50% decrease in pain from baseline—yes/no) from 25 trials. Evidence was available to support the use of tricyclic antidepressants, "strong" opioids, tramadol, topical lidocaine, topical capsaicin, gabapentin, and pregabalin. NNT values were 1.6 and 4.2 (2 trials of amitriptyline); 1.9 (1 trial of desipramine); 3.7 (1 trial of nortriptyline or desipramine); 2.6 (pooled tricyclic antidepressants); 3.2, 5.6, and 5.0 (3 trials of gabapentin); 4.4 (pooled gabapentin); 3.4, 6.2, and 5.6 (3 trials of pregabalin); 4.9 (pooled pregabalin); 2.5 (1 trial of oxycodone); 2.8 (1 trial of morphine or methadone); 2.7 (pooled opioids); 4.8 (1 trial of tramadol); 2.0 (1 trial of topical lidocaine); 2.3 and 3.8 (2 trials of topical capsaicin); and 3.3 (pooled topical capsaicin). Major versus minor harm was distinguished by whether or not the patient was required by an adverse effect to withdraw from the trial (major). NNH (minor/major) values were 8, 6.2, 4.8, −/24, 37, 13, 14.2 (4 trials of tricyclic antidepressants); 5.7/16.9 (pooled tricyclic antidepressants); 3.7, 4.8, 3.9/15.4, 4.8, 8.9 (3 trials of gabapentin); 4.1/12.3 (pooled gabapentin); 4.3, −, −/4.9, 8.1, 27.5 (2 trials of pregabalin, where 8.1 refers to 150 mg/day and 27.5 refers to 300 mg/day in same trial); 3.6/50 (1 trial of oxycodone); −/3.7 (1 trial of morphine or methadone), −/6.3 (pooled opioids); −/10.8 (1 trial of tramadol); 5.3, 3.6/−, 4.7 (2 trials of topical capsaicin); and 3.9/− (pooled topical capsaicin). The authors suggested tricyclic antidepressants as the systemic therapeutic class of first choice followed by gabapentin/pregabalin, then the strong opioids (160).

In September 2004, the practice parameter for the treatment of postherpetic neuralgia was published by the Quality Standards Subcommittee of the American Academy of Neurology. Decisions were based upon absolute pain reduction rate, NNT (plus 95% CI for NNT), and NNH data. Effective agents were limited to tricyclic antidepressants, opioids, topical lidocaine, gabapentin, and pregabalin. The NNT/NNH data have been already been presented in this section. The practice parameter did not provide a specific algorithm for order of selection of effective agents (161).

CONCLUSION

At the present time among AEDs, only gabapentin and, to a somewhat lesser extent, pregabalin have an adequate evidence base upon which to make educated therapeutic decisions. In most types of chronic peripheral neuropathic pain, the gabapentenoids should be the AEDs of first choice. An obvious exception to this statement is the consideration of oxcarbazepine/carbamazepine as the AEDs of first choice in trigeminal neuralgia. For individuals who do not respond optimally to the gabapentenoids or oxcarbazepine/carbamazepine, there are a number of AEDs which should be considered: lamotrigine, levetiracetam, and topiramate. Further research in the areas of quality of life, cost effectiveness, combination therapy, and head-to-head trials are sorely needed to define scientifically rigorous criteria for the use of AEDs in neuropathic pain.

REFERENCES

1. Gilron I, Watson CP, Cahill CM, et al. Neuropathic pain: a practical guide for the clinician. CMAJ 2006; 175:265–275.
2. Guay DRP. Update on gabapentin in the management of neuropathic pain. Consult Pharm 2003; 18:158–178.
3. Suzuki R, Rahman W, Rygh LJ, et al. Spinal-supraspinal serotonergic circuits regulating neuropathic pain and its treatment with gabapentin. Pain 2005; 117:292–303.
4. Mixcoatl-Zecuatl T, Flores-Murrieta FJ, Granados-Soto V. The nitric oxide-cyclic GMP-protein kinase G-K$^+$ channel pathway participates in the antiallodynic effect of spinal gabapentin. Eur J Pharmacol 2006; 531:87–95.
5. Coderre TJ, Kumar N, Lefebvre CD, et al. Evidence that gabapentin reduces neuropathic pain by inhibiting the spinal release of glutamate. J Neurochem 2005; 94:1131–1139.
6. Imamura Y, Bennett GJ. Felbamate relieves several abnormal pain sensations in rats with an experimental peripheral neuropathy. J Pharmacol Expt Ther 1995; 275:177–182.
7. Dogrul A, Gardell LR, Ossipov MH, et al. Reversal of experimental neuropathic pain by T-type calcium channel blockers. Pain 2003; 105:159–168.
8. Tanabe M, Sakaue A, Takasu K, et al. Centrally mediated antihyperalgesic and anti-allodynic effects of zonisamide following partial nerve injury in the mouse. Naunyn-Schmiedebergs Arch Pharmacol 2005; 372:107–114.
9. Bischofs S, Zelenka M, Sommer C. Evaluation of topiramate as an anti-hyperalgesic and neuroprotective agent in the peripheral nervous system. J Periph Nerve Sys 2004; 9:70–78.
10. Fox A, Gentry C, Patel S, et al. Comparative activity of the anti-convulsants oxcarbazepine, carbamazepine, lamotrigine and gabapentin in a model of neuropathic pain in the rat and guinea pig. Pain 2003; 105:355–362.
11. Gonzalez-Darder JM, Ortego-Alvaro A, Ruz-Franzi I, et al. Antinociceptive effects of phenobarbital in "tail flick" test and deafferentation pain. Anesth Analg 1992; 75:81–86.
12. Ardid D, Lamberty Y, Alloui A, et al. Antihyperalgesic effect of levetiracetam in neuropathic pain models in rats. Eur J Pharmacol 2003; 473:27–33.
13. Hord AH, Denson DD, Chalfoun AG, et al. The effect of systemic zonisamide (Zonegran^{TM}) on thermal hyperalgesia and mechanical allodynia in rats with an experimental mononeuropathy. Anesth Analg 2003; 96:1700–1706.

14. Winkler I, Blotnik S, Shimshoni J, et al. Efficacy of antiepileptic isomers of valproic acid and valpromide in a rat model of neuropathic pain. Br J Pharmacol 2005; 146:198–208.
15. Jang Y, Kim ES, Park SS, et al. The suppressive effects of oxcarbazepine on mechanical and cold allodynia in a rat model of neuropathic pain. Anesth Analg 2005; 101:800–806.
16. Erichsen HK, Hao J-X, Xu X-J, et al. A comparison of the antinociceptive effects of voltage-activated Na$^+$ channel blockers in two rat models of neuropathic pain. Eur J Pharmacol 2003; 458:275–282.
17. Hama AT, Boorsook D. The effect of antinociceptive drugs tested at different times after nerve injury in rats. Anesth Analg 2005; 101:175–179.
18. Barton ME, Eberle EL, Shannon HE. The antihyperalgesic effects of the T-type calcium channel blockers ethosuximide, trimethadione, and mibefradil. Eur J Pharmacol 2005; 521:79–85.
19. Flatters SJL, Bennett GJ. Ethosuximide reverses paclitaxel- and vincristine-induced painful peripheral neuropathy. Pain 2004; 109:150–161.
20. Alves ND, De Castro-Costa C, DeCarvelho AM, et al. Possible analgesic effect of vigabatrin in animal experimental chronic neuropathic pain. Arq Neuropsiquiatr 1999; 57:916–920.
21. Wieczorkiewicz-Plaza A, Plaza P, Maciejewski R, et al. Effect of topiramate on mechanical allodynia in neuropathic pain model in rats. Polish J Pharmacol 2004; 56:275–278.
22. Laughlin TM, Tram KV, Wilcox GL, et al. Comparison of antiepileptic drugs tiagabine, lamotrigine, and gabapentin in mouse models of acute, prolonged, and chronic nociception. J Pharmacol Expt Ther 2002; 302:1168–1175.
23. Winkler I, Sobol E, Yagen B, et al. Efficacy of antiepileptic tetramethylcyclopropyl analogues of valproic acid amides in a rat model of neuropathic pain. Neuropharmacology 2005; 49:1110–1120.
24. Lynch JJ III, Wade CL, Zhong CM, et al. Attenuation of mechanical allodynia by clinically utilized drugs in a rat chemotherapy-induced neuropathic pain model. Pain 2004; 110:56–63.
25. Lindia JA, Kohler MG, Martin WJ, et al. Relationship between sodium channel Na$_v$1.3 expression and neuropathic pain in rats. Pain 2005; 117:145–153.
26. Chen S-R, Pan H-L. Effect of systemic and intrathecal gabapentin on allodynia in a new rat model of postherpetic neuralgia. Brain Res 2005; 1042:108–113.
27. Pederson LH, Blackburn-Munro G. Pharmacological characterization of place escape/avoidance behavior in the rat chronic constriction injury model of neuropathic pain. Psychopharmacology 2006; 185:208–217.
28. Matsumoto M, Inoue M, Hald A, et al. Inhibition of paclitaxel-induced A-fiber hypersensitization by gabapentin. J Pharmacol Exp Ther 2006; 318:735–740.
29. Walczak J-S, Pichette V, Leblond F, et al. Characterization of chronic constriction of the saphenous nerve, a model of neuropathic pain in mice showing rapid molecular and electrophysiological changes. J Neurosci Res 2006; 83:1310–1322.
30. Castane A, Celerier E, Martin M, et al. Development and expression of neuropathic pain in CB1 knockout mice. Neuropharmacology 2006; 50:111–122.
31. Beyreuther B, Callizot N, Stohr T. Antinociceptive efficacy of lacosamide in a rat model for painful diabetic neuropathy. Eur J Pharmacol 2006; 539:64–70.
32. Enggaard TP, Klitgaard NA, Sindrup SH. Specific effect of levetiracetam in experimental human pain models. Eur J Pain 2006; 10:193–198.
33. Odrcich M, Bailey JM, Cahill CM, et al. Chronobiological characteristics of painful diabetic neuropathy and postherpetic neuralgia: diurnal pain variation and effects of analgesic therapy. Pain 2006; 120:207–212.
34. Eisenberg E, Damunni G, Hoffer E, et al. Lamotrigine for intractable sciatica: correlation between dose, plasma concentration and analgesia. Eur J Pain 2003; 7:485–491.
35. Rapeport WG, Rogers KM, McCubbin TD, et al. Treatment of intractable neurogenic pain with carbamazepine. Scot Med J 1984; 29:162–165.
36. Tomson T, Tybring G, Bertilsson L, et al. Carbamazepine therapy in trigeminal neuralgia: clinical effects in relation to plasma concentration. Arch Neurol 1980; 37:699–703.

37. Moosa RS, McFadyen ML, Miller R, et al. Carbamazepine and its metabolites in neuralgias: concentration-effect relations. Eur J Clin Pharmacol 1993; 45:297–301.
38. Tecoma ES. Oxcarbazepine. Epilepsia 1999; 40(suppl 5):S37–S46.
39. Glauser TA. Topiramate. Epilepsia 1999; 40(suppl 5):S71–S80.
40. Leppik IE. Zonisamide. Epilepsia 1999; 40(suppl 5):S23–S29.
41. Perucca E. Clinical pharmacology and therapeutic use of the new antiepileptic drugs. Fund Clin Pharmacol 2001; 15:405–417.
42. Perucca E. The clinical pharmacokinetics of the new antiepileptic drugs. Epilepsia 1999; 40(suppl 9):S7–S13.
43. Hachad H, Ragueneau-Majlessi I, Levy RH. New antiepileptic drugs: review on drug interactions. Ther Drug Monit 2002; 24:91–103.
44. Natsch S, Hekster YA, Keyser A, et al. Newer anticonvulsant drugs. Role of pharmacology, drug interactions and adverse reactions in drug choice. Drug Saf 1997; 17: 228–240.
45. Bertilsson L. Clinical pharmacokinetics of carbamazepine. Clin Pharmacokinet 1978; 3:128–143.
46. Zaccara G, Messori A, Moroni F. Clinical pharmacokinetics of valproic acid-1988. Clin Pharmacokinet 1988; 15:367–389.
47. Ben-Menachem E. Pregabalin pharmacology and its relevance to clinical practice. Epilepsia 2004; 45(suppl 6):13–18.
48. Bialer M. Pharmacokinetic evaluation of sustained release formulations of antiepileptic drugs. Clinical implications. Clin Pharmacokinet 1992; 22:11–21.
49. Divalproex (Depakote ER®) Product Information. Abbott, North Chicago, IL, January 2006.
50. Perucca E. Clinically relevant drug interactions with antiepileptic drugs. Br J Clin Pharmacol 2006; 61:246–255.
51. Gabapentin (Neurontin®) Product Information. Pfizer, New York, NY, December 2005.
52. Barrueto F Jr., Green J, Howland MA, et al. Gabapentin withdrawal presenting as status epilepticus. J Toxicol Clin Toxicol 2002; 40:925–928.
53. Tran KT, Hranicky D, Lark T, et al. Gabapentin withdrawal syndrome in the presence of a taper. Bipolar Disord 2005; 7:302–304.
54. Bookwalter T, Gitlin M. Gabapentin-induced neurologic toxicities. Pharmacotherapy 2005; 25:1817–1819.
55. Almahrezi A, Fitzcharles M-A. Dose-dependent severe arthralgia induced by gabapentin. J Rheumatol 2004; 31:1228 (letter).
56. Scullin P, Sheahan P, Kelly S. Myoclonic jerks associated with gabapentin. Pall Med 2003; 17:717–718.
57. Norton JW, Quarles E. Gabapentin-related dyskinesia. J Clin Psychopharmacol 2001; 21:623–624 (letter).
58. Zylicz Z, Mudde AH. Painful gynecomastia: an unusual toxicity of gabapentin? J Pain Symptom Manage 2000; 20:2–3 (letter).
59. Jacob PC, Chand RP, Omeima E-S. Asterixis induced by gabapentin. Clin Neuropharmacol 2000; 23:53.
60. Jones H, Aguila E, Farber HW. Gabapentin toxicity requiring intubation in a patient receiving long-term hemodialysis. Ann Intern Med 2002; 137:74–75 (letter).
61. Scheschonka A, Beuche W. Treatment of post-herpetic pain in myasthenia gravis: exacerbation of weakness due to gabapentin. Pain 2003; 104:423–424.
62. Bekkelund SI, Lilleng H, Tonseth S. Gabapentin may cause reversible visual field constriction. BMJ 2006; 332:1193.
63. Derbyshire E, Martin D. Neutropenia occurring after starting gabapentin for neuropathic pain. Clin Oncol 2004; 16:575–576.
64. Backonja M, Glanzman RL. Gabapentin dosing for neuropathic pain: evidence from randomized, placebo-controlled clinical trials. Clin Ther 2003; 25:81–104.
65. Pregabalin (Lyrica®) Product Information. Pfizer, New York, NY, March 2006.
66. Randinitis EJ, Posvar EL, Alvey CW, et al. Pharmacokinetics of pregabalin in subjects with various degrees of renal function. J Clin Pharmacol 2003; 43:277–283.

67. Heckmann JG, Ulrich K, Dutsch M, et al. Pregabalin associated asterixis. Am J Phys Med Rehabil 2005; 84:724 (letter).
68. Lamotrigine (Lamictal®) Product Information. GlaxoSmithKline, Research Triangle Park, NC, August 2006.
69. Carbamazepine (Tegretol®, Tegretol-XR®) Product Information. Novartis, East Hanover, NJ, September 2003.
70. Patsalos PN, Elyas AA, Zakrzewska JM. Protein binding of oxcarbazepine and its primary active metabolite, 10-hydroxycarbazepine, in patients with trigeminal neuralgia. Eur J Clin Pharmacol 1990; 39:413–415.
71. Oxcarbazepine (Trileptal®) Product Information. Novartis, East Hanover, NJ, December 2001.
72. Wong ICK, Lhatoo SD. Adverse reactions to new anticonvulsant drugs. Drug Saf 2000; 23:35–56.
73. Besag FMC. Behavioural effects of the new anticonvulsants. Drug Saf 2001; 24:513–536.
74. Kutluay E, McCague K, D'Souza J, et al. Safety and tolerability of oxcarbazepine in elderly patients with epilepsy. Epilepsy Behav 2003; 4:175–180.
75. Adkoli S. Symptomatic hyponatremia in patients on oxcarbazepine therapy for the treatment of neuropathic pain: two case reports. J Pain Pall Care Pharmacother 2003; 17:47–51.
76. Topiramate (Topamax®) Product Information. Ortho-McNeil, Raritan, NJ, December 2001.
77. May TW, Rambeck B, Jurgens U. Serum concentrations of topiramate in patients with epilepsy: influence of dose, age, and comedication. Ther Drug Monit 2002; 24:366–374.
78. Lee S, Sziklas V, Andermann F, et al. The effect of adjunctive topiramate on cognitive function in patients with epilepsy. Epilepsia 2003; 44:339–347.
79. Eggener S, Kim SC, User HM, et al. Urolithiasis associated with topiramate. Int Braz J Urol 2004; 30:29–31.
80. Kuo RL, Moran ME, Kim DH, et al. Topiramate-induced nephrolithiasis. J Endourol 2002; 16:229–231.
81. Wasserstein AG, Rak I, Reife RA. Nephrolithiasis during treatment with topiramate. Epilepsia 1995; 36(suppl 3):S153.
82. Wasserstein AG, Rak I, Reife RA. Investigation of the mechanistic basis for topiramate-associated nephrolithiasis: examination of urinary and serum constituents. Epilepsia 1995; 36(suppl 3):S153.
83. Cereza G, Pedros C, Garcia N, et al. Topiramate in non-approved indications and acute myopia or angle closure glaucoma. Br J Clin Pharmacol 2005; 60:578–579 (letter).
84. Thambi L, Kapcala LP, Chambers W, et al. Topiramate-associated secondary angle-closure glaucoma: a case series. Arch Opthalmol 2002; 120:1108 (letter).
85. Bhattacharyya KB, Basu S. Acute myopia induced by topiramate: report of a case and review of the literature. Neurol India 2005; 53:108–109.
86. Boentert M, Aretz H, Ludemann P. Acute myopia and angle-closure glaucoma induced by topiramate. Neurology 2003; 61:1306 (letter).
87. Sankar PS, Pasquale LR, Grosskreutz CL. Uveal effusion and secondary angle-closure glaucoma associated with topiramate use. Arch Ophthalmol 2001; 119:1210–1211.
88. Ben-Menachem E, Axelsen M, Johanson EH, et al. Predictors of weight loss in adults with topiramate-treated epilepsy. Obes Res 2003; 11:556–562.
89. Zonisamide (Zonegran®) Product Information. Elan, San Diego, CA, June 2002.
90. French J. Use of levetiracetam in special populations. Epilepsia 2002; 42(suppl 4):40–43.
91. Levetiracetam (Keppra®) Product Information. UCB, Smyrna, GA, July 2007.
92. Cernea CR, Hojaij FC, DeCarlucci D, et al. First-bite syndrome after reaction of the styloid process. Laryngoscope 2007; 117:181–182.
93. Cheshire WP. Felbamate relieved trigeminal neuralgia. Clin J Pain 2003; 11:139–142.
94. Heartsill LG, Brown TM. Use of gabapentin for rest pain in chronic critical limb ischemia. Ann Pharmacother 2005; 39:1136 (letter).
95. Villarejo A, Porta-Etessam J, Camacho A, et al. Gabapentin for painful legs and moving toes syndrome. Eur Neurol 2004; 51:180–181.

96. Keskinbora K, Pekel AF, Aydinli I. The use of gabapentin in a 12-year old boy with cancer pain. Acta Anaesthesiol Scand 2004; 48:663–664 (letter).
97. Sloan PA, Kancharla A. Treatment of neuropathic orbital pain with gabapentin. J Pain Pall Care Pharmacother 2003; 17(2):89–94.
98. Levendoglu F, Ogun CO, Ozerbil O, et al. Gabapentin is a first line drug for the treatment of neuropathic pain in spinal cord injury. Spine 2004; 29:743–751.
99. Porta-Etessam J, Benito-Leon J, Martinez-Salio A, et al. Gabapentin in the treatment of SUNCT syndrome. Headache 2002; 42:523–524.
100. Hunt CH, Dodick DW, Bosch EP. SUNCT responsive to gabapentin. Headache 2002; 42:525–526.
101. Chen B, Stitik TP, Foye PE, et al. Central post-stroke pain syndrome. Yet another use for gabapentin? Am J Phys Med Rehabil 2002; 81:718–720.
102. Benito-Leon J, Picardo A, Garrido A, et al. Gabapentin therapy for genitofemoral and ilioinguinal neuralgia. J Neurol 2001; 248:907–908 (letter).
103. Piovesan EJ, Siow C, Kowacs PA, et al. Influence of lamotrigine over the SUNCT syndrome. One patient follow-up for two years. Arq Neuropsiquiatr 2003; 61:691–694.
104. Lalwani K, Shohem A, Koh JL, et al. Use of oxcarbazepine to treat a pediatric patient with resistant complex regional pain syndrome. J Pain 2005; 6:704–706.
105. Criscuolo S, Auletta C, Lippi S, et al. Oxcarbazepine (Trileptal®) monotherapy dramatically improves quality of life in two patients with postherpetic neuralgia refractory to carbamazepine and gabapentin. J Pain Symptom Manage 2004; 28:535–536 (letter).
106. Kline KM, Carroll DG, Malnar KF. Painful diabetic peripheral neuropathy relieved with use of oral topiramate. South Med J 2003; 96:662–605.
107. Dinoff BL, Richards JS, Ness TJ. Use of topiramate for spinal cord injury-related pain. J Spinal Cord Med 2003; 26:401–403.
108. Pandy CK, Raza M, Tripathi M, et al. The comparative evaluation of gabapentin and carbamazepine for pain management in Guillain-Barre syndrome patients in the intensive care unit. Anesth Analg 2005; 101:220–225.
109. Richart de Mesones A, Turon Sans J, Misiego M, et al. Neuropathic pain and dysesthesia of the feet after Himalayan expeditions. High Alt Med Biol 2002; 3:395–399.
110. Tripathi M, Kaushik S. Carbamazepine for pain management in Guillain-Barre syndrome patients in the intensive care unit. Crit Care Med 2000; 28:655–658.
111. Hugel H, Ellershaw JE, Dickman A. Clonazepam as an adjuvant analgesic in patients with cancer-related neuropathic pain. J Pain Symptom Manage 2003; 26:1073–1074 (letter).
112. Chandra K, Shafiq N, Pandhi P, et al. Gabapentin versus nortriptyline in post-herpetic neuralgia patients: a randomized, double-blind clinical trial—the GONIP trial. Int J Clin Pharmacol Ther 2006; 44:358–363.
113. Nikolajsen L, Finnerup NB, Kramp S, et al. A randomized study of the effects of gabapentin on postamputation pain. Anesthesiology 2006; 105:1008–1015.
114. Ross JR, Goller K, Hardy J, et al. Gabapentin is effective in the treatment of cancer-related neuropathic pain: a prospective, open-label study. J Pall Med 2005; 8:1118–1126.
115. Tai Q, Kirshblum S, Chen B, et al. Gabapentin in the treatment of neuropathic pain after spinal cord injury: a prospective, randomized, double-blind, crossover trial. J Spinal Cord Med 2002; 25:100–105.
116. Jean WH, Wu CC, Mok MS, et al. Starting dose of gabapentin for patients with post-herpetic neuralgia: a dose-response study. Acta Anaesthesiol Taiwan 2005; 43:73–77.
117. Weissenbacher S, Ring J, Hofmann H. Gabapentin for the symptomatic treatment of chronic neuropathic pain in patients with late-stage lyme borreliosis: a pilot study. Dermatology 2005; 211:123–127.
118. Caraceni A, Zecca E, Bonezzi C, et al. Gabapentin for neuropathic cancer pain: a randomized controlled trial from the Gabapentin Cancer Study Group. J Clin Oncol 2004; 22:2909–2917.
119. Hahn K, Arendt G, Braun JS, et al. A placebo-controlled trial of gabapentin for painful HIV-associated sensory neuropathies. J Neurol 2004; 251:1260–1266.

120. Medina-Santillin R, Morales-Franno G, Espinoza-Raya J, et al. Treatment of diabetic neuropathic pain with gabapentin alone or combined with Vitamin B complex. Preliminary results. Proc West Pharmacol Soc 2004; 47:109–112.
121. Ahn S-H, Park H-W, Lee B-S, et al. Gabapentin effect on neuropathic pain compared among patients with spinal cord injury and different durations of symptoms. Spine 2003; 28:341–347.
122. Berger A, Dukes E, McCarberg B, et al. Change in opioid use after the introduction of gabapentin therapy in patients with postherpetic neuralgia. Clin Ther 2003; 25:2809–2822.
123. Ries M, Mengel E, Kutschke G, et al. Use of gabapentin to reduce chronic neuropathic pain in Fabry disease. J Inherit Metab Dis 2003; 26:413–414.
124. Bosnjak S, Jelic S, Susnjar S, et al. Gabapentin for relief of neuropathic pain related to anticancer treatment: a preliminary study. J Chemother 2002; 14:214–219.
125. To T-P, Lim TC, Hill ST, et al. Gabapentin for neuropathic pain following spinal cord injury. Spinal Cord 2002; 40:282–285.
126. Serpell MG, Neuropathic Pain Study Group. Gabapentin in neuropathic pain syndromes: a randomized, double-blind, placebo-controlled trial. Pain 2002; 99:557–566.
127. Pandey CK, Bose N, Garg G, et al. Gabapentin for the treatment of pain in Guillain-Barre syndrome: a double-blinded, placebo-controlled, crossover study. Anesth Analg 2002; 95:1719–1723.
128. Rice ASC, Maton S, Postherpetic Neuralgia Study Group. Gabapentin in postherpetic neuralgia: a randomized, double blind, placebo controlled study. Pain 2001; 94:215–224.
129. LaSpina I, Porazzi D, Maggiolo F, et al. Gabapentin in painful HIV-related neuropathy: a report of 19 patients, preliminary observations. Eur Neurol 2001; 8:71–75.
130. Sander-Kiesling A, Rumpold Seitlinger G, Dorn C, et al. Lamotrigine monotherapy for control of neuralgia after nerve section. Acta Anaesthesiol Scand 2002; 46:1261–1264.
131. Dunteman ED. Levetiracetam as an adjunctive analgesic in neoplastic plexopathies: case series and commentary. J Pain Pall Care Pharmacother 2005; 19(1):35–43.
132. Price MJ. Levetiracetam in the treatment of neuropathic pain: three case studies. Clin J Pain 2004; 20:33–36.
133. Rowbotham MC, Manville NS, Ren J. Pilot tolerability and effectiveness study of levetiracetam for postherpetic neuralgia. Neurology 2003; 61:866–867.
134. Erdemoglu AK, Varlibas A. Effectiveness of oxcarbazepine in symptomatic treatment of painful diabetic neuropathy. Neurology (India) 2006; 54:173–177.
135. Criscuolo S, Auletta C, Lippi S, et al. Oxcarbazepine monotherapy in postherpetic neuralgia unresponsive to carbamazepine and gabapentin. Acta Neurol Scand 2005; 111:229–232.
136. Magenta P, Arghetti S, DiPalma F, et al. Oxcarbazepine is effective and safe in the treatment of neuropathic pain: pooled analysis of seven clinical studies. Neurol Sci 2005; 26:218–226.
137. Dogra S, Beydoun S, Mazzola J, et al. Oxcarbazepine in painful diabetic neuropathy: a randomized, placebo-controlled study. Eur J Pain 2005; 9:543–554.
138. Beydoun A, Kobetz SA, Carrazona EJ. Efficacy of oxcarbazepine in the treatment of painful diabetic neuropathy. Clin J Pain 2004; 20:174–178.
139. Cheshire WP. Fosphenytoin: an intravenous option for the management of acute trigeminal neuralgia crisis. J Pain Symptom Manage 2001; 21:506–510.
140. van Seventer R, Feister HA, Young JP Jr., et al. Efficacy and tolerability of twice-daily pregabalin for treating pain and related sleep interference in postherpetic neuralgia: a 13-week, randomized trial. Curr Med Res Opin 2006; 22:375–384.
141. Siddall PJ, Cousins MJ, Otte A, et al. Pregabalin in central neuropathic pain associated with spinal cord injury: a placebo-controlled trial. Neurology 2006; 67:1792–1800.
142. Freynhagen R, Strojek K, Griesing T, et al. Efficacy of pregabalin in neuropathic pain evaluated in a 12-week randomized, double-blind, multicentre, placebo-controlled trial of flexible- and fixed-dose regimens. Pain 2005; 115:254–263.
143. Richter RW, Portenoy R, Sharma U, et al. Relief of painful diabetic peripheral neuropathy with pregabalin: a randomized, placebo-controlled trial. J Pain 2005; 6:253–260.

144. Rosenstock J, Tuchman M, Lamoureux L, et al. Pregabalin for the treatment of painful diabetic peripheral neuropathy: a double-blind, placebo-controlled trial. Pain 2004; 110:628–638.
145. Sabatowski R, Galvez R, Cherry DA, et al. Pregabalin reduces pain and improves sleep and mood disturbances in patients with post-herpetic neuralgia: results of a randomized, placebo-controlled clinical trial. Pain 2004; 109:26–35.
146. Lesser H, Sharma U, Lamoureux L, et al. Pregabalin relieves symptoms of painful diabetic neuropathy: a randomized controlled trial. Neurology 2004; 63:2104–2110.
147. Dworkin RH, Corbin AE, Young JP Jr., et al. Pregabalin for the treatment of post-herpetic neuralgia: a randomized, placebo-controlled trial. Neurology 2003; 60: 1274–1283.
148. Novak V, Kanard R, Kissel JT, et al. Treatment of painful sensory neuropathy with tiagabine: a pilot study. Clin Auto Res 2001; 11:357–361.
149. Raskin P, Donofrio PD, Rosenthal NR, et al. Topiramate vs placebo in painful diabetic neuropathy. Analgesic and metabolic effects. Neurology 2004; 63:865–873.
150. Thienel U, Neto W, Schwabe SK, et al for the Topiramate Diabetic Neuropathic Pain Study Group. Topiramate in painful diabetic polyneuropathy: findings from three double-blind placebo-controlled trials. Acta Neurol Scand 2004; 110:221–231.
151. Kochar DK, Garg P, Bumb RA, et al. Divalproex sodium in the management of post-herpetic neuralgia: a randomized double-blind placebo-controlled study. QJM 2005; 98:29–34.
152. Otto M, Bach FW, Jensen TS, et al. Valproic acid has no effect on pain in poly-neuropathy. A randomized controlled trial. Neurology 2004; 62:285–288.
153. Kochar DK, Jain N, Agarwal RP, et al. Sodium valproate in the management of painful neuropathy in type 2 diabetes—a randomized placebo controlled study. Acta Neurol Scand 2002; 106:248–252.
154. Hardy JR, Rees AJ, Gwilliam B, et al. A phase II study to establish the efficacy and toxicity of sodium valproate in patients with cancer-related neuropathic pain. J Pain Symptom Manage 2001; 21:204–209.
155. Gilron I, Bailey JM, Tu D, et al. Morphine, gabapentin, or their combination for neu-ropathic pain. NEJM 2005; 352:1324–1334.
156. Deshpande MA, Holden RR, Gilron I. The impact of therapy on quality of life and mood in neuropathic pain: what is the effect of pain reduction? Anesth Analg 2006; 102:1473–1479.
157. Vera-Llonch M, Dukes E, Delea TE, et al. Treatment of peripheral neuropathic pain: a simulation model. Eur J Pain 2006; 10:279–285.
158. Attal N, Cruccu G, Haanpaa M, et al. EFNS guidelines on pharmacological treatment of neuropathic pain. Eur J Neurol 2006; 13:1153–1169.
159. Finnerup NB, Otto M, McQuay HJ, et al. Algorithm for neuropathic pain treatment: an evidence based proposal. Pain 2005; 118:289–305.
160. Hempenstall K, Nurmikko TJ, Johnson RW, et al. Analgesic therapy in postherpetic neuralgia: a quantitative systematic review. PLoS Med 2005; 2:E164.
161. Dubinsky RM, Kabbani H, El-Chami Z, et al. Practice parameter: treatment of post-herpetic neuralgia: an evidence-based report of the Quality Standards Subcommittee of the American Academy of Neurology. Neurology 2004; 63:959–965.

The Antiepileptic Drugs and Migraine Prevention

Jan Lewis Brandes
Department of Neurology, Vanderbilt University School of Medicine and Nashville Neuroscience Group, Nashville, Tennessee, U.S.A.

K. M. A. Welch
Rosalind Franklin University of Medicine and Science and Department of Neurology, Chicago Medical School, Chicago, Illinois, U.S.A.

INTRODUCTION

Migraine is a highly prevalent chronic episodic illness. The true cause of migraine has proved elusive, and thus effective treatments, especially preventive, have been slow to emerge. Welch et al. suggested in 1989 that multiple causal factors for migraine converge onto a common hyperexcitable brain state, which constitutes the fundamental susceptibility to migraine attacks (1), underscored by recent genetic findings in familial hemiplegic migraine (FHM), which have introduced three strong but separate causal factors. (2–4) Perhaps the most persuasive argument for brain hyperexcitability constituting the basic susceptibility to migraine is that triggers of an attack initiate a depolarizing electrical and metabolic event originating in brain likened to the spreading depression (SD) of Leão (5). SD is believed to be the underlying mechanism of aura (6), which in turn activates the headache and associated features of the attack. Factors that increase or decrease brain excitability form the threshold for triggering attacks. Prevention of migraine attacks with antiepileptic drugs (AEDs) that decrease excitability of cell membranes thus seems a logical approach toward managing severe and frequent migraine. Evidence for hyperexcitability in the interictal phase of the illness, encompassing clinical observations strengthened by noninvasive electrophysiological and functional brain imaging techniques, is reviewed first, followed by discussion of the effectiveness and current place of AEDs in migraine treatment.

CLINICAL INVESTIGATION

Consonant with migraine aura being predominately visual, the occipital cortex has been the focus of clinical investigations that support brain hyperexcitability (7–11), giving rise to the notion of the occipital cortex being to migraine what the temporal lobe is to epilepsy. Accordingly, we will first review a body of experiments, largely psychophysical in nature, in migraine patients. Attention to altered function of primary visual cortex between and during attacks of migraine aura began with Airy's observations on fortification spectra in the late 19th century (12). Detailed descriptions of migraine aura by Richards (13), and his suggestion that aura began with activation of linear detector neurons in primary visual cortex, was followed by systematic investigation of stripe-induced visual discomfort in migraine sufferers by Marcus and Soso (8). Visual stress, particularly repetitive linear and specifically angulated visual stimuli, may evoke an "exhaustion" phenomenon in hyperexcitable responding susceptible specialized line detector neurons of the visual cortex to account for the illusion of fortification spectra as part of the aura. Earlier electro-physiological studies had demonstrated that stressful linear stimuli could excite visual cortex epileptic discharges (11). In support, psychophysical studies by Wray et al. revealed abnormally sensitive "low-level" visual processing in subjects with migraine with aura that they attributed to hyperexcitability, speculating upon dysfunction of the intracortical GABAergic inhibitory system as its origin (7).

In the context of strong visual stimuli and cortical excitability, Wilkins et al. evaluated visual function in migraine patients with complaints of visual triggering of their attacks, perceptual disturbance and photophobia during headache, or spatial or chromatic distortion of text or blurring during reading (14). First, choosing the color of light that improved such perceptual distortion or discomfort, patients were sub-sequently provided glasses to wear with spectral filters that optimized these con-ditions. A double-masked, randomized controlled study with crossover design revealed reduction in headache frequency when the optimal tint was worn, attributing to the colored filters reducing pattern glare. Neurons in excitable regions of visual cortex fire inappropriately when the excitation is strong, for example, reading texts that evoke pattern glare, leading to perceptual distortion and headache; certain colored tints might redistribute excitation from these hyperexcitable cortical regions, reducing abnormal neuronal firing. In accord, light and glare may cause symptoms that range from mild discomfort to the triggering of an attack. Kowacs et al. submitted migraine patients and healthy controls to pressure algometry before and after light-induced discomfort was elicited by progressive light stimulation (15). Unlike controls, migraine patients experienced significant and persistent drops in pain perception thresholds after light stimulation at all sites tested, indicating that visual afferents influencing trigeminal and cervical nociception are hypersensitive compared with normal controls. Consistent with the hyperexcitability hypothesis, motion coherence perimetry docu-mented decreased ability to detect coherent motion in migraine with and without aura, explained by increased baseline neuronal noise due to cortical hyperexcitability. Similarly, studies of visual contrast gain control indicated hyperexcitability, although not on the basis of loss of inhibition as suggested by Wray et al. (7).

To give a balanced viewpoint, irrespective of the migraine subtype, abnormal visual contrast processing in migraine patients indicated a general disturbance of cortical function, rather than disturbance specific to an occipital cortex locus as many studies indicate. Nevertheless, this experiment was based on some migraine sufferers reporting certain visual patterns reliably triggering a migraine attack, such as high-contrast striped patterns or flickering lights (16). Although cortical visual processing is consistently abnormal in migraine, not all investigators support cortical hyper-excitability. Shepherd explored pattern or contrast adaptation, a uniquely cortical phenomenon (17). Prolonged aftereffects in migraine were interpreted as a lack, or suppression, of cortical excitatory connections, or increased cortical inhibition in migraine. At first pass, this psychophysical study appears at odds with those reviewed above, which emphasized hyperexcitability or a lack of inhibition. Changes in neuronal response following adaptation, however, result from hyperpolarization of cell mem-branes or synaptic connections between neurons that respond to the adapting stimuli. Reduced mitochondria energy reserves associated with migraine, or mutations in neuronal P/Q-type Ca^{2+} channels reviewed later, could delay restorative processes resulting in the enhanced after-effects. Enhanced after effects could also reflect receptor hypersensitivity or altered G protein function reported in migraine (18), reconciling the otherwise contrasting findings with other inferences of this study with respect to excitable cortical function.

NEUROPHYSIOLOGICAL FUNCTION AND BRAIN IMAGING

Sources of information in humans on the true cause of migraine in terms of exploring the basis of susceptibility to triggering SD and why the brain appears primed to permit propagation of this form of abnormal electrical and metabolic event are likely to come from understanding brain function between attacks, nevertheless infrequently studied. Noninvasive electrophysiological and brain imaging techniques heralded major advances in understanding migraine pathogenesis because they could be applied safely to a population that is healthy between attacks. Brain imaging with functional magnetic resonance imaging (FMRI) and magnetoencephalography (MEG) (6,19), particularly, have been able to confirm that an abnormal electrical and metabolic event consistent with the SD of Leão, when triggered in brain, is anatomically and functionally linked with symptoms of migraine aura. To trigger this event, multiple factors may converge on a common pathway, which we believe to be transient or persistently exaggerated excitability of neurons in the cerebral cortex, especially occipital (1).

Neurophysiological studies of migraine, involving standard diagnostic or complex evoked responses, in the past have been seminal in establishing functional abnormalities in migraine, but suffer from being indirect measures limited to specific systems of anatomical and functional interest. Many such studies have supported hyperexcitability, while others have not; Ambrosini et al. have provided an exhaustive review and interpretation of these earlier investigations (20). Contemporary brain imaging techniques have shifted attention away from this approach, possibly because of uncertainties engendered by inconsistent electrophysiological results. Nevertheless, recent advances have enabled more direct probing of brain function, such as with transcranial magnetic stimulation (TMS). TMS of the occipital cortex required to produce phosphene generation akin to the scintillating visual experiences of migraine aura was significantly lower in patients with migraine with aura (MWA) *between* their headaches than it was in normal controls (21) Using the same technology, but with different paradigms, other studies have added consistent data that support cortical hyperexcitability (22–24), also indicating that hyperexcitability of the visual cortex in migraine goes beyond visual area V1. Observing phosphenes is a subjective experience; however, this is a drawback of these studies, leading to understandable controversy, because not all studies agree (25).

Unlike the neurophysiological investigations reviewed above, functional brain imaging appears to have provided the most consistent evidence for brain hyperexcitability between attacks. When subjects with a natural and reproducible history of migraine attacks induced by visual stress were studied, the success rates were high for experimentally induced attacks using checkerboard visual stimulation. Exploiting this opportunity, visual activation monitored by MEG and FMRI-BOLD (blood oxygen–level dependent) study confirmed abnormal excitability of widespread regions of the occipital, occipito-temporal, and occipito-parietal cortex, with consequent triggering of the accompaniments of aura symptoms (6,19). In the FMRI-BOLD study of migraine patients (19), visual stimulation, designed to activate the total occipital cortex, initiated multifocally originating SD of initial activation at rates compatible with cortical spreading depression (CSD); multiple events were evoked bilaterally from different regions of the occipital, occipital-parietal, and occipital-temporal cortex. Vincent et al., also using FMRI-BOLD, confirmed the same enhanced interictal reactivity of the visual cortex (26). MEG results, despite using a stimulus designed to activate primary visual cortex alone, confirmed the multifocality of neuronal excitation throughout occipital cortex and the direct current (DC) shifts that arose from these sites (6). Absence of DC shifts in the MEG recordings after prophylactic valproate therapy indicated that the medication inhibited the migraine patient's cortical hyperexcitability or changed the threshold for induction of CSD. Finally, linking FMRI findings to psychophysical experiments described in a previous section, Huang et al. used FMRI-BOLD to document a hyperexcitable neuronal response in terms of peak magnitude of BOLD signal and visual illusions and distortions when MWA patients viewed square wave gratings at different spatial frequencies (27).

MECHANISMS OF HYPEREXCITABILITY

Excitability of cell membranes, especially in the occipital cortex, seems fundamental to the migraine brain's susceptibility to migraine attacks (1). Different cellular mechanisms may underlie increased neuronal excitability in migraine. Primary disorders of brain mitochondria, for example Mitochondrial Myopathy, Encephalopathy, Lactic Acidosis, and Stroke-like episodes, or MELAS, are associated with symptomatic migraine attacks (28). Presumably, impaired energy metabolism causes cellular ionic in-homeostasis, membrane instability, and readily depolarizable neurons when subjected to triggering stimuli, culminating in CSD. Previously, localized phosphorus spectroscopy performed in MWA patients yielded data on brain energy status, which had suggested dysfunction of brain mitochondria (29); abnormal muscle energetics in the same patients raised the possibility of the disorder being generalized (30). Boska et al. extended these single-voxel studies to include multiple brain regions and larger numbers of patients using multislice (31) phosphorus magnetic resonance spectroscopic imaging (31). MWA, migraine without aura (MwoA), and hemiplegic migraine patients were studied between attacks. Trends toward abnormality in posterior brain regions were found in severe forms of migraine as previously shown by the single-voxel studies reviewed above. In addition, some evidence supported compensatory metabolic shifts in the less severe forms of migraine, for example without aura, raising the issue that neurological features become more severe when cells cannot maintain homeostasis effectively in the presence of underlying pathology, such as an inherited channelopathy. In further support of brain energy deficits, results of an experiment wherein migraine patients and controls were subjected to visual stress with a continuous flashing black-and-white checkerboard between attacks during serial single-voxel proton spectroscopy of the primary visual cortex showed levels of N-acetylaspartate (NAA) fell during this time compared with normal controls and MwoA patients (32). Inasmuch as NAA is indicative of mitochondrial function of neurons, these findings would support the importance of stressing neuronal function and energy status in unmasking any mitochondrial abnormality in migraine patients.

Magnesium imaging by means of phosphorus spectroscopy has revealed consistent and profound changes in posterior brain regions of patients severely compromised with hemiplegic migraine (31). This includes low magnesium in ^{31}phosphorus spectroscopic images of members of families with hemiplegic migraine. In FHM, mutation of a gene, probably a gain of function mutation, involved in production of a brain-specific P/Q-type calcium channel has been identified (2). This channelopathy may result in increased release of excitatory neurotransmitters with consequent neuronal hyperexcitability. The imaged magnesium changes, therefore, could reflect attempts by the brain to maintain homeostasis and counteract hyperexcitability with magnesium fixation in cell membranes and by gating excitatory receptors. In fact, migraine patients without aura showed compensatory changes of intracellular Mg^{2+} and membrane phospholipids, again suggesting that neurological symptoms only occur in migraine susceptible individuals when the brain fails to adjust its function to maintain homeostasis. Low systemic or brain magnesium levels certainly may be fundamental mechanisms of neuronal excitability, but fit with a general as opposed to localized hyperexcitability of specific structures as indicated by the regional changes shown in patients with otherwise normal brain magnesium levels. Curiously, migraine patients have low-circulating magnesium levels, which may stress brain capacity to effectively maintain regional magnesium levels (28). Supplementing magnesium to prevent migraine attacks makes sense under these circumstances and indeed has proven modestly successful (33). With respect to the general thesis of this chapter, magnesium has antiepileptic properties exploited for decades in the management of eclampsia.

Much mechanistic information has yielded to recent genetic investigations. Discovery of missense mutations in the α1A subunit of the P/Q-type calcium channel in patients with FHM type-1 indicated the potential involvement of dysfunctional ion channels in migraine (2). Using a knock-in mouse model carrying the human FMH type 1 R192Q mutation, multiple gain-of-function effects were observed (34). Increased neuronal calcium current density, enhanced neuromuscular junction transmission, and a reduced threshold for SD with an increased rate of spread, all support hyperexcitability as the basis for migraine susceptibility. Also, P/Q-type calcium channels in the periaqueductal gray (PAG) region of the brainstem appear to modulate craniovascular nociception, suggesting a role for dysfunctional P/Q-type calcium channels in altering this descending pain modulation system to bring about migraine headache (35).

FMH type 2 has been linked to a mutation in the gene *ATP1A2* that encodes the α2 subunit of the sodium/potassium pump (3). The α2 subunit distribution on the plasma membrane is abundant on neurons and astrocytes and coincides with the sodium/calcium exchanger in these cells. Loss of function of these subunits and resulting impaired clearance of extracellular potassium may be responsible for cortical depolarization, particularly with repetitive stimulation of the same cellular system as in the visual cortex linear detector neurons discussed above. Commonality with the abnormalities of the P/Q calcium channel gain of function abnormality lies in the intracellular sodium increase, which promotes intracellular calcium increase through the sodium/calcium exchanger. Further possibilities for generating cellular hyperexcitability include increased neuronal glutamate release secondary to astrocyte pump abnormalities.

Finally, in FHM type 3 a heterozygous missense mutation occurs in the α1 subunit (Gln1489Lys) in SCN1A on chromosome 2q24. This defective voltage-gated sodium channel causes accelerated recovery from fast inactivation, leading to a higher neuronal firing rate culminating in excess extracellular glutamate- and potassium-induced CSD (4). Thus, although all three genetic mutations differ in site and mechanistic dysfunction, FHM type 1 and FHM type 3 promotes hyperexcitability by presynaptic mechanisms, while FHM type 2 prevents clearance of excitatory neurotransmitter from the synaptic cleft.

Comorbidity with Epilepsy

Given the evidence for increased excitability of neuronal tissue in migraine, parallels with epilepsy are understandable (36). Clarity of definition is important in understanding the complexity the association (37). For example, brain lesions such as arteriovenous malformations, or diseases of known functional mechanism such as MELAS, can present symptomatically with migraine, epilepsy, or migraine aura progressing into an epileptic attack. Epileptic seizures, especially those originating in occipital cortex, can mimic aura. Migraine-induced epilepsy (sometimes known as migralepsy) can occur during or immediately after aura, particularly in migraine patients with prolonged aura or basilar migraine. Because each condition is common (migraine in 6% of men and 17% of women and epilepsy in half to one percent of the population), a chance coexistence of both conditions is not surprising. Nevertheless, we now consider that migraine may be a progressive condition in some patients, causing altered brain function consequent to severe or repeated migraine attacks; no clear pathogenesis leading to seizures, however, has yet been identified. But a relationship between migraine and stroke is established, especially with recurrent and longstanding illness (38); seizures may occur as a consequence of such ischemic cell damage. In the absence of obvious brain lesions, functional changes of yet unknown origin leading to a common brain state of hyperexcitability alone could form the basis of a migraine-epilepsy comorbidity. In an often-quoted study by Ottman et al. (39), prevalence data for migraine was collected in patients with epilepsy and in their relatives with and with out epilepsy. Of the probands, 24% had a migraine history; in relatives with epilepsy, it was 26%, but 15% in relatives without it. Risk of developing migraine was twice as high in the first two groups compared with the last. The data argued in favor of a common brain state, and an inherited phenotype at one end of a spectrum wherein migraine, seizures, or both occur on the basis, we believe, of increased brain excitability. Further evidence for brain hyperexcitability comes from a prospective 5 to 10 year follow-up of epilepsy in patients with migraine compared with epilepsy patients without migraine. A significantly lower cumulative probability of being seizure free over 10 years was found in patients with migraine and epilepsy. Reduced early treatment responses were also observed along with a higher incidence of intractable epilepsy (40). More recently, MWA proved a risk factor for unprovoked seizures in children. When symptoms were evaluated in a population-based case-control study of all incident epilepsy in Icelandic children and in matched controls, migraine was associated with a fourfold increased risk for developing epilepsy, an association explained by MWA [odds ratio (OR), 8.1; 95% (CI), 2.7–24.3] (41). Finally, in further support of an epilepsy-migraine link, seizures are part of the clinical spectrum of FHM type 2, in which mutations of the gene *ATP1A2* that encodes the α2 subunit of the sodium/potassium pump occur, as discussed above (3).

Leninger et al. questioned whether clinical characteristics of SD were exaggerated in patients with concurrent epilepsy and migraine (42). Although frequency of epilepsy syndromes and seizure types did not differ, migraine aura, worsening of pain with activity, phonophobia, and photophobia were significantly more frequent in comorbid patients compared with those with epilepsy alone or migraine alone. AEDs with proven antimigraine benefit might be the logical first approach to management in the former patients.

Therapeutic Implications of Hyperexcitability

Abnormally increased neuronal excitability seems a reasonable basis for targeting therapy in migraine prevention. In fact, revisiting the actions of drug groups found effective in migraine prevention over the past years, such as serotonin receptor blockers, βblockers, calcium channel blockers, and nonsteroidal anti-inflammatory drugs (NSAIDs), reveals a common property of diminished excitability. Unfortunately, none of this preventive medication has proven more than moderately effective in reducing migraine frequency, likely due to uncertainty of the precise molecular target involved in the susceptibility to migraine.

Before 1990, available anticonvulsant medication was limited to phenobarbital, primidone, phenytoin, carbamazepine, and valproate. Numerous novel AEDs have been developed in recent years, and they are now popular as potential agents for migraine prevention; however, rarely has their use been adequately rationalized. Although historically phenobarbital, phenytoin, and carbamazepine were used for preventing migraine in children and adults, not until the newer generation of AEDs coincident with improvements in clinical trial design became available has the evidence of effectiveness of AEDs been established enough to become first-line therapy to prevent severe and frequent migraine attacks. Even so, the effectiveness of the individual AEDs is again only observed in approximately two thirds of patients. As with other above-mentioned drugs that have been standards in migraine prevention, the mechanisms of the AEDs differ both in molecular site and multiplicity of actions, so that reduction of hyperexcitability becomes the common brain state associated with effectiveness. This is not surprising since the mechanisms of brain hyperexcitability in migraine patients are also multifactorial as reviewed in depth above and best exemplified by the differing genetic mutations associated with FHM. AEDs can have marked analgesic actions in humans, such as gabapentin, lamotrigine, phenytoin, levetiracetam, and sodium valproate, but any such role in migraine attack prevention is uncertain, undoubtedly complex, probably targets the components of headache, and will not be discussed here since we are focusing on the antiexcitability properties of the AEDs.

ANTIEPILEPTIC DRUGS IN THE CONTEMPORARY MANAGEMENT OF MIGRAINE

We will review here the AEDs that have been investigated in migraine prevention, emphasizing the two that have received FDA indications for this use, valproate and topiramate. Of the remainder, tonabersat, the latest drug with antiepileptic potential to emerge as a migraine prevention candidate, is in clinical trials. Zonisamide and leveteracitram either have proven ineffective or have not been subjected to rigorous randomized controlled trials. Lamotrigine and gabapentin have limited or qualified effectiveness.

Tonabersat

Tonabersat, a novel benzoylamino benzopyran compound, is currently being studied for migraine prevention on the basis of its gap junction blockade and inhibition of chemically induced repetitive CSD (43). Inhibition of nitric oxide release and blockade of trigeminal nerve stimulation–evoked inflammation are added potential actions of the drug that might benefit migraine. Earlier, 15 patients with MwoA were given tonabersat in a randomized, double-blind, crossover study with placebo control employing glyceryl trinitrate (GTN) infusion as an experimental migraine trigger; no benefit was noted, but the study was terminated prematurely because of an interaction that caused hypotension between the active drug and GTN (44). Clinical trials examining tonabersat's potential in reducing the severity and frequency of episodic migraine attacks are ongoing.

Zonisamide

Zonisamide is a broad-spectrum AED that has been available in the United States since 2000. It acts by blocking sodium as well as T-type calcium channels. Zonisamide has the advantage of a long half-life that makes once-daily dosing possible and minimal interaction with other medications. In the few studies of zonisamide in migraine prevention available for review, however, little evidence of effectiveness has emerged, although rigorous randomized, placebo-controlled studies have not been reported. In a post hoc chart review of severe and refractory episodic and chronic migraine patients treated for two months to a year in some cases, no reduction of frequency or severity of headache was documented, while the adverse event of severe fatigue occurred in over 40% of patients (45). Nevertheless, this low-ranking study based on evidence-based criteria may have proved a disservice to the drug; because the mechanisms of action of zonisamide are similar to those of AEDs that are effective in migraine prevention, it is possible that this drug has not received the thorough study it deserves.

Levetiracetam

Levetiracetam has an unknown mechanism of action, but does not appear to have the activity of other AEDs, though it may exert inhibitory effects on neuronal-type calcium channels. Rigorous randomized, placebo-controlled studies have not been reported, but an open-label study of MWA prophylaxis indicated a sustained benefit in reduced frequency of attacks over six months (46). One particularly interesting property is the effect of levetiracetam on cortical response to bring about desynchronization to visual stimulus frequency; hypersynchronicity of response to visual stimuli characterizes migraine brain (47).

Lamotrigine

Lamotrigine is a broad-spectrum AED that acts primarily by the blockade of sodium channels and, to a lesser extent, calcium channels. Blockade of voltage-sensitive sodium channels leads to inhibition of neuronal release of glutamate, which likely facilitates propagation of CSD. It causes minimal sedation or drug interactions, but is slow to attain therapeutic maintenance doses. In a trial that compared the safety and efficacy of lamotrigine and placebo in migraine prophylaxis in a double-blind, randomized, parallel-groups design, lamotrigine was ineffective in preventing migraine (48). Also, more adverse events were more frequent with lamotrigine, most commonly rash. This study was disappointing because an earlier study that examined the efficacy of lamotrigine in the prevention of migraine aura alone showed a significant reduction in both frequency of aura and aura duration (49). The open-label nature of this study, however, weakens the evidence base for the drug's effectiveness.

Gabapentin

Gabapentin was approved for use as an AED in 1993. Interestingly, more than 80% of prescriptions for gabapentin are for off-label uses, such as neuropathic pain, spasticity, bipolar disorder, as well as migraine headache. Although structurally related to gamma-aminobutyric acid (GABA), its precise mechanism of action in humans is unknown but is thought to involve alteration in GABA-mediated neurotransmission. Gabapentin has the advantage of safety with good tolerability without substantial drug interactions. Unfortunately, it has only modest efficacy in migraine prevention.

Results of a three-month randomized, double-blind, placebo-controlled study in 63 patients suffering from migraine with or without aura showed a significant reduction of frequency and intensity of migraine in just under half the patients treated with gabapentin 1200 mg/day (50). Gabapentin was said to be well tolerated, although somnolence and fatigue figured prominently in a third of the patients. Most convincing was a placebo-controlled, double-blind study conducted in 143 patients receiving up to 2400 mg/day for three months (51). Despite high dropout rates, a modest but significant reduction in frequency was observed; the median four-week migraine attack rate was 2.7 for active drug compared with 3.5 for placebo. Also, 44% of gabapentin patients showed a greater than 50% reduction in migraine attack frequency compared with 16% of placebo. Adverse events were as mentioned above but in fewer patients. In general, gabapentin appears to have a modest benefit in migraine prevention and is well tolerated.

Valproate

Valproate was the first AED approved by the FDA for migraine prevention, and accordingly, will be reviewed in greater depth than those AEDs that have not been approved. Although its precise mechanism of action remains to be established, valproate targets the GABAergic synapse, enhancing GABAergic inhibitory neurotransmission, and increasing brain concentrations of GABA. The effect on the neuronal membrane is unknown. Valproate is rapidly absorbed after oral administration. Peak serum levels occur approximately one to four hours after a single oral dose. The serum half-life of valproate is typically in the range of 6 to 16 hours. Valproate is rapidly distributed throughout the body and the drug is strongly bound (90%) to human plasma proteins. Increases in dose may result in decreases in the extent of protein binding and variable changes in valproate clearance and elimination. The therapeutic plasma concentration range is believed to be from 50 to 100 µg/mL for seizure management, but for migraine, daily dose, serum levels, and therapeutic effect have not been evaluated. Valproate is primarily metabolized in the liver to the glucuronide conjugate. Teratogenicity in human females receiving the drug during pregnancy is an important concern, and the incidence of neural tube defects in the fetus may be increased during the first trimester of pregnancy.

Sørensen first reported the use of valproate in migraine prevention in 1988 (52). Twenty-two patients with severe migraine with and without aura resistant to previous prophylactic treatments participated in a prospective open trial. The dose of valproate was 600 mg twice a day adjusted to a serum level of about 700 µmol/L. Follow-up was from 3 to 12 months. Eleven patients became free from migraine attacks and six had a significant reduction in frequency. In one patient, there was no effect and four dropped out. In a withdrawal experiment, three patients who experienced relapse after being free from migraine for three months became headache free again after resuming valproate.

In 1992, Hering and Kuritsky followed with the first controlled trial of the efficacy of sodium valproate versus placebo in the treatment of migraine in a double-blind, randomized, crossover study in 29 patients (53). Valproate was effective in preventing migraine or reducing the frequency, severity, and duration of the attacks in 86.2% of the patients. These results were confirmed in a somewhat larger and more rigorously designed trial by Jensen et al., in which the number of days with migraine was 3.5 per four weeks during treatment with sodium valproate and 6.1 during placebo (54). The severity and duration of the migraine attacks that did occur were not affected. Fifty percent of the patients had their initial migraine frequency reduced to 50% or less during valproate compared with 18% during placebo. The number of responders increased during the trial to 65% in the last four weeks of the active treatment period. There were no serious side effects requiring withdrawal of patients from the study.

The first U.S. trial in 1995 was the largest controlled trial reported at that time to compare the efficacy and safety of valproate (using the divalproex sodium formulation) and placebo in the prophylaxis of migraine (55). The trial was a multicenter, double-blind, randomized, placebo-controlled investigation of 107 patients randomized to divalproex or placebo (in a 2:1 ratio) for 12 weeks. During treatment, the mean migraine headache frequency per four weeks was 3.5 in the divalproex group and 5.7 in the placebo group ($p \leq 0.001$). Forty-eight % of divalproex-treated patients and 14% of placebo-treated patients showed a 50% or greater reduction in migraine headache frequency from the baseline phase ($p < 0.001$). Divalproex-treated patients also reported significantly less functional restriction than placebo-treated patients and used significantly less symptomatic medication. No significant differences were observed in severity or duration of individual migraine headaches. Thirteen percent of patients found the active drug intolerant compared with 5% of placebo-treated patients.

Numerous other studies since these seminal trials have supported the original observation of the effectiveness of valproate for migraine prevention, including studies of childhood migraine (56). Although only approved for migraine prevention, intravenous valproate has also been used to abort acute migraine attacks, speculatively via reducing excitability of the trigeminal system or interfering at some point in the molecular cascade underpinning the headache (57–60). No randomized, placebo-controlled clinical trials, however, of intravenous valproate in acute migraine attacks have been performed. Studies to date have been retrospective or open label; although one study did compare intravenous valproate with standard acute parenteral medications and found no difference in effect (60).

Two clinical studies have indicated that valproate is effective in migraine prevention by reducing brain hyperexcitability. In the first, Mulleners et al. measured occipital excitability using TMS in 31 migraine patients who displayed improvement with prophylactic valproate therapy (61). In MWA patients, but not in MwoA patients, excitability as measured by phosphene induction thresholds was reduced. Modest correlations were observed between reduced excitability and decrease in headache in the aura patients. In the second study, Bowyer et al. used DC-MEG to determine the effectiveness of prophylactic valproate therapy on neuronal hyperexcitability in nine patients (62). MEG scans were recorded during visual stimulation before commencing medication and again after 30 days of daily valproate use. Large-amplitude DC-MEG signals, imaged to extended areas of occipital cortex, were seen before therapy. After treatment, DC-MEG shifts were reduced in the occipital cortex coincident with reduced incidence of migraine attacks. Thus, the authors demonstrated that hyperexcitability of widespread regions throughout occipital cortex in migraine was diminished by valproate.

Topiramate

Topiramate is the most recent AED to be approved in the United States for migraine prevention. A broad-spectrum AED, topiramate has multiple mechanisms of action, including state-dependent inhibition of voltage-gated sodium channels, inhibition of high-voltage-activated calcium channels, inhibition of glutamate-mediated neurotransmission at α-amino-3-hydroxy-5 methyl-4-isoxazole-propionic acid (AMPA) and kainite receptor subtypes, and enhancement of GABA receptor–mediated chloride flux (63). The mechanism of action precisely responsible for topiramate's antimigraine effect remains to be established but it may be the broad spectrum of activity at glutamatergic synapses in reducing brain hyperexcitability that is responsible. Topiramate also modulates trigeminal signaling and reduces the numbers of induced CSDs (64,65).

In an early clinical trial, Storey et al. evaluated the efficacy and safety of topiramate 200 mg/day in 40 migraine patients in a single-center, double-blind, placebo-controlled study (66). Topiramate-treated patients experienced a significantly lower 28-day migraine frequency compared with placebo-treated patients (3.31 ± 1.7 vs. 3.83 ± 2.1; $p = 0.002$), irrespective of use of concomitant migraine prevention medications. Twenty-six percent of the patients on topiramate and 9.5% of the patients on placebo achieved a 50% reduction in migraine frequency ($p > 0.05$). Adverse effects occurred more frequently in topiramate-treated patients. These included paresthesias, weight loss, altered taste, anorexia, and memory impairment.

In the seminal study that established topiramate as an approved indication for migraine prevention, Brandes et al. reported that mean monthly migraine frequency decreased significantly for patients receiving topiramate at 100 mg/day and at 200 mg/day compared with placebo in a randomized, double-blind, controlled trial of 483 patients (67). Statistically significant reductions occurred within the first month of treatment in patients on 100 and 200 mg/day. Rescue medication use was also reduced in both groups. The most common adverse events were parasthesias, fatigue, anorexia, weight loss, difficulty with memory, taste perversion, and nausea. Efficacy was maintained for the duration of the 18-week, double-blind phase.

Similar results were obtained from the second pivotal trial (68). Pooled efficacy data from two large, similarly designed, placebo-controlled migraine-prevention trials demonstrated that a statistically significant proportion of patients using topiramate met or exceeded two main outcome guidelines recommended by the International Headache Society ($\geq 50\%$ and $\geq 75\%$ reduction in frequency of monthly attacks). On the basis of efficacy and tolerability, topiramate at a dosage of 100 mg/day (administered 50 mg twice daily) should be the target dosage for most migraine patients (69). When trials were extended to chronic migraine, a condition associated with intractability to most preventive strategies, topiramate treatment at daily doses of approximately 100 mg resulted in statistically significant improvements compared with placebo in mean monthly migraine and migraine headache days (70). Benefits of topiramate prevention have now been documented in childhood migraine (71).

Unlike for valproate, no clinical studies were found, which have investigated the effects of topiramate in reducing brain hyperexcitability in migraine, with the exception of the one quoted above, in which levetiracetam, but not topiramate, promoted desynchronization of the EEG response to visual stimulation in association with effectiveness of migraine prevention (48).

Therapeutic Strategies Influencing the Use of AEDs

The choice of a prophylactic agent for migraine is based on multiple factors, including coexisting medical and psychiatric conditions, likely side effects, and increasingly, cost and availability. With current drug availability affected by insurance restrictions in the United States, clinicians may first be required to offer βblockade for migraine prophylaxis; contraindications, however, may limit the use of these in patients with asthma and diabetes. In young healthy migraine patients who exercise regularly, exercise intolerance may pose another limiting factor in the use of βblockade. The established risk for depression with βblockade may also limit their role, given the high prevalence of comorbid depression in migraine. Tricyclic antidepressants, while not FDA approved, continue to be a first-line therapy on the basis of efficacy, but weight gain, sedation, cardiac side effects, and their associated risk of triggering mania in occult bipolar disease may restrict their use in migraine prevention.

For the episodic migraine patient with no other medical conditions, topiramate and valproate may be considered as first-line therapies; the former would be preferentially chosen in a migraine patient with prediabetes, diabetes, polycystic ovarian syndrome (PCOS), obesity, epilepsy, or tremor. For chronic and intractable migraine, topiramate would be preferred over valproate as a first-line approach. No effect on weight, or even weight loss, increasingly influences the choice of topiramate over other first-line antimigraine drugs that often cause weight gain. In fact, recent data also shows that the risk for developing chronic migraine increases with increasing body mass index (72). Valproate may be a first choice in an underweight patient, a patient with comorbid epilepsy, particularly myoclonic epilepsy, or a patient with comorbid bipolar disorder. Adjunctive use of oral contraceptive agents is acceptable with either topiramate or valproate. Valproate does not influence the efficacy of oral contraceptive pills, but at doses over 200 mg of topiramate, oral contraceptive efficacy may be reduced. Nephrolithiasis and glaucoma would be contraindications to the use of topiramate, and PCOS and pregnancy would be relative contraindications for the use of valproate. Topiramate is classed as C, and valproate as D for use in pregnancy, and other migraine preventives should be considered before either agent if treatment during pregnancy is demanded. Monitoring of both agents is recommended, with baseline and serial bicarbonate levels in patients on topiramate, and platelets and white blood cell counts in patients on valproate.

CONCLUSIONS

Two AEDs have indication for use in adult migraine prevention, and under certain circumstance may be used as first lines of treatment. The basis of AED effectiveness appears to be a common effect, although through different actions, of reducing cortical hyperexcitability or cortical over-responsiveness, the fundament of migraine susceptible brain. Some evidence exists that abnormal synchronicity to certain stimuli, especially visual, is reversed by the AEDs and is compatible with their counteracting the triggering of CSD that underpins migraine aura.

REFERENCES

1. Welch KMA, D'Andrea G, Tepley N, et al. The concept of migraine as a state of central neuronal hyperexcitability. Headache 1990; 8:817–828.
2. Ophoff RA, Terwindt GM, Vergouwe MN, et al. Familial hemiplegic migraine and episodic ataxia type-2 are caused by mutations in the Ca2+ channel gene CACNL1A4. Cell 1996; 87:543–552.

3. De Fusco M, Marconi R, Silvestri L, et al. Haploinsufficiency of ATP1A2 encoding the Na+/K+ pump alpha2 subunit associated with familial hemiplegic migraine type 2. Nat Gen 2003; 33(2):192–196.
4. Dichgans M, Freilinger T, Eckstein G, et al. Mutation in the neuronal voltage-gated sodium channel SCN1A causes familial hemiplegic migraine. Lancet 2005; 366:371–377.
5. Leão AAP. Spreading depression of activity in cerebral cortex. J Neurophysiol 1944; 7: 379–390.
6. Bowyer SM, Aurora SK, Moran JE, et al. Magnetoencephalographic fields from patients with spontaneous and induced migraine aura. Ann Neurol 2001; 50(5):582–587.
7. Wray SH, Mijovic-Prelec D, Kosslyn SM. Visual processing in migraineurs. Brain 1995; 118:25–35.
8. Marcus DA, Soso MJ. Migraine and stripe-induced visual discomfort. Arch Neurol 1989; 46:1129–1132.
9. McColl SL, Wilkinson F. Visual contrast gain control in migraine: measures of visual cortical excitability and inhibition. Cephalalgia 2000; 20:74–78.
10. Mulleners WM, Chronicle EP, Palmer JE, et al. Suppression of perception in migraine: evidence for reduced inhibition in the visual cortex. Neurology 2001; 56(2):178–183.
11. Wilkins AAJ, Binnie CD, Darby CE. Visually induced seizures. Prog Neurobiol 1980; 15: 85–117.
12. Airy H. On a distinct form of transient hemianopsia. Philos Trans R Soc Lond 1870; 160: 247–264.
13. Richards W. The fortification illusions of migraine. Sci Am 1971; 224(5):88–96.
14. Wilkins AJ, Patel R, Adjamian P, et al. Tinted spectacles and visually sensitive migraine. Cephalalgia 2002; 22(9):711–719.
15. Kowacs PA, Piovesan EJ, Werneck LC, et al. Influence of intense light stimulation on trigeminal and cervical pain perception thresholds. Cephalalgia 2001; 21(3):184–188.
16. Shepherd AJ. Visual contrast processing in migraine. Cephalalgia 2000; 20(10):865–880.
17. Shepherd AJ. Increased visual after-effects following pattern adaptation in migraine: a lack of intracortical excitation? Brain 2001; 124(Pt 11):2310–2318.
18. Galeotti N, Ghelardini C, Zoppi M, et al. Hypo functionality of Gi proteins as aetiopathogenic mechanism for migraine and cluster headache. Cephalalgia 2001; 21(1):38–45.
19. Cao Y, Welch KM, Aurora S, et al. Functional MRI-BOLD of visually triggered headache in patients with migraine. Arch Neurol 1999; 56(5):548–554.
20. Ambrosini A, de Noordhout AM, Sandor P, et al. Electrophysiological studies in migraine: a comprehensive review of their interest and limitations. Cephalalgia 2003; 23(suppl. 1):13–31.
21. Aurora SK, Ahmad BK, Welch KMA, et al. Transcranial magnetic stimulation confirms hyper excitability of occipital cortex in migraine. Neurology 1998; 50:1111–1114.
22. Mulleners WM, Chronicle EP, Vredeveld JW, et al. Visual cortex excitability in migraine before and after valproate prophylaxis: a pilot study using TMS. Eur J Neurol 2002; 9(1): 35–40.
23. Young WB, Oshinsky ML, Shechter AL, et al. Consecutive transcranial magnetic stimulation: phosphene thresholds in migraineurs and controls. Headache 2004; 44:131–135.
24. Batelli L, Black KR, Wray SH. Transcranial magnetic stimulation of visual area V5 in migraine. Neurology 2002; 58(7):1066–1069.
25. Afra J, Mascia A, Gerard P, et al. Interictal cortical excitability in migraine: a study using transcranial magnetic stimulation of motor and visual cortices. Ann Neurol 1998; 44: 209–215.
26. Vincent M, Pedra A, Mourao-Miranda J, et al. Enhanced interictal responsiveness of the migrainous visual cortex to incongruent bar stimulation: a functional MRI visual activation study. Cephalalgia 2003; 23(9):860–868.
27. Huang J, Cooper TG, Satana B, et al. Visual distortion provoked by a stimulus in migraine associated with hyperneuronal activity. Headache 200; 43:664–671.
28. Welch KM, Ramadan NM. Mitochondria, magnesium and migraine. J Neurol Sci 1995; 134: 9–14.
29. Welch KMA, Levine SR, D'Andrea G, et al. Preliminary observations on brain energy metabolism in migraine studied by in vivo phosphorus 31 NMR spectroscopy. Neurology 1989; 39:538–554.
30. Barbirolli B, Montagna P, Cortelli P, et al. Abnormal brain and muscle energy metabolism shown by ^{31}P magnetic resonance spectroscopy in patients affected by migraine with aura. Neurology 1992; 42:1209–1214.

31. Boska MD, Welch KM, Barker PB, et al. Contrasts in cortical magnesium, phospholipid and energy metabolism between migraine syndromes. Neurology 2002; 58(8):1227–1233.
32. Brooks WM, Welch KMA, Jung RE, et al. 1H-MRS evidence of a mitochondrial disorder in migraine. Cephalalgia 1999; 19:310.
33. Peikert A, Wilimzig C, Kohne-Volland R. Prophylaxis of migraine with oral magnesium: results from a prospective multi-center, placebo-controlled and double blind randomized study. Cephalalgia 1996; 16:257–263.
34. Van den Maagdenberg A, Pietrobon D, Pizzorusso T, et al. A Cacna1a knockin migraine mouse model with increased susceptibility to cortical spreading depression. Neuron 2004; 41:701–710.
35. Knight YE, Bartsch T, Kaube H, et al. P/Q-type calcium channel blockade in the PAG facilitates trigeminal nociception: a functional genetic link for migraine? J Neurosci 2002; 22(5):RC21
36. Andermann F, Lugaresi E. Migraine and Epilepsy. Boston: Butterworth, 1987.
37. Welch KMA, Lewis D. Migraine and epilepsy. Neurol Clin 1997; 15(1):107–114.
38. Donaghy M, Chang CL, Poulter N. Duration, frequency, recency, and type of migraine and the risk of ischemic stroke in women of childbearing age. J Neurol Neurosurg Psychiatry 2002; 73:747–750.
39. Ottman R, Hong S, Lipton RB. Validity of family history data on severe headaches and migraine. Neurology 1993; 43:1954–1960.
40. Velioğlu SK, Boz C, Ozmenoğlu M. The impact of migraine on epilepsy: a prospective prognosis study. Cephalalgia 2005; 25(7):528–535.
41. Ludvigsson P, Hesdorffer D, Olafsson E, et al. Migraine with aura is a risk factor for unprovoked seizures in children. Ann Neurol 2006; 59:210–213.
42. Leniger T, von den Dreisch S, Isbruch K, et al. Clinical characteristics of patients with comorbidity of migraine and epilepsy. Headache 2003; 43(6):672–677.
43. Bradley DP, Smith MI, Netsiri C, et al. Diffusion-weighted MRI used to detect in vivo modulation of cortical spreading depression: comparison of sumatriptan and tonabersat. Exp Neurol 2001; 172(2):342–353.
44. Tvedskov JF, Iversen HK, Olesen J. A double-blind study of SB-220453 (Tonerbasat) in the glyceryltrinitrate (GTN) model of migraine. Cephalalgia 2004; 24(10):875–882.
45. Ashkenazi A, Benlifer A, Korenblit J, et al. Zonisamide for migraine prophylaxis in refractory patients. Cephalalgia 2006; 26(10):1199–1202.
46. Brighina F, Palermo A, Aloisio A, et al. Levetiracetam in the prophylaxis of migraine with aura: a 6-month open-label study. Clin Neuropharmacol 2006; 29(6):338–342.
47. de Tommaso M, Marinazzo D, Nitti L, et al. Effects of levetiracetam vs topiramate and placebo on visually evoked phase synchronization changes of alpha rhythm in migraine. Clin Neurophysiol 2007; 118(10):2297–2304.
48. Steiner TJ, Findley LJ, Yuen AW. Lamotrigine versus placebo in the prophylaxis of migraine with and without aura. Cephalalgia 1997; 17(2):101–102.
49. Lampl C, Katsarava Z, Diener HC, et al. Lamotrigine reduces migraine aura and migraine attacks in patients with migraine with aura. J Neurol Neurosurg Psychiatry 2005; 76(12):1730–1732.
50. Di Trapani G, Mei D, Marra C, et al. Gabapentin in the prophylaxis of migraine: a double-blind randomized placebo-controlled study. Clin Ter 2000; 151(3):145–148.
51. Mathew NT, Rapoport A, Saper J, et al. Efficacy of gabapentin in migraine prophylaxis. Headache 2001; 41(2):119–128.
52. Sørensen KV. Valproate: a new drug in migraine prophylaxis. Acta Neurol Scand 1988; 78(4):346–348.
53. Hering R, Kuritzky A. Sodium valproate in the prophylactic treatment of migraine. Cephalalgia 1992; 12(2):81–84.
54. Jensen R, Brinck T, Olesen J. Sodium valproate has a prophylactic effect in migraine without aura: a triple-blind, placebo-controlled crossover study. Neurology 1994; 44(4): 647–651.
55. Mathew NT, Saper JR, Silberstein SD, et al. Migraine prophylaxis with divalproex. Arch Neurol 1995; 52(3):281–286.
56. Ashrafi MR, Shabanian R, Zamani GR, et al. Sodium Valproate versus Propranolol in paediatric migraine prophylaxis. Eur J Paediatr Neurol 2005; 9(5):333–338.

57. Kailasam J, Meadors L, Chernyschev O, et al. Intravenous valproate sodium (depacon) aborts migraine rapidly: a preliminary report. Headache 2000; 40(9):720–723.
58. Reiter PD, Nickisch J, Merritt G. Efficacy and tolerability of intravenous valproic acid in acute adolescent migraine. Headache. 2005 Jul-Aug;45(7):899–903.
59. Stillman MJ, Zajac D, Rybicki LA. Treatment of primary headache disorders with intravenous valproate: initial outpatient experience. Headache 2004; 44(1):65–69.
60. Edwards KR, Norton J, Behnke M. Comparison of intravenous valproate versus intra-muscular dihydroergotamine and metoclopramide for acute treatment of migraine headache. Headache 2001; 41(10):976–980.
61. Mulleners WM, Chronicle EP, Vredeveld JW, et al. Visual cortex excitability in migraine before and after valproate prophylaxis: a pilot study using TMS. Eur J Neurol 2002; 9(1): 35–40.
62. Bowyer SM, Mason KM, Moran JE, et al. Cortical hyperexcitability in migraine patients before and after sodium valproate treatment. J Clin Neurophysiol. 2005; 22(1):65–67.
63. Shank RP, Gardocki JF, Streeter AJ, et al. An overview of the preclinical aspects of topiramate pharmacology, pharmacokinetics, and mechanism of action. Epilepsia 2000; 41(suppl 1):53–59.
64. Storer JF, Goadsby PJ. Topiramate inhibits trigeminovascular traffic in the cat: a possible locus of action in the prevention of migraine. Neurology 2003; 60(suppl 1):A238–A239 (abstract).
65. Ayata C, Jin H, Kudo C, et al. Suppression of cortical spreading depression in migraine prophylaxis. Ann Neurol 2006; 59; 652–661.
66. Storey JR, Calder CS, Hart DE, et al. Topiramate in migraine prevention: a double-blind, placebo-controlled study Headache 2001; 41(10):968–975.
67. Brandes JL, Saper JR, Diamond M, et al. Topiramate for Migraine Prevention. A randomized controlled trial. JAMA 2004; 291(8):965–973.
68. Silberstein SD, Netto W, Schmitt J, et al. Topirimate in migraine prevention: results of a large controlled trial. Arch Neurol 2004; 61(4):490–495.
69. Freitag FG, Forde G, Neto W, et al. Analysis of pooled data from two pivotal controlled trials on the efficacy of topiramate in the prevention of migraine. J Am Osteopath Assoc 2007; 107(7):251–258.
70. Silberstein SD, Lipton RB, Dodick DW, et al. Topiramate Chronic Migraine Study Group. Efficacy and safety of topiramate for the treatment of chronic migraine: a randomized, double-blind, placebo-controlled trial. Headache 2007; 47(2):170–180.
71. Lakshmi CV, Singhi P, Malhi P, et al. Topiramate in the prophylaxis of pediatric migraine: a double-blind placebo-controlled trial. J Child Neurol 2007; 22(7):829–835.
72. Scher Ai, Stewart WF, Ricci JA, et al. Factors associated with the onset and remission of chronic daily headache in a population-based study. Pain 2003; 106:81–89.

5 Antiepileptic Medications in the Treatment of Neuropsychiatric Symptoms Associated with Traumatic Brain Injury

Patricia Roy, Hochang Lee, and Vani Rao
Department of Psychiatry, Johns Hopkins School of Medicine, Baltimore, Maryland, U.S.A.

EPIDEMIOLOGY OF TRAUMATIC BRAIN INJURY

Traumatic brain injury (TBI) is a significant cause of morbidity and disability in the United States. The Center for Disease Control (CDC) estimates that an average of 1.4 million people suffer from a TBI in the United States each year (1). Children under the age of 14 years account for 475,000 incidents of TBI each year, while older adults (>65 years) account for 83,000. According to the CDC, males are 1.5 times more likely than females to suffer from a TBI. The severity of TBI can range from mild to severe. Mild TBI is defined as a brief change of consciousness or mental status following injury, while a severe brain injury is defined as an extended period of unconsciousness or amnesia following the incident. Studies by the CDC approximate that the annual death rate secondary to TBI is about 50,000. Approximately 16.8% patients require hospitalization and 79.6% require visits and care in an emergency department. In addition to acute care, many patients require long-term rehabilitation and suffer from chronic sequelae such as posttraumatic epilepsy, impaired cognition, and long-term neuropsychiatric syndromes (1).

MECHANISMS OF TRAUMATIC BRAIN INJURY

TBI encompasses primary and secondary injuries. Primary injury, most often caused by direct mechanical impact, can be focal or diffuse. Focal injury can be the result of a penetrating injury and result in localized damage. The more common closed head injury often results in a contusion injury. Contusion injury is the result of acceleration-deceleration injuries, which cause the brain to impact on the bony protuberances of the skull. This produces coup (at the site of impact) and contrecoup (at the opposite side of initial impact) injuries. This type of injury commonly affects the frontal and occipital lobes. Focal injury can also result from intracerebral hematoma, intracranial hemorrhage, or focal hypoxic-ischemic injury.

Diffuse axonal injury is the most common of the diffuse brain injuries and is caused by angular or rotational acceleration of the head, resulting in shearing and/or tearing of the axons. The severity of the axonal damage can be assessed by duration and severity of coma, presence and length of associated amnesia, and presence of rostral brain stem signs. Other types of diffuse brain injury include hypoxia-ischemia, diffuse vascular, and edema.

Secondary injury occurs at the cellular level as a result of the primary injury. It is a complex process and thought to be associated with a cascade of events starting at the time of injury and continuing for a prolonged period. There is an immediate effect on the cells, which is a transient separation of the lipid bilayers.

This causes a temporary defect in the cell membrane that can damage receptors and transporters. There is a marked increase in extracellular glutamate followed by an increased intracellular release of calcium, free-radical damage, release of cytokines, and inflammation, which can be followed by apoptosis and cell death (2). It is thought that subsequent changes in the cholinergic, catecholaminergic, and serotonergic systems result, which may be contributing factors in the development of post-TBI neuropsychiatric symptoms.

RECOVERY FROM TRAUMATIC BRAIN INJURY

There are little data on the exact duration of recovery from TBI. For both focal and diffuse types of injury, the recovery time is dependent on the severity of injury and can last months. Post-TBI physical sequelae often stabilize with time but neuropsychiatric problems can continue to remit and relapse. The latter are often burdensome to the patient, overwhelming to the caregiver, and difficult to treat.

Posttraumatic Brain Injury Psychiatric Syndromes

Rao and Lyketsoshave proposed classifying the psychiatric complications of TBI into six categories. These include cognitive deficits, mood disorders, anxiety disorders, apathy, psychosis, and behavioral dyscontrol disorder (2). In addition, a common neurological sequela of TBI is posttraumatic epilepsy.

Recent guidelines for the pharmacotherapy of post-TBI psychiatric syndromes suggest that patients with TBI are more sensitive to medication side effects, while often being refractory to traditional treatment (3). A general rule of thumb is to start medication at a low dose and increase slowly, with careful monitoring for potential side effects and treatment response. A holistic approach should be instituted, that includes, in addition to pharmacotherapy, psychotherapy and regular education of the patient and caregiver. Moreover, clinicians should be proactive and have a plan to manage problems as they arise.

This chapter gives an overview of the uses of antiepileptic drug (AED) medications in the management of post-TBI neuropsychiatric syndromes. Common post-TBI neuropsychiatric syndromes to be discussed will include major depression, mania, psychosis, behavioral dyscontrol disorder, sleep disturbances, and epilepsy. This chapter focuses specifically on the use of AEDs in the use of the neurological and psychiatric sequelae of TBI. It is important to emphasize that neuropsychiatric symptoms such as anxiety with depression or manic features are often part of a syndrome and should be evaluated and treated as such, rather than as individual symptoms. This said, there are some specific symptoms such as sleep disturbances, which can occur in isolation and not in the context of a defined psychiatric syndrome and should, therefore, be managed independently.

Major Depression

Major depression is common following TBI with reports of an incidence that is over 40% (4,5). Symptoms include low mood, anhedonia, thoughts of suicide or hopelessness, feelings of worthlessness or inappropriate guilt, changes in sleep, fatigue, decreased concentration, decreased appetite, and apathy. Though apathy is often comorbid with depression, it can also be seen independently following TBI. A study of 83 patients with closed head injury found that approximately 11%

developed apathy without depression compared with the development of apathy with depression in 60% of the patients (6). Other neurovegetative symptoms such as sleep disturbances, concentration difficulties, fatigue, and changes in appetite are also seen independently in TBI. Careful attention must, therefore, be paid to comorbid symptoms while making the diagnosis of post-TBI depression.

Studies in the treatment of post-TBI depression are lacking, and clinicians often look to the studies in idiopathic and poststroke depression for guidance to treat patients with TBI and depression. A meta-analysis evaluating the efficacy of antidepressants in poststroke depression showed that antidepressants improve depressive symptoms in this population (7). Regarding AEDs in post-TBI depression, a study of 37 patients with depression and behavioral disturbances following TBI showed improvement in both behavioral disturbances and depressive symptoms with concurrent treatment with citalopram and carbamazepine (8).

Mania

Mania is relatively rare following TBI, but more common than in the general population. One prospective study showed that 6 (9%) of 66 patients developed mania in the first year following such injury (4). Some reports have indicated a longer period until the development of a secondary mania but data are unclear. Mania following TBI is classified in the DSM IV as a mood disorder due to a medical condition. Clinically, it is often associated with more irritability and dysphoria than classic bipolar mania. Symptoms include persistently expansive or irritable mood, grandiosity, decreased need for sleep, pressured speech, racing thoughts, distractibility, impulsivity, and excessive involvement in pleasurable or goal-directed activities. It is often difficult to distinguish between mania and behavioral dyscontrol. Care must be taken to talk with outside informants such as caregivers and establish whether a persistent personality or behavioral change has occurred, as in behavioral dyscontrol, or if the symptoms are episodic in nature, which would indicate mania.

Valproate is an AED that is an established treatment for bipolar mania and might therefore be one of the first-line agents for secondary mania, but unfortunately, controlled trials are lacking. Pope et al. found a response rate of 90% in 10 patients treated with valproate for secondary mania following TBI in a chart review. These patients had an inadequate response to lithium prior to starting treatment with valproate (9). Valproate has the problematic side effect of weight gain but fortunately a lower propensity for sedation and cognitive difficulties, which are of particular concern with TBI patients.

Carbamazepine is another AED that is an established treatment for bipolar mania. Like valproate, it is used for the treatment of mania associated with TBI, though there is little empirical evidence supporting this use. A case study by Stewart and Hemsath, however, describes the successful treatment with carbamazepine of a woman who developed bipolar disorder after TBI (10). Its use is complicated by adverse side effects of sedation, diploplia, weight gain, benign rash in up to one-third of patients, and Stevens-Johnsons syndrome in 0.1% to 0.5% of patients. Another very concerning side effect is leucopenia in 10% to 20% and rare agranulocytosis. This necessitates frequent blood monitoring. Carbamazepine induces hepatic metabolism and affects the metabolism of many drugs, including its own. As a result of these effects, this drug must be carefully monitored over time (11).

Phenytoin has not commonly been used for mania. A few early open-label trials reported success with phenytoin, but few subsequent studies have been attempted. There is preliminary evidence that phenytoin has antimanic and prophylactic use in patients with bipolar disorder (12), but it has not been studied in mania due to TBI. Phenytoin has been associated with cognitive impairments following severe TBI in the month following injury but not 12 months following injury (3).

Gabapentin has been used with mixed success as an adjunctive agent in patients with bipolar disorder. Although initial studies were negative, a double-blind, randomized, placebo-controlled, prophylaxis study using gabapentin as an adjunct to mood stabilization with valproate, lithium, or carbamazepine showed some benefit to adding gabapentin to prevent mood episodes (13).

Lamotrigine is approved and commonly used for bipolar disorder, particularly bipolar depression, but no studies have addressed its use to treat bipolar symptoms after a TBI. It has a favorable side-effect profile for the TBI population. Importantly, it has no associated cognitive difficulties. The most concerning side effect is rash (10%), which can develop into Stevens-Johnson syndrome. Rapid dose titration increases the risk of this effect.

Barbiturates have had little clinical use in mania. A small study of 27 patients receiving barbituates for mood symptoms refractory toother established mood stabilizers showed improvement in 44% of the patients (14). Another study of primidone (which is metabolized to phenobarbital by the body) in a small sample of patients with treatment refractory bipolar disorder showed a lasting positive response in 31% patients (15). Although these studies did not include TBI patients, they are notable for using patients that were refractory to first- and even second-line medications, which may characterize patients with post-TBI manic symptoms. However, since there is little evidence for the effectiveness of barbituates in secondary mania due to TBI, it is not recommended that these agents be used unless most other therapies have been adequate.

Anxiety

Jorge and Starkstein reported that approximately 60% of TBI patients with major depression also met criteria for an anxiety disorder (16). Generalized anxiety disorder is characterized by excessive anxiety and worry that is difficult to control, restlessness, fatigue, difficulty concentrating, muscle tension, irritability, and sleep disturbances. There is an increased occurrence of posttraumatic stress disorder and panic attacks following TBI as well. Major depression with anxiety tends to have a more prolonged clinical course and greater impact on psychosocial functioning (16,17). Studies on the treatment of anxiety following TBI are lacking, but serotonin-selective reuptake inhibitors (SSRIs) are often the drugs of choice for such symptoms, barring any complicating factors such as concern for lowering the seizure threshold. Benzodiazepines are often avoided in these patients because of sedation, the abuse potential for abuse, and a need for escalating doses. In addition, a paradoxical agitation is often seen in TBI patients.

The newer antiepileptics gabapentin and pregabalin have shown promise in anxiety disorders, presumably through their agonist effects on gamma-aminobutyric acid (GABA) receptors (18). To date, pregabalin has been studied in five randomized, double-blind, placebo-controlled trials in the treatment of generalized anxiety disorder and has been found to be efficacious in all five trials. In these studies, it had a rapid onset of anxiolytic action, evident after 7 to 10 days. It was well tolerated, with dizziness and somnolence being the primary concerning side effects. It has also been shown to prevent relapse and not to be associated with a withdrawal syndrome (19). Although pregabalin has not been studied in patients with TBI, it may be considered for TBI patients with anxiety symptoms, particularly those with comorbid seizure disorders.

Behavioral Dyscontrol Syndrome

The behavioral dyscontrol syndrome is characterized by a disturbance in mood, behavior, and cognition, but the central disturbance is that of a dyscontrol of emotion and behavior. Rao and Leyketsos defined the term and classified it into two variants. A major variant is descriptive of persistent, severe, and chronic symptoms. A minor variant is descriptive of acute and transient symptoms. Behavioral problems and aggression are common complications of TBI and are often chronic. Explosive and violent behaviors are associated with diffuse damage to the brain and with focal lesions (2). A retrospective mixed cross-sectional study looking at patients five years after moderate to severe TBI showed a prevalence of aggression of 25% at any given time. Aggression was consistently associated with depression. The authors concluded that aggression is a common and chronic, although fluctuating, problem for patients living with sequelae from TBI (20). Aggression and irritability are major causes of disability to patients and sources of stress for their families. In severe cases hospitalization, sometimes long-term, or worse, incarceration is required for the protection of the individual and people that he or she encounters (3). Aggression is frequently impulsive and often associated with frontal lobe injuries. It is treated with pharmacological agents as well as behavioral interventions. Many of the AEDs have been used to treat behavioral disturbances following TBI, but unfortunately most studies have not specifically targeted the TBI population. Clinicians must, therefore, rely on case reports and clinical data for impulsive behaviors in other psychiatric populations.

Wroblewski et al. reported on five cases with aggressive behaviors post-TBI who had dramatic improvement with valproate. The identified patients were refractory to other treatments and showed rapid improvement with valproate (21). In addition, valproate has been successfully used to manage agitation and aggression in patients with dementia and other organic brain syndromes (22). Stanford et al. found a significant reduction in impulsive aggression in seven impulsive aggressive men without TBI. The results were comparable to the use of phenytoin and had a slightly faster effect than the use of carbamazepine (23).

Carbamazepine is commonly used for agitation in the acute setting with TBI (24). A small case study explored the use of carbamazepine in mixed frontal lobe and psychiatric disorders and showed a decrease in emotional lability (25). Carbamazepine has been used successfully to treat agitation and aggression in dementia and in patients with mental retardation. Small case studies in the treatment of episodic dyscontrol have shown some success (26,27).

A controlled study on the use of phenytoin in 60 inmates with aggression suggested that phenytoin decreased impulsive aggressive acts but not premeditated aggressive acts (28). In a double-blind, placebo-controlled, crossover study of men with intermittent explosive disorder (IED), phenytoin treatment decreased the frequency of impulsive aggressive acts. Gabapentin has shown promise as an adjunctive agent to valproate for impulse control in patients with mental retardation in a small case series (29). There might be a similar role for adjunctive treatment with gabapentin for TBI as well. Of note, there has been a report of psychomotor agitation in two TBI patients with the use of gabapentin and there have been reports of increased agitation in children with attention-deficit hyperactivity disorder (ADHD) or developmental delay upon exposure to gabapentin. Thus, there may be a paradoxical reaction in TBI to gabapentin similar to benzodiazepines, so patients should be monitored carefully (30).

There are no reports on the use of lamotrigine in patients with TBI. In the developmentally disabled population available data are mixed. There have been descriptions of decreases in self-injurious behavior, irritability, and hyperactivity with lamotrigine, but also reports of increased aggression.

Psychosis

Psychotic symptoms, like mania, are uncommon following TBI but are more common than in the general population. Psychosis generally refers to disordered thought content such as delusions or hallucinations or to disordered thought processes such as loosening of associations, thought blocking, flight of ideas, and neologisms. There are several psychotic syndromes seen in TBI. These occur in the period of posttraumatic amnesia, as a complication of posttraumatic epilepsy, in the context of TBI-related mood disorders such as mania or depression, or as a chronic, schizophrenia-like syndrome (31). The estimated incidence in a retrospective review of 350 patients followed for 1 to 10 years was approximately 3% to 4%. About one-third of these patients had a chronic, schizophrenia-like course (32). Identified risk factors for the development of psychosis included left hemisphere and temporal lobe lesions, closed head injury, and increased severity of head injury with more diffuse damage and coma of greater than 24 hours duration. It is important to note that psychotic symptoms can have a delayed onset of months to years following TBI (31).

Psychotic symptoms related to posttraumatic epilepsy can occur primarily in the peri-ictal period so that they occur either during or immediately after the seizure. They occur most commonly in the postictal period and are similar to posttraumatic delirium with confusion, fluctuating consciousness, agitation, hallucinations, and delusions. This condition generally resolves in a few hours following resolution of the seizure but rarely can persist for several days. Interictal psychotic symptoms are more chronic and most commonly occur in a chronic, schizophrenia-like state. The chronic psychosis tends to be characterized by more positive than negative symptoms, such as hallucinations, delusions, passivity experiences, thought broadcasting, and thought insertion. A chronic course can also be marked by predominant paranoid symptoms (31).

When evaluating psychotic symptoms, it is important to determine whether they are related to a mood episode such as depression or mania due to epilepsy or due to a chronic, schizophrenia-like illness, because this will determine management. Psychotic symptoms associated with mania are best treated with mood stabilizers, as discussed previously, often with an atypical antipsychotic in the acute symptomatic phase. If the symptoms occur in the setting of seizures such as peri-ictally, clinical management should focus on optimizing the treatment of the seizures, which will be briefly discussed in the next section. Chronic schizophrenic–like psychotic symptoms are best managed with atypical antipsychotics and long-term seizure control.

Sleep Problems

Sleep disruption is commonly seen after TBI as an isolated symptom and as part of a mood disorder. It can worsen cognition, mood disorders, anxiety symptoms, aggression, and seizure disorders. Moreover, many of the AEDs have detrimental effects on sleep. Such agents include benzodiazepines, barbiturates, and phenytoin. Barbiturates reduce sleep latency and increase sleep continuity, which may help induce sleep but may also increase daytime drowsiness, worsen obstructive sleep apnea, and, with long-term use, may also lead to insomnia. Barbiturates also depress rapid eye movement (REM) sleep and may, therefore, impair the quality of sleep. Both benzodiazepines and barbiturates are addictive and can cause seizures during withdrawal (33). Regular use of benzodiazepines and barbiturates may cause rebound insomnia, often cause significant side effects the day following use such as sedation, and impaired memory, and are associated with dizziness, falls, and motor vehicle accidents (34). Phenytoin also worsens sleep latency and may increase nocturnal awakenings and light sleep. It is known to reduce REM sleep. Carbamazepine and valproate have mixed effects on sleep. Gabapentin may actually improve the quality of sleep by increasing REM sleep and decreasing nocturnal awakenings in patients with epilepsy. It has not been studied for insomnia in the TBI population (33).

Posttraumatic Epilepsy

Posttraumatic epilepsy is a common consequence of brain injury. It accounts for 20% of all symptomatic epilepsy. There are three classifications of posttraumatic seizures. Immediate seizures occur in less than 24 hours following the initial injury; early seizures occur within seven days; and late seizures occur more than eight days following the injury. A wide range of incidences are reported. The risk of immediate seizures has been reported to be 1% to 4%, while the risk of early seizures has been reported to be 4% to 25%, and the risk of late seizures is reported as 9% to 42%. The risk for seizures with penetrating injuries is greater with an incidence of 50% (35,36).

Several risk factors for the development posttraumatic epilepsy have been reported. The amount of focal tissue damage or contusions is considered to be one of the most important risk factors because it is thought that injured cortex neurons are the origin of seizure activity. Other risk factors include longer duration of unconsciousness, penetrating injuries, intracerebral hemorrhage, diffuse cortical contusions, prolonged amnesia of up to three days or longer, early seizures, depressed skull fractures, and acute subdural hematomas requiring surgical evacuation (37). Brain contusions and subdural hematomas requiring surgical intervention are very strong risk factors with an increased risk documented for up to 20 years (35).

Immediate or early seizures can result in secondary brain damage as a result of increased metabolic demands and increased intracranial pressure. It is preferable to treat immediately. Intravenous phenytoin or valproate have traditionally been the drugs of choice; however, controlled trials are lacking (38). Prophylactic treatment with AEDs prior to evidence of a seizure is often a clinical decision based on the risk factors of the individual patient and the treating clinician's experience. Phenytoin and carbamazepine have been effective in preventing early seizures but are not recommended for the prevention of late seizures. Phenytoin has the most evidence for use in preventing early seizures, but should not be used beyond seven days. Prophylactic treatment is not recommended for low-risk patients beyond seven days (39,40). Temkin et al. reported a randomized, double-blind, placebo-controlled trial of 404 TBI patients who were randomized to receive prophylactic phenytoin or placebo for one year. Results indicated that phenytoin reduced seizures only during the first week following TBI (41). Randomized controlled studies have also failed to show that valproate has any impact on chronic epileptogenesis as a consequence of brain injury (38). For higher-risk patients, such as those with early seizures, dural penetrating injuries, multiple contusions, or subdural hematoma requiring evacuation, longer-term prophylactic medications may be indicated (37,38).

It is important to treat seizures when indicated. Haltiner et al. (42) studied the incidence and risk factors for seizure reoccurrence after the onset of a late posttraumatic seizure in a longitudinal cohort design of 63 patients at a level 1 trauma center. They found that the cumulative incidence of recurrent late seizures was 86% by two years and suggested that patients be treated aggressively after the first unprovoked late seizure (42). It is recommended that if late posttraumatic seizures occur, their management should be determined by the type of seizure (such as partial or generalized) and individual response to medications, similar to idiopathic epilepsy (43).

Posttraumatic seizures have considerable impact on the morbidity of patients with TBI (33). When patients were studied five years after the initial injury, recurrent seizures had an association with an increased number of hospital admissions, psychiatric difficulties, and worsened general health maintenance (44). Unfortunately, prophylactic treatment with AEDs has no long-term benefits for seizure prevention. It decreases the incidence of early seizures and secondary brain damage but does not affect the incidence of late seizures.

MOOD STABILIZERS AS NEUROPROTECTIVE AGENTS

While available AEDs show efficacy in controlling the rate of seizure frequency, there is increasing interest in finding drugs that offer a neuroprotective effect following brain injury or alter the course of a seizure disorder by changing an epileptic focus in some way that permanently reduces seizures. Unfortunately, there has been little progress in this endeavor. Below is a brief summary of the neuroprotective effects of available AEDs see also (Table 1).

Phenytoin, carbamazepine, and phenobarbital have shown some evidence of neuroprotection in the animal model of neuronal hypoxic/ischemic injury (45). This is promising for TBI because the pathway for injury in TBI is a pathway shared with ischemic damage and status epilepticus. Among the newer AEDs, lamotrigine has shown some promise in neuroprotection in ischemia and prevention of excitatory amino acid injury to neurons (46). Levetiracetam has shown a protective effect in measured infarct volume (47). Topiramate has shown some evidence for protective effects in focal and in global ischemia in animal models by preventing excessive activation of glutamate receptors (48–50). Zonisamide has been found to have neuroprotective benefits in animal models of ischemia with lower levels of glutamate, reduced neuronal cell loss, and reduced neurological deficits in rats subjected to ischemic injuries when compared with valproate and carbamazepine. It may work by reducing free radicals (51–53).

TABLE 1 Indications, Dosage, and Side Effects of AEDs in the Treatment of Psychiatric Disturbances

Medication	Indications	Dosages	Side effects
Valproic acid	Mania and mood stabilization, behavioral dyscontrol syndromes, and seizures.	Seizures: loading dose of 10–15 mg/kg/day in 1–3 divided doses; maintenance is generally 30–60 mg/kg/day, measure blood levels and titrate to therapeutic level. Mania/behavioral dyscontrol: generally dosed 250 mg po bid and titrated up to therapeutic levels; can use loading of 20 mg/kg.	GI effects of nausea, vomiting, diarrhea, and dyspepsia (often enteric coated form may ease symptoms). Weight gain, alopecia, elevated transaminases. High doses are rarely associated with thrombocytopenia, platelet dysfunction, and hyponatremia. Hepatotoxicity is rare but has been fatal in children. Pancreatitis is rare but has also been fatal. Associated with neural tube defects when administered to pregnant women. May increase levels of lamotrigine when used together.
Carbamazepine	Mania and prophylaxis for mood stabilization in bipolar disorder, behavioral dyscontrol syndromes, and seizures.	Starting dose 200 mg po bid with titration of up to 200 mg daily to 600 to 1200 mg daily in 3 divided doses.	Induction of hepatic enzymes including induction of its own metabolism. Most adverse effects are correlated with plasma concentrations above 9 µg/mL. Mild GI effects such as nausea, vomiting, diarrhea or constipation, and loss of appetite. CNS effects such as confusion, sedation, ataxia, and clumsiness (usually controlled by slow titration or dose adjustment). Blood dyscrasias are but severe and include aplastic anemia and agranulocytosis. (Initial blood monitoring should occur every 3 mo.) Hepatitis, exfoliative dermatitis, Stevens-Johnsons syndrome,
Phenytoin	Behavioral dyscontrol syndromes, seizures.	Loading dose of 15–20 mg/kg in 3 divided doses given every 2–4 hr. Maintenance dose is generally 300 mg daily or 5–6 mg/kg/day in 3 divided doses.	CNS depression, particularly cerebellum and vestibular system with nystagmus and ataxia, nausea, and vomiting, gingival hyperplasia, coarsening of facial features, confusions, hallucination, drowsiness, inhibition of ADA release, and hyperglycemia. It is an antiarrythmic and should not be stopped abruptly.
Gabapentin	Anxiety symptoms, Seizures.	Starting dose 100 mg po tid with rapid titration up to 1800 mg po tid.	Somnolence, dizziness, ataxia, fatigue, and nystagmus (which are generally transient).

(Continued)

TABLE 1 Indications, Dosage, and Side Effects of AEDs in the Treatment of Psychiatric Disturbances (*Continued*)

Medication	Indications	Dosages	Side effects
Lamotrigine	Bipolar disorder, primarily depressive symptoms, seizures.	Starting dose 25 mg po bid with slow increase of 25 mg po bid every 2 wk.	Dizziness, ataxia, headache, sedation, nausea, and vomiting. Rash, which rarely leads to Steven-Johnsons syndrome. Thought to cause neural tube defects in fetuses. May decrease levels of Valproate and may increase levels of carbamazepine.

Abbreviations: po, orally; bid, twice daily; GI, gastrointestinal; CNS, central nervous system; ADA, adenosine deaminase.

CONCLUSION

TBI is a significant cause of morbidity in the United States. Unfortunately, many of the injuries lead to lasting disability as well as significant neuropsychiatric symptoms that have chronic impact on the quality of life and function of many patients. AEDs may offer relief from a wide array of syndromes, ranging from seizures, mood symptoms, behavioral problems, to anxiety. TBI is a challenging population to treat because patients are more susceptible to side effects, particularly cognitive effects and more often refractory to treatment. It is, therefore, important to educate clinicians, caretakers, and patients about the limitations and benefits of our knowledge and treatment. That this population has been understudied and underrepresented in the scientific literature should be taken into account when offering treatment and drug therapies.

REFERENCES

1. Centers for Disease Control and Prevention (CDC). Traumatic Brain Injury. Available at: http://www.cdc.gov/ncipc/tbi/TBI.htm. Accessed November 2006.
2. Rao V, Lyketsos C. Psychatric aspects of traumatic brain injury. Psychiatr Clin North Am 2002; 25(1):43–69.
3. Warden DL, Gordon B, McAllister TW, et al. Guidelines for the pharmacologic treatment of neurobehavioral sequelae of traumatic brain injury. J Neurotrauma 2006; 23(10): 1468–1501.
4. Jorge RE, Robinson RG, Starkstein SE, et al. Secondary mania following traumatic brain injury. Am J Psychiatry 1993; 150(6):916–921.
5. Kreutzer JS, Seel RT, Gourley E. The prevalence and symptom rates of depression after traumatic brain injury: a comprehensive examination. Brain Inj 2001; 15(7):563–576.
6. Kant R, Duffy JD, Pivovarnik A. Prevalence of apathy following head injury. Brain Inj 1998; 12(1):87–92.
7. Chen Y, Gui JJ, Zhan S, et al. Treatment effects of antidepressants in patients with post-stroke depression: a meta-analysis. Ann Pharmacother 2006; 40(12):2115–2122.
8. Perino C, Rago R, Cicolin A, et al. Mood and behavioural disorders following traumatic brain injury: clinical evaluation and pharmacological management. Brain Inj 2001; 15(2): 139–148.
9. Pope HG, McElroy SL, Satlin A, et al. Head injury, bipolar disorder and response to Valproate. Compr Psychiatry 1988; 29(1):34–38.

10. Stewart JT, Hemsath RH. Bipolar illness following traumatic brain injury: treatment with lithium and carbamazepine. J Clin Psychiatry 1988; 49(2):74–75.
11. Bowden CL, Karren NL. Anticonvulsants in bipolar disorder. Aust NZ J Psychiatry 2006; 40:386–393.
12. Mishory A, Winokur M, Bersudsky Y. Prophylactic effect of phenytoin in bipolar disorder: a controlled study. Bipolar Disord 2003; 5:464–467.
13. Vieta E, Manuel GJ, Martinez-Aran A, et al. A double-blind, randomized, placebo-controlled, prophylaxis study of adjunctive gabapentin for bipolar disorder. J Clin Psychiatry 2006; 67(3):473–477.
14. Hayes SG. Barbiturate anticonvulsants in refractory affective disorders. Ann Clin Psychiatry 1993; 5(1):35–44.
15. Schaffer LC, Schaffer CB, Caretto J. The use of primidone in treatment of refractory bipolar disorder. Ann Clin Pychiatry 1999; 11(2):61–66.
16. Jorge RE, Starkstein SE. Pathophysiologic aspects of major depression following traumatic brain injury. J Head Trauma Rehabil 2005; 20(6):475–487.
17. Jorge R, Robinson RE. Mood disorders following traumatic braininjury. Int Rev Psychiatry 2003; 15(4):317–327.
18. Amerinogen MV, Mancini C, Pipe B, et al. Antiepileptic drugs in the treatment of anxiety disorders. Drugs 2004; 64(19):2199–2220.
19. Frampton JE, Foster RH. Pregabalin in the treatment of generalized anxiety disorder. CNS Drugs 2006; 20(8):685–693.
20. Baguley IJ, Cooper J, Felmingham K. Aggressive behavior following traumatic brain injury. How common is common? J Head Trauma Rehabil 2006; 21(1):45–56.
21. Wroblewski BA, Joseph AB, Kupfer J, et al. Effectiveness of valproic acid on destructive and aggressive behaviors in patients with acquired brain injury. Brain Inj 1997; 11:37–47.
22. Mellow AM, Solano-Lopez C, Davis S. Sodium Valproate in the treatment of behavioral disturbance in dementia. J Geriatr Psychiatry Neurol 1993; 6(4):205–209.
23. Stanford MS, Helfritz LE, Conklin SM, et al. A comparison of anticonvulsants in the treatment of impulsive aggression. Exp Clin Psychopharmacol 2005; 13(1):72–77.
24. Fugate LP, Spacek LA, Kresty LA, et al. Measurement and treatment of agitation following traumatic brain injury: II. A survey of the brain injury Special interest Group of the American Academy of Physical Medicine and Rehabilitation. Arch Phys Med Rehabil 1997; 78(9):924–928.
25. McAllister TW. Carbamazepine in mixed frontal lobe and psychiatric disorders. J Clin Psychiatr 1985; 46(9):393–394.
26. Lewin J, Sumners D. Successful treatment of episodic dyscontrol with carbamazepine. Br J Psychiatry 1992;161:261–262.
27. Payne SD. Carbamazepine and episodic dyscontrol. Br J Psychiatry 1993; 162:425–426.
28. Barraatt ES, Stanford MS, Felthous AR, et al. The effects of phenytoin, impulsive and premeditated aggression: a controlled study. J Clin Psychopharmacol 1997; 17(5):341–349.
29. Hellings JA. Much improved outcome with gabapentin-divalproex combination in adults with bipolar disorders and developmental disabilities. J Clin Psychopharmacol 2006; 26:344–346 (letter to editor).
30. Childers MK, Holland D. Psychomotor agitation following gabapentin use in brain injury. Brain Inj 1997; 11(7):537–540.
31. McAllister TW, Ferrell RB. Evaluation and treatment of psychosis after traumatic brain injury. NeuroRehabilitation 2002; 17(4):357–368.
32. Violon A, deMol J. Psychological sequelae after head trauma in adults. Acta Neurochir Suppl 1987; 85:96–102.
33. Bazil CW. The effects of antiepileptic drugs on sleep structure. CNS Drugs 2003; 17(10):719–728.
34. Flanagan SR, Greenwald B, Wieber S. Pharmacological treatment of insomnia for individuals with brain injury. J Head Trauma Rehabil 2007;22(1):67–70.
35. Annegers JF, Hauser WA, Coan SP, et al. A population-based study of seizures after traumatic brain injury. New England J Med 1998; 338(1):20–24.
36. Annegers JF, Coan SP. The risks of epilepsy after traumatic brain injury. Seizure 2000; 9(7):453–457.

37. Englander J, Bushnik T, Duong TT, et al. Analyzing risk factors for late post-traumatic seizures: a prospective, multicenter investigation. Arch Phys Med Rehabil 2003; 84(3): 365–373.

38. Temkin NR, Dikmen SS, Anderson GD, et al. Valproate therapy for prevention of posttraumatic seizures: a randomized trial. J Neurosurg 1999; 91(4):593–600.

39. Schierhout G, Roberts I. Prophylactic antiepileptic agents after head injury: a systematic review. J Neurol Neurosug Psychiatry 1998; 64(1):108–112.

40. Brain Injury Special Interest Group. Practice Parameter: antiepileptic drug treatment of posttraumatic seizures. Brain Injury Special Interest Group of the American Academy of Physical Medicine and Rehabilitation. Arch Phys Med Rehabil 1998; 79(5):595–597.

41. Temkin NR, Dikmen SS, Wilensky AJ, et al. A randomized, double-blind study of phenytoin for the prevention of post-traumatic seizures. New England J Med 1990; 323 (8):497–502.

42. Haltiner AM, Temkin NR, Dikmen SS. Risk of seizure after the first late posttraumatic seizure. Arch Phys Med Rehabil 1997; 78(8):835–840.

43. Temkin NR, Dikmen SS, Winn HR. Management of head injury. Posttraumatic seizures. Neurosurg Clin N Am 1991; 2(2):425–435.

44. Agrawal A, Timothy J, Pandit L, et al. Post-traumatic epilepsy: an overview. Clin Neurol Neurosurg 2006; 108:433–439.

45. Willmore LJ. Antiepileptic drugs and neuroprotection: current status and future roles. Epilepsy Behav 2005; 7:S25–S28.

46. Lee WT, Shen YZ, Chang C. Neuroprotective effect of lamotrigine and MK-801 on rat brain lesions induced by 3-nitropropionic acid: evaluation by magnetic resonance imaging and in vivo proton magnetic resonance spectroscopy. Neuroscience 2000; 95(1): 89–95.

47. Hanon E, Klitgaard H. Neuroprotective properties of the novel antiepileptic drug levetiracetam in rat middle cerebral artery occlusion model of focal cerebral ischemia. Seizure 2001; 10(4):287–293.

48. Yang Y, Shuaib A, Li Q, et al. Neuroprotection by delayed administration of topiramate in a rat model of middle cerebral artery embolization. Brain Res 1998; 804:169–176.

49. Edmonds HL Jr., Jiang YD, Zhang PY, et al. Topiramate as a neuroprotectant in a rat model of global ischemia-induced neurodegeneration. Life Sci 2001; 69:2265–2277.

50. Rigoulot MA, Koning E, Ferrandon A, et al. Neuroprotective properties of topiramate in the lithium-pilocarpine model of epilepsy. J Pharmacol Exp Ther 2004; 308:787–795.

51. Owen AJ, Ijaz S, Miyashita H, et al. Zonisamide as a neuroprotective agent in adult gerbil model of global forebrain ischemia: a histological, in vivo microdialysis and behavioral study. Brain Res 1997; 770:115–122.

52. Minato H, Kikuta C, Fujitani B, et al. Protective effect of zonisamide, an antiepileptic drug, against transient focal cerebral ischemia with middle cerebral artery occlusion-reperfusion in rats. Epilepsia 1997; 38:975–980.

53. Hayakawa T, Higuchi Y, Nigami H, et al. Zonisamide reduces hypoxic-ischemic brain damage in neonatal rats irrespective of its anticonvulsive effect. Eur J Pharmacol 1994; 257:131–136.

Antiepileptic Drugs in Intellectual Disability and/or Autism

Benjamin L. Handen and Maria McCarthy
Western Psychiatric Institute and Clinic, University of Pittsburgh School of Medicine, Pittsburgh, Pennsylvania, U.S.A.

INTRODUCTION

Psychotropic medication has a long and extensive history in the treatment of behavioral disorders in children and adults with intellectual disability (ID) and autism spectrum disorder (ASD), often referred to as "autism." Recent data on medication-prescribing rates indicate that pharmacologic treatment is provided to a significant proportion of individuals from these two populations. For example, a review of prevalence studies of psychotropic drug use among both children and adults with ID found that, from 1986 to 1995, psychotropic medication use prevalence rates [excluding antiepileptic drugs (AEDs)] in institutions ranged from 12% to 40%; for AEDs, prevalence use rates ranged from 24% to 41%. Medication use prevalence rates in the community were somewhat lower, ranging from 19% to 29% for psychotropics and 18% to 23% for AEDs (1). More recently, Stolker et al. (2) reported that 22.8% of persons with ID residing in group homes in the Netherlands were prescribed psychotropics and that 15.9% were prescribed AEDs.

Among individuals with autism, studies have also found psychotropic prescribing rates to be considerably higher than in the general population. For example, in a survey of over 1500 families in North Carolina, approximately 46% of respondents reported that a family member with autism was prescribed psychotropic medication (excluding AEDs) (3). AEDs were prescribed to 12.4% of the sample. Aman et al. (4) reported the results of a similar survey of 747 families in Ohio. Consistent with the findings of Langworthy-Lam et al. (3), slightly less than 46% of the sample was prescribed psychotropic medication, with 11.5% of the sample being prescribed AEDs.

A number of variables have been found to be positively correlated with rates of psychotropic medication use in persons with ID. These include institutionalization (vs. residing in the community), age (with adults more likely to be prescribed medication than children), and IQ (with individuals with lower IQs more likely to receive medication than those with higher IQs)(1). Psychotropic medication exposure among individuals with autism was found to increase with both age and severity of the disorder (4). In addition to greater use of psychotropic medications among individuals with autism and ID, these populations appear to be at greater risk of experiencing unwanted side effects (5,6).

There are no medications that specifically address cognitive deficits among persons with ID or the core features of autism. Instead, psychotropic medications have been prescribed to treat specific behavioral symptoms and/or co-occurring psychiatric disorders. In fact, it was not until relatively recently that most clinicians believed that children and adults with ID experienced the range of psychiatric disorders that are diagnosed among typically developing persons. Reiss et al. (7) used the term "diagnostic overshadowing" to describe the tendency among professionals to underdiagnose mental health disorders among persons with ID by interpreting psychiatric symptoms as a part of their cognitive deficit. Additionally, underdiagnosis often occurs because many persons with ID have difficulty responding to standard diagnostic interview questions (8).

There are many theoretical reasons for the use of AEDs in autism and ID. Most important among these is the increased prevalence of epilepsy in this population. A recent survey of two large primary care practices (comprising a pool of 58,000 individuals) found the rate of epilepsy to be 25% among adults with ID and those with autism. This finding compared with a rate of 1% among the general population (9). Rates appear to be higher among those with greater cognitive deficits and among those who reside in institutions (10). Among the entire population of individuals with autism, epilepsy estimate rates range from 5 to 38%. The lowest rates are reported in children, with higher rates in adolescents and adults (11). The age distribution of seizures among children with autism appears to be bimodal, with one peak between infancy and five years of age and the second in adolescence (after age 10 years) (11). Among children with ID, rates of epilepsy range from 20% to 30% (12). In addition, there have been reports of epileptiform activity without seizures or *transient cognitive impairment* that are associated with dysfunction in cognition, language, and behavior (13,14). A significant minority of these individuals without epilepsy present epileptiform discharges, especially during sleep. These discharges are predominantly over the perisylvian head regions. Anecdotal reports suggest improvement of communication and behavior among individuals with autism with epileptic discharges when treated with AEDs (15,16). Espie et al. (17) found that greater seizure severity, greater seizure frequency, and lesser loss of consciousness interacted with greater behavioral hyperactivity to predict comorbid psychiatric disorders in patients with ID. There is also evidence that autism, ID, epilepsy, and mood disorders commonly co-occur (17,18). This suggests that these disorders may share a common neurochemical substrate, which may be the target of the psychotropic mechanism of action of some AEDs. Many of the newer AEDs that are also used to treat mood disorders are potent inhibitors of amygdala-kindled seizures. The anatomic location of epileptiform activity over the Sylvian fissure in patients with autism, ID, and psychiatric comorbidity supports this theory, as does the modulation of amygdala kindling by serotonergic mechanisms.

The purpose of this chapter is to provide an overview of the literature regarding the use of AEDs to treat behavioral disorders in patients with ID and autism. Unfortunately, many of our current prescribing practices are based on extrapolation from the general child and adult psychopharmacology literature. Additionally, most of the literature on AED use in ID and autism has involved the treatment of seizure disorders. Consequently, there is a considerable challenge in interpreting the available data. While improved seizure control sometimes leads to increased levels of appropriate behavior, some AEDs have also been found to have deleterious effects on cognitive functioning and behavior in these populations. A considerable amount of work remains to be conducted in this area.

OVERVIEW

While the literature on the use of AEDs in autism and ID goes back decades, the majority of available research is limited to uncontrolled case reports. In addition to controlling seizure disorders, AEDs in these two populations have been used to treat bipolar disorder, self-injurious behavior (SIB), aggression, impulsivity, and conduct problems (19–21). Individuals with ID appear more likely than the general population to have rapid-cycling and mixed bipolar disorder (19,22). Additionally, the ID/autistic population displays higher rates of aggression, SIB, and conduct problems (23,24).

Over the past 10 to 15 years, AEDs have been increasingly used as an alternative to lithium for the treatment of mood instability, aggression, and SIB. While several AEDs have been approved by the U.S. Food and Drug Administration (FDA) for use in adults with bipolar disorder (i.e., divalproex, lamotrigine, and carbamazepine), none have been approved in children and adolescents for this purpose. However, many children with ID or autism have seizure disorders for which they are prescribed approved AEDs. Some of the newer AEDs, such as topiramate (Topamax), oxcarbazepine (Trileptal), lamotrigine (Lamictal), and levetiracetam (Keppra), have also been used to treat a variety of behavioral symptoms. These agents may be preferable for use in children with ID and/or autism because they do not require frequent blood draws to establish and monitor medication levels and blood counts. In terms of the effect of AEDs on seizure frequency, it has been well documented that fewer individuals with ID and seizure disorders become "seizure free" following AED treatment than in the typically developing population. Reported seizure-free rates among the ID population fall well below 50% (25,26), while those among the non-ID population treated with AEDs is around 75% (26). Individuals with ID are also more frequently prescribed multiple AEDs than non-ID individuals (27,28).

Valproic Acid and Divalproex Sodium

Valproid acid has been approved by the FDA for the treatment of multiple seizure types in adults and children over 10 years of age. Divalproex sodium (a combination of sodium valproate and valproic acid) is approved for the treatment of epilepsy, migraine, and mania in adults. Both agents are often considered a treatment of choice (though "off-label") for rapid-cycling bipolar disorder, which is a variant more commonly seen in children and adolescents with ID (29,30). A second common off-label use has been the treatment of aggression and SIB in children and adults with ID (30–32). Childs and Blair (33) presented a case report involving two three-year-old twins with autism and absence seizures treated with valproic acid. Following treatment and improved seizure control, an accelerated rate of language and social skills acquisition was noted. Similar gains in language and social skills were reported by Plioplys (16), following valproic acid treatment of three children with autism. Hollander et al. (34) conducted a retrospective study of 14 children and adults with autism who were treated with divalproex sodium. Seventy-one percent of the sample was rated as improved on core symptoms of autism and associated features of affective instability, impulsivity, and aggression. While the medication was generally well tolerated, weight gain, sedation, and stomach upset were reported and one patient had elevated liver enzymes.

Among the more recent studies, Hollander et al. (35) performed an eight-week, double-blind, placebo-controlled trial of divalproex versus placebo for the treatment of repetitive behaviors in autism. Thirteen subjects (average age 9.5 years) with ASD by the Diagnostic and Statistical Manual of Mental Disorders (DSM)-IV criteria, diagnosed using the Autism Diagnostic Interview—Revised (ADI-R) and the Autism Diagnostic Observation Schedule (ADOS), participated. The mean divalproex dose at end point was 822.9 ± 326.2 mg/day (range = 500–1500 mg/day).

There was a significant group difference in improvement in repetitive behaviors scores as measured by the Children's Yale–Brown Obsessive Compulsive Scale (C-YBOCS) ($P = 0.037$) and a large effect size ($d = 1.616$). In a subsequent study, the authors showed that pretreatment with divalproex was superior to placebo pretreatment in preventing the irritability associated with fluoxetine therapy in 13 subjects with ASD (36). The authors speculated that valproate's potential mechanism(s) of action on mood instability, impulsivity, aggression, and repetitive behaviors might include blocking voltage-gated sodium ion channels; enhancing gamma-aminobutyric acid (GABA) transmission; reducing glutamate; acting on serotonin and norepinephrine systems; as well as inhibition of limbic kindling (34,37). However, in another recent double-blind, placebo-controlled trial of valproate to treat aggression in 30 children and adolescents with pervasive developmental disorders (PDDs) conducted by Hellings et al. (38), no statistically significant differences were found between the placebo and active medication groups on the Clinical Global Impressions of Improvement Scale (CGI) and the irritability subscale of the Aberrant Behavior Checklist (ABC) (as both groups evidenced improvement). In addition, of the 16 subjects receiving valproate, one discontinued the study early because of a rash and two others experienced increased serum ammonia levels.

Despite its potential efficacy, valproate has been associated with a number of problematic side effects. Rare and idiosyncratic but potentially life-threatening side effects include fulminant hepatic failure and hemorrhagic pancreatitis (39). Hepatic failure is most common in children with ID, under two years of age, who are on multiple drug regimens and has not been reported in children over 10 years of age on monotherapy (40). Hematologic disorders (e.g., thrombocytopenia) are also somewhat common. Valproate has been associated with the possible development of polycystic ovary syndrome, which is characterized by multiple ovarian cysts, obesity, irregular menses, increased hair growth, and infertility (20). Other side effects include sedation, gastrointestinal upset, weight gain, tremor, alopecia, and an increase in neural tube defects in children exposed to valproate in utero (31,39). Pylvänen and colleagues (41) have shown that the cause of valproate-related endocrine disorders may be valproate-induced obesity, which in turn causes hyperinsulinemia, reduced serum levels of insulin-like growth factor–binding protein 1, and elevated serum levels of sex hormones. Appropriate monitoring requires premedication liver function tests and hematologic indices (i.e., a complete blood count). It is also important to prevent pregnancy and to supplement with folic acid in the event of accidental pregnancy.

Carbamazepine

Carbamazepine has a structure similar to the tricyclic antidepressants. It has been approved for the treatment of generalized and partial seizures with or without secondary generalization, bipolar acute manic and mixed episodes in adults, and trigeminal and glossopharyngeal neuralgia. Findings from studies of carbamazepine in adults with ID are mixed and few data support its use for treatment of psychiatric disorders in children with ID (19). Vanstraelen and Tyrer (22) published a systemic review in 1999 of rapid-cycling bipolar disorder in persons with ID, which evaluated 14 studies and case reports ($N = 40$ subjects) from the Medline/PsychLit databases. Some studies were purely descriptive, some were pharmacotherapy efficacy studies, and others had both descriptive and pharmacotherapeutic elements. Fifteen of the forty subjects in this review received carbamazepine therapy for rapid-cycling bipolar disorder and/or epilepsy. Twelve of the fifteen subjects showed improvement with carbamazapine treatment. Glue (42) performed a study of 10 ID patients with rapid-cycling bipolar disorder treated with either lithium alone or lithium and carbamazepine. Half of the patients responded to treatment. Those who responded to the lithium-carbamazepine combination had a greater number of mood episodes than those who responded to lithium alone. Finally, Komoto et al. (43) reported improvement in mood lability in two adolescents with autism treated with carbamazepine.

In terms of side effects, carbamazepine use has been associated with rare cases of agranulocytosis and aplastic anemia (39). There have also been rare instances of Stevens-Johnson syndrome and toxic epidermal necrolysis, both of which are life-threatening rashes. Hyponatremia has been documented with both carbamazepine and the related AED oxcarbazepine. The risk of hyponatremia appears to be greater with oxcarbazepine. Its mechanism is believed to involve a direct effect on the kidney tubule cell or stimulation of arginine vasopression. Carbamazepine also has the potential to cause birth defects in infants with in utero exposure. Individuals prescribed carbamazepine therefore require monitoring for these potentially life-threatening reactions.

Carbamazepine is a potent inducer of the cytochrome P450 system, especially cytochromes CYP3A4 and CYP2C8. The metabolism of the compound thereby increases with chronic use through autoinduction, so that, after one month, its half-life decreases by 50%, often resulting in the need for an increased dose. Carbamazepine may also accelerate the metabolism of other AEDs (e.g., valproate, the benzodiazepines, and ethosuximide) and oral contraceptives, resulting in loss of efficacy. Conversely, it may decrease the metabolism of other AEDs, such as phenytoin, resulting in toxicity. Other medications (e.g., erythromycin, isoniazid, oleandromycin, omeprazole, cimetadine, verapamil, and propoxyphene), which directly inhibit the actions of cytochromes (especially CYP3A4 and CYP2C8), may decrease the metabolism of carbamazepine, resulting in toxicity.

Oxcarbazepine

Oxcarbazepine, an analog of carbamazepine, is a relatively new AED that may be effective in the treatment of bipolar disorder among the general adult population (44,45). However, the only randomized, placebo-controlled study of oxcarbazepine in bipolar mania conducted in children and adolescents was negative (46). Oxcarbazepine has been FDA approved for treatment of partial seizures in children and adults and is taken alone or in combination with other AEDs (47). Research suggests that oxcarbazepine may be better tolerated than carbamazepine. For example, there have been no reports of aplastic anemia or neural tube defects associated with oxcarbazepine and rashes appear less likely (44,45). Nonetheless, oxcarbazepine's side-effect profile remains a concern. Electrolyte disturbances have been reported, particularly when oxcarbazepine is initially prescribed (45). However, it is often difficult to determine the individual versus combined effects of oxcarbazepine when it is used with other medications.

There are few reports on the use of oxcarbazepine in children and adults with developmental disorders. No well-controlled studies of oxcarbazepine in ID were identified and no reports of any kind, involving individuals with autism were located. We were able to find three moderate-sized reports (two chart reviews and a prospective single-blind study) and two case reports involving individuals with ID. Most reports included the use of oxcarbazepine in combination with other AEDs and all focused on the drug's ability to control seizures rather than its effect on behavioral targets.

In the first moderate-sized report, Valente et al. (48) reviewed the medical charts of 19 children diagnosed with Angelman Syndrome, a genetic disorder characterized by severe ID and seizures. Parents who were interviewed reported that while some AEDs were associated with improved seizure rate and activity, oxcarbazepine (along with carbamazepine and vigabatrin) tended to aggravate seizures. In the second study, Gaily et al. (49) performed a chart review of 40 patients under 18 years of age (mean age 6.2 years) with seizure disorders and ID treated with oxcarbazepine (mean dose 48 mg/kg). All patients had been nonresponsive to other AEDs, with 29 patients having been nonresponsive specifically to carbamazapine. A minimum 50% reduction in seizures was reported with the addition of oxcarbazepine in 14 of 28 patients with localization-related epilepsy, and in 5 of 12 patients with generalized epilepsy. Most patients continued to take other AEDs while receiving oxcarbazepine. Side effects occurred in 40% of patients (including drowsiness, skin rash, and impaired balance), with 8% requiring oxcarbazepine dose adjustment or discontinuation. The third study was a single-blind trial of oxcarbazepine in 16 inpatients with profound ID conducted by Sillanpaa and Pihlaja (50). Fourteen subjects received carbamazepine with other AEDs at the beginning of the trial. The carbamazepine was subsequently switched to oxcarbazepine, while all other medications remained unchanged. In the other two patients, oxcarbazepine was added to ongoing regimens. The mean oxcarbazepine dose was 30 mg/kg. In 8 of the 16 patients, oxcarbazepine was considered better than the prior treatment regimen. However, seven patients experienced side effects, including status epilepticus in two cases. At three-and-a-half-year follow-up, only three patients remained on oxcarbazepine.

Of the two case reports, the first involved an adolescent with Lennox-Gastaut syndrome (characterized by seizures, ID, and behavioral concerns such as hyperactivity and aggression) in which the patient's complex partial seizures and behavior was only partially controlled with clobazam and oxcarbazepine (51). The second was a 23-year-old woman with ID who developed severe hypocalcemia while receiving oxcarbazepine (52).

Lamotrigine

Lamotrigine is approved by the FDA for treatment of certain types of seizures and to increase the time between mood episodes in patients with bipolar I disorder (53). While lamotrigine can be highly effective in adults, it is not recommended for use in children because of a high rate of potentially life-threatening rashes (20). Despite this, open-label studies of its use as add-on therapy for seizures among children with ID have found fairly good response with no significant side effects (54). By contrast, according to a 2000 review by Sabers and Gram (55), lamotrigine presents a mixed picture when used in individuals with ID for psychiatric and behavioral symptoms. Although a number of studies have documented improved mood, well-being, and functioning with lamotrigine in this population (56–58), there have also been reports of increased aggression and activity level with this agent (57,59). For example, in a retrospective chart review, Gidal et al. (60) found adjunctive lamotrigine to be fairly well tolerated in a group of 44 patients (ages 8–59 years) with profound ID. Over 54% of the sample experienced a decrease in seizure frequency of 50% or greater. However, three of the five patients with SIB at baseline experienced an increase in this behavior, requiring drug discontinuation. Studies of lamotrigine in other populations in which there is associated ID (e.g., Lennox-Gastaut syndrome, Rett syndrome) have generally found improved behavior and quality of life (61–64).

Only two studies involving individuals with autism were located. A study of lamotrigine in 13 children with autism and refractory seizure disorders found both improved seizure control and decreased autistic symptoms in 61% of the group (65). Conversely, in one of the few randomized, placebo-controlled, parallel-group studies in this area, Belsito et al. (66) found no significant differences between lamotrigine and placebo on measures of core features of autism and behavior problems in a group of 28 children, aged 3 to 11 years. The most frequently reported side effects were insomnia and hyperactivity.

Levetiracetam

Levetiracetam is FDA approved for the treatment of partial seizures in children (4 years and older) and adults, and for myoclonic seizures in adolescents (12 years and older) and adults. It is typically taken with other seizure medications (67). A fairly new AED, initial reports found levetiracetam to be effective as an add-on therapy for individuals with refractory epilepsy. The most common side effects were somnolence, lethargy, dizziness, headache, and tiredness (68). However, there have been recent reports of increased aggression and mood lability (69). Individuals with ID appear to be at particular risk for side effects, although there is a considerable amount of inconsistency across published studies (70,71).

Studies of levetiracetam in children and adults with ID have generally focused on its effect on seizure frequency. The drug has rarely been used solely to address behavioral concerns in the ID population. Indeed, most studies of levetiracetam in ID have reported the development of behavioral side effects and/or the worsening of any preexisting challenging behaviors. For example, Kossoff et al. (72) described the development of psychosis in four children (ages 5–17 years) with cognitive deficits and/or learning problems and prior behavioral deficits who were treated with levetiracetam for seizure control. Ben-Menachem and Gilland (70) reported that increased behavioral concerns tended to occur among individuals with a prior history of behavioral disturbances or those with ID in a study of 98 adult patients who had been placed on levetiracetam (as an add-on therapy) for a one-year period. Opp et al. (71) conducted a prospective, multicenter survey of 285 children with refractory generalized and focal seizures who were placed on levetiracetam as an adjunctive therapy. Over 90% of the sample had ID. ID was found to be associated with poorer response, a greater number of side effects, and earlier discontinuation of therapy (with a higher likelihood among individuals with more severe ID). While somnolence was the most frequently reported side effect, "general behavioral changes" and increased aggression were the next most common concerns. Similarly, Brodtkorb et al. (73) followed 184 adult patients who were prescribed levetiracetam, 56 of whom had ID. Both the ID and non-ID patients had similar positive response rates to levetiracetam (37% and 40%, respectively) and rates of side effects. However, the individuals with ID experienced considerably more behavioral problems (23% vs. 10%). A recent study by Neuwirth et al. (74) found adults with ID displaying a greater number of side effects when prescribed levetiracetam than typically developing patients. Finally, a study by Kelly et al. (69) found significant reductions in seizure frequency with adjunctive levetiracetam in 66% of a sample of 64 individuals (ages 12–66 years) with ID. However, 11% of the sample discontinued treatment because of adverse events, such as somnolence, aggression, and mood swings.

There have been few studies of levetiracetam among individuals with autism. Interestingly, the high rates of behavioral side effects noted among children and adults with ID receiving levetiracetam are not reported among children with autism. Rugino and Samsock (75) conducted an open-label trial (average duration of 4 weeks) of levetiracetam in 10 males with autism (ages 4–10 years) who did not have seizure disorders. Significant improvement was noted on a number of behavior problem checklists assessing areas such as hyperactivity, impulsivity, and mood instability. Significant gains on ratings of aggression, however, were only observed for subjects who remained on concomitant therapy targeting this behavior. In one of the few randomized, placebo-controlled studies, Wasserman et al. (76) conducted a 10-week trial in 20 children and adolescents with autism (ages 5–17 years) who did not have seizure disorders. While levetiracetam was well tolerated, no significant group differences were found on the CGI, ABC, or C-YBOCS.

Topiramate

Topiramate has been approved by the FDA for monotherapy and adjunctive treatment of seizures, including those associated with Lennox-Gastaut syndrome. It is also indicated for the prophylaxis of migraine headache. There have been a number of studies of topiramate among individuals with ID, and many of them have provided information on both the antiepileptic and behavioral effects of this agent in this population. Most studies involved topiramate as an add-on therapy to other AEDs. Interestingly, the open-label and retrospective studies appear to have found more positive results than the only available randomized, double-blind, placebo-controlled study. In the latter, Kerr et al. (77) compared adjunctive topiramate with placebo in 74 adolescents and adults (12 years and older) with ID and epilepsy. The most common adverse events reported by the active medication group were anorexia (24.3%) and somnolence (32.4%). Seven (18.9%) subjects in the topiramate group and six (16.2%) in the placebo group discontinued medication because of adverse events. There was no statistically significant difference between groups regarding mean total seizure frequency or number of responders (although there was a strong trend in favor of topiramate for both outcome measures). Additionally, a range of tools were used to assess psychosocial effects (e.g., the Adaptive Behavioral Scale, the Epilepsy Outcome Scale, and the ABC), but none demonstrated significant group differences.

Among the open-label studies, Arvio and Sillanpaa (78) conducted a retrospective chart review of 57 patients (children and adults) with ID who had been placed on topiramate as an add-on therapy. Over one-half of the sample had a 50% or greater decease in the rate of seizures, with 10% of patients experiencing side effects that necessitated topiramate discontinuation. Some patients reportedly became more alert with improved seizure control and 25% of the responders reported either decreased rates of aggression ($N = 8$ subjects) or weight loss ($N = 6$ subjects). Similar to the findings of Arvio and Sillanpaa (78), Singh and White-Scott (79) reported improved alertness with adjunctive topiramate in 59% of a group of

20 adults with ID (as well as a significant reduction in seizures in 44% of patients). Finally, Kelley et al. (80) conducted a prospective study of add-on topiramate in 64 individuals with ID (ages 16–65 years). Sixteen subjects were seizure free for six months or more, and 29 subjects experienced a 50% or greater reduction in seizure frequency after six months of treatment. Nine subjects discontinued the trial because of a range of side effects, including weight loss, confusion, and aggression.

Some additional studies have focused on the use of topiramate as an add-on therapy in specific ID populations. For example, Alva-Moncayo and Ruiz-Ruiz (81) treated a group of 15 children (ages 2–15 years) who were diagnosed with Lennox-Gastaut syndrome. Seizure rates decreased by 50% or greater in over half of the cases. Glauser et al. (82) used topiramate as an add-on treatment in 11 children who had been diagnosed with West syndrome, characterized by infantile spasms and ID. Nine of the 11 children evidenced a 50% or greater reduction in infantile spasms and seven children were gradually weaned from concomitant AEDs. While all patients remained in the study, a number of side effects were reported, including increased irritability ($N = 9$) and sleep disturbance ($N = 3$).

Taking advantage of topiramate's tendency to cause appetite suppression, some researchers have examined the agent's effect on individuals with Prader-Willi syndrome. This condition is characterized by short stature, obesity, mild-to-moderate ID, and behavior problems such as SIB and compulsive eating. A case series of add-on topiramate in three adults with Prader-Willi syndrome found a significant decrease in SIB in all three patients, including skin picking (83). A subsequent prospective, open-label study of add-on topiramate by this same research team in eight adults with Prader-Willi syndrome found no significant change in calories consumed, body mass index, or on the five subscales of the ABC (84). However, a clinically significant decrease in skin picking was again noted, as well as a statistically significant decrease in the total number of items endorsed on the ABC. Conversely, Smathers et al. (85) reported reductions in SIB and aggression, improved mood, and more stable weight in seven of eight children and adolescents (ages 10–19 years) with Prader-Willi syndrome who had been clinically treated with topiramate. Four patients lost weight. The medication was well tolerated, with somnolence as the only significant side effect (occurring in three patients).

There has been some recent interest in topiramate as a treatment for behavioral disorders in children with autism. For example, Hardan et al. (86) published an open-label, retrospective study of topiramate in 15 children with PDD. Eight patients were rated as responders (based on a CGI rating of 1 or 2) and significant improvement between baseline and end of trial was noted on parental ratings of conduct, hyperactivity, and inattention. However, three patients discontinued medication because of cognitive difficulties (speech and word finding problems) and one because of a skin rash. Subsequent reports have found less positive results among individuals with autism. Mazzone and Ruta (87) reported that only two of five children with autism (ages 9–13 years) responded to topirimate, based on a CGI of 1 or 2 and improvement on behavior rating scales (the Anxious/Depressed and Attention Problems subscales of the CBCL). Side effects were mild, with one child reporting sedation. Because one of the common side effects of topiramate is decreased appetite, some clinicians and researchers have suggested that it be used in combination with atypical antipsychotics (e.g., risperidone, olanzapine) to counter the weight gain that is often associated with these agents. However, Canitano (88) found topiramate to have mixed effects on weight in a group of

10 children and adolescents with PDDs (eight of whom were also prescribed risperidone) in a prospective, open-label study. In fact, 4 of 10 subjects dropped out of the study within the first two weeks (three due to agitation, psychomotor agitation, and hyperactivity, and the fourth due to lack of response). Of the subjects who remained, four evidenced mild-to-moderate weight loss and two gained weight during the course of the study.

SUMMARY AND RECOMMENDATIONS

Relatively little is known about many of the medications used to treat psychiatric disorders in both children and adults with ID and/or autism. This is due both to a tendency to believe that persons with developmental disabilities are less likely to have such disorders and the fact that children and adults with ID or autism have been excluded in many medication-efficacy studies. However, with increasing evidence that individuals with ID or autism can have the full range of psychiatric disorders and are at three to five times greater risk than the general population for behavioral and emotional problems, there has been a gradual increase in the number of drug studies in both populations. Yet, the majority of studies continue to be open trials and case reports. Large, randomized clinical trials are the exception. The available data suggest that persons with ID and/or autism respond to various psychotropic medications in ways similar to the typically developing population, but response rates tend to be poorer and more variable and side effects appear to be more frequent. This requires even greater monitoring and the use of lower doses and slower dosage increases than in the general population.

Regarding AED use in the ID and autism populations, most studies have focused on these agents to treat comorbid seizure disorders. Both positive and negative behavioral effects are often of secondary concern. The majority of studies of AEDs in managing psychiatric and behavioral syndromes in ID and/or autism are case reports or open trials. The few available double-blind, placebo-controlled trials have produced equivocal results. As a result, few definitive recommendations can be made regarding the use of AEDs to treat psychiatric and behavioral disorders in individuals with ID and/or autism and caution is advised.

REFERENCES

1. Singh N, Ellis C, Wechsler H. Psychopharmacoepidemiology of mental retardation: 1966 to 1995. J Child Adolesc Psychopharmacol 1997; 7:255–266.
2. Stolker JJ, Koedoot PJ, Heerdink ER, et al. Psychotropic drug use in intellectually disabled group-home residents with behavioural problems. Pharmacopsychiatry 2002; 35: 19–23.
3. Langworthy-Lam KS, Aman MG, Van Bourgondien ME. Prevalence and patterns of use of psychoactive medicines in individuals with autism in the Autism Society of North Carolina. J Child Adolesc Psychopharmacol 2002; 12:311–322.
4. Aman MG, Lam KS, Collier-Crespin A. Prevalence and patterns of use of psychoactive medicines among individuals with autism in the Autism Society of Ohio. J Autism Dev Disord 2003; 33:527–534.
5. Handen BL, Gilchrist R. Treatment of mental retardation. In: Mash E, Barkley RA, eds. Treatment of Childhood Disorders. 3rd ed. New York, NY: The Guilford Press, 2006.
6. Handen B, Lubetsky M. Pharmacotherapy in autism and related disorder. Sch Psychol Q 2005; 20:155–171.
7. Reis S, Leventhal DW, Szyszko K. Emotional disturbance and mental retardation: diagnostic overshadowing. Am J Ment Defic 1982; 86:567–574.

8. DesNoyers Hurley A, Reiss S, Aman MG, et al. Instruments for assessing effects in psychotropic medication. In: Reiss S, Aman MG, eds. The International Consensus Handbook: Psychotropic Medications and Developmental Disabilities. Columbus, Ohio: Nisonger Center, 1998:85–94.

9. McDermott S, Moran R, Platt T, et al. Prevalence of epilepsy in adults with mental retardation and related disabilities in primary care. Am J Ment Retard 2005; 110:36–47.

10. Harris JC. Intellectual Disability: Understanding Its Development, Causes, Classification, Evaluation, and Treatment. New York, NY: Oxford University Press, 2006.

11. Tuchman R, Rapin I. Epilepsy in autism. Lancet Neurology 2002; 1:352–358.

12. Alvarez N. Epilepsy in children with mental retardation. eMedicine from WebbMD, 2007. Available at: http://www.emedicine.com/NEURO/topic550.htm. Updated on August 29, 2007.

13. Binnie CD. Cognitive impairment during epileptiform discharges: is it ever justifiable to treat the EEG? Lancet Neurol 2003; 2:725B–730B.

14. Tuchman R, Rapin I. Regression in pervasive developmental disorders: seizures and epileptiform electroencephalogram correlates. Pediatrics 1997; 99:560–566.

15. Nass R, Petrucha D. Acquired aphasia with convulsive disorder: a pervasive developmental disorder variant. J Child Neurol 1990; 5:327–328.

16. Plioplys AV. Autism: electroencephalogram abnormalities and clinical improvement with valproic acid. Arch Pediatr Adolesc Med 1994; 148:220–222.

17. Espie CA, Watkins J, Curtice L, et al. Psychopathology in people with epilepsy and intellectual disability; an investigation of potential explanatory variables. J Neurol Neurosurg Psychiatry 2003; 74:1485–1492.

18. Di Martino A, Tuchman RF. Antiepileptic drugs: affective use in autism spectrum disorders. Pediatr Neurol 2001; 25:199–207.

19. Aman MG, Collier-Crespin A, Lindsay RL. Pharmacotherapy of disorders in mental retardation. Eur Child Adolesc Psychiatry 2000; (suppl 1):198–107.

20. Green WH. Child and Adolescent Clinical Psychopharmacology. Philadelphia, PA: Lippincott Williams & Wilkins, 2001.

21. Santosh PJ, Baird G. Psychopharmacotherapy in children and adults with intellectual disability. Lancet 1999; 354:233–242.

22. Vanstraelen M, Tyrer SP. Rapid cycling bipolar affective disorder in people with intellectual disability: a systematic review. J Intellect Disabil Res 1999; 43:349–359.

23. Emerson E. Prevalence of psychiatric disorders in children and adolescents with and without intellectual disability. J Intellect Disabil Res 2003; 47:51–58.

24. Stromme P, Diseth TH. Prevalence of psychiatric diagnoses in children with mental retardation: data from a population-based study. Dev Med Child Neurol 2000; 42:266–270.

25. Kelly K, Stephen LJ, Brodie MJ. Pharmacological outcomes in people with mental retardation and epilepsy. Epilepsy Behav 2004; 5:67–71.

26. Huber B, Hauser I, Horstmann V, et al. Long-term course of epilepsy in a large cohort of intellectually disabled patients. Seizure 2007; 16:35–42.

27. Hogg J. The administration of psychotropic and anticonvulsant drugs to children with profound intellectual disability and multiple impairments. J Intellect Disabil Res 1992; 36:473–488.

28. Singh BK, Towle PO. Antepilieptic drug status in adult outpatients with mental retardation. Am J Ment Retard 1993; 98(suppl):41–46.

29. Hellings JA. Psychopharmacology of mood disorders in persons with mental retardation and autism. Ment Retard Dev Disabil Res Rev 1999; 5:270–278.

30. Antochi R, Stavrakaki C, Emery PC. Psychopharmacological treatments in persons with dual diagnosis of psychiatric disorders and developmental disabilities. Postgrad Med J 2003; 9:139–146.

31. Kowatch RA, Bucci JP. Mood stabilizers and anticonvulsants. Pediatr Clin North Am 1998; 45:1173–1186.

32. Ruedrich S, Swalesm TP, Fossaceca C, et al. Effect of divalproex sodium on aggression and self-injurious behaviour in adults with intellectual disability: a retrospective review. J Intellect Disabil Res 1999; 43:105–111.

33. Childs JA, Blair JL. Valproic acid treatment of epilepsy in autistic twins. J Neurosci Nurs 1997; 29:244–248.
34. Hollander E, Dolgoff-Kasper R, Cartwrigth C, et al. An open trial of divalproex sodium in autism spectrum disorders. J Clin Psychiatry 2001; 62:530–534.
35. Hollander E, Soorya L, Wasserman S, et al. Divalproex sodium vs. placebo in the treatment of repetitive behaviours in autism spectrum disorder. Int J Neuropsychopharmacol 2006; 9:209–213.
36. Anagnostou E, Esposito K, Soorya L, et al. Divalproex versus placebo for the prevention of irritability associated with fluoxetine treatment in autism spectrum disorder. J Clin Psychopharmacol 2006; 26:444–446.
37. Soderpalm B. Anticonvulsants: aspects of their mechanisms of action. Eur J Pain. 2002; 6(suppl A):3–9.
38. Hellings JA, Weckbaugh M, Nickel EJ, et al. A double-blind, placebo-controlled study of valproate for aggression in youth with pervasive developmental disorders. J Child Adolesc Psychopharmacol 2005; 15:682–692.
39. Physicians' Desk Reference. Oradell, NJ: Medical Economics Co, 2004.
40. Fenichel GM. Clinical Pediatric Neurology: A Signs and Symptoms Approach. Philadelphia, PA: WB Saunders, 1997.
41. Pylvänen V, Pakarinen A, Knip M, et al. Insulin-related metabolic changes during treatment with valproate in patients with epilepsy. Epilepsy Behav 2006; 8:643–648.
42. Glue P. Rapid cycling affective disorders in the mentally retarded. Biol Psychiatry 1989; 26:250–256.
43. Komoto J, Usui S, Hirata J. Infantile autism and affective disorder. J Autism Dev Disord 1984; 14:81–84.
44. Centorrino F, Albert MJ, Berry JM, et al. Oxcarbazepine: clinical experience with hospitalized psychiatric patients. Bipolar Disord 2003; 5:370–374.
45. Ketter TA, Wang PW, Becker OV, et al. The diverse roles of anticonvulsants in bipolar disorders. Ann Clin Psychiatry 2003; 15:95–108.
46. Wagner KD, Kowatch RA, Emslie GJ, et al. A double-blind, randomized, placebo-controlled trial of oxcarbazepine in the treatment of bipolar disorder in children and adolescents. Am J Psychiatry 2006; 163:1179–1186.
47. Food and Drug Administration. CDER Patient Information Sheet Levetiracetam (marketed as Keppra). Available at: http://www.fda.gov/cder/drug/InfoSheets/patient/levetiracetamPIS.htm. Updated on March 22, 2007.
48. Valente KD, Koiffmann CP, Fridman C, et al. Epilepsy in patients with angelman syndrome caused by deletion of the chromosome 15q11-13. Arch Neurol 2006; 63:122–128.
49. Gaily E, Granstrom ML, Liukkonen E. Oxcarbazepine in the treatment of epilepsy in children and adolescents with intellectual disability. J Intellect Disabil Res 1998; 42(suppl 1):41–45.
50. Sillanpaa M, Pihlaja T. Oxcarbazepine (GP 47 680) in the treatment of intractable seizures. Acta Paediatr Hung 1988–89; 29:359–364.
51. Agapejev S, Padula NA, Morales NM, et al. Neurocysticercosis and Lennox-Gastaut syndrome: case report. Arq Neuropsiquiatria 2000; 58:538–547.
52. Zdrojewicz Z, Dubiski A, Jonek A, et al. Tetanic crisis and antiepileptic drugs. A case report. Neuro Endocrinol Lett 2005; 26:317–319.
53. Food and Drug Administration. CDER Patient Information Sheet Lamotrigine (marketed as Lamictal). Available at: http://www.fda.gov/cder/drug/InfoSheets/patient/lamotriginePIS.htm. Updated on September 28, 2006.
54. Buchanan N. The efficacy of lamotrigine on seizure control in 34 children, adolescents and young adults with intellectual and physical disability. Seizure 1995; 4:233–236.
55. Sabers A, Gram L. Newer anticonvulsants: comparative review of drug interactions and adverse effects. Drugs 2000; 60:23–33.
56. Betts T, Goodwin G, Winthers RM, et al. Human safety of lamotrigine. Epilepsia 1991; 32 (suppl 2):S17–S21.
57. Ettinger AB, Weisbrot DM, Saracco J, et al. Positive and negative psychotropic effects of lamotrigine in patients with epilepsy and mental retardation. Epilepsia 1998; 39:874–877.

58. Smith D, Baker G, Davis G, et al. Outcomes of add-on treatment with lamotrigine in partial epilepsy. Epilepsia 1993; 34:312–322.
59. Beran RG, Gibson RJ. Aggressive behaviour in intellectually challenged patients with epilepsy treated with lamotrigine. Epilepsia 1998; 39:280–282.
60. Gidal BE, Walker JK, Lott RS, et al. Efficacy of lamotrigine in institutionalized, developmentally disabled patients with epilepsy: A retrospective evaluation. Seizure 2000; 9:131–136.
61. Buchanan N. Lamotrigine use in twelve patients with the Lennox-Gastaut syndrome. Eur J Neurol 1995; 2:501–503.
62. Mullens L, Gallagher J, Manasco P. Improved neurological function accompanies effective control of the Lennox-Gastaut syndrome with Lamictal: results of a multinational, placebo-controlled trial. Epilepsia 1996; 37(suppl 5):S163.
63. Jacoby A, Baker G, Bryant-Comstock L, et al. Lamotrigine add-on therapy is associated with improvement in mood in patients with severe epilepsy. Epilepsia 1996; 37(suppl 5): S202.
64. Uldall P, Hansen FJ, Tonnby B. Lamotrigine in Rett syndrome. Neuropediatrics 1993; 24: 339–340.
65. Uvebrant P, Bauziene R. Intractable epilepsy in children: the efficacy of lamotrigine treatment, including non-seizure related benefits. Neuropediatrics 1994; 25:284–289.
66. Belsito KM, Law PA, Kirk KS, et al. Lamotrigine therapy for autistic disorder: a randomized, double-blind, placebo-controlled trial. J Autism Dev Disord 2001; 31: 175–181.
67. Food and Drug Administration. CDER Patient Information Sheet Oxcarbazepine (marketed as Trileptal). Available at http://www.fda.gov/cder/drug/InfoSheets/patient/oxcarbazepinePIS.htm. Updated on March 16, 2007.
68. Hurtado B, Koepp M, Sander J, et al. The impact of levetiracitem on challenging behavior. Epilepsy Behav 2006; 588–592.
69. Kelly K, Stephen LJ, Brodie MJ. Levetiracetam for people with mental retardation and refractory epilepsy. Epilepsy Behav 2004b; 5:878–883.
70. Ben-Menachem E, Gilland E. Efficacy and tolerability of levetiracetam during 1-year follow-up in patients with refractory epilepsy. Seizure 2003; 12:131–135.
71. Opp J, Tuxhorn I, May T, et al. Levetiracetam in children with refractory epilepsy: a multicenter open label study in Germany. Seizure 2005; 14:476–484.
72. Kossoff EH, Bergey GK, Freeman J, et al. Levetiracetam psychosis in children with epilepsy. Epilepsia 2001; 42:1611–1613.
73. Brodtkorb E, Klees TM, Nakken KO, et al. Levetiracetam in adult patients with and without learning disability: focus on behavioral adverse effects. Epilepsy Behav 2004; 5: 231–235.
74. Neuwirth M, Saracz J, Hegyi M, et al. Experience with levetiracetam in childhood epilepsy. Ideggyogy Sz 2006; 59:179–182.
75. Rugino TA, Samsock TC. Levetiracetam in autistic children: an open-label study. J Dev Behav Pediatr 2002; 23:225–230.
76. Wasserman S, Iyengar R, Chaplin WF. Levetiracetam versus placebo in childhood and adolescent autism: a double-blind placebo-controlled study. Int Clin Psychopharmacol 2006; 21:363–367.
77. Kerr MP, Baker GA Brodie MJ. A randomized, double-blind, placebo-controlled trial of topiramate in adults with epilepsy and intellectual disability: impact on seizures, severity, and quality of life. Epilepsy Behav 2005; 7:472–480.
78. Arvio M, Sillanpaa M. Topiramate in long-term treatment of epilepsy in the intellectually disabled. J Intellect Disabil Res 2005; 49:183–189.
79. Singh BK, White-Scott S. Role of topiramate in adults with intractable epilepsy, mental retardation, and developmental disabilities. Seizure 2002; 11:47–50.
80. Kelly K, Stephen LJ, Sills GJ, et al. Topiramate in patients with learning disability and refractory epilepsy. Epilepsia 2002; 43:399–402.
81. Alva-Moncayo E, Ruiz-Ruiz A. The value of topiramate used with conventional schemes as an adjunctive therapy in the treatment of Lennox-Gastaut syndrome. Rev Neurol 2003; 36:453–457.

82. Glauser TA, Clark PO, Strawsburg R. A pilot study of topiramate in the treatment of infantile spasms. Epilepsia 1998; 39:1324–1328.
83. Shapira NA, Lessig MC, Murphy TK, et al. Topiramate attenuates self-injurious behaviour in Prader-Willi Syndrome. Int J Neuropsychopharmacol 2002; 5:141–145.
84. Shapira NA, Lessig MC, Lewis MH, et al. Effects of topiramate in adults with Prader-Willi syndrome. Am J Ment Retard 2004; 109:301–309.
85. Smathers S, Wilson J, Nigro M. Topiramate effectiveness in Prader-Willi syndrome. Pediatr Neurol 2003; 28:130–133.
86. Hardan AY, Jou RJ, Handen BL. A retrospective assessment of topiramate in children and adolescents with pervasive developmental disorders. J Child Adolesc Psychopharmacol 2005; 14:426–432.
87. Mazzone L, Ruta L. Topiramate in children with autistic spectrum disorders. Brain Dev 2006; 28:668.
88. Canitano R. Clinical experience with topiramate to counteract neuroleptic induced weight gain in 10 individuals with autistic spectrum disorders. Brain Dev 2005; 27:228–232.

7 Treatment of Acute Manic and Mixed Episodes

Paul E. Keck, Jr., Susan L. McElroy, and Jeffrey R. Strawn
*Lindner Center of HOPE, Mason, and Department of Psychiatry, University
of Cincinnati College of Medicine, Cincinnati, Ohio, U.S.A.*

INTRODUCTION

Antiepileptic agents have been used to treat bipolar manic and mixed episodes
since early investigational pilot trials dating back to the 1960s (1). Research into the
potential efficacy of antiepileptic agents in the treatment of bipolar disorder has
been based on empirical observations of the efficacy of specific agents as well as
heuristic models of the potential pathogenesis of bipolar disorder, such as the
kindling hypothesis (2). Antiepileptic agents include a broad group of compounds
with diverse pharmacological properties and differential efficacy in various forms
of epilepsy. In this chapter, we review the evidence to date regarding the efficacy of
antiepileptic agents in the treatment of bipolar manic and mixed episodes, with
particular attention to agents studied in randomized, controlled trials.

VALPROIC ACID

Various formulations of valproic acid (valproate, divalproex sodium, valpromide)
have been shown to be efficacious for the treatment of acute manic and mixed
episodes in a number of randomized, controlled trials (Table 1). In three, three-
week, placebo-controlled, monotherapy trials among hospitalized patients, divalproex (3,4) and divalproex extended release (ER) (5) were superior to placebo in
reduction of manic symptoms. These large trials confirmed the findings of smaller,
placebo-controlled, crossover pilot studies (6,7).

The efficacy of the divalproex formulation in acute bipolar mania has also
been studied in direct comparator trials against olanzapine (8,9) and lithium (10,11)
in adults and against quetiapine in adolescents (12). Most of these latter, comparator trials were not powered sufficiently to detect potential differences in efficacy among agents and generally yielded comparable efficacy results. However,
one of the olanzapine comparator trials included a sufficiently large sample of
patients to detect a potential difference in efficacy between agents and found a
slight difference in favor of olanzapine over divalproex (8). In both olanzapine
comparator trials, divalproex had better overall tolerability (8,9).

A number of studies have specifically examined the efficacy, safety, and
tolerability of divalproex oral loading, which has been administered either as
20 mg/kg/day (13–15), 25 mg/kg/day (ER formulation) (5), or 30 mg/kg/day for
two days, followed by 20 mg/kg/day (9,11).

Although none of these trials was adequately powered to detect a significant
difference in efficacy of the oral loading strategy, this approach was nevertheless
found to be well tolerated. In addition, in a study comparing this strategy with
haloperidol specifically in patients with psychotic mania, divalproex-treated
patients had comparable reductions in psychotic as well as manic symptoms (15).

Divalproex has also been used as a comparator in adjunctive treatment trials
(16–23). All but one of such studies (16) compared the acute efficacy of placebo added

TABLE 1 Randomized, Controlled Trials of Divalproex in Bipolar Manic and Mixed Episodes

Study	Diagnostic criteria	Design	Results
Bowden et al., 2006	Bipolar I, manic or mixed episode (DSM-IV)	DBPC, LOCF (3-wk), DVPX ER 25 mg/kg, increased by 500 mg on day 3, and adjusted to serum concentrations of 85–125 µg/mL	DVPX ER > placebo, mean MRS[3] DVPX ER (48%) > placebo (34%), response
DelBello et al., 2006	Bipolar I, manic or mixed episode (DSM-IV)	DBC, LOCF (4-wk), DVPX vs. QTP in adolescents	QTP = DVPX
Sachs et al., 2004	Bipolar I, manic episode (DSM-IV)	DBPC (3-wk), QTP + Li or DVPX vs. Li or DVPX monotherapy Lithium target levels: 0.7–1.0 mEq/L; valproic acid serum concentrations 50–100 µg/mL. QTP dosed 100 mg (day 1) and increased 100 mg/day until day 4 and optimized to between 200 and 800 mg/day by day 21	QTP + Li (56%) or + DVPX (53%) > Li (27%) or DVPX (36%) monotherapy, YMRS response
Yatham et al., 2004	Bipolar I, manic episode (DSM-IV)	DBPC (3 or 6 wk), QTP + Li or DVPX. Li and DVPX dosed to serum levels of 0.7–1.0 mEq/L and 50–100 µg/mL, respectively. QTP flexibly dosed to 800 mg/day	QTP + DVPX/Li (15.9) > Li/DVPX alone (12.2), improvement in YMRS score
Muller-Oerlinghausen et al., 2003	Acute manic episode (ICD-10 criteria)	DBPC (3-wk) of adjunctive VPA (20 mg/kg, fixed-dose) in patients treated with neuroleptic therapy	VPA > placebo, neuroleptic dose (primary outcome measure) DVPX (70%) > placebo (46%), YMRS[4] 50% reduction.
Tohen et al., 2002	Bipolar I, manic or mixed episode (DSM-IV)	DBC of flexable-dose OLZ (5–20 mg/day) and DVPX (500–2500 mg/day).	OLZ (54%) > DVPX (42%), YMRS[4] 50% reduction
Zajecka et al., 2002	Bipolar I, manic episode (DSM-IV)	DBC (3-wk) of flexable-dose olanzapine and DVPX with 12 week follow-up	No difference between DVPX and OLZ, MRS[3] score.
Bowden et al., 1994	Research Diagnostic Criteria for manic disorder	DBPC, LOCF (3-wk), Li (adjusted to 1.5 mmol/L) vs. DVPX	DVPX 48%, Li 49%, placebo 25%, MRS[3] 50% reduction
Freeman et al., 1992	Bipolar I, manic episode or "mixed state" (DSM-IIIR)	DBPC (3-wk). Li vs. VPA	Li = DVPX, on MRS, GAS, BPRS
Pope et al., 1991	Bipolar I, manic or mixed (DSM-IIIR)	DBPC (3-wk), Li nonresponders. DVPX dose adjusted to serum concentration of 50–125 µg/mL	DVPX (54%) > placebo (5%), YMRS score DVPX (20 point improvement) > placebo (0 point improvement), GAS

Abbreviations: ICD, International Classification of Diseases; DSM, Diagnostic And Statistical Manual Of Mental Disorders; DBPC, double-blind, placebo-controlled trial; DBC, double-blind, controlled trial; DVPX, divalproex; LCOF, last observation carried forward; MRS, Mania Rating Scale; YMRS, Young Mania Rating Scale; ER, extended release; QTP, quetiapine; Li, lithium; OLZ, olanzapine; GAS, Global Assessment Scale; BPRS, Brief Psychiatric Rating Scale.

to divalproex or lithium with a second-generation (atypical) antipsychotic (SGA) added to divalproex or lithium in patients with bipolar mania with or without psychotic symptoms. SGAs, either begun in combination with divalproex or lithium or added adjunctively to pre-existing and usually only partially successful mono-therapy with divalproex or lithium, were superior to placebo in these trials. One study addressed whether the addition of valproate was superior to placebo in patients receiving first-generation antipsychotics for patients with acute mania (16). Significantly, more valproate-treated patients displayed a decrease in the need for concomitant antipsychotic medication by the three-week study end point.

A number of post hoc analyses have been conducted to examine potential predictors of response to valproate in patients with acute mania (24,25). These analyses indicated that patients with manic and mixed episodes had comparable response rates to valproate and that the number of prior mood episodes did not adversely affect valproate response. In addition, the presence or absence of psychosis did not appear to affect response either (9,11). A post hoc analysis of pooled intent-to-treat data from three randomized, placebo-controlled studies of divalproex studies in patients with acute mania found a linear relationship between serum valproate concentration and response and that the target serum concentration of valproate for optimal response was above 94 mg/L (26). In summary, data from the controlled trials reviewed above indicate that valproate has a broad spectrum of efficacy in both acute manic and mixed episodes, with or without psychosis, and appears to be comparable to lithium and antipsychotics in overall acute antimanic efficacy.

CARBAMAZEPINE

Although 14 double-blind, controlled trials provided preliminary evidence of carbamazepine's efficacy in the treatment of acute mania (27), these findings were only recently replicated in two large, multicenter, randomized, placebo-controlled, parallel-group trials (Table 2) (28,29). In the first of these two trials (28), there was no significant difference in mean reduction of manic symptoms in patients with

TABLE 2 Selected Randomized Controlled Trials of Carbamazepine in Bipolar Manic and Mixed Episodes

Study	Diagnostic criteria	Design	Results
Zhang et al., 2007	Bipolar I, mixed or manic episode (DSM-IV)	DBPC (12-wk), LOCF. CBZ+ FEWP vs. CBZ or placebo	CBZ (93%) > placebo (57%), YMRS 50% reduction No efficacy difference between CBZ+ FEWP and CBZ
Weisler et al., 2005	Bipolar I, mixed or Manic episode (DSM-IV)	DBPC (3-wk) LOCF, CBZ beaded-extended release) 200 mg BID increased (as necessary, tolerated) by 200 mg/day to 1600 mg/day	CBZ > placebo, YMRS total score reduction and CGI score
Weisler et al., 2004	Bipolar I, mixed or manic episode (DSM-IV)	DBPC (3-wk) LOCF, CBZ (beaded-extended release) 400 mg/day increased to 1600 mg/day	CBZ (42%) > placebo (22%), YMRS 50% reduction

Abbreviations: BID, twice a day; CBZ, carbamazepine; DBPC, double-blind, placebo-controlled trial; DBC, double-blind, controlled trial; LOCF, last observation carried forward; YMRS, Young Mania Rating Scale; FEWP, Free and Easy Wanderer Plus (Jia-wey Shiau-Yau San, Chinese herbal remedy).

mixed episodes treated with carbamazepine compared with placebo, due in part to a high placebo response in the subgroup. However, in the second trial (29), response rates were significantly higher in both manic and mixed patients receiving carbamazepine compared with placebo. Aside from the subgroup analyses in these two trials, there are no consistent data regarding clinical predictors of acute response to carbamazepine.

Carbamazepine had previously been compared with lithium (30,31) and chlorpromazine (32,33) in head-to-head studies without a placebo group. These studies, although individually limited by small sample sizes, in aggregate found comparable antimanic efficacy among patients receiving carbamazepine, lithium, or chlorpromazine.

There are few controlled studies involving carbamazepine as adjunctive or combination treatment in patients with acute bipolar mania. In an eight-week, double-blind comparison trial of carbamazepine with lithium versus haloperidol with lithium involving 33 patients with acute mania, both treatment groups had comparable mean reductions in both manic and psychotic symptoms as well as similar response rates at end point (34). Risperidone was compared with placebo in combination with carbamazepine, lithium, or divalproex in patients with acute mania in another trial (35). Interestingly, risperidone was superior to placebo in combination with lithium of divalproex, but not with carbamazepine. This may have been due to induction of risperidone metabolism in the carbamazepine group, leading to subtherapeutic risperidone serum concentrations. Finally, carbamazepine was utilized as the principal antimanic agent in a study comparing a Chinese herbal medicine formulation with placebo in patients with acute mania (36). In this trial, the herbal medicine in combination with carbamazepine was no more efficacious than placebo with carbamazepine.

OXCARBAZEPINE

Oxcarbazepine, the 10-keto analogue of carbamazepine, has been studied in five controlled trials as monotherapy for patients with acute bipolar mania (37–41). The first double-blind study was a small pilot trial involving six patients in an A-B-A crossover design (37). The improvement seen during the oxcarbazepine component of this trial led to two double-blind comparison trials versus haloperidol and lithium, respectively (38,39).

In both studies, oxcarbazepine and the respective comparator agent were of similar efficacy. However, both studies were limited by small samples, the use of chlorpromazine as an as-needed adjunctive medication, and the absence of a placebo control group (42). In more recent controlled trials, the efficacy of oxcarbazepine in the treatment of acute bipolar mania has not yet been convincingly established. For example, in an open-label on-off-on study, four (33%) of 12 patients were classified as responders to oxcarbazepine, and antimanic effects were evident primarily in patients with mild-to-moderate symptoms (40). In the only large, randomized, double-blind, placebo-controlled, parallel-group trial of oxcarbazepine reported to date, a seven-week study conducted in children and adolescents with acute bipolar manic or mixed episodes, oxcarbazepine was not superior to placebo in reduction of manic symptoms (41).

PHENYTOIN

Two small controlled trials of phenytoin in the treatment of manic symptoms have recently been reported (43,44). The first trial compared the combination of phenytoin and haloperidol with placebo and haloperidol in a five-week study of patients with bipolar or schizoaffective disorder with manic symptoms (43). Significantly, more improvement in manic symptoms was evident in patients receiving the combination of phenytoin and haloperidol. The second trial examined the use of phenytoin in the prevention of manic symptoms in patients with allergies, pulmonary, or rheumatological illnesses receiving corticosteroid treatment (44). Thus, this trial was designed to prevent the occurrence of manic symptoms due to corticosteroids and not in patients with bipolar disorder per se.

The phenytoin-treated group displayed significantly smaller increases on patient self-report measures of manic symptoms compared with patients receiving placebo. Taken together, these findings are intriguing and suggest that phenytoin may have antimanic properties. However, these initial findings require confirmation in placebo-controlled studies of phenytoin monotherapy in patients with acute bipolar manic and mixed episodes.

TOPIRAMATE

In four randomized, placebo-controlled, parallel-group, three-week trials in adult patients with bipolar mania, two of which also included a lithium comparison group, topiramate was not found to have significant antimanic efficacy compared with placebo (45). These results could not be explained by a high placebo response. Moreover, the lithium groups were superior to placebo in the two trials utilizing a lithium control group. A placebo-controlled trial of topiramate monotherapy in children and adolescents with acute bipolar mania was discontinued upon analysis of the adult trial data described above (46). Thus, the results of this study, which was limited by a small sample, were inconclusive. Lastly, topiramate was also compared with placebo as an adjunct to lithium or valproate in patients with acute bipolar I mania (47). As in the monotherapy trials, there was no significant reduction in manic symptoms in patients receiving topiramate compared with placebo. Of note, topiramate treatment was associated with a significant reduction in body weight compared with placebo. This secondary finding is consistent with observations of topiramate's weight loss effects in other studies in patients with bipolar disorder (48,49), epilepsy (50), migraine (51), diabetic neuropathy (52), obesity (53), and binge-eating disorder associated with obesity (54).

GABAPENTIN

Two placebo-controlled trials of gabapentin in the treatment of acute bipolar mania failed to find significant efficacy of gabapentin over placebo (55,56). These included a large, multicenter, parallel-group trial of gabapentin as adjunctive therapy in patients with bipolar I manic or mixed episodes (55) and a small crossover trial in patients with rapid cycling bipolar disorders refractory to previous trials of mood stabilizing agents (56). In an interesting analysis of a sample of 43 patients with bipolar disorder who were treatment refractory to mood stabilizers and who received gabapentin in an open-label trial, significant improvement was observed in a subgroup of patients with comorbid anxiety and/or alcohol abuse (57). These preliminary observations suggest that gabapentin may have utility in the treatment of patients with bipolar disorder with comorbid anxiety or alcohol-use disorders.

LAMOTRIGINE

In three randomized, controlled trials, lamotrigine was not found to be significantly superior to placebo in the treatment of bipolar manic symptoms (56,58,59). In the first of these studies, a series of six-week crossover trials comparing lamotrigine, gabapentin, and placebo in patients with treatment-refractory rapid-cycling bipolar disorders, there was no significant difference in reduction of manic symptoms during the lamotrigine trials compared with the placebo trials (56). However, manic symptoms were low at baseline in this study, raising the possibility that treatment effects may have been obscured among the treatment groups in this pole of the illness. In the second lamotrigine bipolar mania trial, lamotrigine or placebo was added to ongoing lithium treatment in patients who were inadequately responsive to lithium or was administered as monotherapy in patients who could not tolerate lithium side effects (58). Again, there were no significant differences in reduction of manic symptoms among the patients receiving lamotrigine or placebo.

The third lamotrigine study in patients with bipolar mania was a small comparison trial with lithium in which both treatments produced significant reductions in manic symptoms (59). However, the small sample size ($N = 30$), low mean lithium levels (0.7 mEq/L), and absence of a placebo group limit interpretation of these results. Thus, although lamotrigine has demonstrated efficacy as a maintenance treatment for patients with bipolar I disorder (60,61), there are no compelling data to indicate that it exerts acute antimanic efficacy.

SUMMARY

Although a number of antiepileptic agents have been studied in the treatment of bipolar manic and mixed episodes, only two, valproic acid and carbamazepine, have established efficacy in rigorous randomized, placebo-controlled, parallel-group trials. Topiramate, lamotrigine, and gabapentin have not been shown to be superior to placebo in controlled trials. Phenytoin and oxcarbazepine have not been studied adequately in definitive trials and thus must be regarded as unproven in their efficacy in manic and mixed episodes.

REFERENCES

1. Bowden CL. Anticonvulsants in bipolar disorder. Aust N Z J Psychiatry 2006; 40: 386–393.
2. Post RM, Weiss SR. Convergences in course of illness and treatments of the epilepsies and recurrent affective disorders. Clin EEG Neurosci 2004; 35:14–24.
3. Pope HG Jr., McElroy SL, Keck PE Jr. Valproate treatment of acute mania: a placebo-controlled study. Arch Gen Psychiatry 1991; 48:62–68.
4. Bowden CL, Brugger AM, Swann AC, et al. Efficacy of divalproex versus lithium and placebo in the treatment of mania. JAMA 1994; 271:918–924.
5. Bowden CL, Swann AC, Calabrese JR, et al. A randomized, placebo-controlled, multicenter study of divalproex extended release in the treatment of acute mania. J Clin Psychiatry 2006; 67:1501–1510.

6. Emrich HM, Von Zerssen D, Kissling W. On a possible role of GABA in mania: therapeutic efficacy of sodium valproate. In: Costa E, Dicharia G, Gessa GL, eds. GABA and Benzodiazepine Receptors. New York, NY: Raven Press, 1981:287–296.
7. Brennan MIW, Sandyk R, Borsook D. Use of sodium valproate in the management of affective disorders: basic and clinical aspects. In: Emrich HM, Okuma T, Muller AA, eds. Anticonvulsants in Affective Disorders. Amsterdam, The Netherlands: Exerpta Medica, 1984:56–65.
8. Tohen M, Baker RW, Altshuler LL, et al. Olanzapine versus divalproex in the treatment of acute mania. Am J Psychiatry 2002; 159:1011–1017.
9. Zajecka JM, Weisler R, Sachs G, et al. A comparison of the efficacy, safety, and tolerability of divalproex sodium and olanzapine in the treatment of bipolar disorder. J Clin Psychiatry 2002; 63:1148–1155.
10. Freeman TW, Clothier JL, Pazzaglia P, et al. A double-blind comparison of valproic acid and lithium in the treatment of acute mania. Am J Psychiatry 1992; 149:247–250.
11. Hirschfeld RM, Allen MH, McEvoy J, et al. Safety and tolerability of oral loading of divalproex in acutely manic bipolar patients. J Clin Psychiatry 1999; 60:815–818.
12. DelBello MP, Kowatch RA, Adler CM, et al. A double-blind randomized pilot study comparing quetiapine and divalproex for adolescent mania. J Am Acad Child Adolesc Psychiatry 2006; 45:305–313.
13. Keck PE Jr., McElroy SL, Tugrul KC, et al. Valproate oral loading in the treatment of acute mania. J Clin Psychiatry 1993; 54:305–308.
14. McElroy SL, Keck PE Jr., Tugrul KC, et al. Valproate as a loading treatment in acute mania. Neuropsychobiol 1993; 27:146–149.
15. McElroy SL, Keck PE Jr., Stanton SP, et al. A randomized comparison of divalproex oral loading versus haloperidol in the initial treatment of acute psychotic mania. J Clin Psychiatry 1998; 59:142–146.
16. Müller-Oerlinghausen B, Retzow A, Henn FA, et al. Valproate as an adjunct medication for the treatment of acute mania: a prospective, randomized, double-blind, placebo-controlled trial. European Valproate Mania Study Group. J Clin Psychopharmacol 2000; 20:195–203.
17. Yatham LN, Paulsson B, Mullen J, et al. Quetiapine versus placebo in combination with lithium or divalproex for the treatment of bipolar mania. J Clin Psychopharmacol 2004; 24:599–606.
18. Sachs G, Chengappa KNR, Suppes T, et al. Quetiapine with lithium or divalproex for the treatment of bipolar mania: a randomized, double-blind, placebo-controlled study. Bipolar Disord 2004; 6:213–223.
19. Yatham LN, Binder C, Kusumaker V, et al. Risperidone plus lithium versus risperidone plus valproate in acute and continuation treatment of mania. Int Clin Psychopharmacol 2004; 19:103–109.
20. Sachs GS, Grossman F, Ghaemi SN, et al. Combination of a mood stabilizer with risperidone or haloperidol for the treatment of acute mania: a double-blind, placebo-controlled comparison of efficacy and safety. Am J Psychiatry 2002; 159:1146–1154.
21. Tohen M, Chengappa KNR, Suppes T, et al. Efficacy of olanzapine in combination with valproate or lithium in the treatment of mania in patients partially nonresponsive to valproate or lithium monotherapy. Arch Gen Psychiatry 2002; 59:62–69.
22. Bahk WM, Shin YC, Woo JM, et al. Topiramate and divalproex in combination with risperidone for acute mania: a randomized open-label study. Prog Neuropsychopharmacol Biol Psychiatry 2005; 29:115–121.
23. DelBello MP, Schweirs ML, Rosenberg HL, et al. A double-blind, randomized, placebo-controlled study of quetiapine as adjunctive treatment for adolescent mania. J Am Acad Child Adolesc Psychiatry 2002; 41:1216–1223.
24. Swann AC, Bowden CL, Calabrese JR, et al. Differential effects of number of previous episodes of affective disorder in response to lithium or divalproex in acute mania. Am J Psychiatry 1999; 156:1264–1266.
25. Swann AC, Bowden CL, Morris D, et al. Depression during mania: treatment response to lithium or divalproex. Arch Gen Psychiatry 1997; 54:37–42.

26. Allen MH, Hirschfeld RM, Wozniak PJ, et al. Linear relationship of valproate serum concentration to response and optimal serum levels for acute mania. Am J Psychiatry 2006; 163:272–275.
27. Keck PE Jr., McElroy SL, Nemeroff CB. Anticonvulsants in the treatment of bipolar disorder. J Neuropsychiatr Clin Neurosci 1992; 4:595–605.
28. Weisler RH, Kalali AH, Ketter TA, et al. A multicenter, randomized, double-blind, placebo-controlled trial of extended release carbamazepine capsules as monotherapy for bipolar patients with manic or mixed episodes. J Clin Psychiatry 2004; 65:478–484.
29. Weisler RH, Keck PE Jr., Swann AC, et al. Extended release carbamazepine capsules as monotherapy for acute mania in bipolar disorder: a multicenter, randomized, double-blind, placebo-controlled trial. J Clin Psychiatry 2005; 66:323–330.
30. Lerer B, Moore N, Meyendorff E, et al. Carbamazepine versus lithium in mania: a double-blind study. J Clin Psychiatry 1987; 48:89–93.
31. Small JG. Anticonvulsants in affective disorders. Psychopharmacol Bull 1990; 26:25–36.
32. Grossi E, Sacchetti E, Vita A. Carbamazepine vs. Chlorpromazine in mania: a double-blind trial. In: Emrich HM, Okuma T, Muller AA, eds. Anticonvulsants in Affective Disorders. Amsterdam, The Netherlands: Exerpta Medica, 1984:184–194.
33. Okuma T, Inanga K, Otsuki S, et al. Comparison of the antimanic efficacy of carbamazepine and chlorpromazine. Psychopharmacol 1979; 66:211–217.
34. Small JG, Klapper MH, Marhenke JD, et al. Lithium combined with carbamazepine or haloperidol in the treatment of mania. Psychopharmacol Bull 1995; 31:265–272.
35. Yatham LN, Grossman F, Augustyns I, et al. Mood stabilizers plus risperidone or placebo in the treatment of acute mania. Br J Psychiatry 2003; 182:141–147.
36. Zhang ZJ, Kang WH, Tan QR, et al. Adjunctive herbal medicine with carbamazepine for bipolar disorders: a double-blind, randomized, placebo-controlled study. J Psychiatr Res 2007; 41(3–4):360–369.
37. Emrich HM, Altmann H, Dose M, et al. Therapeutic effects of GABA-ergic drugs in affective disorders: a preliminary report. Pharmacol Biochem Behav 1983; 19:369–373.
38. Emrich HM. Studies with oxcarbazepine (Trileptal) in acute mania. Int Clin Psychopharmacol 1990; 5(suppl 1):83–88.
39. Muller AA, Stoll KD. Carbamazepine and oxcarbazepine in the treatment of manic syndromes: studies in Germany. In: Emrich HM, Okuma T, Muller AA, eds. Anticonvulsants in Affective Disorders. Amsterdam, The Netherlands: Experta Medica, 1984:222–229.
40. Hummel B, Walden J, Stampfer R, et al. Acute antimanic efficacy and safety of oxcarbazepine in an open trial with on-off-on design. Bipolar Disord 2002; 4:412–417.
41. Wagner KD, Kowatch RA, Emslie GJ, et al. A double-blind, randomized, placebo-controlled trial of oxcarbazepine in the treatment of bipolar disorder in children and adolescents. Am J Psychiatry 2006; 163:1179–1186.
42. Jefferson JW. Oxcarbazepine in bipolar disorder. J Clin Psychiatry 2001; 3:181.
43. Mishory A, Yaroslavsky Y, Bersudsky Y, et al. Phenytoin as an antimanic anticonvulsant. Am J Psychiatry 2000; 157:463–465.
44. Brown ES, Stuard G, Liggin JD, et al. Effect of phenytoin on mood and declarative memory during prescription corticosteroid therapy. Biol Psychiatry 2005; 57:543–548.
45. Kushner SF, Khan A, Lane R, et al. Topiramate monotherapy in the management of acute mania: results of four double-blind placebo-controlled trials. Bipolar Disord 2006; 8:15–27.
46. DelBello MP, Findling RL, Kushner S, et al. A pilot controlled trial for mania in children and adolescents with bipolar disorder. J Am Acad Child Adolesc Psychiatry 2005; 44:539–547.
47. Chengappa KNR, Schwarzman LK, Hulihan JF, et al. Adjunctive topiramate therapy in patients receiving a mood stabilizer for bipolar I disorder: a randomized, placebo-controlled trial. J Clin Psychiatry 2006; 67:1698–1706.
48. McElroy SL, Suppes T, Keck PE Jr., et al. Open-label adjunctive topiramate in the treatment of bipolar disorders. Biol Psychiatry 2000; 47:1025–1033.

49. Chengappa KNR, Levine J, Rathore D, et al. Long-term effects of topiramate on bipolar mood instability, weight change and glycemic control: a case-series. Eur Psychiatry 2001; 16:186–190.
50. Biton V. Effect of antiepileptic drugs on bodyweight: overview and clinical implications for the treatment of epilepsy. CNS Drugs 2003; 17:781–791.
51. Brandes JL, Saper JR, Diamond M, et al. Topiramate for migraine prevention: a randomized controlled trial. JAMA 2004; 291:965–973.
52. Raskin P, Donofrio PD, Vinik AI, et al. Efficacy, safety, and metabolic effects of topiramate in a multicenter, controlled trial of painful diabetic neuropathy. Neurol 2004; 63:865–873.
53. Wilding J, Van Gaal L, Rissanen A, et al. A randomized double-blind placebo-controlled study of the long-term efficacy and safety of topiramate in the treatment of obese subjects. Int J Obesity 2004; 28:1399–1410.
54. McElroy SL, Arnold LM, Shapira NA, et al. Topiramate in the treatment of binge eating disorder associated with obesity: a randomized, placebo-controlled trial. Am J Psychiatry 2003; 160:255–261.
55. Pande AC, Crockatt JG, Janney CA, et al. Gabapentin in bipolar disorder: a placebo-controlled trial of adjunctive therapy. Bipolar Disord 2000; 2:249–255.
56. Frye MA, Ketter TA, Kimbrell TA, et al. A placebo-controlled study of lamotrigine and gabapentin monotherapy in refractory mood disorders. J Clin Psychopharmacol 2000; 20:607–614.
57. Perugi G, Toni C, Frare F, et al. Effectiveness of adjunctive gabapentin in resistant bipolar disorder: is it due to anxious-alcohol abuse comorbidity? J Clin Psychopharmacol 2002; 22:584–591.
58. Anand A, Oren DA, Berman RM, et al. Lamotrigine treatment of lithium failure in oupatient mania: a double-blind, placebo-controlled trial. Third International Conference on Bipolar Disorder, Pittsburgh, Pennsylvania, June 16, 1999 (abstr).
59. Ichim L, Berk M, Brook S. Lamotrigine compared with lithium in mania: a double-blind, placebo-controlled trial. J Affect Disord 2000; 12:5–10.
60. Bowden CL, Calabrese JR, Sachs GS, et al. A placebo-controlled 18-month trial of lamotrigine and lithium maintenance treatment in recently manic or hypomanic patients with bipolar I disorder. Arch Gen Psychiatry 2003; 60:392–400.
61. Calabrese JR, Bowden CL, Sachs GS, et al. A placebo-controlled 18-month trial of lamotrigine and lithium maintenance treatment in recently depressed patients with bipolar I disorder. J Clin Psychiatry 2003; 64:1013–1024.

8 The Role of Antiepileptic Drugs in Long-Term Treatment of Bipolar Disorder

Charles L. Bowden and Vivek Singh
Department of Psychiatry, University of Texas Health Science Center at San Antonio, San Antonio, Texas, U.S.A.

INTRODUCTION

Long-term management of bipolar disorder is complex and challenging, largely because of the inherent complexity of the disorder and the multitude of interacting psychosocial stressors and supports that interweave over time. Bipolar disorder comprises four to six behavioral/symptomatic domains, and each requires unique attention psychopharmacologically when present. Studies consistently report factors for depression, mania, irritability, anxiety, and psychosis. Impulsivity and affective/mood instability are the closest to a universal symptom complex in bipolar disorder, appearing to some degree in all phases of the illness and even in patients recovered with continuing care (1,2). No drug, neither a single lifestyle modification nor a form of psychotherapy effectively eliminates all symptoms. Because of the persisting expression of symptomatology of bipolar illness in even the best functioning individuals, treatment needs to be continued over the lifetime and periodically modified to target symptoms that may emerge during the course of long-term treatment. Tolerability and consequently adherence, factors that translate efficacious into effective treatments, should drive drug selection and continuation in maintenance treatment of bipolar disorder.

Mood stabilizers are considered the foundation of treatment of bipolar disorder. Although definitions of the phrase mood stabilizer vary, all of the definitions emphasize that the drug must benefit one or more primary mood states of bipolar illness, be effective in acute and maintenance phase treatment and not worsen any aspect of the illness (3,4).

Antiepileptic drugs (AEDs), also called anticonvulsants, are mainstays of long-term treatment of bipolar disorder. A paradigm shift in long-term management of bipolar disorder has been an increased focus on the aggressive management of interepisode symptomatology and related psychosocial dysfunction, with less but certainly still important attention to syndromal mood states.

We present the evidence for efficacy, safety, and practical guidelines for long-term use in bipolar disorder of all approved AEDs, including those AEDs for which clear evidence indicates that they have no primary roles in treatment of bipolar disorder. Although the emphasis is on long-term treatment since acute episodes occur in the course of illness, this aspect of AED use is also addressed.

VALPROATE

Divalproex, a stable formulation of sodium valproate and valproic acid with delayed release properties, was approved by the United States Food and Drug Administration (FDA) in 1995 for the treatment of acute mania following a large randomized, double blind, parallel-group clinical trial of divalproex versus lithium versus placebo published in 1994 (5). Although the mechanism of action of valproate in bipolar disorder is unclear, more is known about its and lithium's central nervous system (CNS) related actions than any other treatments employed in bipolar disorder. Principally from animal studies, but in some cases human investigations, it is known to reduce protein kinase C (PKC) activity in manic patients (6), inhibit glycogen synthase kinase 3 (GSK-3), activate the extracellular signal-regulated kinase (ERK) pathway (7), increase the expression of the cyto-protective protein B-cell lymphoma/leukemia-2 gene (bcl-2) (8), reduce inositol biosynthesis, lengthen the period of circadian rhythms and increase arrhythmicity in *Drosophila*, and reverse early DNA damage caused by amphetamine in an animal model of mania (9). The impact on circadian rhythms is of particular interest given in recent data, implicating sets of genes associated with circadian rhythmicity in bipolar disorder (10). For most of the above-summarized effects, similar results have been observed with both valproate and lithium. Each of the above systems has been associated with manic states and animal models for mania (11). However, valproate's mechanisms of action are unique, resulting from decreased myo-inositol 1-phosphate synthase inhibition (12) and inhibition of histone deacetylase (13).

Profile of Actions

In short-term studies, both divalproex and lithium significantly decreased impulsivity and hyperactivity, whereas divalproex, but not lithium, improved irritability (1). Neither drug was superior to placebo in alleviating anxiety components. In a recent study indicating efficacy of a sustained release formulation of divalproex in mania, the specific areas of superiority of divalproex over placebo were for racing thoughts, decreased need for sleep, and items reflecting hyperactivity (14). Of interest in the study, extended release divalproex showed greater benefits in more seriously ill manic patients (14). In other monotherapy studies in acute mania, valproate was equivalent in efficacy to haloperidol in patients with psychotic mania (15), to olanzapine in two studies (16,17), and superior to carbamazepine (18).

The efficacy of valproate in combination with other agents with proven efficacy as monotherapy in the treatment of mania has been demonstrated by several randomized, double-blind, placebo controlled studies. These studies also indicate that when antipsychotics are used in combination with lithium or valproate, patients receiving combination therapy regimens can be effectively treated with lower doses than are used for antipsychotic drug monotherapy (19–21). Analysis of the data from the Sachs et al. study did not demonstrate any advantage of the combination treatment in the cotherapy group (patients in a manic state without any treatment in whom risperidone and either lithium or valproate were initiated concomitantly), whereas in the add-on therapy group (patients nonresponsive to monotherapy with lithium or valproate at an adequate dose for two weeks or more in whom risperidone was then added), there was a distinct advantage to the addition of risperidone. Each of the other studies required some degree of failure with monotherapy prior to initiation of combination treatment. In another study, the addition of valproate to a typical antipsychotic (haloperidol) led to greater improvement in manic symptomatology than using haloperidol alone (21). These findings suggest that combination therapy should be initiated in patients who have either failed to respond or have responded partially to a monotherapeutic approach at an adequate dosage for an adequate duration of time.

Maintenance Efficacy

In patients with bipolar I disorder who were randomized to one year of maintenance treatment with divalproex, lithium, or placebo following meeting recovery criteria within three months of an index manic episode, divalproex showed a trend for superiority over lithium ($P = 0.06$) on the primary efficacy measure, time to a full mood episode, with neither drug significantly superior to placebo, due to a lower than expected rate of relapse among placebo-treated subjects (22). On most secondary measures, divalproex was superior to placebo. These included rate of early discontinuation for onset of any mood episode, onset of a depressive episode, and dropout for any reason (23,24). Divalproex was superior to lithium in prolonging the duration of successful prophylaxis in the study and improvement in global assessment function (GAF) scores. Similar results were reported in an earlier randomized, open study comparing valpromide with lithium (25). Divalproex also appeared better than lithium with regard to depressive outcomes. Compared with those randomized to lithium, patients randomized to divalproex had lesser worsening of depressive symptomatology, a lower probability of relapse into depression (particularly if they had demonstrated a response to divalproex when manic), and better response if a selective serotonin reuptake inhibitor (SSRI) was added following the development of a depressive episode (23).

Maintenance Outcome Comparisons with Placebo

Smith et al. recently conducted a thorough meta-analysis of all randomized control trials in the maintenance phase of bipolar disorder. The rate of study withdrawal for any reason was 18% [95% confidence interval (CI) 4–30%] less with valproate than with placebo (24,26). The rate of relapse to any mood episode was 18% less with valproate than with placebo with the rate of relapse to a manic episode being 27% less with valproate than with placebo. The relapse rate to a depressive episode was 60% less (CI 18–80%) in the valproate group than with placebo. The risk ratio for withdrawal for adverse effects was higher with valproate than with placebo (4.19, 95% CI 1.3–13.5%).

Maintenance Outcome Comparisons with Lithium

In comparisons with lithium, the withdrawal rate was 48% higher with lithium than with valproate (27). Combining the Bowden et al. and Calabrese et al. studies, the risk ratio withdrawal rate was 21% higher for lithium than for valproate (4,26). The relapse rates for any mood episode were 34% greater for lithium than for valproate. The relapse rates due to a manic episode did not differ significantly between the two agents (3% more for lithium than valproate) but the rate of relapse due to a depressive episode was 50% higher for lithium than for valproate. The withdrawal rate due to an adverse event was 81% higher for lithium than for valproate. Taken in the aggregate, these analyses indicate a broader spectrum of efficacy for valproate compared with both placebo and lithium, substantially better tolerability for valproate than for lithium, and evidence of at least as much benefit on depressive as for manic recurrences.

Maintenance Effectiveness in Adjunct Therapy

One small study with 99 subjects compared adjunctive olanzapine with mood stabilizer monotherapy, either valproate or lithium (28). The only outcome reported for all randomized subjects was time to relapse for any mood episode. There were nonsignificantly fewer relapses in the monotherapy group than in the adjunctive olanzapine group (13%, CI 45% fewer to 131% more). An even smaller subgroup of the acutely enrolled patients who were defined post hoc as in both sympto-matic and syndromal remission had significantly longer time to mania relapse, but not depression relapse, with mood stabilizer monotherapy than with adjunctive olanzapine.

A second small study of 12 participants compared valproate plus lithium with lithium alone (29). Although the difference was reported as significantly favoring valproate plus lithium over lithium alone, the possibility of no benefit of the com-bination was not excluded. In the aggregate, the two studies suggest that adjunctive regimens including valproate may be more effective than monotherapy regimens with either lithium or other mood stabilizers, but more systematic, adequately designed studies are needed for this aspect.

A 47-week maintenance study comparing divalproex and olanzapine (17) in bipolar patients with an index episode of acute mania did not meet criteria for inclusion in the Smith et al. meta-analysis (26), because patients were randomized during the acute episode and not following achievement of mood stability. Rates of completion were low for both treatments (15% vs. 16%), and though symptomatic remission occurred earlier with olanzapine, efficacy was equivalent for the two drugs over the latter portion of the study. The two drugs did not differ in the rates of manic relapse and the median time to a manic relapse (19). Patients who attained remission at the end of acute treatment were more likely to complete the 47-week trial than those who did not (divalproex 26% vs. 11%; olanzapine 20% vs. 11%, $P = 0.001$), indicating that acute treatment response, while manic, for both val-proate and olanzapine, is predictive of more effective treatment with the same drug during maintenance therapy. In addition, long-term treatment with divalproex was associated with significant reductions in both total and low-density cholesterol, compared with increases with olanzapine. Weight gain was greater with olanzapine than with divalproex (17).

In a 20-month, randomized, double-blind maintenance study of valproate or lithium monotherapy in bipolar patients with rapid cycling, only one quarter of patients enrolled, met criteria for an acute bimodal response to either drug and less than 25% of those randomized maintained benefits without relapse (27). These findings indicate that monotherapy regimens have limited efficacy in the treatment of rapid-cycling patients.

Efficacy in the Young and the Elderly

Open studies of valproate have demonstrated moderate to marked sustained improvement in over half of manic youth aged 8 through 18 years (30–33). An open-label, randomized 6-week study ($N = 42$) assessing the efficacy of divalproex, lithium, and carbamazepine in bipolar I and II patients experiencing manic or mixed manic episodes did not show any significant difference in rates of response between the three treatment groups, though the effect size for improvement was largest with divalproex (divalproex 1.63, lithium 1.06, carbamazepine 1.00) (34).

A randomized, placebo-controlled study ($N = 56$) reported significant ben-efits for valproate on irritability and agitation associated with dementia (35). These findings were consistent with open studies that have demonstrated benefit on some aspects of irritability and agitation in elderly patients with varying symptomatology (36–38). More systematic, controlled studies are needed to draw conclusions on valproate's effectiveness in these age groups.

Dosage and Serum Level Monitoring

Placebo-controlled trials have shown that acutely manic patients with valproate serum levels ≥45 µg/mL are significantly more likely to have at least a 20% improvement in their manic symptomatology (24,39–41). During maintenance treatment, valproate levels between 75 and 99 µg/mL were more likely to maintain prophylaxis than serum levels above or below this range and provided significantly superior outcomes than those observed with placebo (Table 1) (42).

Tolerability

Valproate is generally well tolerated as evidenced in the largest maintenance trial of divalproex in bipolar disorder, in which weight gain and tremors were the only adverse events more common with divalproex than placebo (22). Common dose/serum level related side effects seen with valproate include tremors, nausea, and related gastrointestinal distress, sedation, and reduction in platelets and white blood cell count (43,44). Alopecia can occur, in part consequent to chelation of trace elements, such as selenium and zinc, by valproic acid in the gut. Therefore the time of valproate dosing should be separated by several hours from that of taking a multivitamin preparation containing zinc and selenium. Low rates of hepatotoxicity (1/49,000) and pancreatitis (<1%) have been reported with valproate. Hepatic impairment, almost limited to children less than two years of age treated for epilepsy, may be a consequence of the interference of valproate with rapidly dividing cells in the immature liver. A similar mechanism is plausibly linked to neural tube defects and hair loss. In long-term studies, including the 12-month maintenance study of divalproex, valproate has not been associated with worsening of any hepatic indices by laboratory assessments, and in some instances, small but significant improvements in indices occurred (24). Routine monitoring of hepatic function and amylase levels is not indicated, unless active hepatic or pancreatic dysfunction is present (Table 1). Weight gain (about 3–24 pounds) is seen in 3% to 20% of patients on valproate. Valproate serum levels greater than 125 µg/mL are more likely to cause weight gain than levels below 125 mg/mL (24).

Valproate is an FDA Pregnancy Category D drug and has been associated with neural tube defects (1–4%) (24). The risk of CNS abnormalities is dose and serum level dependent, with the higher doses customarily employed in treating epilepsy associated with higher rates than those clinically utilized for bipolar disorder.

LAMOTRIGINE

Lamotrigine is FDA approved and recommended for the maintenance treatment of bipolar disorder, principally for the depressive manifestations of the illness. Although the specific mechanisms by which lamotrigine prevents recurrent depressive episodes in bipolar disorder are unknown, lamotrigine has several recognized mechanisms that distinguish it from other mood-stabilizing as well as antiepileptic drugs. Lamotrigine inhibits use-dependent voltage-sensitive sodium

TABLE 1 Characteristics of Antiepileptics Evaluated in Bipolar Disorder[a]

	VPA	CBZ	OXC	LAM	GBP	TMP	ZON	LEV	PHT
Time to steady state (days)	1–3	21–28[b]	2	3–15	1–2	4–5	5–15	2	7–28
Half-life (hr)	9–16	12–17[c]	2–9[d]	25–30	5–7	19–23	63	6–8	7–22
Bioavailability (%)	>95	85	100	98	60–27[e]	80	100	100	100[f]
Protein binding (%)	90–95	40–90	40	40–50	0–3	13–17	40	<10	93–98
Metabolism	Liver	Liver	Liver/biliary	Liver	None	Minimal	Liver	Liver	Liver
Clinically relevant metabolite	2-propyl-4-pentenoic acid (may cause toxicity)	10,11-epoxide (clinically active and may cause toxicity)	10-hydroxy carbazepine (clinically active)	None	None	None	None	None	None
Dosage range (mg/day)	200–2500	200–1200	300–2400	50–400	600–3600	100–600	100–600	1000–3000	100–400
Target blood levels (µg/mL)	50–125	6–12	10–35	N	N	N	10–40	N	10–20
Monitoring of drug levels	RB	R	NR	NR	NR	NR	NR	NR	NR
Monitoring of liver functions	R	R	NR	NR	NR	NR	NR	NR	NR
Monitoring of renal functions	NR	NR	NR	NR	NR	R[g]	NR	NR	NR
Monitoring of blood counts	R	R	NR	NR	NR	NR	NR	NR	NR
Monitoring of lipids	NR	NR	NR	NR	NR	NR	NR	NR	NR
Monitoring of blood sugar	NR	NR	NR	NR	NR	NR	NR	NR	NR
US-FDA pregnancy category	D	D	C	C	C	C	C	C	D

[a]Ref. 52.
[b]After completion of autoinduction.
[c]Due to autoinduction.
[d]Two hours for parent compound, nine hours for active metabolite.
[e]60% at 900 mg/day in divided doses and progressively decreases to 27% at 4800 mg/day in divided doses.
[f]Ref. 70.
[g]Ref. 71.

Abbreviations: VPA, valproate or divalproex; CBZ, carbamazepine; OXC, oxcarbazepine; LAM, lamotrigine; GBP, gabapentin; TMP, topiramate; ZON, zonisamide; LEV, levetiracetam; PHT, phenytoin or fosphenytoin; NR, not required; RB, required at baseline; R, required; N, not required; D, not defined.

channel activity. It also modulates presynaptic release of excitatory amino acid neurotransmitters such as glutamate. These effects reduce rates of repetitive neuronal after-discharges.

Maintenance Efficacy

Lamotrigine was the second agent after lithium to be approved by the FDA for maintenance treatment of bipolar disorder. This approval was based on findings from two paired, randomized, parallel-group, placebo-controlled, multicenter studies that demonstrated its prophylactic efficacy in patients with bipolar I disorder (45,46). These studies were designed to assess the safety and efficacy of lamotrigine and lithium for preventing relapse or recurrence of any mood episode in patients with bipolar I disorder. Both studies consisted of a screening of up to 2 weeks: an open-label phase of up to 8 to 16 weeks during which lamotrigine (dosage range of 100–200 mg/day) was started as monotherapy or as adjunctive treatment to ongoing treatment and an 18-month, double-blind phase wherein patients were randomized to receive lamotrigine (100–400 mg/day), lithium (flexibly dosed to achieve blood levels of 0.8–1.1 mEq/L), or placebo. Since all subjects received and adequately tolerated lamotrigine, and met randomization criteria while receiving lamotrigine alone, these studies qualified as enriched design trials (i.e., both selected for patients who benefited acutely from lamotrigine). The first study ($n = 175$) consisted of patients who were in the midst of or had experienced a recent episode of mania/hypomania (45), while the second study included patients who were experiencing or had recently experienced a major depressive episode ($n = 463$) (46). On the primary efficacy measure, time to intervention for any mood episode, lamotrigine and lithium were each superior to placebo in both studies. Lamotrigine, but not lithium, in both studies demonstrated superiority over placebo in delaying time to intervention for depression, whereas lithium, but not lamotrigine, was superior to placebo in time to delaying mania. In a pooled combined analysis of the two studies, both lamotrigine and lithium demonstrated superior efficacy than placebo on the primary efficacy measure, time to intervention for any mood episode. While lamotrigine, but not lithium, demonstrated superiority to placebo in prolonging time to intervention for a depressive episode, both lamotrigine and lithium were more efficacious than placebo in prolonging time to intervention for a manic, hypomanic, or mixed episode. Patients on lamotrigine were more likely to experience a recurrence or relapse to an episode of the same polarity than of an opposite one (47). The risk of switching to mania, hypomania, or a mixed state was similar between lamotrigine and lithium (5% vs. 7%).

In a large, 26-week, placebo-controlled study in 182 patients with rapid cycling bipolar disorder, lamotrigine (dosage range 100–500 mg/day) did not demonstrate superiority to placebo on the primary efficacy measure, time to intervention with additional pharmacotherapy for any mood episode, in the general cohort of patients and those with bipolar I disorder, but did show a trend toward superiority in patients with bipolar II disorder (48). Moreover, survival analysis (time to dropout for any reason) showed lamotrigine's superiority over placebo in the general group of patients and those with bipolar II disorder, but showed no significant separation from placebo in bipolar I patients.

The Smith et al. meta-analysis provides an important comparative data from these three studies (26).

Maintenance Outcome Comparisons with Placebo

Participants were 29% less likely to withdraw for any reason with lamotrigine than with placebo (26). The rate of relapse due to any mood episode was 32% lower with lamotrigine than with placebo (CI 15–45%). The rate of relapse due to a manic episode was nonsignificantly lower with lamotrigine (25%) but did not exclude the possibility of an increased risk (95% CI 51% fewer to 11% more). The relapse rate due to a depressive episode was 35% lower (CI 9–54%) with lamotrigine than with placebo. There were 5% fewer withdrawals due to an adverse event with lamotrigine than with placebo, although the upper confidence interval did not exclude an increased risk.

Maintenance Outcome Comparisons with Lithium

Hazard rate estimates indicated 9% more withdrawals for any reason with lithium than lamotrigine (26). Rates of relapse due to any mood episode were 7% lower with lithium than with lamotrigine (CI 30% fewer to 25% more). Relapse rates due to mania were 44% lower with lithium than with lamotrigine while relapse rates due to depression were 22% higher for lithium than for lamotrigine. Withdrawal rates due to an adverse event were 120% higher for lithium than for lamotrigine (CI 31–270%). In the aggregate, these results indicate that lamotrigine has marked efficacy compared with both placebo and lithium for prophylaxis of depression, but not mania. They also indicate superior tolerability to lithium.

Dosing

Lamotrigine should be titrated gradually to minimize the emergence of adverse events, particularly serious rash. Clinicians should initiate lamotrigine at 25 mg/day for the first two weeks, titrate to 50 mg/day for weeks 3 and 4, and then increase the dosage by 50 to 100 mg/wk to a target dose of 200 mg/day or as clinically indicated (Table 2) (49). If lamotrigine is part of a combination regimen involving carbamazepine, a powerful inducer of lamotrigine's clearance, the initiating dose of lamotrigine should be doubled and lamotrigine titration accelerated. When lamotrigine is added to ongoing treatment with valproate, an inhibitor of lamotrigine's clearance, lamotrigine should be initiated at 12.5 mg/day or 25 mg every other day for weeks 1 and 2 and the rate of titration should be slower.

Tolerability

Lamotrigine has a high tolerability profile and, in placebo controlled studies, did not appear to cause the switching or cycle acceleration associated with antidepressants (47). The most commonly reported adverse events in these studies included headache, ataxia, dizziness, tremors, nausea, somnolence, diplopia, and blurred vision (50–53). Lamotrigine is not associated with weight gain or sexual

TABLE 2 Initial Dosing Regimens of Lamotrigine

	Lamotrigine alone	Lamotrigine + valproate	Lamotrigine + carbamazepine
Weeks 1 and 2	25 mg q.d.	25 mg q.o.d. or 12.5 mg/day	25 mg b.i.d.
Weeks 3 and 4	50 mg q.d.	25 mg q.d.	50 mg b.i.d.
Week 5	100 mg q.d.	50 mg q.d.	100 mg b.i.d.
Week 6	200 mg q.d.	100 mg q.d.	150 mg b.i.d.
Week 7	—	—	200 mg b.i.d.

dysfunction and does not negatively impact cognitive functioning (47,54). In a published analysis of the rates of rash in 12 multicenter clinical trials involving 3,153 patients exposed to lamotrigine, 11.6% developed a benign rash while less than 0.1% developed a serious rash (47). The risk of developing a rash is increased with a dosage titration rate that is more rapid than recommended. In a recent study, there was no evidence that the risk of rash, either benign or serious, was increased when lamotrigine was added to ongoing valproate treatment, or when valproate was added to ongoing lamotrigine treatment if patients had been taking a steady dose of lamotrigine for at least two weeks prior to valproate addition (55). Oral contraceptives (e.g., ethinylestradiol and levonorgestrel) cause a significant decrease in serum trough levels of lamotrigine via estrogenic induction of glucuronidation (AUC by 52%, C_{max} by 39%) during the 21 days that the oral contraceptives are administered. The serum trough concentration of lamotrigine increases rapidly by twofold by the end of the "pill free" period (56). Consequently, the prophylactic efficacy of lamotrigine may be compromised when oral contraceptives are initiated in patients on a steady dose of lamotrigine. In addition, the risk of rash may be increased during the "pill free" period."

The FDA lists lamotrigine as a Pregnancy Category C drug. Category C refers to drugs that have not been studied. The 2005 Interim Report of the International Lamotrigine Pregnancy Registry reported data on the teratogenic potential of lamotrigine based on the frequency of birth defects seen in patients who were exposed to lamotrigine monotherapy during the first trimester of pregnancy (2.6%, 95% CI 1.7–3.8%) compared with a background rate estimated at 2% to 3% for patients with epilepsy (57). There was a significant increase in the rate of birth defects (11.9%, 95% CI 6.6–20.2%) among patients who were exposed to a combination regimen of lamotrigine and valproate. However, in those exposed to lamotrigine polytherapy that did not include valproate, the rate was 2.6% (05% CI 1.2–6.5%). These preliminary data indicate that lamotrigine exposure during the first trimester of pregnancy does not increase teratogenicity beyond 2% to 3% baseline rate seen in patients with epilepsy (2–3%). Since most data on teratogenicity for AEDs are derived from patients with epilepsy where AEDs dosages tend to be higher compared with dosages used in patients with bipolar disorder, extrapolations to the latter should be interpreted with caution (57).

CARBAMAZEPINE

Carbamazepine is a trycyclic compound with a broad spectrum of efficacy in epilepsy. Similar to valproate, its antimanic properties were noted through serendipitous observation. Less is known about its mechanisms of action, which do not appear to encompass most of those of lithium or valproate. Carbamazepine enhances GABAergic transmission and possesses antiglutamatergic properties (58). Two recent large randomized, placebo-controlled studies have established its efficacy in mania, though neither study included an active comparator (59,60). In addition, in the first study, carbamazepine was superior to placebo on change in mania score at day 21 only. No acute data beyond three weeks are available from randomized studies. One small, randomized, blind study provides comparative data. Valproate yielded significantly greater and earlier improvement than carbamazepine and proved superior to carbamazepine on four mania scale items— elevated mood, irritability, speech disturbance, and thought disturbance (18). Carbamazepine did not prove superior to valproate on any of the manic items and more carbamazepine-treated patients required rescue medications. Rates of adverse events were four times higher for carbamazepine than those for valproate.

Maintenance Treatment

One maintenance study enrolled 94 bipolar patients who were randomized to carbamazepine or lithium either during an acute mood episode ("acutely randomized," $N = 41$) or at entry into the maintenance phase of the study ("prophylactically randomized," $N = 53$). Lithium was significantly superior to carbamazepine in delaying time to treatment for a new episode in both patient groups (61). In an open randomized study, time to a new episode or discontinuation for other reasons was significantly longer for lithium than for carbamazepine (62). Among patients with bipolar II disorder, with small samples of 28 and 29 subjects treated with lithium and carbamazepine respectively, there was no significant differences in time to discontinuation for any protocol defined reason (63). One small study of 22 subjects compared carbamazepine with placebo. No differences in rates of efficacy between carbamazepine and placebo were found (64). One study compared rates of withdrawal for any reason for carbamazepine or lithium-treated patients, and found 32% fewer withdrawals for any reason with lithium than with carbamazepine (65). Taken in the aggregate, there are insufficient data to recommend carbamazepine for maintenance treatment of bipolar disorder unless other treatments with more robust evidence have failed. Additionally, although the studies are of limited methodological clarity, the available data suggest that carbamazepine is inferior to lithium and valproate.

Dosage and Serum Level Monitoring

Dosing of carbamazepine is essentially empirical, based on patient tolerability and response. Carbamazepine's induction of its own metabolism and its adverse effects on the CNS, particularly in the early course of treatment, warrants that it be started at low doses, in the treatment of both bipolar disorder and epilepsy, and increased gradually until response or adverse events ensue. Initial dosing is generally started at 100 to 200 mg b.i.d. and increased as needed to a dosage up to 1200 mg/day, usually given in divided dosages (Table 1). The recent availability of extended release formulations (e.g., Equetro) offers the advantages of less frequent dosing and fewer side effects (e.g., psychomotor disturbances), which are partially linked to peak serum levels. No studies specifically focused on dosing or correlating serum level and response in the maintenance treatment of bipolar disorder, however, have been published.

Tolerability

Carbamazepine's role, both in the acute and maintenance treatment phases of bipolar disorder, is significantly limited by its adverse event profile. The side effects associated with carbamazepine are attributed to its major metabolite, carbamazepine-epoxide (16,66). The discontinuation rate due to adverse events in a randomized, double-blind, crossover maintenance study was higher in the carbamazepine group (22%) than in the lithium group (4%) (67). Dose related side effects with carbamazepine include dizziness, sedation, ataxia, diplopia, and nystagmus (68). Agranulocytosis and aplastic anemia, both idiosyncratic in nature, are seen in 1 per 10,000 to 100,000 patients treated with carbamazepine. Benign and transient leucopenia are observed in 10% of patients; thrombocytopenia and sustained leucopenia are both seen in 2% of patients. Mild hyponatremia caused by carbamazepine may manifest more seriously in the geriatric or medically ill patient subgroups. Carbamazepine is associated with a benign rash in 10% of patients, which may be the harbinger of a life threatening Stevens-Johnson syndrome. By inducing the cytochrome P450 enzymes, particularly P450-3A4, carbamazepine lowers the plasma levels of other drugs, including other AEDs (valproate, lamotrigine, zonisamide, topiramate, phenytoin, and oxcarbazepine), antipsychotics (aripiprazole, clozapine, haloperidol, olanzapine, risperidone, and ziprasidone), antidepressants (bupropion, citalopram, and tricyclic antidepressants), anxiolytics/sedatives (buspirone, clonazepam, and alprazolam), stimulants (methylphenidate, modafinil), and oral contraceptives (68,69). As a result, higher doses of some medications, such as oral contraceptives, need to be administered when they are taken concomitantly with carbamazepine to maintain continued efficacy.

Other AEDs with Reported use in Bipolar Disorder

Several other AEDs have had case reports and/or small open-label studies suggesting long-term effectiveness in bipolar disorder. These include phenytoin, oxcarbazepine, topiramate, levetiracetam, gabapentin, vigabatrin, and zonisamide. Unless future evidence of long-term efficacy and tolerability in bipolar disorder are published, the use of any of these agents for maintenance treatment of bipolar disorder is not recommended.

CONCLUSION

In recent years, several AEDs have been investigated for their potential mood-stabilizing properties. These drugs are characterized by heterogeneity, both in regards to mechanisms of action and possessing differential efficacy in the various mood states of bipolar disorder. Among the AEDs, only valproate, lamotrigine, and carbamazepine have been rigorously studied for prophylaxis in bipolar disorder. Evidence from well-controlled studies support the role of valproate and lamotrigine for specific, but not necessarily broad, use in maintenance treatment of bipolar disorder. Importantly, both drugs show better tolerability than lithium in randomized blind studies.

The last decade has seen significant improvement in our understanding of bipolar disorder. A wider therapeutic armamentarium is needed as a large proportion of bipolar patients have frequent relapses and recurrences during long-term treatment. As additional AEDs become available, rigorously designed studies examining the safety and efficacy of monotherapeutic and combination strategies of these agents in the long-term treatment of bipolar disorder should be employed to better guide the practicing clinician in providing evidence-based treatments for patients with this disabling illness.

REFERENCES

1. Swann AC, Bowden CL, Calabrese JR, et al. Pattern of response to divalproex, lithium, or placebo in four naturalistic subtypes of mania. Neuropsychopharmacology 2002; 26(4): 530–536.
2. Janowsky DS, Morter S, Hong L, et al. Myers Briggs Type Indicator and tridimensional personality questionnaire differences between bipolar patients and unipolar depressed patients. Bipolar Disord 1999; 1(2):98–108.

3. Sachs GS. Bipolar mood disorder: practical strategies for acute and maintenance phase treatment. J Clin Psychopharmacol 1996; 16(suppl 1):32S–47S.
4. Bowden CL, Swann AC, Calabrese JR, et al. Maintenance clinical trials in bipolar disorder: design implications of the divalproex-lithium-placebo study. Psychopharmacol Bull 1997; 33(4):693–699.
5. Bowden CL, Brugger AM, Swann AC, et al. Efficacy of divalproex vs. lithium and placebo in the treatment of mania. JAMA 1994; 271:918–924.
6. Hahn CG, Umapathy, Wang HY, Koneru R, et al. Lithium and valproic acid treatments reduce PKC activation and receptor-G protein coupling in platelets of bipolar manic patients. J Psychiatr Res 2005; 39(4):355–363.
7. Einat H, Yuan P, Gould TD, et al. The role of the extracellular signal-regulated kinase signaling pathway in mood modulation. J Neurosci 2003; 23(19):7311–7316.
8. Gray NA, Zhou R, Du J, et al. The use of mood stabilizers as plasticity enhancers in the treatment of neuropsychiatric disorders. J Clin Psychiatry 2003; 64(suppl 5):3–17.
9. Andreazza AC, Frey BN, Stertz L, et al. Effects of lithium and valproate on DNA damage and oxidative stress markers in an animal model of mania. Bipolar Disord 2007; 9(S1):16.
10. Dokucu ME, Yu L, Taghert PH. Lithium- and valproate-induced alterations in circadian locomotor behavior in Drosophila. Neuropsychopharmacology 2005; 30(12):2216–2224.
11. Einat H, Manji HK. Cellular plasticity cascades: genes-to-behavior pathways in animal models of bipolar disorder. Biol Psychiatry 2006; 59(12):1160–1171.
12. Shaltiel G, Shamir A, Shapior J, et al. Valproate decreases inositol biosynthesis. Biol Psychiatry 2004; 56:868–874.
13. Harwood AJ, Agam G. Search for a common mechanism of mood stabilizers. Biochem Pharmacol 2003; 66(2):179–189.
14. Bowden CL. Valproate in mania: from Pierre Lambert to New Delhi Study. Neuropsychopharmacology 2006; 16(S4):S587.
15. McElroy SL, Keck PE, Stanton SP, et al. A randomized comparison of divalproex oral loading versus haloperidol in the initial treatment of acute psychotic mania. J Clin Psychiatry 1996; 57:142–146.
16. Zajecka JM, Weisler R, Sachs G, et al. A comparison of the efficacy, safety, and tolerability of divalproex sodium and olanzapine in the treatment of bipolar disorder. J Clin Psychiatry 2002; 63:1148–1155.
17. Tohen M, Ketter TA, Zarate CA. Olanzapine versus divalproex sodium for the treatment of acute mania and maintenance of remission: a 47-week study. Am J Psychiatry 2003; 160:1263–1271.
18. Vasudev K, Goswami U, Kohli K. Carbamazepine and valproate monotherapy: feasibility, relative safety and efficacy, and therapeutic drug monitoring in manic disorder. Psychopharmacology 2000; 150:15–23.
19. Sachs G, Grossman F, Okamoto A, et al. Risperidone plus mood stabilizer versus. placebo plus mood stabilizer for acute mania of bipolar disorder: a double-blind comparison of efficacy and safety. Am J Psychiatry 2002; 159:1146–1156.
20. Yatham LN, Grossman F, Augustyns I, et al. Mood stabilisers plus risperidone or placebo in the treatment of acute mania. International, double-blind, randomised controlled trial. Br J Psychiatry 2003; 182:141–147.
21. Muller-Oerlinghausen B, Retzow A, Henn FA, et al. Valproate as an adjunct to neuroleptic medication for the treatment of acute episodes of mania: a prospective, randomized, double-blind, placebo-controlled, multicenter study. J Clin Psychopharmacol 2000; 20(2):195–203.
22. Bowden CL, Calabrese JR, McElroy SL, et al. A randomized, placebo-controlled 12-month trial of divalproex and lithium in treatment of outpatients with bipolar I disorder. Arch Gen Psychiatry 2000; 57:481–489.
23. Gyulai L, Bowden CL, McElroy SL, et al. Maintenance efficacy of divalproex in the prevention of bipolar depression. Neuropsychopharmacology 2003; 28(7):1374–1382.
24. Bowden CL. Valproate. Bipolar Disord 2003; 5:189–202.

25. Lambert PA, Venaud G. Comparative study of valpromide versus. lithium as prophylactic treatment in affective disorders. Nervure 1992; 5(2):57–65.
26. Smith LA, Cornelius V, Warnock A, et al. Effectiveness of mood stabilizers and anti-psychotics in the maintenance phase of bipolar disorder: a systematic review of randomized controlled trials. Bipolar Disord 2007; 9(4):394–412.
27. Calabrese JR, Shelton MD, Rapport DJ, et al. A 20-month, double-blind, maintenance trial of lithium versus divalproex in rapid-cycling bipolar disorder. Am J Psychiatry 2005; 162(11):2152–2161.
28. Tohen M, Chengappa KN, Suppes T, et al. Relapse prevention in bipolar I disorder: 18-month comparison of olanzapine plus mood stabiliser vs mood stabiliser alone. Br J Psychiatry 2004; 184(4):337–345.
29. Solomon DA, Ryan CE, Keitner GI, et al. A pilot study of lithium carbonate plus divalproex sodium for the continuation and maintenance treatment of patients with bipolar I disorder. J Clin Psychiatry 1997; 58(3):95–99.
30. Deltito JA, Levitan J, Damore J, et al. Naturalistic experience with the use of divalproex sodium on an in-patient unit for adolescent psychiatric patients. Acta Psychiatr Scand 1998; 97(3):236–240.
31. Mandoki MW. Valproate-lithium combination and verapamil as treatments of bipolar disorder in children and adolescents. Neuropsychopharmacology 1993; 9(suppl):183S.
32. Papatheodorou G, Kutcher SP. Divalproex sodium treatment in late adolescent and young adult acute mania. Psychopharmacol Bull 1993; 29:213–219 (abstr).
33. Wagner KD, Weller E, Carlson G, et al. An open-label trial of divalproex in children and adolescents with bipolar disorder. J Am Acad Child Adolesc Psychiatry 2002; 41(10): 1224–1230.
34. Kowatch RA, Suppes T, Carmody TJ, et al. Effect size of lithium, divalproex sodium, and carbamazepine in children and adolescents with bipolar disorder. J Am Acad Child Adolesc Psychiatry 2000; 39(6):713–720.
35. Porsteinsson AP, Tariot PN, Erb R, et al. Placebo-controlled study of divalproex sodium for agitation in dementia. Am J Geriatr Psychiatry 2001; 9(1):58–66.
36. McFarland BH, Miller MR, Straumfjord AA. Valproate use in the older manic patient. J Clin Psychiatry 1990; 51:479–481.
37. Narayan N, Nelson J. Treatment of dementia with behavioral disturbance using divalproex or a combination of divalproex and a neuroleptic. J Clin Psychiatry 1997; 58(8): 351–354.
38. Niedermier JA, Nasrallah HA. Clinical correlates of response to valproate in geriatric inpatients. Ann Clin Psychiatry 1998; 10(4):165–168.
39. Bowden CL, Janicak PG, Orsulak P, et al. Relation of serum valproate concentration to response in mania. Am J Psychiatry 1996; 153(6):765–770.
40. Petty F, Davis LL, Nugent AL, et al. Valproate therapy for chronic, combat-induced postraumatic stress disorder. J Clin Psychopharmacol 2002; 22(1):100–101.
41. Pope HG Jr., McElroy SL, Keck PE Jr., et al. Valproate in the treatment of acute mania: a placebo-controlled study. Arch Gen Psychiatry 1991; 48:62–68.
42. Keck PE Jr., Bowden CL, Meinhold JM, et al. Relationship between serum valproate and lithium levels and efficacy and tolerability in bipolar maintenance therapy. Int J Psychiatry Clin Pract 2005; 9(4):271–277.
43. DeVane CL. Pharmacokinetics, drug interactions, and tolerability of valproate. Psychopharmacol Bull 2003; 37(S2):25–42.
44. Acharya S, Bussel JB. Hematologic toxicity of sodium valproate. J Pediatr Hematol Oncol 2000; 22(1):62–65.
45. Bowden CL, Calabrese JR, Sachs G, et al. A placebo-controlled 18-month trial of lamotrigine and lithium maintenance treatment in recently manic or hypomanic patients with bipolar I disorder. Arch Gen Psychiatry 2003; 60:392–400.
46. Calabrese JR, Bowden CL, Sachs G, et al. A placebo-controlled 18-month trial of lamotrigine and lithium maintenance treatment in recently depressed patients with bipolar I disorder. J Clin Psychiatry 2003; 64:1013–1024.

47. Calabrese JR, Vieta E, Shelton MD. Latest maintenance data on lamotrigine in bipolar disorder. Eur Neuropsychopharmacol 2003; 13:S57–S66.
48. Calabrese JR, Suppes T, Bowden CL, et al. A double-blind placebo-controlled prophylaxis study of lamotrigine in rapid cycling bipolar disorder. J Clin Psychiatry 2000; 61: 841–850.
49. GlaxoSmithKline. 2001. GlaxoSmithKline, Five Moore Drive, RTP, North Carolina 27709.
50. Wang PW, Ketter TA, Becker OV, et al. New anticonvulsant medication uses in bipolar disorder. CNS Spectr 2003; (12):941–947.
51. Muzina DJ, El-Sayegh S, Calabrese JR. Antiepileptic drugs in psychiatry-focus on randomized controlled trial. Epilepsy Res 2002; 50(1–2):195–202.
52. Physicians' Desk Reference. 59th ed. Montvale, NJ: Thomson PDR, 2005.
53. Van Parys JA, Meinardi H. Survey of 260 epileptic patients treated with oxcarbazepine (Trileptal) on a named-patient basis. Epilepsy Res 1994; 19(1):79–85.
54. Bowden CL, Calabrese JR, Ketter TA, et al. Impact of lamotrigine and lithium on weight in obese and nonobese patients with bipolar I disorder. Am J Psychiatry 2006; 163(7): 1199–1201.
55. Singh V, Bowden C. Mixed states (MS) as predictors of polarity of relapse in bipolar disorder (BD). Presented at the American College of Neuropsychology in Hollywood, Florida, 2006 (abstr).
56. Johannessen SI, Battino D, Berry DJ, et al. Therapeutic drug monitoring of the newer antiepileptic drugs. Ther Drug Monit 2003; 25(3):347–363.
57. GlaxoSmithKline. 2007. Lamotrigine Pregnancy Registry. Interim Report. 1 September 1992 through 31 March 2007, issued July 2007. Available at: http://pregnancyregistry .gsk.com/index.html.
58. Bowden CL. Carbamazepine in bipolar disorder. In: Goodnick PJ, ed. Predictors of Treatment Response in Mood Disorders. Washington, DC: American Psychiatric Press, 1996:119–132.
59. Weisler RH, Keck PE Jr., Swann AC, et al. Extended-release carbamazepine capsules as monotherapy for acute mania in bipolar disorder: a multicenter, randomized, double-blind, placebo-controlled trial. J Clin Psychiatry 2005; 66(3):323–330.
60. Weisler RH, Kalali AH, Ketter TA, and SPD417 Study Group. A Multicenter, Randomized, Double-Blind, Placebo-Controlled Trial of extended-release carbamazepine capsules as monotherapy for bipolar disorder patients with manic or mixed episodes. J Clin Psychiatry 2004; 65:478–484.
61. Hartong EG, Moleman P, Hoogduin CA, et al. Prophylactic efficacy of lithium versus carbamazepine in treatment-naive bipolar patients. J Clin Psychiatry 2003; 64(2):144–151.
62. Greil W, Kleindienst N. The comparative prophylactic efficacy of lithium and carbamazepine in patients with bipolar I disorder. Int Clin Psychopharmacol 1999; 14(5):277–281.
63. Greil W, Kleindienst N. Lithium versus carbamazepine in the maintenance treatment of bipolar II disorder and bipolar disorder not otherwise specified. Int Clin Psychopharmacol 1999; 14(5):283–285.
64. Okuma T, Inanage K, Otsuki S, et al. A preliminary double-blind study on the efficacy of carbamazepine in prophylaxis of manic-depressive illness. Psychopharmacology 1981; 73: 95–96.
65. Greil W, Ludwig-Mayerhofer W, Erazo N, et al. Lithium versus carbamazepine in the maintenance treatment of bipolar disorders—a randomised study. J Affect Disord 2007; 43(2):151–161.
66. Freeman TW, Clothier JL, Pazzaglia P, et al. A double-blind comparison of valproate and lithium in the treatment of acute mania. Am J Psychiatry 1992; 149:108–111.
67. Denicoff KD, Smith-Jackson EE, Disney ER, et al. Preliminary evidence of the reliability and validity of the prospective life-chart methodology (LCM-p). J Clin Psychiatry 1997; 58: 470–478.
68. Ketter TA, Wang PW, Post RM. Carbamazepine and oxcarbazepine. In: Schatzberg AF, Nemeroff CB, eds. The American Psychiatric Publishing Textbook of Psychopharmacology 3rd ed. Washington, DC, London, England: American Psychiatric Publishing, Inc., 2004:581–606.

69. Hellewell JS. Oxcarbazepine (Trileptal) in the treatment of bipolar disorders: review of efficacy and tolerability. J Affect Disord 2002; 72(S1):S23–S34.
70. Fischer JH, Patel TV, Fischer PA. Fosphenytoin: clinical pharmacokinetics and comparative advantages in the acute treatment of seizures. Clin Pharmacokinet 2003; 42(1): 33–58.
71. Chengappa KN, Gerhson S, Levine J. The evolving role of topiramate among other mood stabilizers in the management of bipolar disorder. Bipolar Disord 2001; 3(5):215–232.

9 | Antiepileptic Drugs in the Treatment of Rapid-Cycling Bipolar Disorder and Bipolar Depression

David E. Kemp, Keming Gao, and Joseph R. Calabrese
Bipolar Disorders Center for Intervention and Services Research, Case Western Reserve University, Cleveland, Ohio, U.S.A.

David J. Muzina
Cleveland Clinic Psychiatry and Psychology, Cleveland, Ohio, U.S.A.

INTRODUCTION

In 1974, Dunner and Fieve described a variant of bipolar disorder marked by extensive mood fluctuations, giving rise to the concept of rapid cycling (1). Now incorporated into our current diagnostic nomenclature, rapid cycling is defined by the DSM-IV (Diagnostic and Statistical Manual of Mental Disorders, 4th Edition) as the occurrence of four or more mood episodes during a 12-month period, inclusive of mixed episodes, mania, hypomania, or major depression. Over the past 30 years, rapid cycling as a modifier of the course of bipolar disorder has been substantiated by differences in gender, bipolar subtype, propensity for thyroid dysfunction, and prospectively defined outcomes (2–6). It is now recognized that patients with rapid cycling must contend with an earlier age of mood disorder onset, a higher lifetime number of mood episodes, and greater mood episode severity (2). In fact, compared with their non-rapid-cycling counterparts, patients with rapid-cycling experience eight times more depressive and nine times more hypomanic/manic episodes over a 12-month period (4).

Given the increased affective morbidity associated with rapid cycling, at-risk patients should be identified and treated with interventions intended to stabilize mood from both the manic and depressive poles. Considered the hallmark of rapid cycling, major depressive episodes are the most prevalent, persistent, and difficult-to-treat illness dimension (7). Although antiepileptic drugs (AEDs) have traditionally been regarded as "mood stabilizers," the rationale to support their use in bipolar disorder has primarily been derived from the treatment of mania. However, there is growing evidence to support the use of certain AEDs in the acute and long-term treatment of bipolar depression. This chapter will review both rapid-cycling bipolar disorder and bipolar depression, highlighting their often-coupled clinical presentation and more treatment refractory course. The results of randomized clinical trials involving AEDs will be reviewed in order to translate research findings into clinically meaningful approaches to patient care.

RAPID-CYCLING BIPOLAR DISORDER

The occurrence of rapid cycling is neither rare nor inconsequential. Approximately one in five patients presents with a rapid-cycling pattern, and its prevalence is estimated to range from 13% to 56% (8). Historically, females and individuals with bipolar II disorder were believed to account for the majority of rapid-cycling cases

(3,5,7–9), though recent studies have begun to question the higher association with bipolar II disorder (2,4). A Systematic Treatment Enhancement Program for Bipolar Disorder (STEP-BD) report found equal rates of rapid cycling occurring among patients diagnosed with either bipolar subtype (4), while a prospective study of 539 outpatients found a higher occurrence of rapid cycling in patients with bipolar I (41.3%) as compared with bipolar II (27.9%) disorder (2). Regardless of subtype predominance, the continuous mood cycling uniformly suggests greater illness severity, including a heightened risk for attempted suicide. Data from our prospectively collected cohort of 564 patients with rapid-cycling bipolar disorder demonstrate that 41% have attempted suicide, with the highest prevalence among those with comorbid substance use disorders (10). Although there is no direct evidence to substantiate higher rates of completed suicide in rapid-cycling patients, longitudinal data from the National Institute of Mental Health Collaborative Depression Study indicate that patients with rapid-cycling bipolar disorder are more than twice as likely as non-rapid-cycling patients to attempt suicide (11).

Antiepileptic Drugs in the Treatment of Rapid Cycling
Lithium and Carbamazepine
In 1980, Kukopulos et al. (12) identified one of the earliest disease features to be associated with rapid cycling, namely, a poor response to lithium prophylaxis. In this report, inadequate lithium response occurred in 84% (42/50) of patients who received treatment for more than one year. Likewise, a five-year prospective study of patients with bipolar I disorder found an absence of rapid cycling in good responders to lithium but a 26% incidence among nonresponders (13). Over time, accumulating reports revealed that more than 70% of patients respond poorly or only partially to lithium (14), and a need was realized for pharmacologic agents more effective at managing the rapid-cycling variant.

To meet this need, investigators shifted from the study of lithium and began to explore agents in the anticonvulsant drug class. Endeavoring to find more effective treatments, carbamazepine was selected as the first anticonvulsant to be specifically studied in rapid cycling. One early report suggested carbamazepine possessed antimanic properties (15). However, a year later, results from an open-label study showed that while carbamazepine was effective for a select group of rapid-cycling patients, the majority did not demonstrate a robust response (16). Furthermore, a retrospective study of 215 bipolar patients identified that a history of rapid cycling or circular continuous cycling was a predictor of poor response not only to lithium but to carbamazepine as well (17).

In contrast, to use in monotherapy, carbamazepine may be better suited for the treatment of rapid cycling when used in conjunction with another mood stabilizer. When used alone, carbamazepine has demonstrated a 19% rate of response, but when combined with lithium, the response rate rose to 56% (18). In this same study, lithium monotherapy was associated with a disappointing 28% rate of response. Despite the added improvement when using carbamazepine in combination with lithium, this drug regimen remains limited in its ability to achieve mood stabilization for nearly half of all subjects.

Valproate
On the basis of preliminary open data, Calabrese et al. hypothesized that the AED valproate may be efficacious for the treatment of rapid cycling. In order to test this

theory, a homogenous cohort of 101, prospectively defined rapid-cycling bipolar outpatients were administered valproate either as monotherapy or adjunctive therapy for up to 17.2 months (14,19). Seventy-seven percent of patients were found to demonstrate a marked antimanic response with valproate. However, only 38% showed a prophylactic effect against new depressive episodes. In total, marked prophylactic responses were seen in 72% of manic, 94% of mixed-state, and 33% of depressed patients. These results suggest that valproate is better suited to treat mania and mixed states in rapid cycling and offers only minimal to moderate efficacy in treating depression.

For the next 12 years, the belief that valproate and other AEDs were superior to lithium at treating rapid cycling was commonplace, but it was not until 2005 that a head-to-head, randomized, double-blind, parallel-group trial of lithium and valproate (as divalproex) was conducted to objectively compare outcomes (20). In this trial, patients were eligible for enrollment if they were diagnosed with rapid-cycling bipolar I or II disorder and had a history of at least one episode of mania, hypomania, or a mixed state within the past three months. Patients were first stabilized for up to six months with the open-label combination of lithium and divalproex, and any additional psychotropic medications were slowly weaned over a three-month period. Subjects were then eligible for randomization into the double-blind, maintenance phase upon meeting the following criteria: a 24-item Hamilton Depression Rating Scale (HAM-D) score less than or equal to 20, a Global Assessment Scale score greater than of equal to 51, a Young Mania Rating Scale (YMRS) score less than or equal to 12, lithium levels greater than or equal to 0.8 mEq/L, and valproate levels greater than or equal to 50 µg/mL for a minimum of four consecutive weeks. This trial design ensured that patients tolerated both treatments and were experiencing only mild-to-moderate symptoms of hypomania and/or depression prior to entering the maintenance phase; by definition, they were in partial remission. Upon meeting these eligibility criteria, patients were randomly assigned to treatment with either lithium or divalproex monotherapy and were followed for up to 20 months.

Of the 254 patients entering the initial stabilization phase of the trial, 65 (26%) did not respond to the combination of lithium and divalproex, with the majority exhibiting symptoms of refractory depression. Sixty patients (24%) completed the stabilization phase and underwent randomization to double-blind maintenance monotherapy (lithium: $N = 32$, divalproex: $N = 28$). For these patients, the mean lithium level was 0.92 mEq/L (dose range 900–2100 mg/day) and the mean valproate level was 77 µg/mL (dose range 750–2750 mg/day), respectively.

No significant difference between the lithium and divalproex groups was found on the primary outcome measure of time to treatment for emerging symptoms of relapse (Fig. 1). Likewise, no significant difference was observed in time to premature discontinuation for any reason, time to treatment for depression, or time to treatment for a manic/hypomanic/mixed episode.

Divalproex-treated patients experienced lower rates of tremors and polyuria/polydipsia, but no difference in discontinuations due to adverse events was found between treatment groups. Overall survival in the study was low, with only 16% of lithium-treated and 29% of divalproex-treated patients completing the 20-month maintenance phase. For a monotherapy study conducted over 20 months' duration, the low completion rates were surprising but consistent with a 12-month maintenance study comparing divalproex and lithium monotherapy, where 38% of divalproex-treated and 24% of lithium-treated patients completed the trial (21).

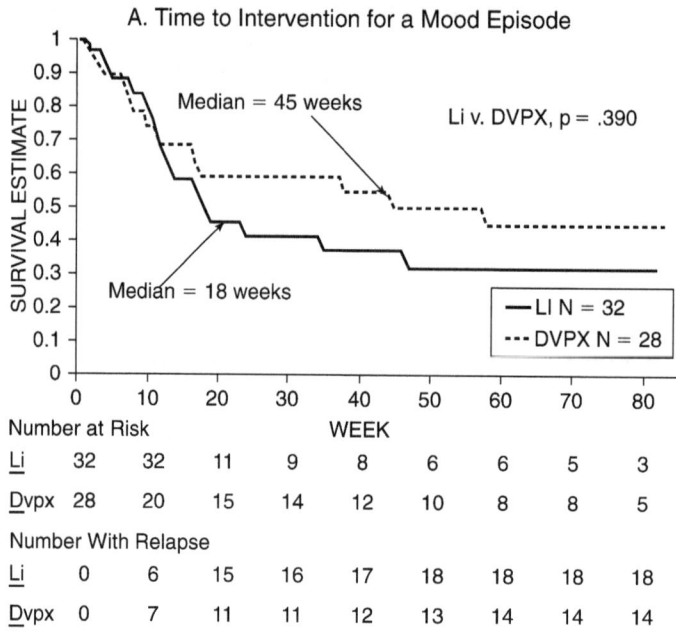

Number at Risk

Li	32	32	11	9	8	6	6	5	3
Dvpx	28	20	15	14	12	10	8	8	5

Number With Relapse

Li	0	6	15	16	17	18	18	18	18
Dvpx	0	7	11	11	12	13	14	14	14

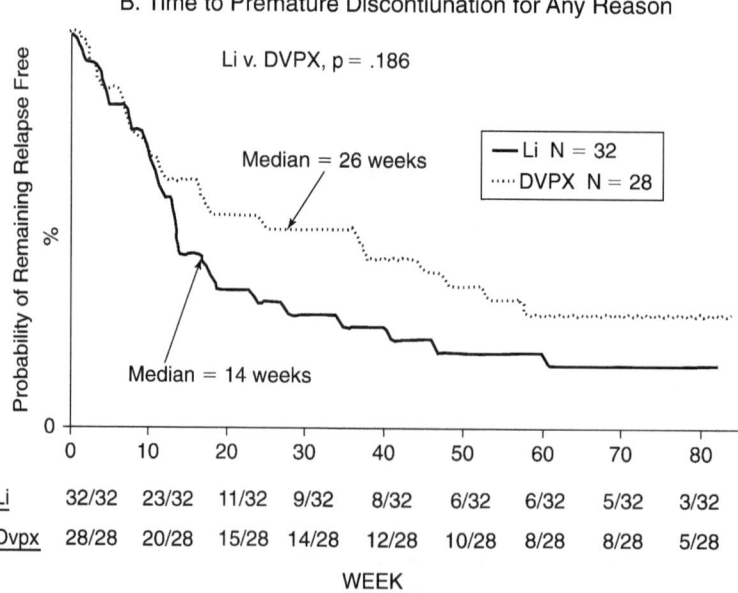

Li	32/32	23/32	11/32	9/32	8/32	6/32	6/32	5/32	3/32
Dvpx	28/28	20/28	15/28	14/28	12/28	10/28	8/28	8/28	5/28

WEEK

FIGURE 1 (**A**) and (**B**) Time to treatment intervention for any mood episode and time to study discontinuation among stabilized rapid-cycling bipolar disorder patients randomly assigned to double-blind maintenance monotherapy with lithium or divalproex. *Source*: From Ref. 20.

The results of this study did not confirm prior notions that valproate would be more effective than lithium in rapid-cycling bipolar disorder. As the observed treatment effect between valproate and lithium was small, the study was underpowered to detect a significant difference between agents. The estimated hazard ratio of 0.74 (95% CI = 0.36 to 1.49) reflected a need for 364 patients per study arm, substantially higher than the cumulative enrollment of 60 patients in the actual study.

Despite this limitation, the results pertain to treatment with two commonly used mood stabilizers and are generalizable to clinical practice. The up to six-month stabilization period and requirement that patients demonstrate continued improvement over four consecutive weeks prior to maintenance-phase randomization ensured that results would represent a true prophylactic effect of lithium or valproate monotherapy, as opposed to the effect of discontinuation of prestudy medications or relapse back into the index mood episode. The 20-month maintenance phase is the longest duration ever studied in a population of rapid cyclers and allowed for the assessment of recurrence over a meaningful time period. Perhaps of greatest relevance to clinicians is the realization that the combination of valproate and lithium will not be adequate for the majority of rapid-cycling patients. Most cases of mood episode nonresponse were due to refractory depressive symptoms. This reinforces observations that depression is the most common presentation of rapid-cycling bipolar disorder and raises awareness that novel compounds to treat and prevent rapid-cycling depressive states continue to be urgently needed.

With the results of this trial in hand, it becomes more apparent that the early studies of lithium suffered a design flaw by comparing lithium only to placebo. In order to truly gauge lithium's efficacy in the treatment of rapid cycling, it would need to be contrasted with an active comparator as accomplished in the Calabrese et al. study (20). Thus, the early lithium trials were accurate in detecting that rapid cycling is an indicator of difficult-to-treat illness, but lacked adequate assay sensitivity by not comparing lithium to agents within the anticonvulsant drug class (17,22). In support of this conclusion, a post hoc analysis of a 47-week maintenance study comparing the atypical antipsychotic olanzapine to divalproex in manic or mixed rapid-cycling patients found no difference in efficacy between treatments (23). Among the divalproex-treated patients, improvement in YMRS scores were initially better in rapid- than non-rapid-cycling patients, but this difference was only maintained during the first two study weeks.

Lamotrigine

During its clinical development for epilepsy, the AED lamotrigine was shown to exert positive effects on mood (24). Reports of efficacy in treatment-resistant bipolar disorder (25), bipolar depression (26), and open-label data suggesting benefit in rapid cycling (27) led to the evaluation of lamotrigine monotherapy for the long-term prophylaxis of mood episodes in patients with rapid-cycling bipolar disorder (28). This study was the first placebo-controlled assessment of any medication in a prospectively defined group of patients with rapid-cycling bipolar disorder.

The trial consisted of two phases: a preliminary, open-label stabilization phase and a randomized, double-blind continuation phase. Initially, patients received the addition of lamotrigine (titrated to between 100 and 300 mg/day) to their current psychotropic medication regimen. After four to eight weeks of lamotrigine exposure, all concomitant medications were tapered and discontinued. Subjects tolerating open-label lamotrigine with a HAM-D score less than or equal to 14 and a Mania Rating Scale (MRS) score less than or equal to 12 over a two-week period were randomized to lamotrigine or placebo for up to 26 weeks. Of 342 patients entering the preliminary phase, 182 patients were randomized to the continuation phase.

Time to additional pharmacotherapy to treat an emerging mood episode, the primary outcome measure, did not differ between groups. Median survival times were 18 weeks for lamotrigine-treated and 12 weeks for placebo-treated subjects (Fig. 2). However, when overall survival in the study was examined, lamotrigine-treated subjects remained in treatment significantly longer than those taking placebo (lamotrigine = 14 weeks vs. placebo = 8 weeks; p = 0.036). For patients requiring additional pharmacotherapy, 80% necessitated treatment for depressive symptoms. A comparison between patients with bipolar I and II disorder found that the bipolar II subgroup treated with lamotrigine survived significantly longer; namely 17 weeks, in contrast to 7 weeks for placebo-treated patients (p = 0.015). No drug-placebo difference in survival was detected for patients with bipolar I disorder. When assessing patients who remained stable without relapse for six months, a greater percentage were treated with lamotrigine (41%, 37/90) compared with placebo (26%, 23/87; p = 0.04). Once again, a statistical difference was observed among the bipolar II (46% vs. 18%; p = 0.04), but not the bipolar I, cohort.

A statistical difference favoring lamotrigine over placebo in both study survival and prevention of relapse suggests a differential effectiveness in patients with bipolar II compared to bipolar I disorder. The finding is intriguing, given that a controlled trial found lamotrigine to be superior to placebo for treating depressive symptoms in bipolar I disorder (26). Part of the difference may be attributable to the high placebo response observed in the patients with bipolar I disorder. Another explanation is that the lack of strong prophylactic antimanic effects with lamotrigine undermines its usefulness as a monotherapy in patients with rapid cycling. Overall, the results of this study support the use of lamotrigine as monotherapy for the treatment of rapid-cycling bipolar disorder, but primarily for patients with the bipolar II subtype.

Lamotrigine has also been evaluated in a double-blind, randomized, placebo-controlled, crossover study with the AED gabapentin (29). The sample consisted of 31 patients with refractory mood disorders treated successively with lamotrigine, gabapentin, or placebo for six weeks. Rapid-cycling patients composed 92% of the population, most of whom were diagnosed with bipolar I (11/31) or bipolar II (14/31) disorder. A significantly greater percentage of patients responded to lamotrigine compared to gabapentin or placebo as indicated by a Clinical Global Impressions Scale modified for bipolar disorder (CGI-BP) score of much or very much improved. Fifty-two percent (16/31) of lamotrigine-treated patients met

---

FIGURE 2 Survival curves indicating length of study participation for bipolar I (N = 125) and II (N = 52) subtypes treated with lamotrigine compared with placebo. **(A)** Bipolar I patients who withdrew when they required additional pharmacotherapy for emerging mood symptoms. **(B)** Bipolar I patients who prematurely withdrew from the study for any reason (including additional pharmacotherapy for emerging mood symptoms). **(C)** Bipolar II patients who withdrew when they required additional pharmacotherapy for emerging mood symptoms. **(D)** Bipolar II patients who prematurely withdrew from the study for any reason (including additional pharmacotherapy for emerging mood symptoms). *Source*: From Ref. 28.

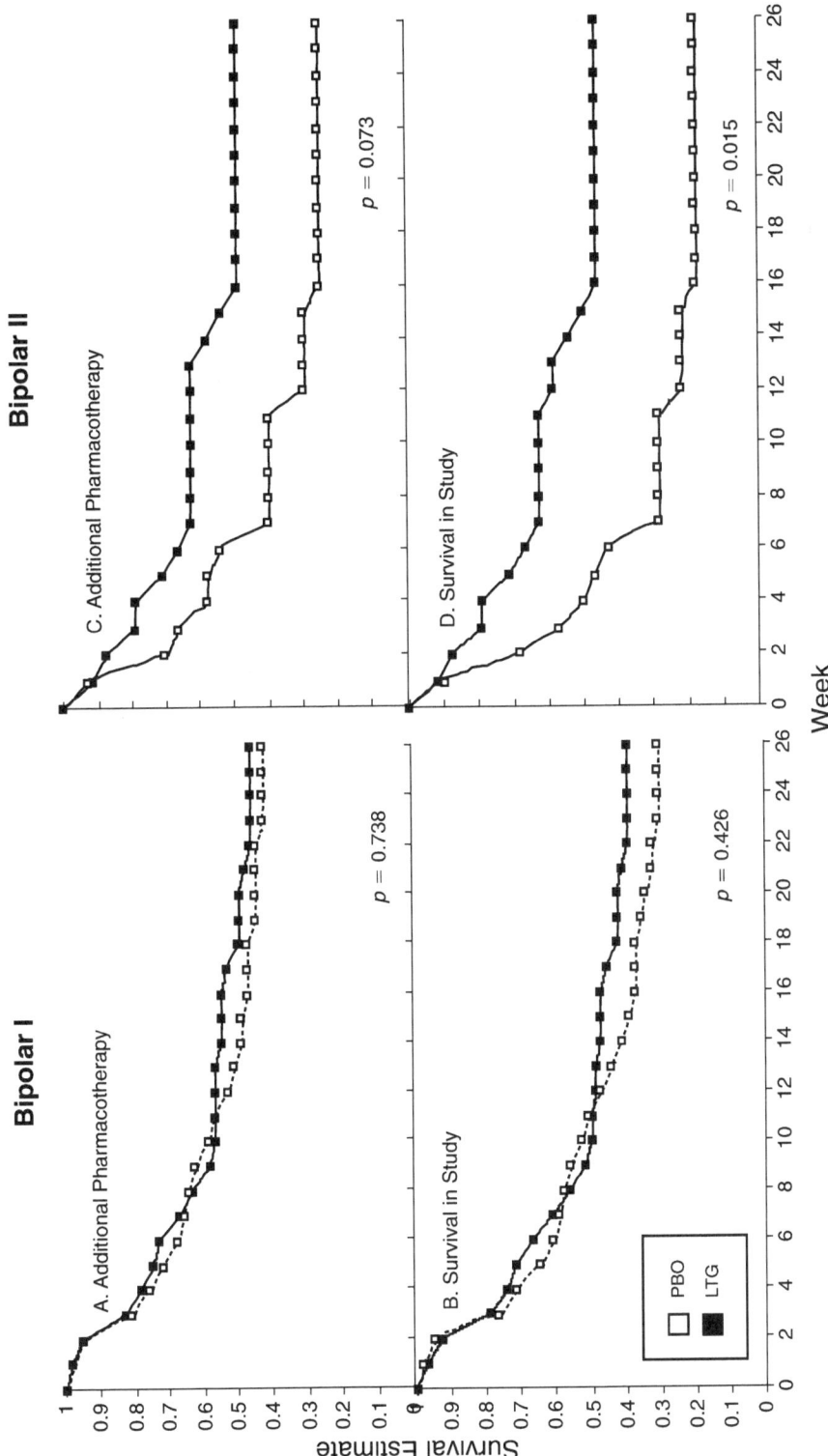

response criteria, compared with 26% (8/31) treated with gabapentin and 23% (7/31) treated with placebo.

Newer AEDs in the Treatment of Rapid Cycling

Less commonly used AEDs in the treatment of rapid-cycling bipolar disorder include tiagabine (30–32), levetiracetam (33,34), and topiramate (35,36). Topiramate has been evaluated in a study of 27 female rapid-cycling outpatients as an adjunctive treatment to lithium or divalproex (36). Fifteen patients achieved a significant improvement in mood as assessed by the 21-item HAM-D and YMRS, reaching a state of euthymia by 10 weeks of treatment. Eight (53%) of these 15 patients completed 40 weeks of treatment and remained euthymic. Weight loss of greater than or equal to 5% was experienced by nine (33%) patients; other side effects included ataxia, confusion, drowsiness, and the re-emergence of psychosis. A case report exists of a 38-year old woman with a 22-year history of rapid-cycling bipolar I disorder refractory to multiple treatments. The patient demonstrated a remarkable improvement with the combination of clozapine and topiramate, experiencing sustained remission for a period of three years (35). Despite these favorable reports, four separate placebo-controlled trials of topiramate mono-therapy in bipolar I mania or mixed states have failed to demonstrate efficacy. The lack of randomized, double-blind evidence for the use of topiramate in bipolar depression or rapid cycling speaks for restraint in its routine use as a mood stabilizer (37).

Levetiracetam has been reported to disrupt the sequence of rapid cycling in two cases, improving symptoms of depression and mania/mixed mania (33) One patient with a history of rapid-cycling bipolar disorder and comorbid substance abuse reportedly responded to levetiracetam monotherapy after failing 15 different psychotropic medications and remained well for one year (34).

Case studies suggest that some patients may benefit from the gamma-aminobutyric acid (GABA) reuptake inhibitor tiagabine as an add-on therapy during the long-term treatment of rapid-cycling bipolar disorder (31). However, other case series report tiagabine to be poorly tolerated and to offer little evidence of effectiveness in refractory bipolar illness (32). With rapid dose escalation, tia-gabine has been associated with possible seizure induction and should be used extremely cautiously (30).

Rapid-Cycling Bipolar Disorder and Comorbid Alcohol and Substance Use Disorders

A substantial area of unmet need involves the management of bipolar disorder and co-occurring substance use disorders (38). Perhaps not surprisingly, bipolar I and II disorder are the Axis I conditions observed to have the highest lifetime prevalence rates of alcohol abuse or dependence (46.2% and 39.2%, respectively) (39). Nega-tively influencing the course of bipolar disorder, comorbid alcoholism results in more frequent mood episodes and a shorter duration of remission between epi-sodes (40). Indeed, a lifetime history of drug abuse has been shown to be an independent predictor of rapid-cycling status (2).

To compare differences in treatment response among patients with active substance use disorders, our group recently completed enrollment in the first maintenance trial that compared lithium monotherapy with the combination of lithium plus divalproex in 149 rapid-cycling bipolar I or II patients with an alcohol or drug use disorder (41). In this trial, all patients met DSM-IV criteria for alcohol, cannabis, and/or cocaine abuse or dependence and were required to have had an episode of hypomania or mania within three months preceding study entry. Patients were also integrated into a 12-step-based intensive outpatient chemical dependency treatment program. Initially, patients were treated with a combination of lithium and divalproex ($N = 149$); responders were then randomized to double-blind treatment with lithium alone or lithium plus divalproex for up to six months. Thirty-eight subjects (25%) did not respond to open-label treatment with the combination of lithium and divalproex, and thus were not randomly assigned. Approximately equal numbers of these patients were experiencing refractory depressive or manic/hypomanic/mixed states. A total of 31 (21%) patients demonstrated a bimodal response to the treatment combination and were randomized to the maintenance phase.

On the primary outcome measure of time to treatment for a new mood episode, the median survival for combination-treated patients was 17.8 weeks compared with 15.9 weeks for lithium monotherapy-treated patients ($p = 0.6$). No significant difference in time to treatment intervention for a depressive or manic episode was evidenced between either group. Interestingly, among randomized subjects, more than half no longer met abuse criteria or had entered into early full remission of their respective substance use disorder. This suggests that in acutely symptomatic patients who are actively abusing alcohol or other substances, treatment with appropriate mood stabilizer therapy can treat not only the acute mood episode, but can also be beneficial in managing the co-occurring substance use disorder.

RAPID CYCLING AND DEPRESSION: A COMMON GROUND

Accumulating data suggest a distinct relationship between depression and rapid cycling. Nearly two decades ago, depression was identified as the index episode for the majority of patients with rapid cycling (42). Newer studies also report a high frequency of depression as the index episode, including the previously described placebo-controlled maintenance trial of lamotrigine (28) and the maintenance study comparing lithium with divalproex (20). Moreover, during the course of each of these trials, depression emerged as the most frequently recurring mood state. The spectrum of prophylactic efficacy of valproate, possessing substantial antimanic but only modest antidepressant activity, further supports the prominence of depression in rapid cycling (14,19). A meta-analysis of patients enrolled in the former Stanley Foundation Bipolar Network identified that rapid-cycling patients spend more days depressed than non-rapid-cycling patients (145 vs. 121 days) (2). Throughout the one-year assessment, patients experienced depression 35.6% of the time, considerably greater than the 12.6% of the time spent manic/hypomanic or the 3.3% of the time spent cycling or in a mixed state.

Depression is a substantial cause of morbidity and mortality in bipolar I and II disorders, and remains the primary clinical challenge in treating bipolar disorder in general and rapid cycling in particular. Patients with bipolar I disorder followed an average of 12.8 years spent 31.9% of the time depressed, in comparison with 8.9% of the time manic/hypomanic and 5.9% of the time cycling/mixed (43). Results indicate that depressive symptoms are even more predominant in patients with bipolar II disorder, occurring almost 40 times as frequently as hypomanic symptoms (44). The observation that depression is the primary morbidity in bipolar disorder has also been confirmed by a naturalistic, prospective study of outpatients followed daily for one year. Patients spent three times as many days depressed as manic, with depressive episodes lasting four times as long as manic episodes (45). Not surprisingly, the negative impact depression extols on psychosocial functioning leads to suicide in approximately 20% of patients (46). Nearly 30% of bipolar patients attempt suicide (47,48), a rate double than that observed in unipolar depression (47). Depression could also be considered as a marker of chronicity. At intake, patients presenting with a purely depressive episode are expected to have greater symptom persistence than patients presenting with a purely manic episode (43). Coryell et al. (49) noted that depressive symptoms occurring early in the course of bipolar disorder predicted depression at 15-year follow-up. No such relationship was identified for the persistence of manic symptoms.

Depression in bipolar disorder has not been studied as extensively as has mania. Lithium, divalproex, carbamazepine, and every second-generation antipsychotic with the exception of clozapine, is FDA approved for the treatment of mania. There are only two FDA approved treatments for bipolar depression, an olanzapine-fluoxetine combination and quetiapine. Additional research is needed to develop agents effective for all aspects of bipolar depression, including subsyndromal symptoms and phase-specific (acute, continuation, and maintenance) interventions. A summary of acute bipolar depression trials involving AEDs is provided in Table 1.

AEDs in the Treatment of Bipolar Depression
Carbamazepine

Developed in 1957, carbamazepine was one of the earliest anticonvulsants to be investigated for the relief of acute bipolar depression. Using a double-blind, placebo-controlled, off-on-off again design, carbamazepine was shown to result in response for 63% (15/24) of bipolar subjects at an average dose of 971 mg/day (50) Studies demonstrating the antidepressant properties of carbamazepine are limited by the use of heterogeneous samples, which combined patients with unipolar and bipolar disorder along with those suffering from treatment-refractory illness (51) Adding to carbamazepine's complexity of use is the requirement for routine monitoring of hematological and hepatic parameters. The incidence of agranulocytosis with carbamazepine use is around 1:100,000 (52). Although perhaps less likely to result in weight gain than valproate (53), patients receiving carbamazepine for the treatment of depression may be more susceptible to weight gain than those treated for mania (54). Given the limited study of carbamazepine in depressive states and the significant potential for adverse effects, it is not regarded as a first-line agent for the treatment of bipolar depression.

A related compound, oxcarbazepine, differs from carbamazepine by the addition of a ketone substitution. However, it does not require routine blood monitoring, does not cause induction of its own metabolism, and is associated with less prominent drug interactions (55). There are no published controlled trials of oxcarbazepine in bipolar depression. The only published controlled study of oxcarbazepine monotherapy in bipolar disorder involves the treatment of mania or mixed states in youths with bipolar I disorder. In this trial, no difference was evidenced between oxcarbazepine and placebo (56).

Valproate/Divalproex

Initial support for the use of valproate in the treatment of acute bipolar depression was noted by Winsberg et al. (57) in a 12-week open-label study of bipolar II

TABLE 1 Blinded, Controlled, Trials of Anticonvulsants in the Treatment of Acute Bipolar Depression

Agent	Design	Subjects	Number randomized	Duration	Primary outcome measure	Primary outcome results	Key findings
Divalproex Davis et al. (2005) 58	DB, PC	BP I	DVX (N = 13) PBO (N = 12)	8 wk	Percentage change from baseline to end point on HAMD	DVX Δ = 43.5% PBO Δ = 27.0% $p < 0.001$	DVX superior to PBO at reducing depression and anxiety
Divalproex extended release	DB, PC	BP I, II, NOS	DVP (N = 10)	6 wk	Change from baseline to end point on MADRS	DVX Δ = −13.6	DVX superior to PBO at reducing depression
Ghaemi et al. (2007) 60			PBO (N = 8)			PBO Δ = −1.4 $p = 0.003$	No difference in response[a] rates between DVX and PBO
Lamotrigine	DB, PC	BP I	LTG 50 mg/day (N = 66)	7 wk	Change from baseline to end point on MADRS[d]	LTG 200 mg/day	Greater rates of response[a] on LTG 50 and 200 mg/day than on PBO
Calabrese et al. (1999) 26			LTG 200 mg/day (N = 63) PBO (N = 66)			Δ = −13.3 LTG 50 mg/day Δ = −11.2 PBO Δ = −7.8 $p < 0.05$ for LTG 200 mg/day vs. PBO	LTG 200 mg/day showed greater efficacy than 50 mg/day
Lamotrigine/ Citalopram	Adjunctive, DB, CIT active comparator	BP I, II	LTG (N = 10)	12 wk	Change from baseline to end point on MADRS	LTG Δ = −13.3	LTG and CIT equally effective at reducing depression
Schaffer et al. (2006) 75			CIT (N = 10)			CIT Δ = −14.2 $p = $ NS	Combined response[a] rose from 31.6% at wk 6 to 52.6% at wk 12

(Continued)

TABLE 1 Blinded, Controlled, Trials of Anticonvulsants in the Treatment of Acute Bipolar Depression (*Continued*)

Agent	Subjects	Design	Number randomized	Duration	Primary outcome measure	Primary outcome results	Key findings
Lamotrigine/gabapentin	BPI, II	DB, PC, crossover	LTG (N = 31)	6 wk	Responder[b] analysis based on CGI-BP	LTG = 52%	LTG superior to both GBP and PBO in the treatment of refractory mood disorders
Frye et al. (2000) 29	MDD		GBP (N = 31)			GBP = 26%	
			PBO (N = 31)			PBO = 23%	
						p = 0.031	
Lamotrigine/olanzapine-fluoxetine combination	BP I	DB, OFC active comparator	LTG (N = 205)	7 wk	Change from baseline to end point on CGI-S	OFC showed greater improvement than LTG on CGI-S	OFC modestly superior to LTG in reducing depression
Brown et al. (2006) 86			OFC (N = 205)			p = 0.002	OFC associated with greater weight gain and metabolic abnormalities
Topiramate/bupropion SR	BP I, II	Adjunctive, SB, BUP active comparator	TOP (N = 18)	8 wk	Responder[c] analysis based on HAMD-17	TOP = 56%	TOP and BUP equally effective at reducing depression as adjunctive therapy
McIntyre et al. (2002) 69			BUP (N = 18)			BUP = 59%	Most patients in both treatment groups experienced weight loss
						p = NS	

[a] ≥50% reduction in MADRS score.
[b] Rated as much or very much improved.
[c] ≥50% reduction in Hamilton Depression Rating Scale (HAMD-17) score.
[d] Primary outcome measure not defined a priori.

Abbreviations: Δ, change; BP I, bipolar I disorder; BP II, bipolar II disorder; BP NOS, bipolar disorder not otherwise specified; BUP, bupropion SR; CIT, citalopram; CGI-BP, Clinical Global Impressions scale for Bipolar Illness; CGI-S, Clinical Global Impressions Severity of Illness Scale; DB, double-blind; DVX, divalproex sodium; GBP, gabapentin; HAMD, Hamilton Depression Scale; Li, lithium; LTG, lamotrigine; MADRS, Montgomery-Åsberg Depression Rating Scale; MDD, unipolar major depressive disorder; OFC, olanzapine-fluoxetine combination; PBO, placebo; PC, placebo-controlled; SB, single-blind; TOP, topiramate.

outpatients. A mean divalproex dose of 882 mg/day resulted in a 63% response rate (12/19) as assessed by the 17-item HAM-D. The highest rate of response tended to be in medication naïve (82%) compared with mood-stabilizer naïve (38%) patients, but this difference did not reach statistical significance ($p < 0.08$). One published trial by Davis et al. of 25 bipolar I–depressed patients randomized to double-blind treatment with divalproex or placebo found the rate of improvement in depressive symptoms over time to be twice as great with divalproex than placebo (58). In this study, a significant reduction in anxiety symptoms was also noted in divalproex-treated subjects. Divalproex was well tolerated, with only one patient withdrawing from the study because of adverse effects. An unpublished, multisite trial of divalproex in bipolar depression (I, II, or NOS) found no significant difference in the rate of response compared with placebo (43% vs. 27%) (59). Similar to the Davis et al. trial, this study enrolled a relatively small number of subjects ($N = 45$) and utilized the HAM-D as the primary outcome measure. However, the Davis et al. study was conducted at a single site, perhaps accounting for the detectable difference with divalproex as opposed to the negative multisite trial conducted by Sachs et al. A placebo-controlled study involving divalproex extended release (ER) in the treatment of bipolar depression was recently reported, enrolling 18 patients with bipolar I, II, or NOS disorders (60). Change from baseline to end point score on the Montgomery-Åsberg Depression Rating Scale (MADRS) was significant for a time by treatment interaction favoring divalproex ER over placebo ($p = 0.0078$). The absolute improvement in MADRS total score over time was 13.6 points with divalproex versus 1.4 points with placebo ($p = 0.003$).

A post hoc analysis to assess the efficacy of divalproex in the prevention of bipolar depression was carried out by Gyulai et al. in recently manic bipolar I patients ($N = 571$) enrolled in a 52-week maintenance trial (61). After completing an open-label stabilization phase, eligible patients were randomized to divalproex ($N = 187$), lithium ($N = 91$), or placebo ($N = 94$) in a 2:1:1 ratio. Divalproex-treated patients were less likely to discontinue early for depression than placebo-treated patients ($p < 0.05$). Divalproex was also more effective than lithium in delaying the time to depressive relapse among patients who responded to divalproex in the open-period and in those with a past history of psychiatric hospitalization.

In this trial, paroxetine or sertraline could be added for breakthrough depression. The combination of divalproex and a selective serotonin reuptake inhibitor (SSRI), but not lithium and an SSRI, was more effective than SSRI monotherapy in prophylaxing against depressive symptoms. Interestingly, this was the first time a randomized, controlled maintenance trial found antidepressant monotherapy to be inferior to an antidepressant plus a mood stabilizer in preventing breakthrough depression.

Lamotrigine

Treatment of acute bipolar depression. Lamotrigine was the first monotherapy agent to be investigated in a randomized, double-blind, parallel-group trial in bipolar I depression (26). A total of 195 subjects were enrolled in an equivalent fashion to lamotrigine 50 mg/day, lamotrigine 200 mg/day, or placebo for seven weeks. The sample was moderately ill; 50% of patients had prior hospitalizations and 30% had previously attempted suicide. Significant improvement from placebo began to emerge at week 3 when patients were taking lamotrigine 50 mg/day. At study end point, significant improvement was noted for lamotrigine 200 mg/day on the MADRS ($p < 0.05$) and approached significance for the 50 mg/day group $p = 0.058$). Significantly more patients in both groups demonstrated a response ($\geq 50\%$ improvement on MADRS total score), but only the lamotrigine 200 mg/day dose performed significantly better on the CGI-I. Neither dose of lamotrigine showed improvement over placebo on the HAM-D, perhaps reflecting the greater weighting toward somatic symptoms (e.g., insomnia, anxiety, and agitation) with this instrument. The low incidence of somnolence as a side effect may also have contributed to the limited improvement on HAM-D scores with lamotrigine in comparison with placebo.

A double-blind crossover study similarly found lamotrigine to be more effective than placebo in patients with refractory mood disorders, the majority of whom were diagnosed with bipolar disorder (29). However, four other double-blind, placebo-controlled trials of lamotrigine conducted in the acute treatment of bipolar depression failed to show drug-placebo separation on the primary outcome measures (62). In each of the four studies, the effect size was small on measures such as the MADRS and 31-item HAM-D, falling consistently below 0.2 (the lower limits of a small treatment effect). A large placebo response appeared to contribute to the inability of lamotrigine to demonstrate superiority over placebo in treating acute bipolar depression in these trials.

Prophylaxis against recurrent depression.   In addition to the acute relief of depressive symptoms, the prevention of recurrence is of paramount concern in the longitudinal treatment of bipolar disorder. Over 90% of patients with bipolar disorder will experience a recurrence at some point in their lifetime (63). Even when following a guideline-based treatment algorithm, over the course of two years almost half of patients will suffer a recurrence, with most being depressive in nature (64).

To assess the prevention of relapse or recurrence of mood episodes in bipolar I disorder, a randomized, double-blind, placebo-controlled trial of lamotrigine was conducted in patients who recently experienced a manic or hypomanic episode (65). Lithium served as the active comparator arm, given its proven efficacy in the maintenance treatment of bipolar disorder. Patients who were currently or recently manic or hypomanic were enrolled into an initial 8- to -16-week open-label phase. During this period, lamotrigine was titrated to at least 100 mg/day and other psychotropic medications were gradually withdrawn. Patients demonstrating response entered into the double-blind, maintenance phase and were randomized to lamotrigine (100–400 mg/day, $N = 59$), lithium (serum level = 0.8–1.1 mEq/L, $N = 46$), or placebo ($N = 70$). Regarding the primary outcome measure, both lithium and lamotrigine were significantly superior to placebo on time to intervention for any mood episode. Lamotrigine, but not lithium, was superior to placebo at prolonging the time to treatment for a depressive episode (lamotrigine vs. placebo $p = 0.02$; lithium vs. placebo $p = 0.17$). Conversely, lithium, but not lamotrigine, was superior to placebo at prolonging the time to treatment for a manic, hypomanic, or mixed episode (lithium vs. placebo $p = 0.006$; lamotrigine vs. placebo $p = 0.28$). In this study, lamotrigine was well tolerated, with headache emerging as the only adverse event occurring more commonly than with lithium in the double-blind phase, while lithium was associated with a higher incidence of diarrhea.

In conjunction with the 18-month maintenance trial assessing lamotrigine in recently hypomanic or manic patients, an analogous trial was performed in recently depressed patients (66). Again, results showed that both lamotrigine and lithium monotherapy were superior to placebo at delaying the time to intervention for a mood episode. A complementary pattern of efficacy was also observed, with lithium significantly delaying the time to intervention for manic but not depressive episodes, and lamotrigine significantly delaying the time to intervention for depressive but not manic episodes. These trials employed moderately enriched designs, requiring patients to initially tolerate and respond to lamotrigine. Although this method will generally lead to decreased variance throughout the randomization phase, it may limit generalizability of results. The enriched design may also have led to exaggeration of the ineffectiveness of lithium in preventing recurrent episodes of depression. Collectively, however, the results of these two studies strongly support the use of lamotrigine for the prophylaxis of depressive episodes in bipolar disorder.

It has been proposed that in order to assess the true performance of a drug in preventing recurrence, relapses should be excluded by requiring patients to experience sustained relief of mood symptoms for at least two months prior to evaluating a drug's prophylactic efficacy (67). To assess whether lamotrigine exhibited pure maintenance efficacy, a post hoc analysis was performed on both of the lamotrigine 18-month maintenance studies (65,66) in which all potential relapses (mood episodes of same polarity as the index episode) that occurred within 90 and 180 days of randomization were excluded (68) Similar to results of the original analyses, lamotrigine was found to be superior to placebo in terms of overall study survival. Both lithium and lamotrigine were superior to placebo in delaying time to onset of a new mood episode, supporting the pure-maintenance effects of these agents.

Emerging Treatments for Bipolar Depression

In small, underpowered, preliminary studies, the mood stabilizers topiramate and zonisamide have demonstrated putative antidepressant properties. Topiramate was compared with bupropion slow release (SR) under single-blind conditions as an add-on treatment for bipolar I or II depression (69). After eight weeks of treatment, both agents resulted in comparable reductions in depressive symptoms, with 56% of topiramate-treated and 58% of bupropion SR-treated patients meeting response criteria ($\geq$50% reduction in HAM-D score). Weight loss was apparent in both treatment groups, but was statistically greater with topiramate. Zonisamide, one of the newest AEDs on the market, has been evaluated in small open-label studies for the treatment of mania (70) and bipolar depression (71,72). Mixed results were seen in a trial of 20 depressed patients who were administered open-label zonisamide as an adjunctive therapy (72). Twenty-five percent of patients (5/20) were deemed treatment responders based on a greater than or equal to 50% decline in MADRS score over eight weeks. However, 50% (10/20) of patients discontinued treatment mainly because of side effects. The most common adverse effects were sedation, nausea, dizziness, and cognitive dysfunction. It appears that zonisamide, similar to topiramate, may also be associated with weight loss in some patients. Zonisamide may prove promising as a treatment for bipolar disorder with mood stabilizing effects from below baseline, but until placebo-controlled trials are undertaken, evidence for its efficacy is limited at best and it should likely be considered for use only when patients have failed more established therapies.

Combination Therapy

For patients already taking a mood stabilizer but who continue to display depressive symptoms, it is unclear whether the next-step treatment should be to add an antidepressant or another mood stabilizer, such as an AED. Combining two or more mood stabilizing agents is becoming common practice and may be more efficacious than monotherapy (73,74). A small trial by Young et al. (74) found no difference in efficacy when a second mood stabilizer or an antidepressant was added to an existing mood stabilizer—both were equally useful in managing depressive symptoms. However, the addition of an antidepressant resulted in fewer dropouts. Likewise, in a separate trial evaluating the addition of lamotrigine or citalopram to depressed bipolar I or II patients taking divalproex, lithium, or carbamazepine, no significant difference in antidepressant efficacy was observed between study drugs (75). Both lamotrigine and citalopram resulted in similar reductions in depressive severity.

Lithium and divalproex are the most commonly prescribed drugs for bipolar disorder; yet when the two are used in combination they are ineffective at stabilizing mood in nearly 75% of rapid-cycling patients (18,19). Most of the refractory episodes are due to depression, or mood states "below baseline," as opposed to mania, hypomania, or subsyndromal mood elevation that would be characterized as episodes "above baseline." Ketter and Calabrese have offered that an agent effective at "stabilizing mood from below" would possess considerable antidepressant properties but would not worsen the course of illness by inducing (hypo) mania or cycle acceleration (76). Such treatment options are limited, and none of the AEDs have demonstrated consistently strong evidence to meet this definition. This suggests that future trials should aim at combining agents that work well at preventing episodes from above baseline with agents that prevent episodes from below baseline. Until such time, the current evidence base does not robustly support a front-line monotherapy role for any AED for acute bipolar depression, whether or not there is associated rapid cycling.

Treatment Guidelines for Bipolar Depression

A host of professional organizations and consensus panels have established guidelines for the treatment of bipolar depression, and there are considerable variations in their recommendations (see Table 2). Lithium is generally regarded as an acceptable monotherapy agent (77–81). The majority of guidelines also support the use of lamotrigine monotherapy for the depressed phase of bipolar disorder (77,79–82), primarily on the basis of positive results from one placebo-controlled acute depression trial (26) and two 18-month maintenance trials (65,66). With combination treatments becoming more common, several guidelines also recommend combined treatment with two mood stabilizers or a mood stabilizer plus an antidepressant as a first-line therapy (78,81–84). Although not an anticonvulsant, compelling evidence supports the use of quetiapine in bipolar depression. The most recent series of recommendations, published in 2006 by the Canadian Network for Mood and Anxiety Treatments, have newly included quetiapine monotherapy as an acceptable initial treatment and continue to recommend use of the antipsychotic olanzapine in combination with an SSRI (81).

TABLE 2 Summary of First-Line Recommended Treatments for Acute Bipolar Depression

Study	Monotherapy				Combination therapy					
	Li	LTG	QUE	VPA	Antimanic[a] + AD	Antimanic[a] + LTG	Li + LTG	Li + AD	LTG + AD	Li + VPA
APA (Hirschfeld et al. 2002) 77	Yes	Yes	No	No	No	No	No	No	No	No
World Federation of SBP (Grunze et al. 2002) 82	No	No	No	No	No	No	No	Yes	Yes	No
British Association for Psychopharmacology (Goodwin et al. 2003) 83	No	No	No	No	Yes	No	No	Yes	No	No
Expert Consensus Guidelines (Keck et al., 2004) 78	Yes	No	No	No	No	No	Yes	Yes	No	No
Australian and New Zealand Guidelines (Mitchell et al. 2004) 79	Yes	Yes	No	No	No	No	No	No	No	No
International Consensus Group (Calabrese et al. 2004) 80	Yes	Yes	No	No	No	No	No	No	No	No
Texas Medication Algorithms (Suppes et al. 2005) 84	No	Yes[b]	No	No	No	Yes	Yes	No	No	No
Canadian Network for Mood and Anxiety (Yatham et al. 2006) 81	Yes	Yes	Yes	No	Yes[c]	No	No	Yes	No	Yes

[a] An antimanic agent includes any medication that has evidence of being an effective treatment for mania.
[b] Only recommended if there is no history of severe or recent mania.
[c] Only Li, VPA, and Olanzapine are recommended as antimanic agents for use in combination with an AD.
Abbreviations: AD, antidepressant; APA, American Psychiatric Association; Li, lithium; LTG, lamotrigine; QUE, quetiapine; SBP, Societies of Biological Psychiatry; VPA, valproate.

CONCLUSIONS

AEDs have played an integral role in the management of rapid-cycling bipolar disorder and bipolar depression. Lamotrigine, the first agent ever studied in prospective, double-blind, placebo-controlled trials in both conditions, has established a rigorous standard of evidence for the maintenance treatment of bipolar disorder by which emerging therapies will be compared. The AEDs are not equivalent and clearly possess variant efficacy and tolerability profiles. For acute bipolar depression, despite some conflicting data, lamotrigine is the AED most supported by treatment guidelines and the extant literature; though for rapid cycling, lamotrigine's forte may be confined to patients with the bipolar II subtype. Valproate appears suited for the management of rapid cycling, and its modest antidepressant effects may make it most useful as an adjunctive therapy, perhaps in combination with an antidepressant or lamotrigine. There remains little evidence to recommend zonisamide, oxcarbazepine, gabapentin, levetiracetam, or topiramate in bipolar depression or rapid cycling, or, for that matter, any phase of bipolar disorder. However, these agents are not known to exacerbate manic switching and may be employed for the management of co-occurring anxiety (e.g., gabapentin) or substance use (e.g., topiramate) disorders or to offset weight loss associated with traditional mood stabilizer therapy (e.g., topiramate and zonisamide).

The AEDs have brought numerous benefits to the field, but their application has principally been evaluated in monotherapy studies. Long aware that monotherapy often falls short of improving symptom control and reducing relapse, clinicians often rely on multiple drug regimens. It is here that evidence is most limited to guide prescribing practices. On the horizon are trials aimed at assessing combination strategies to treat the most complex manifestations of bipolar disorder. Data collection in a group of rapid-cycling bipolar patients with comorbid substance use disorders is nearing completion and will compare the combination of divalproex and lithium with the triple therapy combination of divalproex, lithium, and lamotrigine. These results are highly anticipated and should help resolve whether exposure to multiple agents merely adds to the side-effect burden and treatment cost or rather provides greater efficacy and improved well-being for the estimated 169 million existing individuals worldwide that suffer from bipolar disorder (85).

Although not developed specifically to ease the burden of psychiatric illness, AEDs are a staple for patients with some of the most chronic and refractory variations of bipolar illness. Their expansion into the management of bipolar disorder will likely continue, and with that growth, bring promise for patients with rapid cycling, bipolar depression, and other states of unmet need.

REFERENCES

1. Dunner DL, Fieve RR. Clinical factors in lithium carbonate prophylaxis failure. Arch Gen Psychiatry 1974; 30(2):229–233.
2. Kupka RW, Luckenbaugh DA, Post RM, et al. Comparison of rapid-cycling and non-rapid-cycling bipolar disorder based on prospective mood ratings in 539 outpatients. Am J Psychiatry 2005; 162(7):1273–1280.
3. Bauer MS, Calabrese J, Dunner DL, et al. Multisite data reanalysis of the validity of rapid cycling as a course modifier for bipolar disorder in DSM-IV. Am J Psychiatry 1994; 151 (4):506–515.

4. Schneck CD, Miklowitz DJ, Calabrese JR, et al. Phenomenology of rapid-cycling bipolar disorder: data from the first 500 participants in the Systematic Treatment Enhancement Program. Am J Psychiatry 2004; 161(10):1902–1908.

5. Maj M, Magliano L, Pirozzi R, et al. Validity of rapid cycling as a course specifier for bipolar disorder. Am J Psychiatry 1994; 151(7):1015–1019.

6. Kupka RW, Luckenbaugh DA, Post RM, et al. Rapid and non-rapid cycling bipolar disorder: a meta-analysis of clinical studies. J Clin Psychiatry 2003; 64(12):1483–1494.

7. Calabrese JR, Shelton MD, Bowden CL, et al. Bipolar rapid cycling: focus on depression as its hallmark. J Clin Psychiatry 2001; 62(suppl 14):34–41.

8. Tondo L, Baldessarini RJ. Rapid cycling in women and men with bipolar manic-depressive disorders. Am J Psychiatry 1998; 155(10):1434–1436.

9. Coryell W, Solomon D, Turvey C, et al. The long-term course of rapid-cycling bipolar disorder. Arch Gen Psychiatry 2003; 60(9):914–920.

10. Gao K, Bilali S, Conroy C. Clinical impacts of comorbid anxiety disorder or substance use disorder on patients with rapid cycling bipolar disorder. Paper presented at: American Psychiatric Association Annual Meeting, May 20–25, 2006, Toronto, Canada.

11. Coryell W, Endicott J, Keller M. Rapidly cycling affective disorder. Demographics, diagnosis, family history, and course. Arch Gen Psychiatry 1992; 49(2):126–131.

12. Kukopulos A, Reginaldi D, Laddomada P, et al. Course of the manic-depressive cycle and changes caused by treatment. Pharmakopsychiatr Neuropsychopharmakol 1980; 13 (4):156–167.

13. Maj M, Pirozzi R, Magliano L, et al. Long-term outcome of lithium prophylaxis in bipolar disorder: a 5-year prospective study of 402 patients at a lithium clinic. Am J Psychiatry 1998; 155(1):30–35.

14. Calabrese JR, Woyshville MJ, Kimmel SE, et al. Predictors of valproate response in bipolar rapid cycling. J Clin Psychopharmacol 1993; 13(4):280–283.

15. Post RM, Uhde TW, Roy-Byrne PP, et al. Correlates of antimanic response to carbamazepine. Psychiatry Res 1987; 21(1):71–83.

16. Joyce PR. Carbamazepine in rapid cycling bipolar affective disorder. Int Clin Psychopharmacol 1988; 3(2):123–129.

17. Okuma T. Effects of carbamazepine and lithium on affective disorders. Neuropsychobiology 1993; 27(3):138–145.

18. Denicoff KD, Smith-Jackson EE, Disney ER, et al. Comparative prophylactic efficacy of lithium, carbamazepine, and the combination in bipolar disorder. J Clin Psychiatry 1997; 58(11):470–478.

19. Calabrese JR, Delucchi GA. Spectrum of efficacy of valproate in 55 patients with rapid-cycling bipolar disorder. Am J Psychiatry 1990; 147(4):431–434.

20. Calabrese JR, Shelton MD, Rapport DJ, et al. A 20-month, double-blind, maintenance trial of lithium versus divalproex in rapid-cycling bipolar disorder. Am J Psychiatry 2005; 162(11):2152–2161.

21. Bowden CL, Calabrese JR, McElroy SL, et al. A randomized, placebo-controlled 12-month trial of divalproex and lithium in treatment of outpatients with bipolar I disorder. Divalproex Maintenance Study Group. Arch Gen Psychiatry 2000; 57(5)481–489.

22. Di Costanzo E, Schifano F. Lithium alone or in combination with carbamazepine for the treatment of rapid-cycling bipolar affective disorder. Acta Psychiatr Scand 1991; 83 (6):456–459.

23. Suppes T, Brown E, Schuh LM, et al. Rapid versus non-rapid cycling as a predictor of response to olanzapine and divalproex sodium for bipolar mania and maintenance of remission: post hoc analyses of 47-week data. J Affect Disord 2005; 89(1–3):69–77.

24. Smith D, Chadwick D, Baker G, et al. Seizure severity and the quality of life. Epilepsia 1993; 34(suppl 5):S31–S35.

25. Calabrese JR, Bowden CL, McElroy SL, et al. Spectrum of activity of lamotrigine in treatment-refractory bipolar disorder. Am J Psychiatry 1999; 156(7):1019–1023.

26. Calabrese JR, Bowden CL, Sachs GS, et al. A double-blind placebo-controlled study of lamotrigine monotherapy in outpatients with bipolar I depression. Lamictal 602 Study Group. J Clin Psychiatry 1999; 60(2):79–88.

27. Calabrese JR, Fatemi SH, Woyshville MJ. Antidepressant effects of lamotrigine in rapid cycling bipolar disorder. Am J Psychiatry 1996; 153(9):1236.
28. Calabrese JR, Suppes T, Bowden CL, et al. A double-blind, placebo-controlled, prophylaxis study of lamotrigine in rapid-cycling bipolar disorder. Lamictal 614 Study Group. J Clin Psychiatry 2000; 61(11):841–850.
29. Frye MA, Ketter TA, Kimbrell TA, et al. A placebo-controlled study of lamotrigine and gabapentin monotherapy in refractory mood disorders. J Clin Psychopharmacol 2000; 20 (6):607–614.
30. Grunze H, Erfurth A, Marcuse A, et al. Tiagabine appears not to be efficacious in the treatment of acute mania. J Clin Psychiatry 1999; 60(11):759–762.
31. Schaffer LC, Schaffer CB, Howe J. An open case series on the utility of tiagabine as an augmentation in refractory bipolar outpatients. J Affect Disord 2002; 71(1–3):259–263.
32. Suppes T, Chisholm KA, Dhavale D, et al. Tiagabine in treatment refractory bipolar disorder: a clinical case series. Bipolar Disord 2002; 4(5):283–289.
33. Braunig P, Kruger S. Levetiracetam in the treatment of rapid cycling bipolar disorder. J Psychopharmacol 2003; 17(2):239–241.
34. Kaufman KR. Monotherapy treatment of bipolar disorder with levetiracetam. Epilepsy Behav 2004; 5(6):1017–1020.
35. Chen CK, Shiah IS, Yeh CB, et al. Combination treatment of clozapine and topiramate in resistant rapid-cycling bipolar disorder. Clin Neuropharmacol 2005; 28(3):136–138.
36. Kusumakar V, Yatham L, Kutcher S, et al. Preliminary, open-label study of topiramate in rapid-cycling bipolar women. Eur Neuropsychopharmacol 1999; 9:S357.
37. Kushner SF, Khan A, Lane R, et al. Topiramate monotherapy in the management of acute mania: results of four double-blind placebo-controlled trials. Bipolar Disord 2006; 8(1):15–27.
38. McElroy SL, Altshuler LL, Suppes T, et al. Axis I psychiatric comorbidity and its relationship to historical illness variables in 288 patients with bipolar disorder. Am J Psychiatry 2001; 158(3):420–426.
39. Regier DA, Farmer ME, Rae DS, et al. Comorbidity of mental disorders with alcohol and other drug abuse. Results from the Epidemiologic Catchment Area (ECA) Study. JAMA 1990; 264(19):2511–2518.
40. Brady KT, Lydiard RB. Bipolar affective disorder and substance abuse. J Clin Psychopharmacol 1992; 12(suppl 1):17S–22S.
41. Kemp DE, Gao K, Ganocy SJ, et al. Lithium monotherapy versus the combination of lithium and divalproex for rapid cycling bipolar disorder comorbid with substance abuse or dependence: a 6-month, double-blind, maintenance trial. Neuropsychopharmacology 2006; 31(suppl 1):S106.
42. Wehr TA, Sack DA, Rosenthal NE, et al. Rapid cycling affective disorder: contributing factors and treatment responses in 51 patients. Am J Psychiatry 1988; 145(2):179–184.
43. Judd LL, Akiskal HS, Schettler PJ, et al. The long-term natural history of the weekly symptomatic status of bipolar I disorder. Arch Gen Psychiatry 2002; 59(6):530–537.
44. Judd LL, Akiskal HS, Schettler PJ, et al. A prospective investigation of the natural history of the long-term weekly symptomatic status of bipolar II disorder. Arch Gen Psychiatry 2003; 60(3):261–269.
45. Post RM, Leverich GS, Nolen WA, et al. A re-evaluation of the role of antidepressants in the treatment of bipolar depression: data from the Stanley Foundation Bipolar Network. Bipolar Disord 2003; 5(6):396–406.
46. Goodwin FK, Jamison K. Manic-Depressive Illness. New York, NY: Oxford University Press, 1990.
47. Chen YW, Dilsaver SC. Lifetime rates of suicide attempts among subjects with bipolar and unipolar disorders relative to subjects with other Axis I disorders. Biol Psychiatry 1996; 39(10):896–899.
48. Fagiolini A, Kupfer DJ, Rucci P, et al. Suicide attempts and ideation in patients with bipolar I disorder. J Clin Psychiatry 2004; 65(4):509–514.
49. Coryell W, Turvey C, Endicott J, et al. Bipolar I affective disorder: predictors of outcome after 15 years. J Affect Disord 1998; 50(2–3):109–116.

50. Post RM, Uhde TW, Roy-Byrne PP, et al. Antidepressant effects of carbamazepine. Am J Psychiatry 1986; 143(1):29–34.
51. Ballenger JC, Post RM. Carbamazepine in manic-depressive illness: a new treatment. Am J Psychiatry 1980; 137(7):782–790.
52. Schatzberg AF, Cole JO, DeBattista C. Manual of Clinical Psychopharmacology. 4th ed. Washington, DC: American Psychiatric Publishing, Inc., 2003.
53. Mattson RH, Cramer JA, Collins JF. A comparison of valproate with carbamazepine for the treatment of complex partial seizures and secondarily generalized tonic-clonic seizures in adults. The Department of Veterans Affairs Epilepsy Cooperative Study No. 264 Group. N Engl J Med 1992; 327(11):765–771.
54. Joffe RT, Post RM, Uhde TW. Effect of carbamazepine on body weight in affectively ill patients. J Clin Psychiatry 1986; 47(6):313–314.
55. Baruzzi A, Albani F, Riva R. Oxcarbazepine: pharmacokinetic interactions and their clinical relevance. Epilepsia 1994; 35(suppl 3):S14–S19.
56. Wagner KD, Kowatch RA, Emslie GJ, et al. A double-blind, randomized, placebo-controlled trial of oxcarbazepine in the treatment of bipolar disorder in children and adolescents. Am J Psychiatry 2006; 163(7):1179–1186.
57. Winsberg ME, DeGolia SG, Strong CM, et al. Divalproex therapy in medication-naive and mood-stabilizer-naive bipolar II depression. J Affect Disord 2001; 67(1–3):207–212.
58. Davis LL, Bartolucci A, Petty F. Divalproex in the treatment of bipolar depression: a placebo-controlled study. J Affect Disord 2005; 85(3):259–266.
59. Sachs GS, Altshuler LL, Ketter T, et al. Divalproex versus placebo for the treatment of bipolar depression. Poster session presented at: The American College of Neuropsychopharmacology 40th Meeting, December 9–13, 2001, Waikoloa, Hawaii.
60. Ghaemi SN, Gilmer WS, Goldberg JF, et al. Divalproex in the treatment of acute bipolar depression: a preliminary double-blind, placebo-controlled pilot study. J Clin Psychiatry 2007; 68(12):1840–1844.
61. Gyulai L, Bowden CL, McElroy SL, et al. Maintenance efficacy of divalproex in the prevention of bipolar depression. Neuropsychopharmacology 2003; 28(7):1374–1382.
62. Calabrese JR, Huffman RF, White RL, et al. Lamotrigine in the acute treatment of bipolar depression: results of five double-blind, placebo-controlled clinical trials. Bipolar Disord 2008; 10(2):323–333.
63. Solomon DA, Keitner GI, Miller IW, et al. Course of illness and maintenance treatments for patients with bipolar disorder. J Clin Psychiatry 1995; 56(1):5–13.
64. Perlis RH, Ostacher MJ, Patel JK, et al. Predictors of recurrence in bipolar disorder: primary outcomes from the Systematic Treatment Enhancement Program for Bipolar Disorder (STEP-BD). Am J Psychiatry 2006; 163(2):217–224.
65. Bowden CL, Calabrese JR, Sachs G, et al. A placebo-controlled 18-month trial of lamotrigine and lithium maintenance treatment in recently manic or hypomanic patients with bipolar I disorder. Arch Gen Psychiatry 2003; 60(4):392–400.
66. Calabrese JR, Bowden CL, Sachs G, et al. A placebo-controlled 18-month trial of lamotrigine and lithium maintenance treatment in recently depressed patients with bipolar I disorder. J Clin Psychiatry 2003; 64(9):1013–1024.
67. Prien RF, Caffey EM Jr., Klett CJ. Prophylactic efficacy of lithium carbonate in manic-depressive illness. Report of the Veterans Administration and National Institute of Mental Health collaborative study group. Arch Gen Psychiatry 1973; 28(3):337–341.
68. Calabrese JR, Goldberg JF, Ketter TA, et al. Recurrence in bipolar I disorder: a post hoc analysis excluding relapses in two double-blind maintenance studies. Biol Psychiatry 2006; 59(11):1061–1064.
69. McIntyre RS, Mancini DA, McCann S, et al. Topiramate versus bupropion SR when added to mood stabilizer therapy for the depressive phase of bipolar disorder: a preliminary single-blind study. Bipolar Disord 2002; 4(3):207–213.
70. Kanba S, Yagi G, Kamijima K, et al. The first open study of zonisamide, a novel anticonvulsant, shows efficacy in mania. Prog Neuropsychopharmacol Biol Psychiatry 1994; 18(4): 707–715.
71. Anand A, Bukhari L, Jennings SA, et al. A preliminary open-label study of zonisamide treatment for bipolar depression in 10 patients. J Clin Psychiatry 2005; 66(2):195–198.

72. Ghaemi SN, Zablotsky B, Filkowski MM, et al. An open prospective study of zonisamide in acute bipolar depression. J Clin Psychopharmacol 2006; 26(4):385–388.
73. Solomon DA, Ryan CE, Keitner GI, et al. A pilot study of lithium carbonate plus divalproex sodium for the continuation and maintenance treatment of patients with bipolar I disorder. J Clin Psychiatry 1997; 58(3):95–99.
74. Young LT, Joffe RT, Robb JC, et al. Double-blind comparison of addition of a second mood stabilizer versus an antidepressant to an initial mood stabilizer for treatment of patients with bipolar depression. Am J Psychiatry 2000; 157(1):124–126.
75. Schaffer A, Zuker P, Levitt A. Randomized, double-blind pilot trial comparing lamotrigine versus citalopram for the treatment of bipolar depression. J Affect Disord 2006; 96(1–2):95–99.
76. Ketter TA, Calabrese JR. Stabilization of mood from below versus above baseline in bipolar disorder: a new nomenclature. J Clin Psychiatry 2002; 63(2):146–151.
77. Practice guideline for the treatment of patients with bipolar disorder (revision). Am J Psychiatry 2002; 159(suppl 4):1–50.
78. Keck PE, Perlis RH, Otto MW, et al. The expert consensus guideline series: treatment of bipolar disorder 2004. Postgraduate Med 2004; 1–19.
79. Australian and New Zealand clinical practice guidelines for the treatment of bipolar disorder. Aust N Z J Psychiatry 2004; 38(5):280–305.
80. Calabrese JR, Kasper S, Johnson G, et al. International consensus group on bipolar I depression treatment guidelines. J Clin Psychiatry 2004; 65(4):571–579.
81. Yatham LN, Kennedy SH, O'Donovan C, et al. Canadian Network for Mood and Anxiety Treatments (CANMAT) guidelines for the management of patients with bipolar disorder: update 2007. Bipolar Disord 2006; 8(6):721–739.
82. Grunze H, Kasper S, Goodwin G, et al. World Federation of Societies of Biological Psychiatry (WFSBP) guidelines for biological treatment of bipolar disorders. Part I: Treatment of bipolar depression. World J Biol Psychiatry 2002; 3(3):115–124.
83. Goodwin GM, Young AH. The British Association for Psychopharmacology guidelines for treatment of bipolar disorder: a summary. J Psychopharmacol 2003; 17(4 suppl):3–6.
84. Suppes T, Dennehy EB, Hirschfeld RM, et al. The Texas implementation of medication algorithms: update to the algorithms for treatment of bipolar I disorder. J Clin Psychiatry 2005; 66(7):870–886.
85. Kessler RC, Berglund P, Demler O, et al. Lifetime prevalence and age-of-onset distributions of DSM-IV disorders in the National Comorbidity Survey Replication. Arch Gen Psychiatry 2005; 62(6):593–602.
86. Brown EB, McElroy SL, Keck PE, et al. A 7-week, randomized, double-blind trial of olanzapine/fluoxetine combination versus lamotrigine in the treatment of bipolar I depression. J Clin Psychiatry 2006; 67(7):1025–1033.

10 Role of Antiepileptic Drugs in the Treatment of Major Depressive Disorder

Erik Nelson
Department of Psychiatry, University of Cincinnati Medical Center, Cincinnati, Ohio, U.S.A.

ANTIEPILEPTICS IN THE TREATMENT OF MAJOR DEPRESSIVE DISORDER

The effectiveness of antiepileptic drugs (AEDs), particularly valproate, carbamazepine, and lamotrigine, as mood stabilizers in bipolar disorder has been thoroughly documented over the past 30 years (1). However, the value of these agents in unipolar major depression is less well established and no AED is currently approved for this indication. Moreover, very few rigorous controlled trials have been conducted with these agents in samples of patients with unipolar depression (2). Nevertheless, the results of a number of studies suggest that some AEDs, including carbamazepine, valproate, phenytoin, lamotrigine, topiramate, gabapentin, and tiagabine, may have antidepressant effects in unipolar patients.

Carbamazepine

Carbamazepine is one of the three AEDs approved for the treatment of bipolar disorder. Its anticonvulsant effects appear to be, in part, mediated by a reduction in glutamate release due to the inhibition of voltage-gated sodium channels, although mood stabilization may depend on other mechanisms that occur with chronic administration, such as modulation of monoamine and gamma-aminobutryric acid (GABA) neurotransmission (1). Evidence that carbamazepine decreases the frequency of depressive episodes in bipolar disorder sparked interest in the possibility that it may have acute antidepressant effects in both bipolar and unipolar mood disorders (3). There is, however, only a single double-blind, placebo-controlled study of carbamazepine published to date that included a significant number of patients with unipolar depression (3). In this crossover study, 5 (45%) of 11 treatment-resistant unipolar depressed inpatients responded to carbamazepine monotherapy as indicated by an improvement of one point or more ("mild response") on the Bunney-Hamburg scale. Only two patients (18%) met the more stringent response criterion of improvement by two points or more on this 15-point scale ("good response"). In the bipolar depressed patients, 15 of 24 (63%) had a mild response and 10 (42%) had a good response. Although a greater percentage of bipolar patients responded to carbamazepine in this study, the difference in response rates between the diagnostic groups was not statistically significant. The difference between the mean depression rating score from the two weeks of placebo treatment and the rating from the four weeks of carbamazepine treatment, however, was significant only in the bipolar depressed group.

Nonetheless, several open-label studies suggest that carbamazepine may benefit patients with unipolar depression. In an open-label trial of carbamazepine monotherapy in patients with chronic depression, 11 out of 12 patients were described as "responders" to carbamazepine 400 to 600 mg/day, although the criterion for determining response was not given (4). Moreover, there was a significant improvement in the mean score on the Montgomery-Åsberg Depression Rating Scale (MADRS) (from 36.3 to 22.1) after carbamazepine therapy. Other studies report benefits with carbamazepine when used to augment the effects of antidepressants. Rybakowski et al. (5) randomized 59 patients with treatment-resistant depression, 18 of whom had unipolar depression, to either lithium or carbamazepine augmentation of ongoing antidepressant therapy. There was no significant difference between the two treatments; 16 (57.1%) of the 28 patients who received carbamazepine responded, with 9 (32.1%) reaching full remission. Although the response of the unipolar patients was not analyzed separately, there was no significant effect of unipolar/bipolar diagnosis on the response to either drug. In a series of patients with unipolar depression who had failed to respond to open-label venlafaxine, four out of six treated with carbamazepine augmentation were considered responders (6). Another study investigated the effects of carbamazepine augmentation in six patients who had failed to respond to four weeks of treatment with citalopram (7). In this open-label trial, there was a significant reduction in MADRS score after four weeks of adjunctive carbamazepine. The authors, however, warned that a reduction in the mean citalopram plasma concentration was observed after the addition of carbamazepine.

A retrospective chart review of 16 treatment-resistant depressed patients (13 of whom were unipolar) treated with carbamazepine also reported benefits with this agent (8). Seven patients out of the total sample had a moderate or marked response to the medication, despite the fact that only two patients in this group received concomitant antidepressant therapy. The authors noted that the rate of adverse effects in this study was rather high, which may have been related to the relatively older age of the patient sample (mean age 63.9 ± 10.5 years). Several case reports also describe antidepressant effects with carbamazepine when used as an adjunct to treatment with an antidepressant (9,10) or lithium (11). Moreover, two case reports point to potential benefits of carbamazepine therapy in the treatment of major depression with psychotic features. In one case, a patient with psychotic depression who was refractory to numerous medication trials responded to carbamazepine monotherapy (12). In the other case, a patient with "rapid cycling" psychotic depression benefited from a combination of carbamazepine and lithium (13).

Another potential role for carbamazepine therapy in the management of patients with unipolar depression is the prophylaxis of depressive episodes. Stuppaeck et al. (14,15) reported on a group of unipolar depressed patients treated with carbamazepine at two and five years of therapy. At the two-year time point, 17 out of the 24 patients described were diagnosed with unipolar depression, and all but four received carbamazepine monotherapy. Eleven of these patients were completely free of depressive episodes while on carbamazepine; two of these were taking concomitant lithium. An additional two patients were noted as having a decrease in episode frequency, while four patients had no change with carbamazepine prophylaxis. The mean number of depressive episodes per year decreased from 2.45 to 0.77 with carbamazepine treatment, a statistically significant change. In the report on longer-term carbamazepine prophylaxis, Stuppaeck et al. (15) describe the treatment of 17 patients with "major depression with melancholia" using 200 to 600 mg/day. Fifteen of these patients were treated with carbamazepine monotherapy, while two patients were treated with lithium as well. Five patients stopped taking carbamazepine during the five-year study, three because of lack of efficacy and two because of patient preference despite a good response to the drug. Seven of the fifteen patients were completely free of depression during the observation period. Of the remaining patients, five demonstrated a moderate decrease in episode frequency, two had no change in episode frequency, and one had an increase in episode frequency. As in the shorter prophylaxis study, there was a significant decrease in the mean number of episodes with prophylactic carbamazepine treatment, from 2.11 to 0.7 episodes per year. The mean prophylactic dose in this study was 480 mg and the mean carbamazepine plasma concentration was 6.2 μg/mL.

Lamotrigine

Like carbamazepine, lamotrigine appears to reduce excitatory glutamate release through its actions on voltage-gated sodium channels. Also, like carbamazepine, lamotrigine was first identified as having potential antidepressant effects when it was noted that patients taking it for epilepsy experienced an improvement in mood symptoms (16). It is currently approved for maintenance treatment of bipolar disorder, and the results of one double-blind, placebo-controlled study suggest that it has antidepressant properties in patients with bipolar I disorder (17). However, there are currently no published studies of lamotrigine as monotherapy for unipolar depression. Several studies have investigated the effects of lamotrigine as an adjunct to antidepressants in patients with major depression. Two randomized, placebo-controlled studies evaluated lamotrigine augmentation of antidepressants in samples predominantly consisting of unipolar depressed patients. In one study, 40 patients (33 of whom were unipolar) received lamotrigine or placebo added to ongoing paroxetine treatment (18). Although there was no significant difference compared with placebo in the change in Hamilton Depression Rating Scale (HAM-D) score, a significantly greater decrease in the Clinical Global Impression-Severity (CGI-S) score was reported in lamotrigine-treated patients. Moreover, the lamotrigine group demonstrated greater improvement compared with placebo-treated patients on the following HAM-D items: depressed mood, guilt, work nonproductivity, and lack of interest. In the other placebo-controlled augmentation study, patients who had failed at least one prior antidepressant trial were treated concurrently with fluoxetine 20 mg and either lamotrigine or placebo for six weeks (19). Again, there was no significant difference in the change in depression scores between patients treated with lamotrigine or placebo. However, there was a significantly greater improvement in the lamotrigine-treated group on the CGI-S and Clinical Global Impression-Improvement (CGI-I) scales.

Open-label studies also suggest potential benefits of the addition of lamotrigine to antidepressant therapy. Schindler et al. (20) conducted an eight-week, open-label comparison of lamotrigine and lithium augmentation of antidepressant therapy in 34 treatment-resistant unipolar patients. Both drugs produced a statistically significant improvement in symptom ratings, and the degree of change in scores was not significantly different between the two treatment groups. Specifically, 23% of the lamotrigine-treated patients met criteria for remission of the depressive episode, while 53% were considered responders on the basis of at least a 50% reduction in HAM-D score from baseline. In contrast, 18% of lithium-treated patients remitted, and 47% were considered responders. The mean dose of lamotrigine in this study was 153 mg. A smaller six-month trial also evaluated the effectiveness of lamotrigine added to antidepressants in 14 treatment-resistant unipolar patients (21). The addition of lamotrigine (dose range 50–200 mg) produced a significant improvement in depressive symptoms at both eight weeks and six months of therapy. At the end of the trial, four patients were rated as very much improved and seven much improved on the CGI-I scale. Furthermore, retrospective chart reviews (22–24) and case reports (25) also support the benefits of adjunctive lamotrigine in patients with treatment-resistant unipolar depression.

Valproate

Valproate, a broad spectrum AED that has effects on voltage-gated sodium channels and GABA neurotransmission, was the first anticonvulsant to be FDA approved for use in bipolar disorder. A few studies suggest that valproate therapy has acute and maintenance antidepressant effects in bipolar patients, (26,27), although its effects on depressive symptoms may be less robust than its antimanic properties. However, a dearth of studies has assessed the effectiveness of valproate in patients with unipolar depression. In fact, there are currently no published placebo-controlled trials of valproate monotherapy or valproate augmentation of antidepressants in nonbipolar depressed patients. Davis et al. (28) conducted the only prospective study of valproate monotherapy in unipolar patients, an eight-week open-label trial. At the end of the trial, 19 of the 22 study completers demonstrated a clinically significant response to the drug. The intent-to-treat analysis, which included 32 patients, demonstrated a statistically signficant improvement in overall depressive symptoms from baseline, which corresponded to an 11.9 point decrease in the mean HAM-D score (a decrease of 55%) from baseline. Debattista et al. (29) conducted an open-label study of valproate augmentation of antidepressants in 12 patients with major depression who were experiencing agitation as a symptom of their depressive episode. At the end of this four-week trial, patients displayed a statistically significant decrease in HAM-D scores (baseline 23.7 ± 5.9, end point 18.1 ± 8.1). Patients also exhibited a significant reduction in agitation during the trial that was independent of the overall antidepressant response. The authors commented that the antidepressant response observed was only modest compared with the effects on agitation, although it is important to note that the observation period of valproate therapy in this study was only four weeks, with up to two weeks for titration to the final dose. Although two to three weeks on a therapeutic dose of valproate may be sufficient for agitation effects to be optimized, this is generally not enough time for a complete antidepressant response to evolve.

Hayes et al. (30) conducted a retrospective chart review of long-term valproate use in psychiatric illness that included nine patients with major depression. Seven of these patients demonstrated improvement in Global Assessment of Functioning (GAF) scale scores after at least one year of treatment. The mean increase in GAF score was 27.7 ± 21.7 points for the depressed group (baseline GAF = 41.7 ± 14.7), which approximated that of the mixed bipolar group and resulted in the majority of the patients reaching the "mild symptom range or the virtually asymptomatic state." A few individual case reports also support the hypothesis that valproate has antidepressant properties in patients with unipolar major depression (31–33).

Phenytoin

Like lamotrigine and carbamazepine, phenytoin's anticonvulsant effects appear to be mediated by decreased glutamate release secondary to inhibition of voltage-gated sodium channels. Unlike these other AEDs, phenytoin is not approved for use in bipolar disorder, and there are relatively few studies investigating its therapeutic potential in bipolar patients. However, two controlled studies of phenytoin have been conducted in unipolar depression, one assessing its potential as monotherapy and the other evaluating its efficacy in augmenting SSRI antidepressants. The former study was a six-week trial comparing fluoxetine 20 mg and phenytoin 200 to 400 mg in patients with major depression (there was no placebo arm) (34). Twelve of fourteen patients in the phenytoin-treated group responded on the basis of a 50% or greater reduction in HAM-D score. There was no difference in the mean change in HAM-D score from baseline between the groups (−18.6 points for the fluoxetine group; −18.2 points for phenytoin). The mean blood level of phenytoin was 10.9 ± 2.0 μg/mL at week 6. It should be noted that a relatively low dose of fluoxetine was used, raising the concern that both treatments might have failed to demonstrate superiority over a placebo, had one been used in this study.

In the second controlled study, phenytoin was compared with placebo in patients who had received at least three weeks of treatment with adequate doses of fluvoxamine, fluoxetine, or paroxetine, but still had a score of 18 or higher on the HAM-D, 24 item version (35). After four weeks of double-blind treatment, there was no difference in change on the HAM-D between the phenytoin- and placebo-treated groups. The authors point out that a relatively high placebo response was observed in this study, which may have obscured any potential benefit of phenytoin augmentation. However, only 2 of 11 patients demonstrated a 30% or greater improvement in HAM-D score in the phenytoin group compared with seven of nine in the placebo group, making it unlikely that there was any clinically significant benefit of phenytoin augmentation in this trial.

Topiramate

Topiramate appears to modulate glutamatergic and GABA neurotransmission and is approved for the treatment of epilepsy and migraine headaches. Four double-blind, placebo-controlled studies have shown that topiramate is not efficacious for acute bipolar manic or mixed episodes (36). However, improvement in depressive symptoms after topiramate therapy has been reported in bipolar patients (37). There is currently one published double-blind, placebo-controlled study assessing topiramate as monotherapy for unipolar major depression (38). This trial compared the effects of 10 weeks of treatment with topiramate 200 mg or placebo in 64 women diagnosed with recurrent major depressive disorder. The change in mean depressive symptom scores from baseline to end point was significantly greater for the topiramate compared with the placebo group, though the total decrease in symptom scores was small for both groups (−3.9 points for topiramate, −1.1 for placebo). The authors also reported a decrease in expressed anger, improved attention, and increased health-related quality of life in the topiramate compared with the placebo group.

Several studies support the effectiveness of topiramate as a treatment for obesity and binge eating disorder (39). Accordingly, open-label studies and case reports have focused on the use of topiramate in depressed patients with comorbid obesity. Carpenter et al. (40) reviewed the charts of 16 women diagnosed with a major depressive episode (12 were unipolar) and mild-to-moderate obesity who received adjunctive topiramate. Although the response in unipolar patients was not analyzed separately, 4 of 11 (36%) patients were judged responders after treatment in the acute phase (4–8 weeks) and 7 of 16 (44%) responded at the end of extended treatment (mean duration 17.7 ± 13.4 weeks), according to the criterion of a CGI-I score at end point of much or very much improved. Despite a significant decrease in the Inventory of Depressive Symptoms-Self Rated Version score, only 2 of the 11 patients (18%) who completed this assessment demonstrated a decrease of 50% or more after acute-phase topiramate treatment, prompting the authors to qualify the antidepressant effect as "modest." Mean body weight decreased significantly with topiramate treatment in this trial (6.1 ± 8.2%), but interestingly, weight loss was not correlated with change in depressive symptoms. In addition to this larger retrospective study in depressed patients with obesity, there are two published case reports of successful topiramate augmentation in patients diagnosed with treatment-resistant depression and both comorbid binge eating disorder (41) and obesity (42).

Gabapentin

Gabapentin, a GABA-modulating drug that is approved for use in epilepsy and postherpetic neuralgia, was once thought to have significant potential as a mood-stabilizing agent. However, the results of controlled clinical trials suggest that it is not an effective monotherapy for bipolar disorder, although it may still have a role as an adjunct in treatment-resistant patients (43). There are no published placebo-controlled trials of gabapentin in either bipolar or unipolar depressed patients. However, a small number of open-label studies suggest that gabapentin may have antidepressant effects in bipolar patients (44,45). There are currently only two published studies, both retrospective chart reviews that addressed the response of unipolar depressed patients to adjunctive gabapentin therapy. In the first study, 2 of 10 patients were considered responders on the basis of a CGI-I score, reflecting moderate-to-marked improvement (46). The mean maximum dose of gabapentin in this review was 1699 ± 1237 mg/day. In the second study (47), 24 of the total 27 patients studied had a unipolar depressive disorder (20 with major depression). Although the response of the unipolar patients was not analyzed separately, there was a statistically significant improvement in CGI scores at study end point, and 10 (37%) patients met CGI-I response criteria after gabapentin augmentation. The mean final gabapentin dose was 904 ± 445 mg/day.

Oxcarbazepine

Oxcarbazepine is structurally similar to carbamazepine and appears to share its property of inhibiting voltage-gated sodium channels and subsequently reducing glutamate release. Unlike carbamazepine, it is not approved for use in bipolar disorder, although a number of smaller studies suggest that it is useful in this patient population, including patients who are in the depressed phase of the illness. To date, only two retrospective chart reviews have assessed the effectiveness of oxcarbazepine in unipolar depression by including a small number of such patients (48,49). Both studies reported significant improvement in patients who were depressed at the time of treatment but did not separately report the response of unipolar depressed patients. No other studies of oxcarbazepine in unipolar depression are available at this time.

Tiagabine

Tiagabine is a GABA reuptake inhibitor that is approved for adjunctive therapy in the treatment of partial seizures. A few studies have evaluated tiagabine in patients with bipolar disorder with mixed results (50,51), although no studies specifically address its effectiveness in bipolar depression. Only one study of tiagabine has been conducted in unipolar depression, an eight-week, open-label prospective trial of tiagabine monotherapy in patients with depression and signficant anxiety symptoms (52). In this trial, there was a statistically significant change in HAM-D and Hamilton Anxiety Rating Scale scores (−14.9 points and −10.2 points, respectively). Seven out of 15 patients met the criteria for antidepressant response (CGI-I rating of much improved and ≥50% improvement in HAM-D score) at the study end point, while four met criteria for full remission of symptoms (score of ≤7 on the HAM-D).

ANTIEPILEPTICS AND SUICIDALITY

A higher rate of depression and suicidality has been reported in patients with epilepsy (53). This phenomenon has been attributed to various factors, including the pathophysiology of epilepsy (54), psychosocial factors related to this illness, and the effects of AEDs (55). Kalinin (56), in his review of AEDs and suicidality, concluded that some AEDs, particularly phenobarbital, appear to be associated with increased suicidality in patients with epilepsy, while others, such as valproate and carbamazepine, may be protective for some patients. The results regarding suicidal thoughts and behaviors for other AEDs are either mixed or inconclusive. Studies conducted in mood disorder patients confirm that certain AEDs, such as valproate and carbamazepine, may decrease the risk of suicidality (57). Some studies suggest that lithium offers greater protection against suicidality than AEDs (58,59), although not all studies have reported a greater benefit with lithium in this regard (57). There are currently no studies that specifically have addressed the effect of AEDs on suicidal behavior in unipolar depressed patients.

Importantly, a recent FDA analysis of 199 placebo-controlled trials of 11 AEDs found that patients receiving AEDs had approximately twice the risk of suicidal behavior or ideation (0.43%) compared with patients receiving placebo (0.22%) (60). The AEDs assessed were carbamazepine, felbamate, gabapentin, lamotrigine, levetiracetam, oxcarbazepine, pregabalin, tiagabine, topiramate, valproate, and zonisamide. The studies examined the effectiveness of these drugs in epilepsy, psychiatric disorders (e.g., bipolar disorder, depression, and anxiety), and other conditions (e.g., migraine and neuropathic pain syndromes). The increased risk of suicidal behavior and suicidal ideation was observed as early as one week after starting the AED and continued through 24 weeks. The results were generally consistent among the 11 drugs. Patients who were treated for epilepsy, psychiatric disorders, and other conditions were all at increased risk for suicidality when compared with placebo, and there did not appear to be a specific demographic subgroup of patients to which the increased risk could be attributed. However, the relative risk for suicidality was higher in patients with epilepsy (3.6) compared with patients with psychiatric (1.6) or other disorders (2.3) (60).

REFERENCES

1. Post RM, Ketter TA, Uhde T, et al. Thirty years of clinical experience with carbamazepine in the treatment of bipolar illness, principles and practice. CNS Drugs 2007; 21 (1):47–71.
2. Shelton RC. Mood-stabilizing drugs in depression. J Clin Psychiatry 1999; 60(suppl 5): 37–40.
3. Post RM, Uhde TW, Roy-Byrne PP, et al. Antidepressant effects of carbamazepine. Am J Psychiatry 1986; 143(1):29–34.

4. Prasad AJ. Efficacy of carbamazepine as an antidepressant in chronic resistant depressives. J Indian Med Assoc 1985; 83(7):235–237.
5. Rybakowski JK, Suwalska A, Chlopocka-Wozniak M. Potentiation of antidepressants with lithium or carbamazepine in treatment-resistant depression. Neuropsychobiology 1999; 40(3):134–139.
6. Ciusani E, Zullino DF, Eap CB, et al. Combination therapy with venlafaxine and carbamazepine in depressive patients not responding to venlafaxine, pharmacokinetic and clinical aspects. J Psychopharmacol 2004; 18(4):559–566.
7. Steinacher L, Vandel P, Zullino DF, et al. Carbamazepine augmentation in depressive patients non-responding to citalopram, a pharmacokinetic and clinical pilot study. Eur Neuropsychopharmacol 2002; 12(3):255–260.
8. Cullen M, Mitchell P, Brodaty H, et al. Carbamazepine for treatment-resistant melancholia. J Clin Psychiatry 1991; 52(11):472–476.
9. De la Fuente JM, Mendlewicz J. Carbamazepine addition in tricyclic antidepressant-resistant unipolar depression. Biol Psychiatry 1992; 32(4):369–374.
10. Otani K, Yasui N, Kaneko S, et al. Carbamazepine augmentation therapy in three patients with trazodone-resistant unipolar depression. Int Clin Psychopharmacol 1996; 11(1):55–57.
11. Kramlinger KG, Post RM. The addition of lithium to carbamazepine. Antidepressant efficacy in treatment-resistant depression. Arch Gen Psychiatry 1989; 46(9):794–800.
12. Schaffer CB, Mungas D, Rockwell E. Successful treatment of psychotic depression with carbamazepine. J Clin Psychopharmacol 1985; 5(4):233–235.
13. Arana GW, Santos AB, Knax EP, et al. Refractory rapid cycling unipolar depression responds to lithium and carbamazepine treatment. J Clin Psychiatry 1989; 50(9):356–357.
14. Stuppaeck C, Barnas C, Miller C, et al. Carbamazepine in the prophylaxis of mood disorders. J Clin Psychopharmacol 1990; 10(1):39–42.
15. Stuppaeck CH, Barnas C, Schwitzer J, et al. Carbamazepine in the prophylaxis of major depression, a 5-year follow-up. J Clin Psychiatry 1994; 55(4):146–150.
16. Edwards KR, Sackellares JC, Vuong A, et al. Lamotrigine monotherapy improves depressive symptoms in epilepsy, a double-blind comparison with valproate. Epilepsy Behav 2001; 2(1):28–36.
17. Calabrese JR, Bowden CL, Sachs GS, et al. A double-blind placebo-controlled study of lamotrigine monotherapy in outpatients with bipolar I depression. Lamictal 602 Study Group. J Clin Psychiatry 1999; 60(2):79–88.
18. Normann C, Hummel B, Scharer LO, et al. Lamotrigine as adjunct to paroxetine in acute depression, a placebo-controlled, double-blind study. J Clin Psychiatry 2002; 63(4): 337–344.
19. Barbosa L, Berk M, Vorster M. A double-blind, randomized, placebo-controlled trial of augmentation with lamotrigine or placebo in patients concomitantly treated with fluoxetine for resistant major depressive episodes. J Clin Psychiatry 2003; 64(4):403–407.
20. Schindler F, Anghelescu IG. Lithium versus lamotrigine augmentation in treatment resistant unipolar depression, a randomized, open-label study. Int Clin Psychopharmacol 2007; 22(3):179–182.
21. Gabriel A. Lamotrigine adjunctive treatment in resistant unipolar depression, an open, descriptive study. Depress Anxiety 2006; 23(8):485–488.
22. Barbee JG, Jamhour NJ. Lamotrigine as an augmentation agent in treatment-resistant depression. J Clin Psychiatry 2002; 63(8):737–741.
23. Rocha FL, Hara C. Lamotrigine augmentation in unipolar depression. Int Clin Psychopharmacol 2003; 18(2):97–99.
24. Gutierrez RL, McKercher RM, Galea J, et al. Lamotrigine augmentation strategy for patients with treatment-resistant depression. CNS Spectr 2005; 10(10):800–805.
25. Maltese TM. Adjunctive lamotrigine treatment for major depression. Am J Psychiatry 1999; 156(11):1833.
26. Davis LL, Bartolucci A, Petty F. Divalproex in the treatment of bipolar depression, a placebo-controlled study. J Affect Disord 2005; 85(3):259–266.
27. Gyulai L, Bowden CL, McElroy SL, et al. Maintenance efficacy of divalproex in the prevention of bipolar depression. Neuropsychopharmacology 2003; 28(7):1374–1382.

28. Davis LL, Kabel D, Patel D, et al. Valproate as an antidepressant in major depressive disorder. Psychopharmacol Bull 1996; 32(4):647–652.
29. Debattista C, Solomon A, Arnow B, et al. The efficacy of divalproex sodium in the treatment of agitation associated with major depression. J Clin Psychopharmacol 2005; 25(5):476–479.
30. Hayes SG. Long-term use of valproate in primary psychiatric disorders. J Clin Psychiatry 1989; 50(suppl):35–39.
31. Mitchell P, Cullen MJ. Valproate for rapid-cycling unipolar affective disorder. J Nerv Ment Dis 1991; 179(8):503–504.
32. Pies R, Adler DA, Ehrenberg BL. Sleep disorders and depression with atypical features, response to valproate. J Clin Psychopharmacol 1989; 9(5):352–357.
33. Sharma V. Lithium augmentation of valproic acid in treatment resistant depression. Lithium 1994; 5:99–103.
34. Nemets B, Bersudsky Y, Belmaker RH. Controlled double-blind trial of phenytoin vs. fluoxetine in major depressive disorder. J Clin Psychiatry 2005; 66(5):586–590.
35. Shapira B, Nemets B, Trachtenberg A, et al. Phenytoin as an augmentation for SSRI failures, a small controlled study. J Affect Disord 2006; 96(1–2):123–126.
36. Kushner SF, Khan A, Lane R, et al. Topiramate monotherapy in the management of acute mania: results of four double-blind placebo-controlled trials. Bipolar Disord 2006; 8(1):15–27.
37. McIntyre RS, Mancini DA, McCann S, et al. Topiramate versus bupropion SR when added to mood stabilizer therapy for the depressive phase of bipolar disorder, a preliminary single-blind study. Bipolar Disord 2002; 4(3):207–213.
38. Nickel C, Lahmann C, Tritt K, et al. Topiramate in treatment of depressive and anger symptoms in female depressive patients, a randomized, double-blind, placebo-controlled study. J Affect Disord 2005; 87(2–3):243–252.
39. McElroy SL, Hudson JI, Capece JA, et al. Topiramate for the treatment of binge eating disorder associated with obesity, a placebo-controlled study. Biol Psychiatry 2007; 61 (9):1039–1048.
40. Carpenter LL, Leon Z, Yasmin S, et al. Do obese depressed patients respond to topiramate? A retrospective chart review. J Affect Disord 2002; 69(1–3):51–255.
41. Schmidt do Prado-Lima PA, Bacaltchuck J. Topiramate in treatment-resistant depression and binge-eating disorder. Bipolar Disord 2002; 4(4):271–273.
42. Dursun SM, Devarajan S. Accelerated weight loss after treating refractory depression with fluoxetine plus topiramate, possible mechanisms of action? Can J Psychiatry 2001; 46(3):287–288.
43. Carta MG, Hardoy MC, Hardoy MJ, et al. The clinical use of gabapentin in bipolar spectrum disorders. J Affect Disord 2003; 75(1):83–91.
44. Wang PW, Santosa C, Schumacher M, et al. Gabapentin augmentation therapy in bipolar depression. Bipolar Disord 2002; 4(5):296–301.
45. Young LT, Robb JC, Patelis-Siotis I, et al. Acute treatment of bipolar depression with gabapentin. Biol Psychiatry 1997; 42(9):851–853.
46. Ghaemi SN, Katzow JJ, Desai SP, et al. Gabapentin treatment of mood disorders, a preliminary study. J Clin Psychiatry 1998; 59(8):426–429.
47. Yasmin S, Carpenter LL, Leon Z, et al. Adjunctive gabapentin in treatment-resistant depression, a retrospective chart review. J Affect Disord 2001; 63(1–3):243–247.
48. Centorrino F, Albert MJ, Berry JM, et al. Oxcarbazepine, clinical experience with hospitalized psychiatric patients. Bipolar Disord 2003; 5(5):370–374.
49. Raja M, Azzoni A. Oxcarbazepine vs. valproate in the treatment of mood and schizoaffective disorders. Int J Neuropsychopharmacol 2003; 6(4):409–414.
50. Suppes T, Chisholm KA, Dhavale D, et al. Tiagabine in treatment refractory bipolar disorder, a clinical case series. Bipolar Disord 2002; 4(5):283–289.
51. Schaffer LC, Schaffer CB, Howe J. An open case series on the utility of tiagabine as an augmentation in refractory bipolar outpatients. J Affect Disord 2002; 71(1–3): 259–263.
52. Carpenter LL, Schecter JM, Tyrka AR, et al. Open-label tiagabine monotherapy for major depressive disorder with anxiety. J Clin Psychiatry 2006; 67(1):66–71.

53. Hawton K, Fagg J, Marsack P. Association between epilepsy and attempted suicide. J Neurol Neurosurg Psychiatry 1980; 43(2):168–170.
54. Harden CL. The co-morbidity of depression and epilepsy, epidemiology, etiology, and treatment. Neurology 2002; 59(6 suppl 4):S48–S55.
55. Suicide and epilepsy (no author listed). Br Med J 1980; 281(6239):530.
56. Kalinin VV. Suicidality and antiepileptic drugs, is there a link? Drug Saf 2007; 30(2): 123–142.
57. Yerevanian BI, Koek RJ, Mintz J. Bipolar pharmacotherapy and suicidal behavior. Part I, Lithium, divalproex and carbamazepine. J Affect Disord 2007; 103(1–3):5–11.
58. Goodwin FK, Fireman B, Simon GE, et al. Suicide risk in bipolar disorder during treatment with lithium and divalproex. JAMA 2003; 290(11):1467–1473.
59. Collins JC, McFarland BH. Divalproex, lithium and suicide among Medicaid patients with bipolar disorder. J Affect Disord. 2007 (in press) (epub ahead of print).
60. U.S. Food and Drug Administration (FDA). Information for healthcare professionals suicidality and antiepileptic drugs. Available at: http://www.fda.gov/cder/drug/ InfoSheets/HCP/antiepilepticsHCP.htm. Accessed January 5, 2008.

11 Antiepileptics in the Treatment of Schizophrenia

Leslie Citrome
New York University School of Medicine, New York, New York, and Clinical Research and Evaluation Facility, Nathan S. Kline Institute for Psychiatric Research, Orangeburg, New York, U.S.A.

INTRODUCTION

In the absence of knowledge about the precise pathophysiology of schizophrenia, pharmacological treatments have been limited to symptoms. Although the reduction of positive symptoms such as hallucinations or delusions are important, particularly when they intrude on self-care or interactions with other people, there is growing appreciation of the importance of treating other symptom domains such as negative symptomatology, cognitive function, and persistent aggressive behavior. In this context, clinicians routinely turn to augmentation strategies when faced with the observation that antipsychotic monotherapy can be inadequate for many patients with schizophrenia. Prime medication candidates for use in combination with antipsychotics are those agents with a different mechanism of action so that there is the possibility of pharmacodynamic synergy, perhaps leading to a faster, better, or more sustainable therapeutic response. Antiepileptic drugs (AEDs) and lithium, medications used for bipolar disorder, are also commonly used in combination with antipsychotics to treat schizophrenia.

The evidence base supporting the use of adjunctive AEDs for patients with schizophrenia is mixed. Initial positive case reports and open-label studies have not always been followed by successful randomized clinical trials (Table 1). This chapter will review the utilization patterns of AEDs in patients with schizophrenia, the evidence base supporting this use, and end with pragmatic advice for the clinician on when and how to consider augmentation with a specific AED for an individual patient.

EXTENT OF USE

The use of adjunctive AEDs in patients with schizophrenia is extensive, especially among inpatients in intermediate and long-term care settings. Within the inpatient facilities operated by the New York State Office of Mental Health (NYSOMH), the percentage of inpatients with schizophrenia receiving adjunctive AEDs or lithium has leveled off at approximately 50% during the last five years (Fig. 1, lithium not shown). Although valproate is the most commonly used adjunctive anticonvulsant, others appear to be increasing in their popularity, albeit more slowly (1–3). Some AEDs are being used less often over time, such as adjunctive gabapentin or adjunctive carbamazepine.

The mean dose of AEDs used is substantial. Data available from NYSOMH inpatient facilities in 2006 reveals that among 7154 patients receiving antipsychotics (76.5% of whom had a diagnosis of schizophrenia or schizoaffective disorder), the average daily dose of valproate was 1677 mg ($N = 2813$), gabapentin 1552 mg ($N = 363$), oxcarbazepine 1183 mg ($N = 306$), carbamazepine 781 mg ($N = 178$), topiramate 237 mg ($N = 357$), and lamotrigine 225 mg ($N = 528$) [unpublished data updated from (4)]. Moreover, combinations of mood stabilizers are also

TABLE 1 Evidence for Adjunctive Use of Antiepileptics for the Treatment of Schizophrenia

Agent	Year introduced in United States	Case reports and open studies	Controlled clinical trials[a] (number of reports)	Utility (benefit?)
Carbamazepine	1974	Yes	Yes (7)	Maybe
Valproate	1978	Yes	Yes (8)	Maybe
Gabapentin	1993	Yes (±)	None	Probably not
Lamotrigine	1994	Yes (±)	Yes (6)	Maybe
Topiramate	1997	Yes (±)	Yes (3)	Probably not
Oxcarbazepine	2000	Yes (±)	None	Too early to tell

Note: ±, both positive and negative results.
[a]English-language reports.

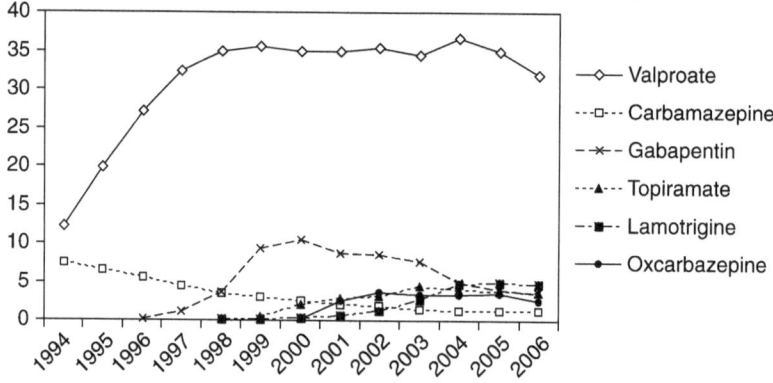

FIGURE 1 Percent inpatients with schizophrenia receiving adjunctive antiepileptics within the New York State Office of Mental Health from 1994 (*N* = 8405) to 2006 (*N* = 3132). *Source*: From unpublished data updated from Ref. 4.

used. Approximately half of all patients receiving a mood stabilizer received more than one, with the exception of patients receiving valproate where the rate of coprescribing of another AED or lithium was about 25% (4).

Somewhat lower utilization rates for adjunctive mood stabilizers are observed in other parts of the world. The overall trend over time, however, has been for increased use. In the treatment of acute episodes of schizophrenia in a German university hospital, adjunctive mood stabilizer use increased from 15% in 1998 to 26% in 2001 and 28% in 2004 (5). For all inpatients with schizophrenia at the same hospital, adjunctive use of AEDs specifically increased from approximately 3% in 1998 to 12% in 2003, while that for adjunctive lithium decreased from 13% to 4% (6). In the 10 hospitals participating in a drug surveillance program in Germany and Switzerland, among 745 patients with schizophrenia in 1995, 9.5% received AEDs, increasing to 15% of 1015 patients in 2001 (7).

Adjunctive AED use in outpatient populations has also been described. In a cross-sectional study of 456 outpatients with schizophrenia, in Rochester, New York (8), 39% of white patients and 25% of black patients received adjunctive lithium or AEDs in 2003 or 2004. The percentage is lower in China, where in a randomly selected sample of 250 stable outpatients with schizophrenia, 10% received a mood stabilizer (actual medications in this category were not defined) (9).

In an analysis of database data for both inpatient and outpatient encounters contained in the National Psychosis Registry of the U.S. Department of Veterans Affairs (10), among 77,243 patients with a diagnosis of schizophrenia or schizo-affective disorder in 1999 and 2000, concurrent treatment with a mood stabilizer was observed among 37% ($N = 2148$) of patients given prescriptions for antipsychotic polypharmacy and 27% ($N = 10,797$) of patients given prescriptions for antipsychotic monotherapy.

Thus, the use of adjunctive AEDs in both inpatients and outpatients with schizophrenia is extensive. There are international variations in practice, but overall use has increased with time.

EVIDENCE SUPPORTING AUGMENTATION WITH ANTIEPILEPTIC DRUGS

Table 1 outlines the variability in quality and quantity of the evidence supporting the use of adjunctive AEDs in the treatment of schizophrenia. Although uncontrolled case reports or case series provide relatively weak supporting evidence, they do provide a rationale for follow-up double-blind and/or randomized clinical trials. However, not all AEDs in use as adjunctive agents in the treatment of schizophrenia have been tested in controlled trials, and many of the published studies suffer from a variety of methodological flaws such as an inadequate number of subjects (insufficient statistical power to detect differences), lack of control of confounds such as affective symptomatology (seen when studies include patients with schizoaffective disorder), inadequate duration (usually too short), or inappropriate target populations (acute exacerbations of schizophrenia rather than treatment-refractory schizophrenia with persistent residual symptoms).

Carbamazepine

Carbamazepine was introduced in the United States in 1974 for the treatment of epilepsy. Initial reports from Finland on the possible use of carbamazepine in the treatment of violent patients with schizophrenia with and without EEG abnormalities (11) led to further investigations with carbamazepine in patients with schizophrenia with normal EEGs (12). The available controlled studies of adjunctive carbamazepine in the treatment of schizophrenia (double-blind and/or randomized) for which English-language reports are available are included in Table 2 (13–19). In the largest of these studies ($N = 162$) (15), a double-blind clinical trial of carbamazepine in patients with Diagnostic and Statistical Manual of Mental Disorders III (DSM-III) schizophrenia or schizoaffective disorder, there was a failure to detect significant improvement on the total Brief Psychiatric Rating Scale (BPRS) with adjunctive carbamazepine compared with adjunctive placebo. However, differences did emerge among the BPRS items of suspiciousness, uncooperativeness, and excitement. The other studies listed in Table 2 were substantially smaller in terms of sample size, and with the exception of an early crossover design study (13), they failed to detect any meaningful advantage for adjunctive carbamazepine use. Moreover, a recent comparison with a second-generation antipsychotic, olanzapine, demonstrated superiority of that agent over a combination of perazine and carbamazepine, particularly with positive symptoms (19). A comprehensive Cochrane Library Review meta-analysis (20) concluded on the basis of eight studies ($N = 182$), which compared adjunctive carbamazepine

TABLE 2 Controlled Studies of Adjunctive Carbamazepine in Schizophrenia

Author and year (reference)	N	Length (days)	Target daily dose of CBZ (mg)[a]	Design	Diagnosis	Outcome
Neppe 1983 (13)	11	42	600	AP + CBZ vs. AP + placebo (crossover)	Inpatients, 8 with schizophrenia (and EEG abnormalities)	Improvement in "overall clinical rating" with CBZ
Dose 1987 (14)	22	28	600–1200	HAL + CBZ vs. HAL + placebo	Inpatients with schizophrenia or schizoaffective disorder	No difference on BPRS
Okuma 1989 (15)	162	28	200–1200	AP + CBZ vs. AP + placebo (although double-blind, the study was not randomized)	Inpatients or outpatients with schizophrenia or schizoaffective disorder	No difference on BPRS; Possible improvement on suspiciousness, uncooperative-ness and excitement with CBZ
Nachshoni 1994 (16)	28	49	600	AP + CBZ vs. AP + placebo	Inpatients with "residual schizophrenia with negative symptoms"	No difference on BPRS or SANS
Simhandl 1996 (17)	42	42	15–42 μmol/L	AP + CBZ vs. AP + Li vs. AP + placebo	Schizophrenia (treatment-nonresponsive)	No difference on BPRS; within groups CBZ and Li improved on CGI from baseline
Hesslinger 1998 (18)	27	28	Mean 567	HAL vs. HAL + CBZ vs. HAL + VAL (although randomized, the study was not double-blind)	Inpatients with schizophrenia or schizoaffective disorder	CBZ was associated with significantly lower HAL plasma levels and with a worse clinical outcome compared with antipsychotic monotherapy
Ohlmeier 2007 (19)	33	21	Mean 404	Perazine + CBZ vs. olanzapine (although randomized, the study was not double-blind)	Inpatients with schizophrenia	Olanzapine monotherapy was superior to perazine plus CBZ on positive symptoms on PANSS and BPRS

[a]If unavailable mean daily dose or target plasma level is provided.
Abbreviations: HAL, Haloperidol; CBZ, Carbamazepine; Li, Lithium; VAL, Valproate; AP, Antipsychotic; BPRS, Brief Psychiatric Rating Scale; SANS, Scale for the Assessment of Negative Symptoms; CGI, Clinical Global Impression; PANSS, Positive and Negative Syndrome Scale.

with adjunctive placebo, that adding carbamazepine to antipsychotic treatment was as acceptable as adding placebo with no difference between the numbers leaving the study early from each group and that carbamazepine augmentation was superior compared with antipsychotics alone in terms of overall global improvement. However, there were no differences in the outcome of 50% reduction in BPRS scores. The authors concluded that carbamazepine cannot be recommended for routine clinical use for treatment or augmentation of antipsychotic treatment of schizophrenia, but that large, simple, well-designed, and reported trials are justified, especially if focusing on those populations for which data is especially scant: patients with schizophrenia with violent episodes and/or EEG abnormalities. Although the frequency of use of carbamazepine in psychiatric practice appears to have decreased in patients with bipolar disorder, schizophrenia, or schizoaffective disorder during the 1990s in the United States (2,21), this trend may reverse itself now that an extended-release formulation of carbamazepine received approval in December 2004 by the U.S. Food and Drug Administration (FDA) for the indication of bipolar mania (22). An important obstacle to the use of carbamazepine is that it induces its own metabolism (and that of other agents being administered), and hence dose adjustments are often needed for both carbamazepine and the antipsychotic being prescribed. For example, a recent study of the second-generation antipsychotic, aripiprazole, given with carbamazepine demonstrated substantially reduced plasma levels of the antipsychotic in the presence of carbamazepine cotherapy (23).

Valproate

Valproate is the active moiety of both valproic acid and divalproex sodium and is currently the most commonly used adjunctive AED in the treatment of schizophrenia. Valproic acid was introduced as a treatment for epilepsy in France in 1967 and was approved in the United States by the FDA in 1978 for the monotherapy and adjunctive therapy of complex partial seizures and simple or complex absence seizures. For patients with mental disorders, the pivotal year was 1995, when divalproex sodium was approved by the FDA for the indication of manic episodes associated with bipolar disorder. The first signals indicating the use of adjunctive valproate in the treatment of schizophrenia came from case reports and open-label studies. Early reports from 1976 (24) and 1979 (25) demonstrated reduced psychopathology in general, as measured by the BPRS, and improvement on emotional withdrawal, respectively. An open-label study of valproate and haloperidol in 30 patients with schizophrenia suggested that augmentation with valproate can result in improvements in suspiciousness, hallucinations, unusual thought content, and emotional withdrawal, as well as in fewer inpatient days (26). A report of the combination of valproate with the second-generation antipsychotic, risperidone, demonstrated clinical improvement in an otherwise treatment-resistant patient with schizophrenia (27).

The available controlled studies of adjunctive valproate in the treatment of schizophrenia (double-blind and/or randomized) for which English-language reports are available are included in Table 3 (18,28–34). Initial controlled studies of adjunctive valproate in patients with schizophrenia have been limited in terms of the number of subjects. In the first, Ko and colleagues (28) found no additional benefit with adjunctive valproate in a 28-day crossover study with six neuroleptic-resistant patients with chronic schizophrenia (not experiencing an exacerbation). In

TABLE 3 Controlled Studies of Adjunctive Valproate in Schizophrenia

Author and year (reference)	N	Length (days)	Target daily dose of VAL (mg)[a]	Design	Diagnosis	Outcome
Ko 1985 (28)	6	28	1600–2400	AP + VAL vs. AP + placebo (crossover)	Inpatients with neuroleptic-resistant chronic schizophrenia (not exacerbation)	No valproate effect noted
Fisk 1987 (29)	62	42	1200 or 1500	AP + VAL vs. AP + placebo	Inpatients with chronic psychosis and tardive dyskinesia	No differences in mental state and behavior as measured by the "Krawiecka scale" (85)[b]
Dose 1998 (30)	42	28	900–1200	HAL + VAL vs. HAL + placebo	Inpatients with acute, nonmanic schizophrenic or schizoaffective psychosis	No difference on BPRS; Possible effect on hostile belligerence
Hesslinger 1998 (18)	27	28	Mean 757	HAL vs. HAL + CBZ vs. HAL + VAL (although randomized, the study was not double-blind)	Inpatients with schizophrenia or schizoaffective	VAL had no significant effect on either plasma levels of HAL or on psychopathology
Wassef 2000 (31)	12	21	75–100 µg/mL	HAL + VAL vs. HAL + placebo	Inpatients with acute exacerbation of chronic schizophrenia	Significant Improvement in CGI and SANS but not BPRS
Casey 2003 (32)	249	28	Mean ~2300	RIS + VAL vs. OLZ + VAL vs. RIS + placebo vs. OLZ + placebo	Inpatients with acute schizophrenia	Improvement on PANSS
Abbott 2006 (33)	402	84	Mean ~2900	RIS + VAL vs. OLZ + VAL vs. RIS + placebo vs. OLZ + placebo	Inpatients with acute schizophrenia	No advantage for combination treatment with adjunctive VAL
Citrome 2007 (34)	33	56	50–100 µg/mL	RIS vs. RIS + VAL (although randomized, the study was not double-blind)	Inpatients with schizophrenia and hostile behavior	Although significantly fewer patients randomized to monotherapy completed the study, no significant differences between monotherapy and combination treatment were observed in change of the rating instruments used, including the PANSS

[a]If unavailable mean daily dose or target plasma level is provided.
Abbreviations: AP, antipsychotic; HAL, haloperidol; VAL, valproate; RIS, risperidone; OLZ, olanzapine; BPRS, Brief Psychiatric Rating Scale; SANS, Scale for the Assessment of Negative Symptoms; CGI, Clinical Global Impression; PANSS, Positive and Negative Syndrome Scale.

another study, this time among 42 patients with acute, nonmanic schizophrenic or schizoaffective psychosis comparing haloperidol and placebo versus haloperidol and valproate over 28 days, no difference on the BPRS was observed, but a possible effect on "hostile belligerence" was noted (30). In another study of acute patients with schizophrenia ($N = 12$) comparing adjunctive valproate with placebo in patients receiving haloperidol, a significant improvement was observed in the Clinical Global Impression (CGI) scale as well as on the Schedule for Assessment of Negative Symptoms (SANS) but not on the BPRS (31). Two other controlled studies found no meaningful advantage for adjunctive valproate (29,30). These initial randomized studies enrolled relatively small number of subjects, hence differences between the groups might have been difficult to detect because of lack of sufficient statistical power. They also included different types of patients—neuroleptic-resistant patients in one (28), chronic patients with tardive dyskinesia in another (29), and acute patients in the other three reports (18,30,31).

The published study with the largest number of subjects ($N = 249$) is that of a multicenter, randomized, double-blind, 28-day clinical trial of adjunctive divalproex in hospitalized patients with an acute exacerbation of schizophrenia conducted by the manufacturer of divalproex (32). Schizoaffective and treatment-refractory patients were specifically excluded, thus the study did answer the question whether or not adjunctive valproate has an effect on acute psychotic symptoms rather than on mood. However, this study did not answer the question whether or not adjunctive valproate would be useful in treatment-refractory patients with persistent symptoms of schizophrenia. The study design consisted of receiving one of four treatments for four weeks: olanzapine and divalproex, olanzapine and placebo, risperidone and divalproex, or risperidone and placebo. Doses of risperidone 6 mg/day or olanzapine 15 mg/day were reached by day 6. Divalproex was started at 15 mg/kg and titrated to a maximum of 30 mg/kg by day 14. The mean dose of divalproex achieved was approximately 2300 mg/day with a mean plasma level of approximately 100 µg/mL. The Positive and Negative Syndrome Scale (PANSS) was the primary outcome measure. Ratings were done at baseline, days 3, 5, 7, 10, 14, 21, and 28. PANSS total score significantly improved in the combination therapy group compared with the monotherapy group at specific time points (days 3, 5, 7, 10, 14, and 21) and throughout the study period [repeated measures analysis of variance (ANOVA), $P = 0.020$]. Significant treatment differences occurred as early as day 3. The major effect was on the positive symptoms of schizophrenia. No new safety concerns were observed; the combination therapy was as well tolerated as monotherapy. A post hoc analysis also revealed that patients receiving adjunctive divalproex had greater reductions in hostility on days 3 and 7 (as measured by the Hostility item in the Positive Subscale of the PANSS) compared with antipsychotic monotherapy and that this effect was independent of the effect on the positive symptoms of schizophrenia or sedation (35).

The above 28-day study provided the strongest evidence so far for a real effect of adjunctive AED treatment for schizophrenia and provided the impetus for the manufacturer to conduct a second study, this time with the extended-release preparation of divalproex with 402 patients with acute schizophrenia (33). The principal results of this 84-day multicenter, double-blind, randomized clinical trial have been publicly disclosed on the Web site clinicalstudyresults.org (www .clinicalstudyresults.org) and revealed that the study failed to demonstrate any benefit with combination treatment versus monotherapy with risperidone or olanzapine. This failure to replicate the earlier study (32) is consistent with the results of another recently reported clinical trial of adjunctive valproate in the treatment of patients with schizophrenia and hostility (34). This was an eight-week, open-label, rater-blinded, randomized, parallel-group clinical trial in hospitalized adults where patients were randomly assigned to receive risperidone alone ($N = 16$) or risperidone plus valproate ($N = 17$). Although significantly fewer patients randomized to monotherapy completed the study, no significant differences between monotherapy or combination treatment were observed in change of any of the rating instruments used, including the PANSS.

Evidence supporting the use of adjunctive valproate in the treatment of schizophrenia is thus limited. There remains active interest in this combination treatment, and small uncontrolled studies continue to be published showing advantages for combination treatment, such as the use of this strategy with older adults in a prospective, 12-week open-label study ($N = 20$) (36), a retrospective six-month study examining adjunctive divalproex ($N = 15$) or lithium ($N = 9$) added to clozapine and compared with clozapine monotherapy in treatment-resistant schizophrenia patients ($N = 25$) (37), and a four-week study of the effect of valproic acid on plasma levels of risperidone and its active metabolite ($N = 12$) (38). Pharmacoepidemiological evidence published includes the results of a large ($N = 10,262$) retrospective analysis of persistence of treatment with valproate augmentation versus switching antipsychotic medication (39). Diagnostic categories were not available. Valproate led to longer persistence of treatment than switching antipsychotics, but the average doses of valproate were small (<425 mg/day), as were the doses of the antipsychotics (risperidone < 1.7 mg/day, quetiapine < 120 mg/day, and olanzapine < 7.5 mg/day).

Although the use of an extended-release preparation may be particularly helpful when encouraging medication adherence for patients who are otherwise prescribed complicated medication regimens, different formulations of valproate may have different effects, as suggested by a prospective "quasi-experimental" clinical trial involving over 9000 psychiatric admissions over six years (40). Inpatients who initially received divalproex sodium had a 32.7% longer hospital stay and 3.8% higher readmission rate than did patients who initially received valproic acid. After other variables were controlled, the hospital stay of patients who continued the initial medication was 15.2% longer (2 days) for divalproex than valproic acid. Medication intolerance occurred in approximately 6.4% more patients taking valproic acid than divalproex. However, switching from valproic acid to divalproex did not significantly prolong length of stay over that for continuous divalproex or increase the rehospitalization rate. The authors concluded that lower peak valproate concentrations with divalproex sodium may have enhanced tolerability but may also explain the lower effectiveness, and that extended-release divalproex could lower effectiveness further and require higher doses. They suggested that inpatients should start with generic valproic acid and then change to delayed-release divalproex only if intolerance occurs. Switching to the extended-release preparation from the regular (delayed-release) preparation of divalproex does involve consideration of bioavailability differences; the average bioavailability of the extended-release preparation is 81% to 89% relative to delayed-release tablets given twice daily (41,42). The consequences of this difference were assessed in 30 patients with schizophrenia who were switched in a four-week open-label treatment trial (43). Patients were converted from divalproex delayed release to extended release on a 1.0:1.0 mg basis (rounded up to the nearest 500-mg increment), if baseline valproate plasma levels were at least 85 μg/mL; otherwise, the conversion rate was 1.0:1.2 mg (rounded up). Patients who converted on a 1:1 mg basis had lower end point valproate trough plasma levels than at baseline but did not experience deterioration in their psychopathology, presumably because they had a higher plasma level of valproate to begin with.

A comprehensive Cochrane Library Review meta-analysis (44) concluded on the basis of five studies ($N = 379$) that compared adjunctive valproate with adjunctive placebo that adding valproate did not demonstrate a significant effect on the participants' global state or general mental state at end point. The reviewers noted that subjects receiving valproate more frequently experienced sedation than those in the placebo group. Given this limited evidence, further large, simple, well-designed, and reported trials were thought necessary.

In reviewing all of the studies described above, larger and focused controlled trials examining the use of adjunctive valproate in specific subpopulations of patients with schizophrenia would be helpful, such as treatment-refractory patients and the more chronically ill.

Lamotrigine

Lamotrigine was commercialized in the United States as an AED in 1994, and the FDA approved it for the indication of maintenance treatment of bipolar I disorder in 2003. A report was published in 1999 of a case series of six patients with treatment-resistant schizophrenia who benefited from lamotrigine being added to their regimen of clozapine (45). In another open trial, patients receiving lamotrigine augmentation of clozapine had a significant decrease in BPRS scores after two weeks of treatment, but there was no significant improvement when lamotrigine was added to risperidone, haloperidol, olanzapine, or fluphenthixol (46). In contrast, others have found benefit in adding lamotrigine to regimens of antipsychotics other than clozapine, notably, zuclopenthixol, risperidone, and haloperidol in patients with treatment-resistant schizophrenia (47). These positive results are tempered by reports of other cases where a benefit of adjunctive lamotrigine with clozapine was not observed (48), a report of worsening of psychotic symptoms in a patient with schizophrenia when lamotrigine was added to quetiapine (49), and a case of remission of positive symptoms of schizophrenia when a regimen of lamotrigine and olanzapine was switched to carbamazepine and olanzapine in a patient with schizophrenia and EEG abnormalities (50). Additional case reports are available regarding the use of lamotrigine to augment clozapine in patients with both schizophrenia and alcohol dependence, where an anticraving effect may be observed (51).

The available controlled studies of adjunctive lamotrigine in the treatment of schizophrenia (double-blind and/or randomized) for which English-language reports are available are included in Table 4 (52–57). The first was conducted in Finland by Tiihonen and colleagues (52), where adjunctive lamotrigine was added to clozapine in patients with treatment-resistant schizophrenia in a small ($N = 34$), double-blind, placebo-controlled crossover trial. Patients who had failed clozapine monotherapy received lamotrigine (200 mg/day) for up to 12 weeks. Adjunctive lamotrigine resulted in the improvement of positive, but not negative, symptoms. Similarly, in a 10-week, double-blind, parallel-group clinical trial ($N = 38$) by Kremer and colleagues (53), administering adjunctive lamotrigine to treatment-resistant inpatients with schizophrenia resulted in improvement in the PANSS positive, general psychopathology, and total symptoms scores in completers ($N = 31$);

TABLE 4 Controlled Studies of Adjunctive Lamotrigine in Schizophrenia

Author and year (reference)	N	Length (days)	Target daily dose of LAM (mg)	Design	Diagnosis	Outcome
Tiihonen 2003 (52)	34	84	200	CLO + LAM vs. CLO + placebo (crossover)	Male inpatients with CLO-resistant chronic schizophrenia (not exacerbation)	Improvement in BPRS, PANSS positive, and PANSS general psychopathology; Most robust effect seen in the most ill patients ($N = 10$) (BPRS $\geq$ 45); No improvement in negative symptoms
Kremer 2004 (53)	38	70	400	AP + LAM vs. AP + placebo	Inpatients with treatment-resistant schizophrenia	Improvement in PANSS positive, general psychopathology, and total symptoms scores in completers; No difference in negative symptoms or total BPRS; No difference with intent-to-treat analyses
Akhondzadeh 2005 (54)	36	56	150	RIS + LAM vs. RIS + placebo	Inpatients with schizophrenia	Superiority over RIS alone in the treatment of negative symptoms, general psychopathology, and PANSS total scores; patients' attention improved on the Stroop color-naming subtest (time and error)
Zoccali 2007 (55)	60	168	200	CLO + LAM vs. CLO + placebo	Outpatients with treatment-resistant schizophrenia	Improvement on negative, positive, and general psychopathological symptomatology
Glaxo-Smith-Kline 2005 (56)	209	84	100–400	AP + LAM vs. AP + placebo	Inpatients or outpatients with schizophrenia and with stable, residual psychotic symptoms	SANS total score and CGI improved more with placebo than LAM
Glaxo-Smith-Kline 2006 (57)	210	84	100–400	AP + LAM vs. AP + placebo	Inpatients or outpatients with schizophrenia and with stable, residual psychotic symptoms	Cognitive composite score improved more with LAM than with placebo

Abbreviations: CLO, clozapine; LAM, lamotrigine; AP, antipsychotic; BPRS, Brief Psychiatric Rating Scale; SANS, Scale for the Assessment of Negative Symptoms; PANSS, Positive and Negative Syndrome Scale; CGI, Clinical Global Impression.

however, no differences were observed in negative symptoms or total BPRS scores, and no differences were found in the intent-to-treat (ITT) analysis. Response to lamotrigine did not differ between patients treated with first-generation compared with second-generation antipsychotics. In a third inpatient study conducted in Iran (54), 36 patients with schizophrenia were randomized to receive risperidone plus lamotrigine or risperidone plus placebo for eight weeks. Advantages for combination treatment were observed for negative symptoms, general psychopathology, and total PANSS but not for positive symptoms. Some additional cognitive effect was noted on a subtest assessing color naming. An outpatient study involving 60 patients with treatment-resistant schizophrenia assessed double-blind over a 24-week period (55) found improvement of positive and negative symptoms as well as improvement in measures of cognitive performance when lamotrigine was added to clozapine compared with placebo added to clozapine among the 51 completers.

The initial signals from the uncontrolled studies by Dursun (45,46) and the randomized clinical trial by Tiihonen (52) spurred the launch of two 12-week large-scale ($N = 209$ and $N = 210$) studies by the manufacturer of lamotrigine in patients with schizophrenia who had not responded adequately to second-generation antipsychotics alone (56–58). Patients were randomized to receive either adjunctive lamotrigine or adjunctive placebo. Results from these two trials did not support the effectiveness of lamotrigine as an add-on treatment for patients with residual psychotic symptoms of schizophrenia. Secondary objectives that evaluated additional measures of global response, negative symptoms, depressive symptoms, and quality of life also failed to support clinical effectiveness. The only indication of a possible therapeutic effect of lamotrigine was the improvement in the cognitive composite score in one study (57), but this effect was neither found in the other study (56) nor was it a primary hypothesis. These results are clearly at odds with the other published controlled trials (52–55). It is possible that the patients enrolled in the large multicenter studies conducted by the manufacturer were not as ill as the patients who participated in the other studies. In addition, placebo response in both of the manufacturer's studies was substantial, diminishing the ability to observe a therapeutic effect with lamotrigine.

A comprehensive Cochrane Library Review meta-analysis (59) concluded on the basis of five studies ($N = 537$) that compared adjunctive lamotrigine versus adjunctive placebo that the data are not robust and the effect sizes showing an advantage for combination therapy are small.

Topiramate

Topiramate was introduced in the United States in 1997 as an antiseizure medication. It does not have FDA approval for any psychiatric disorder per se. However, topiramate is one of the few medications that have been associated with weight loss. Thus this agent has attracted a great deal of interest among clinicians as an adjunct to second-generation antipsychotics to address the adverse event of weight gain. An early case report from 2000 described a patient with schizophrenia being treated with clozapine who lost 21 kg over five months when receiving adjunctive topiramate 125 mg/day (60). In a two-year retrospective case series analysis, weight loss was observed in 10 patients with schizophrenia and schizoaffective disorder with antipsychotic-induced weight gain and who received adjunctive topiramate at a mean daily dose of approximately 200 mg (61). Adjunctive topiramate limited the amount of weight gain observed among 60 male outpatients with schizophrenia receiving olanzapine in a 12-week, randomized, open-label, parallel-group trial conducted in Korea (62). The strongest evidence to date supporting the use of adjunctive topiramate for the treatment of excess weight in patients with schizophrenia is a 12-week, randomized, placebo-controlled prospective study of 66 hospitalized patients conducted in Korea (63). Patients were randomized to receive adjunctive topiramate at doses of 100 mg/day or 200 mg/day, or a placebo. Body weight, body mass index, waist measurement, and hip measurement decreased significantly in the 200-mg/day topiramate group compared with the 100-mg/day topiramate and placebo groups over 12 weeks. The waist-to-hip ratio did not change in any group.

The use of adjunctive topiramate in treating the symptoms of schizophrenia has also been studied. A case report from 2001 describes how adjunctive topiramate can attenuate the severity of negative symptoms of schizophrenia (64). However, negative reports also exist. In an open trial, no significant improvement was observed in nine patients receiving topiramate augmentation of clozapine, olanzapine, haloperidol, or fluphenthixol (46). Deterioration has also been described. For example, when using adjunctive topiramate up to the range of 200 to 300 mg/day to treat five patients with treatment-refractory schizophrenia (4 patients were taking clozapine), two patients deteriorated to the point that the investigators could not obtain reliable post-treatment PANSS scores, and for the remaining three patients, the PANSS total score deteriorated substantially (including both positive and negative symptoms) (65). In another case report, a patient with schizophrenia originally treated with clozapine and valproate experienced a worsening of psychosis in the context of replacing valproate with topiramate, which remitted when valproate was resumed (66). The cognitive side effects of topiramate have been suggested as one of the reasons patients with schizophrenia may deteriorate with adjunctive topiramate (67). Other case reports of adjunctive topiramate in treating schizophrenia have examined the potential role topiramate may play in reducing alcohol abuse (68).

The available controlled studies of adjunctive topiramate in the treatment of schizophrenia (double-blind and/or randomized) for which English-language reports are available are included in Table 5 (62,63,69). The sole extant study targeting psychopathology was conducted in Finland in 26 patients with treatment-resistant schizophrenia (69). The study was a randomized, double-blind, placebo-controlled trial in which 300 mg/day of topiramate was gradually added to the patient's ongoing treatment (clozapine, olanzapine, risperidone, or quetiapine) over two 12-week crossover treatment periods. In the ITT analysis, topiramate was more effective than placebo in reducing PANSS general psychopathological symptoms, but no significant improvement was observed in positive or negative symptoms.

Gabapentin

Although introduced in the United States in 1993, there is very limited published data on the use of adjunctive gabapentin for the treatment of schizophrenia. It does not have FDA approval for any psychiatric disorder per se. No controlled studies are available regarding adjunctive gabapentin for the treatment of schizophrenia. There is an early report of favorable long-term antianxiety and hypnotic effects of adjunctive gabapentin in patients with comorbid anxiety-related disorders (70). Among the 18 patients described in that naturalistic study, 10 were diagnosed with

TABLE 5 Controlled Studies of Adjunctive Topiramate in Schizophrenia

Author and year (reference)	N	Length (days)	Target daily dose of TOP (mg)	Design	Diagnosis	Outcome
Ko 2005 (63)	66	84	100 or 200	AP + TOP 100 mg vs. AP + TOP 200 mg vs. AP + placebo	Inpatients with schizophrenia and overweight	With TOP 200 mg, body weight, body mass index, waist measurement, and hip measurement decreased significantly compared with TOP 100-mg and placebo groups. Waist-to-hip ratio did not change in any group. BPRS decreased by 0.4%, 3.2%, and 2.9% in the placebo, TOP 100-mg, and TOP 200-mg groups, respectively
Tiihonen 2005 (69)	26	84	300	AP+TOP vs. AP + placebo (crossover)	Male inpatients with treatment-resistant chronic schizophrenia (on CLO, OLZ, or QUE)	Improvement in PANSS general; no difference in total PANSS, PANSS positive, or PANSS negative
Kim 2006 (62)	60	84	100	OLZ vs. OLZ + TOP (although randomized, the study was not double-blind)	Outpatients with schizophrenia	TOP was associated with less weight gain at weeks 4, 8, and end point. Improvement on the PANSS total were observed in both groups and not significantly different

Abbreviations: AP, antipsychotic; TOP, topiramate; CLO, clozapine; OLZ, olanzapine; QUE, quetiapine; PANSS, Positive and Negative Syndrome Scale.

schizophrenia and 4 with schizoaffective disorder. In a chart review of 11 patients in a state-operated psychiatric hospital (4 with schizophrenia and 4 with schizoaffective disorder), adjunctive gabapentin was associated with a reduction in agitation (71). Negative reports exist, including a case report of a patient with schizophrenia who experienced increased hallucinations and delusions when gabapentin was added to his regimen of clozapine, procyclidine, divalproex, and fluoxetine (72). There is some interest regarding the use of gabapentin for movement disorders associated with schizophrenia treatments, including akathisia (73) and tardive dyskinesia (74).

Oxcarbazepine

Oxcarbazepine was launched in the United States in 2000 for the management of seizures. It does not have FDA approval for any psychiatric disorder per se. No controlled studies are available regarding adjunctive oxcarbazepine for the treatment of schizophrenia. Because it is an analogue of carbamazepine, it was anticipated that it would have a similar efficacy profile and yet not be as problematic in terms of liver enzyme induction as carbamazepine. A retrospective medical record review of the use of oxcarbazepine in 56 hospitalized psychiatric patients (14 with schizophrenia or "other idiopathic psychotic disorders" and 6 with schizoaffective disorder) found the agent to be well tolerated and simpler to use than carbamazepine (75). There is an open-label case series of six male inpatients where oxcarbazepine was added to antipsychotic treatment, starting with 300 mg/day and ending with a final dose of 900 to 2100 mg/day (76). After 42 days of combination treatment, BPRS scores decreased substantially. A negative case report is also available where worsening of dysphoria and irritability was observed with adjunctive oxcarbazepine in a patient with schizophrenia and obsessive-compulsive traits (77). The patient's clinical deterioration was attributed to pharmacokinetic interactions (77).

ANTIEPILEPTIC DRUGS FOR AGGRESSION?

A common rationale for using adjunctive AEDs in patients with schizophrenia is to manage persistent aggressive behavior (78,79). In a prior iteration of a set of guidelines for the treatment of schizophrenia, adjunctive valproate was ranked first for the problem of aggression/violence and for agitation/excitement (with a history of substance abuse) (80). The above discussions of carbamazepine and valproate have described some of the evidence supporting this use of AEDs, but there remains little in the way of controlled clinical trials that specifically study patients with hostile behavior. These studies are logistically difficult to conduct given the imprecise definitions of aggression, the difficulty of measuring outcome because of the relative rarity of aggressive events, and the challenges of selecting appropriate patients for study, which includes determining allowable comorbidities and concomitant medications (81). Since the usual outcome measure is the aggressive event rate, a large sample size and lengthy baseline and trial periods are required when this rate is low (81). Furthermore, formidable practical and ethical obstacles interfere with the many sound techniques (e.g., randomization) used in typical designs of psychopharmacological clinical trials (81). Thus, most of the evidence supporting the notion that adjunctive AEDs are helpful in managing aggressive behavior in patients with schizophrenia comes from uncontrolled observations or is generalized from studies of other disorders (82).

The use of combinations of AEDs in patients with schizophrenia and aggression has also been reported in the literature. A retrospective study was carried out in a sample of 45 patients with schizophrenia, schizoaffective and bipolar disorder, and hospitalized in a forensic psychiatric facility in Canada (83). Patients were placed on adjunctive AEDs only if they failed to respond adequately to antipsychotic agents alone. Patients treated with topiramate, valproate, or the combination of topiramate and valproate showed a decrease in Overt Aggression Scale scores and a decrease in the number of episodes of agitation. However, valproate therapy, but not topiramate therapy, decreased the intensity of agitation episodes as measured by the Agitation-Calmness Evaluation Scale.

CLINICAL RECOMMENDATIONS

Unlike for the treatment of bipolar mania (84), combinations of antipsychotics and AEDs are not FDA approved for the treatment of schizophrenia. Such "off-label" use makes it imperative for the clinician to be able to articulate a solid rationale for choosing the combination therapy and to document that reason in the medical record. Diagnostic reassessment is also worthwhile to "rule in" a mood disorder (as per DSM-IV-TR, a diagnosis of schizophrenia cannot be made if there is evidence of the presence of schizoaffective disorder or a mood disorder with psychotic features). Another diagnostic possibility is the presence of a comorbid psychiatric or somatic disorder that is complicating treatment response. A common example is that of comorbid alcohol abuse. Before prescribing combination treatment, adherence to the current therapy must be assessed. If lack of response to treatment is due to noncompliance, adding another medication is unlikely to help.

Not all AEDs have the same evidence base for the treatment of schizophrenia. Data supporting the use of augmentation strategies is not robust to begin with, but a lack of controlled trials in patients with schizophrenia for the use of adjunctive gabapentin or for oxcarbazepine, and weak support for topiramate, make the choice of these agents less compelling than for carbamazepine, valproate, or lamotrigine. The data for carbamazepine and valproate make those agents a possible choice for patients with aggressive or impulsive behavior, and that for lamotrigine as a possible adjunctive medication for use with clozapine in patients with treatment-refractory schizophrenia. Special considerations include the need for plasma level monitoring of carbamazepine and possible dose adjustment of the antipsychotic prescribed with it. Worsening with adjunctive lamotrigine has been reported and may necessitate discontinuation of that agent even before an adequate dose of lamotrigine has been achieved.

The use of adjunctive AEDs in patients with schizophrenia can be considered as a mini-clinical trial with that patient. Specific target symptoms need to be identified and measured before starting the combination treatment and then periodically reassessed. If both the clinician and the patient cannot conclude that a substantial benefit is accruing, then that combination needs to be expeditiously discontinued. The ongoing additional risk of multiple medication treatment cannot be justified unless there is tangible and documentable therapeutic benefit.

SUMMARY

The coprescribing of AEDs with antipsychotics among patients with schizophrenia is common practice. Clinicians resort to combination therapies when monotherapies are inadequate in controlling symptoms or maintaining response.

The evidence base supporting the use of augmentation strategies with AEDs in the treatment of schizophrenia is limited. Although case reports and open uncontrolled studies have been published for carbamazepine, valproate, gabapentin, lamotrigine, topiramate, and oxcarbazepine, these have not always led to the conduct of double-blind and/or randomized clinical trials. Carbamazepine has been assessed in several small controlled studies, but the overall number of patients who have participated in published augmentation studies over the past 25 years is only approximately 300. It is possible that the best use of carbamazepine with antipsychotics is for patients with schizophrenia and aggression, but no adequately powered studies have been conducted to specifically test this. Adjunctive valproate has been widely used as a treatment strategy for patients with residual symptoms, but the largest reported trials have focused on patients with acute exacerbations of schizophrenia rather than on the more refractory patient. For both valproate and lamotrigine, the industry-conducted clinical trials have essentially failed to support the use of combination treatment.

There remains a need for the clinician to be nimble enough to consider novel combinations of medications in an effort to reduce persistent symptoms of schizophrenia. "Absence of evidence" is not the same as "evidence of absence" for the possibility that an individual patient may benefit from adjunctive AEDs. However, this means the clinician must make an attempt to quantify improvement, help the patient assess the value of the treatment while balancing benefits and adverse effects, and be prepared to abandon the combination if substantial advantages for the use of the combination are not forthcoming.

REFERENCES

1. Citrome L, Levine J, Allingham B. Utilization of valproate: extent of inpatient use in the New York State Office of Mental Health. Psychiatr Q 1998; 69(4):283–300.
2. Citrome L, Levine J, Allingham B. Changes in use of valproate and other mood stabilizers for patients with schizophrenia from 1994 to 1998. Psychiatr Serv 2000; 51(5): 634–638.
3. Citrome L, Jaffe A, Levine J. Datapoints - mood stabilizers: utilization trends in patients diagnosed with schizophrenia 1994–2001. Psychiatr Serv 2002; 53(10):1212.
4. Citrome L. Antipsychotic polypharmacy versus augmentation with anticonvulsants: the US Perspective. Paper presented at: XXIV CINP Congress, Paris, France, 2004, June 20–24. Int J Neuropsychopharmacol 2004, 7(suppl 1):S69 (abstr).
5. Wessels T, Grunler D, Bunk C, et al. Changes in the treatment of acute psychosis in a German public hospital from 1998 to 2004. Psychiatr Q 2007; 78(2):91–99.
6. Davids E, Bunk C, Specka M, et al. Psychotropic drug prescription in a psychiatric university hospital in Germany. Prog Neuropsychopharmacol Biol Psychiatry 2006; 30(6): 1109–1116.
7. Grohmann R, Engel RR, Geissler KH, et al. Psychotropic drug use in psychiatric inpatients: recent trends and changes over time-data from the AMSP study. Pharmacopsychiatry 2004; 37(suppl 1):S27–S38.
8. Mallinger JB, Lamberti JS. Racial differences in the use of adjunctive psychotropic medications for patients with schizophrenia. J Ment Health Policy Econ 2007; 10(1):15–22.
9. Xiang YT, Weng YZ, Leung CM, et al. Clinical and social determinants of psychotropic drug prescription for schizophrenia outpatients in China. Prog Neuropsychopharmacol Biol Psychiatry 2007; 31(3):756–760.
10. Kreyenbuhl JA, Valenstein M, McCarthy JF, et al. Long-term antipsychotic polypharmacy in the VA health system: patient characteristics and treatment patterns. Psychiatr Serv 2007; 58(4):489–495.

11. Hakola HP, Laulumaa VA. Carbamazepine in treatment of violent schizophrenics. Lancet 1982; 1(8285):1358.
12. Luchins DL. Carbamazepine in violent non-epileptic schizophrenics. Psychopharmacol Bull 1984; 20(3):569–571.
13. Neppe VM. Carbamazepine as adjunctive treatment in nonepileptic chronic inpatients with EEG temporal lobe abnormalities. J Clin Psychiatry 1983; 44(9):326–331.
14. Dose M, Apelt S, Emrich HM. Carbamazepine as an adjunct of antipsychotic therapy. Psychiatry Res 1987; 22(4):303–310.
15. Okuma T, Yamashita I, Takahashi R, et al. A double-blind study of adjunctive carbamazepine versus placebo on excited states of schizophrenic and schizoaffective disorders. Acta Psychiatr Scand 1989; 80(3):250–259.
16. Nachshoni T, Levin Y, Levy A, et al. A double-blind trial of carbamazepine in negative symptom schizophrenia. Biol Psychiatry 1994; 35(1):22–26.
17. Simhandl C, Meszaros K, Denk E, et al. Adjunctive carbamazepine or lithium carbonate in therapy-resistant chronic schizophrenia. Can J Psychiatry 1996; 41(5):317.
18. Hesslinger B, Normann C, Langosch JM, et al. Effects of carbamazepine and valproate on haloperidol plasma levels and on psychopathologic outcome in schizophrenic patients. J Clin Psychopharmacol 1999; 19(4):310–315.
19. Ohlmeier MD, Jahn K, Wilhelm-Gossling C, et al. Perazine and carbamazepine in comparison to olanzapine in schizophrenia. Neuropsychobiology 2007; 55(2):81–88.
20. Leucht S, Kissling W, McGrath J, et al. Carbamazepine for schizophrenia. Cochrane Database Syst Rev 2007; 3:CD001258.
21. Fenn HH, Robinson D, Luby V, et al. Trends in pharmacotherapy of schizoaffective and bipolar affective disorders: a 5-year naturalistic study. Am J Psychiatry 1996; 153(5):711–713.
22. Weisler RH, Hirschfeld R, Cutler AJ, et al. Extended-release carbamazepine capsules as monotherapy in bipolar disorder: pooled results from two randomised, double-blind, placebo-controlled trials. CNS Drugs 2006; 20(3):219–231.
23. Citrome L, Macher JP, Salazar DE, et al. Pharmacokinetics of aripiprazole and concomitant carbamazepine. J Clin Psychopharmacol 2007; 27(3):279–283.
24. Linnoila M, Viukari M, Kietala O. Effect of sodium valproate on tardive dyskinesia. Br J Psychiatry 1976; 129):114–119.
25. Nagao T, Ohshimo T, Mitsunobu K, et al. Cerebrospinal fluid monoamine metabolites and cyclic nucleotides in chronic schizophrenic patients with tardive dyskinesia or drug-induced tremor. Biol Psychiatry 1979; 14(3):509–523.
26. Wassef AA, Hafiz NG, Hampton D, et al. Divalproex sodium augmentation of haloperidol in hospitalized patients with schizophrenia: clinical and economic implications. J Clin Psychopharmacol 2001; 21(1):21–26.
27. Chong SA, Tan CH, Lee EL, et al. Augmentation of risperidone with valproic acid. J Clin Psychiatry 1998; 59(8):430.
28. Ko GN, Korpi ER, Freed WJ, et al. Effect of valproic acid on behavior and plasma amino acid concentrations in chronic schizophrenia patients. Biol Psychiatry 1985; 20(2):209–215.
29. Fisk GG, York SM. The effect of sodium valproate on tardive dyskinesia revisited. Br J Psychiatry 1987; 150:542–546.
30. Dose M, Hellweg R, Yassouridis A, et al. Combined treatment of schizophrenic psychoses with haloperidol and valproate. Pharmacopsychiatry 1998; 31(4):122–125.
31. Wassef AA, Dott SG, Harris A, et al. Randomized, placebo-controlled pilot study of divalproex sodium in the treatment of acute exacerbations of chronic schizophrenia. J Clin Psychopharmacol 2000; 20(3):357–361.
32. Casey DE, Daniel DG, Wassef AA, et al. Effect of divalproex combined with olanzapine or risperidone in patients with an acute exacerbation of schizophrenia. Neuropsychopharmacology 2003; 28(1):182–192.
33. Abbott Laboratories. ABT-711 M02-547 Clinical Study Report. Available at: http://www.clinicalstudyresults.org/documents/company-study_782_0.pdf. Accessed November 20, 2006.
34. Citrome L, Shope CB, Nolan KA, et al. Risperidone alone versus risperidone plus valproate in the treatment of patients with schizophrenia and hostility. Int Clin Psychopharmacol 2007; 22(6):356–362.

35. Citrome L, Casey DE, Daniel DG, et al. Effects of adjunctive valproate on hostility in patients with schizophrenia receiving olanzapine or risperidone: a double-blind multicenter study. Psychiatr Serv 2004; 55(3):290–294.

36. Sajatovic M, Coconcea N, Ignacio RV, et al. Adjunct extended-release valproate semisodium in late life schizophrenia. Int J Geriatr Psychiatry 2008; 23(2):142–147.

37. Kelly DL, Conley RR, Feldman S, et al. Adjunct divalproex or lithium to clozapine in treatment-resistant schizophrenia. Psychiatr Q 2006; 77(1):81–95.

38. Yoshimura R, Shinkai K, Ueda N, et al. Valproic acid improves psychotic agitation without influencing plasma risperidone levels in schizophrenic patients. Pharmacopsychiatry 2007; 40(1):9–13.

39. Cramer JA, Sernyak M. Results of a naturalistic study of treatment options: switching atypical antipsychotic drugs or augmenting with valproate. Clin Ther 2004; 26(6): 905–914.

40. Wassef AA, Winkler DE, Roache AL, et al. Lower effectiveness of divalproex versus valproic acid in a prospective, quasi-experimental clinical trial involving 9,260 psychiatric admissions. Am J Psychiatry 2005; 162(2):330–339.

41. Abbott Laboratories. Depakote ER Divalproex Sodium Extended-Release Tablets, Formulary Information. Abbott Park, IL: Abbott Laboratories, 2000.

42. Dutta S, Zhang Y, Selness DS, et al. Comparison of the bioavailability of unequal doses of divalproex sodium extended-release formulation relative to the delayed-release formulation in healthy volunteers. Epilepsy Res 2002; 49(1):1–10.

43. Citrome L, Tremeau F, Wynn PS, et al. A study of the safety, efficacy, and tolerability of switching from the standard delayed release preparation of divalproex sodium to the extended release formulation in patients with schizophrenia. J Clin Psychopharmacol 2004; 24(3):255–259.

44. Basan A, Leucht S. Valproate for schizophrenia. Cochrane Database Syst Rev 2003; 3: CD004028.

45. Dursun SM, McIntosh D, Milliken H. Clozapine plus lamotrigine in treatment-resistant schizophrenia. Arch Gen Psychiatry 1999; 56(10):950.

46. Dursun SM, Deakin JF. Augmenting antipsychotic treatment with lamotrigine or topiramate in patients with treatment-resistant schizophrenia: a naturalistic case-series outcome study. J Psychopharmacol 2001; 15(4):297–301.

47. Thomas R, Howe V, Foister K, et al. Adjunctive lamotrigine in treatment-resistant schizophrenia. Int J Neuropsychopharmacol 2006; 9(1):125–127.

48. Heck AH, de Groot IW, van Harten PN. Addition of lamotrigine to clozapine in inpatients with chronic psychosis. J Clin Psychiatry 2005; 66(10):1333.

49. Chan YC, Miller KM, Shaheen N, et al. Worsening of psychotic symptoms in schizophrenia with addition of lamotrigine: a case report. Schizophr Res 2005; 78(2–3):343–345.

50. Stuve W, Wessels A, Timmerman L. Remission of positive symptomatology of a schizophrenic psychosis after withdrawing lamotrigine: a case report. Eur Psychiatry 2004; 19(1):59–61.

51. Kalyoncu A, Mirsal H, Pektas O, et al. Use of lamotrigine to augment clozapine in patients with resistant schizophrenia and comorbid alcohol dependence: a potent anti-craving effect? J Psychopharmacol 2005; 19(3):301–305.

52. Tiihonen J, Hallikainen T, Ryynanen OP, et al. Lamotrigine in treatment-resistant schizophrenia: a randomized placebo-controlled crossover trial. Biol Psychiatry 2003; 54 (11):1241–1248.

53. Kremer I, Vass A, Gorelik I, et al. Placebo-controlled trial of lamotrigine added to conventional and atypical antipsychotics in schizophrenia. Biol Psychiatry 2004; 56(6): 441–446.

54. Akhondzadeh S, Mackinejad K, Ahmadi-Abhari SA, et al. Does the addition of lamotrigine to risperidone improve psychotic symptoms and cognitive impairments in chronic schizophrenia? Therapy 2005; 2(3):399–406.

55. Zoccali R, Muscatello MR, Bruno A, et al. The effect of lamotrigine augmentation of clozapine in a sample of treatment-resistant schizophrenic patients: a double-blind, placebo-controlled study. Schizophr Res 2007; 93(1–3):109–116.

56. Glaxo-Smith-Kline. A multicenter, double-blind, placebo-controlled, randomized, parallel group evaluation of the efficacy of a flexible dose of lamotrigine versus placebo as

add-on therapy in schizophrenia. Study No. SCA30926. Available at: http://ctr.gsk.co. uk/Summary/lamotrigine/III_SCA30926.pdf. Accessed November 5, 2005.

57. Glaxo-Smith-Kline. A multicenter, randomized, double-blind, parallel group study to evaluate the efficacy and safety of a flexible dose of lamotrigine compared to placebo as an adjunctive therapy to an atypical antipsychotic agent(s) in subjects with schizophrenia. Study No. SCA101464. Available at: http://ctr.gsk.co.uk/Summary/lamotrigine/III_ SCA101464.pdf. Accessed May 27, 2006.

58. Goff DC, Keefe R, Citrome L, et al. Lamotrigine as add-on therapy in schizophrenia: results of two placebo-controlled trials. J Clin Psychopharmacol 2007; 27(6):582–589.

59. Premkumar TS, Pick J. Lamotrigine for schizophrenia. Cochrane Database Syst Rev 2006; 4:CD005962.

60. Dursun SM, Devarajan S. Clozapine weight gain, plus topiramate weight loss. Can J Psychiatry 2000; 45(2):198.

61. Lévy E, Agbokou C, Ferreri F, et al. Topiramate-induced weight loss in schizophrenia: a retrospective case series study. Can J Clin Pharmacol 2007; 14(2):E234–E239.

62. Kim JH, Yim SJ, Nam JH. A 12-week, randomized, open-label, parallel-group trial of topiramate in limiting weight gain during olanzapine treatment in patients with schizophrenia. Schizophr Res 2006; 82(1):115–117.

63. Ko YH, Joe SH, Jung IK, et al. Topiramate as an adjuvant treatment with atypical anti-psychotics in schizophrenic patients experiencing weight gain. Clin Neuropharmacol 2005; 28(4):169–175.

64. Drapalski AL, Rosse RB, Peebles RR, et al. Topiramate improves deficit symptoms in a patient with schizophrenia when added to a stable regimen of antipsychotic medication. Clin Neuropharmacol 2001; 24(5):290–294.

65. Millson RC, Owen JA, Lorberg GW, et al. Topiramate for refractory schizophrenia. Am J Psychiatry 2002; 159(4):675.

66. Hofer A, Fleischhacker WW, Hummer M. Worsening of psychosis after replacement of adjunctive valproate with topiramate in a schizophrenia patient. J Clin Psychiatry 2003; 64(10):1267–1268.

67. Duggal HS. Psychotic symptoms associated with topiramate: cognitive side effects or worsening of psychosis? J Clin Psychiatry 2004; 65(8):1145.

68. Huguelet P, Morand-Collomb S. Effect of topiramate augmentation on two patients suffering from schizophrenia or bipolar disorder with comorbid alcohol abuse. Pharmacol Res 2005; 52(5):392–394.

69. Tiihonen J, Halonen P, Wahlbeck K. Topiramate add-on in treatment-resistant schizophrenia: a randomized, double-blind, placebo-controlled, crossover trial. J Clin Psychiatry 2005; 66(8):1012–1015.

70. Chouinard G, Beauclair L, Belanger MC. Gabapentin: long-term antianxiety and hypnotic effects in psychiatric patients with comorbid anxiety-related disorders. Can J Psychiatry 1998; 43(3):305.

71. Megna JL, Devitt PJ, Sauro MD, et al. Gabapentin's effect on agitation in severely and persistently mentally ill patients. Ann Pharmacother 2002; 36(1):12–16.

72. Jablonowski K, Margolese HC, Chouinard G. Gabapentin-induced paradoxical exacerbation of psychosis in a patient with schizophrenia. Can J Psychiatry 2002; 47(10):975–976.

73. Pfeffer G, Chouinard G, Margolese HC. Gabapentin in the treatment of antipsychotic-induced akathisia in schizophrenia. Int Clin Psychopharmacol 2005; 20(3):179–181.

74. Hardoy MC, Carta MG, Carpiniello B, et al. Gabapentin in antipsychotic-induced tardive dyskinesia: results of 1-year follow-up. J Affect Disord 2003; 75(2):125–130.

75. Centorrino F, Albert MJ, Berry JM, et al. Oxcarbazepine: clinical experience with hospitalized psychiatric patients. Bipolar Disord 2003; 5(5):370–374.

76. Leweke FM, Gerth CW, Koethe D, et al. Oxcarbazepine as an adjunct for schizophrenia. Am J Psychiatry 2004; 161(6):1130–1131.

77. Baird P. The interactive metabolism effect of oxcarbazepine coadministered with tricyclic antidepressant therapy for OCD symptoms. J Clin Psychopharmacol 2003; 23(4): 419.

78. Citrome L. Use of lithium, carbamazepine, and valproic acid in a state-operated psychiatric hospital. J Pharm Technol 1995; 11(2):55–59.

79. Citrome L, Volavka J. Clinical management of persistent aggressive behavior in schizophrenia. Part II: Long-term pharmacotherapeutic strategies. Essent Psychopharmacol 2002; 5(1):17–30.
80. McEvoy JP, Scheifler PL, Frances A. The expert consensus guideline series, treatment of schizophrenia. J Clin Psychiatry 1999; 60(suppl 11):43.
81. Volavka J, Citrome L. Atypical antipsychotics in the treatment of the persistently aggressive psychotic patient: methodological concerns. Schizoph Res 1999, 35(suppl): S23–S33.
82. Citrome L. Schizophrenia and valproate. Psychopharmacol Bull 2003; 37(suppl 2):74–88.
83. Gobbi G, Gaudreau PO, Leblanc N. Efficacy of topiramate, valproate, and their combination on aggression/agitation behavior in patients with psychosis. J Clin Psychopharmacol 2006; 26(5):467–473.
84. Citrome L, Goldberg JF, Stahl SM. Toward convergence in the medication treatment of bipolar disorder and schizophrenia. Harv Rev Psychiatry 2005; 13(1):28–42.
85. Krawiecka M, Goldberg D, Vaughan M. A standardized psychiatric assessment scale for rating chronic psychotic patients. Acta Psychiatr Scand 1977; 55(4):299–308.

12 Antiepileptic Drugs in the Treatment of Anxiety Disorders: Role in Therapy

Michael Van Ameringen and Catherine Mancini
Department of Psychiatry and Behavioural Neurosciences, McMaster University and Anxiety Disorders Clinic, McMaster University Medical Centre—HHS, Hamilton, Ontario, Canada

Beth Patterson and Christine Truong
Anxiety Disorders Clinic, McMaster University Medical Centre—HHS, Hamilton, Ontario, Canada

INTRODUCTION

Pharmacological treatments for anxiety disorders have been evolving rapidly. A variety of drug groups have been shown to be effective. Benzodiazepines have long been used to treat anxiety; however, the development of tolerance to these drugs has made them less favorable treatments (1,2). Serotonin selective reuptake inhibitors (SSRIs) and serotonin-norepinephrine reuptake inhibitors (SNRIs) have emerged to become the current gold standard. Despite such widespread use, these agents are only effective in approximately 50% to 60% of patients and can be associated with significant side effects (3). There is a clinical need for alternative medication treatments for anxiety disorders, in the form of either monotherapy or as augmentation agents.

Antiepileptic drugs (AEDs) have been widely used in the treatment of mood disorders and have become first-line treatments for bipolar disorder (4,5). The successful use of AEDs in mood disorders has led clinicians and researchers to investigate their potential efficacy in other psychiatric disorders, in particular, in anxiety disorders.

This chapter attempts to review the small but emerging literature on the use of AEDs in anxiety disorders. Information for this review was obtained from a MEDLINE search and a review of abstracts from major psychiatric congresses (including the Annual Meeting of the American Psychiatric Association, the National Conference of the Anxiety Disorders Association of America, the Annual Meeting of the American College of Neuropsychopharmacology, and the International Forum on Mood and Anxiety Disorders). Each anxiety disorder will be reviewed, focusing on available data that have been presented or published for each AED that has been studied in that disorder.

The notion of using AEDs in anxiety disorders can find a basis in emerging constructs, describing fear circuits in the brain. Numerous brain regions are likely involved in the expression of fear; however, the amygdala is thought to play a key role because of its ability to link sensory stimuli with affective outcomes and initiate emotionally appropriate behaviors (6). Various pathologies, such as anxiety disorders and addiction, could be a manifestation of an "overexpression" of these amygdala-based, conditioned emotional associations (7). This overexpression may result from a failure of proper inhibitory control in the amygdala.

Gamma-aminobutyric acid (GABA) is the primary inhibitory neurotransmitter in the central nervous system (CNS). The inhibitory action of GABA counterbalances the excitatory activity of the neurotransmitter glutamate. The homeostasis between GABA and glutamate controls CNS arousal and neuronal excitability. Maintaining this balance prevents overexcitability, which is known to occur in seizure disorders but is also thought to play a role in pathological anxiety (8), potentially through the overexpression of conditioned fear associations, as previously mentioned.

Abnormalities in both the GABAergic and glutamatergic systems have been associated with various anxiety disorders. For example, decreased occipital GABA levels in panic disorder patients, by as much as 22% compared with healthy controls, have been found (9). A dysfunction in GABA-A receptor binding is also thought to play a role in anxiety disorders, stemming from the observation of diminished response to exogenous benzodiazepines in individuals with anxiety (10). A potential glutamatergic dysfunction has recently been associated with obsessive-compulsive disorder (OCD) on the basis of a neuroimaging study describing an increased level of caudate glutamatergic concentrations in treatment-naïve pediatric OCD patients (11). It has also been hypothesized that a glutamatergic abnormality in social anxiety may be a key component in the dysfunctional neurocircuitry. Increased levels of glucocorticoids in response to stress are thought to stimulate the release of hippocampal glutamate, which may inhibit neurogenesis. A decrease in neurogenesis may be associated with social phobia, as found in animal models of social dominance with subordinate status being linked with a marked decrease in new cells in the dentate gyrus (12).

Various AEDs are thought to modulate GABA and glutamate function, and treating anxious patients with such agents may therefore restore the homeostasis between these two neurotransmitters and decrease neuronal overexcitability, particularly in the amygdala. The following is a summary of the AEDs that have been examined in the treatment of anxiety disorders.

Carbamazepine is indicated for epilepsy and is useful in treating partial and complex seizures. It is also indicated for treatment of acute mania and prophylaxis in bipolar disorder. Its primary mechanism of action is through blockade of voltage-gated sodium channels in neuronal cell membranes, thus preventing the release of excitatory neurotransmitters from nerve terminals (13–16).

Gabapentin is an AED that increases the release of nonsynaptic GABA from glial cells, thereby decreasing neuronal overexcitability (8). Although it was initially synthesized as a GABA analogue, its exact mechanism of action is unclear (17). A gabapentin-binding site has been demonstrated in neocortical and hippocampal areas with unclear functional significance (17).

Lamotrigine is used as either an adjunct or monotherapy agent for epilepsy. It is thought to produce antiseizure effects by its action on voltage-sensitive sodium channels, and subsequent inhibition of the release of glutamate and aspartate. It has been studied in mood disorders and has been found to be effective for the treatment of bipolar depression (18).

Levetiracetam reduces currents through high-voltage-activated calcium channels, and acts via unique binding sites on CNS membranes. Although the exact mechanism of action is unknown, levetiracetam does not have a direct effect on GABA concentrations or GABA receptors, but promotes chloride influx at $GABA_A$ receptors by inhibiting zinc and β-carbolines in the same manner as valproate and clonazepam (19).

Oxcarbazepine is structurally related to carbamazepine; however, it is not metabolized to the 10,11-epoxide, which is thought to be responsible for a decrease in the side effects typically seen with carbamazepine. Its primary mechanism of action is thought to involve blockade of voltage dependent sodium channels (20–22).

Phenytoin is used to control generalized tonic-clonic and psychomotor seizures. It appears to inhibit seizure activity through its action on the motor cortex. Its anticonvulsive effects likely come from its promotion of sodium efflux thus stabilizing firing thresholds against hyperexcitability (23,24).

Pregabalin is a structural analogue to GABA, although it is not active at GABA receptors, nor does it acutely alter GABA uptake or degradation (25). It may have a novel mechanism of action by binding to a subunit of voltage-dependent calcium channels in CNS tissues (26) and acts as a presynaptic modulator of several excitatory neurotransmitters (25).

Tiagabine is the only selective GABA reuptake inhibitor (SGRI). It increases synaptic GABA availability by selective inhibition of the GABA transporter-1, the most abundant GABA transporter (26,27). It has been indicated for add-on treatment of partial seizures.

Topiramate appears to have several mechanisms of action. It has been shown to enhance the activity of GABA at non-benzodiazepine sites, to inhibit glutamate via α-amino-3 hydroxy-5-methyl-4-isoxazole propionic acid (AMPA)/kainate subreceptors, and to block voltage-gated sodium channels. It is also a weak inhibitor of carbonic anhydrase isoenzymes CAII and CAIV (28).

Valproate is primarily used as sole or adjunctive therapy for the treatment of simple or complex absence seizures and generalized seizures with tonic-clonic manifestations. It is used adjunctively for patients with multiple seizure types. Valproate is also indicated for the treatment of mania in bipolar disorder. Although its exact mechanism of action is unknown, it has been suggested that valproate increases brain concentrations of GABA by promoting chloride influx at $GABA_A$ receptors, in turn, by inhibiting the $GABA_A$ receptor modulators zinc and β-carbolines (19).

Vigabatrin, a specific GABA transaminase inhibitor, is used as an anticonvulsant and also to treat hyperekplexia (startle disease) in neonates (29,30).

SOCIAL PHOBIA

Social phobia (social anxiety disorder) is characterized by a marked and persistent fear of social or performance situations due to an excessive fear of embarrassment or humiliation (31). Individuals with social phobia typically fear and avoid public speaking, participating in small groups, dating, speaking to authority figures, attending parties, and speaking with and meeting strangers.

Numerous drug classes have been found to be efficacious in social phobia, including SSRIs (32,33), SNRIs (34), monoamine oxidase inhibitors (MAOIs) (35–37), reversible inhibitors of monoamine oxidase-A (RIMAs) (38,39), and benzodiazepines, as well as AEDs.

Topiramate

Van Ameringen et al. (40) evaluated the effectiveness of topiramate in treating social phobia in a 16-week open-label trial of 23 patients with generalized social phobia. The mean dose of topiramate at end point was 222.8 ± 141.8 mg/day, with a dose range of 25 to 400 mg/day. In the intent-to-treat (ITT) sample, 12(45.1%) patients were responders [defined as a Clinical Global Impression of Improvement (CGI-I) scale score of ≤2] and significant improvement was found from baseline to end point on the Liebowitz Social Anxiety Scale (LSAS). Significant changes in self-report measures of social anxiety were also demonstrated. However, no changes were found on measures of depression or generalized anxiety. Six of the twenty-three participants (26.1%) achieved remission status, defined as an end point LSAS score less than or equal to 30. The most common adverse events included weight loss, paresthesia, and headache, with only five patients dropping out of the study as a result of them. Although this was an open-label design, these results suggest that topiramate may have a specific effect on symptoms of social phobia. This finding is particularly intriguing given the purported mechanism of action of topiramate involving both glutamate and GABA neurotransmitter systems. The remission rate in this study was similar to that found in a recent placebo-controlled trial of venlafaxine in the treatment of social phobia (41). However, a major drawback with topiramate may be individuals' ability to tolerate its bothersome side effects, particularly cognitive impairment.

Gabapentin

The effectiveness of gabapentin in treating social phobia was examined in a placebo-controlled study by Pande et al. (42). Sixty-nine patients were randomly assigned to a 14-week double-blind treatment of either gabapentin, with a varying dose of 900 to 3600 mg/day or a placebo. The treatment group demonstrated significantly more symptom reduction then the control group, as measured by the LSAS ($p = 0.008$), the Brief Social Phobia Scale (BSPS; $p = 0.007$), and the Social Phobia Inventory (SPIN; $p = 0.008$). In the ITT analysis, twice as many patients taking gabapentin were considered responders (32% for gabapentin vs. 14% for placebo), defined as a decrease of at least 50% on the LSAS; however, this difference in response rate did not reach significance ($p = 0.08$). The Clinical Global Impression of Change (CGI-C) scale response rate (defined as "much" or "very much improved") was 38.2% for the gabapentin group as compared with 17.1% for the placebo group. Adverse events that occurred significantly more in the gabapentin group included dizziness, somnolence, nausea, flatulence, and decreased libido. Of the 44% of individuals who withdrew from this study before completion, 21% of those taking gabapentin withdrew because of adverse events, compared with 11% of the placebo group. Although gabapentin did not separate for placebo on the primary outcome measure (≥50% decrease in LSAS baseline scores), there was a suggestion from secondary outcome measures that there may be a treatment effect of gabapentin on social phobic symptoms, though moderate.

The effects of gabapentin on anxiety induced by simulated public speaking were investigated in 32 normal male volunteers, aged 17 to 30 years, who were randomly assigned to gabapentin 400 mg/day ($N = 11$), 800 mg/day ($N = 10$), or placebo ($N = 11$) (43). The self-rated Visual Analogue Mood Scale (VAMS) and Profile of Mood States (POMS) were used as primary outcome measures along with physiological measures of heart rate and blood pressure and were obtained at five time points throughout the procedure. Two hours after receiving study treatment, subjects were given two minutes to prepare a four-minute improvised speech that would be recorded on video camera. Subjects were given their choice of several sensitive topics to speak about. Treatment with gabapentin at 800 mg/day attenuated the anxiety of subjects that had a decrease on the VAMS item calm-excited ($p < 0.05$) as compared with gabapentin 400 mg/day and to placebo ($p = 0.036$). In addition, volunteers receiving both doses of gabapentin showed a decrease in the hostility score on the POMS. No significant drug effect was found in differences between physiological measures. These results are in agreement with other studies, suggesting an anxiolytic potential of gabapentin.

Pregabalin

The effectiveness of pregabalin in treating social phobia was demonstrated by a double-blind, placebo-controlled study conducted by Pande et al. (44). In this study, 135 patients with social phobia were randomly assigned to 10 weeks of high-dose pregabalin (600 mg/day; $N = 47$), low-dose pregabalin (150 mg/day; $N = 42$), or a placebo ($N = 46$). Using the ITT sample, pregabalin 600 mg/day was found to be significantly better than placebo on the primary outcome measure of change from baseline to end point in the LSAS total score ($p = 0.024$), as well as on the secondary measures the LSAS subscales of total fear, total avoidance, social fear, and social avoidance, and the BSPS fear subscale. The rate of response (defined as a CGI-I rating of much or very much improved) was 43% (20 of 47) for the high-dose group, compared with 22% (10 of 46) for the placebo group. The low-dose group showed greater improvement over the placebo group, but the difference did not reach statistical significance. Pregabalin was also found to be relatively well tolerated, with mild-to-moderate somnolence and dizziness being the most common side effects associated with the high-dose group. Of the 30.4% of patients who withdrew from the study, 23.4% of those in the high-dose pregabalin group withdrew because of adverse events, compared with 9.5% in the low-dose group and 8.7% in the placebo group. The results of this study suggest that pregabalin may be a promising new agent in the treatment of social phobia.

Valproate

Valproate has shown mixed results in the treatment of social phobia, as described in two reports. Nardi et al. treated 16 generalized social phobics in an open trial of valproate with doses of 500 to 1500 mg/day (mean dose = 1071 ± 75 mg/day) for one to nine months. All patients were considered to be nonresponders (45). In another study, Kinrys et al. treated 17 social phobics in a 12-week open trial of valproate with doses of 500 to 2500 mg/day (mean dose = 1985 ± 454 mg/day). In the ITT analysis, 41.1% were considered responders by the CGI-I, with a mean drop in the LSAS of 19.1 points. Adverse events included nausea, somnolence, dizziness, and fatigue. Only 1 of 17 participants dropped out because of adverse events (46). Conclusions that can be drawn from this study are limited because of the small sample size and open-label design. The contradicting results of these two studies suggest the need for further investigations of valproate in social phobia.

Tiagabine

Tiagabine monotherapy (mean dose = 10 mg/day) for social phobia was investigated by Dunlop et al. (47) in a 12-week open-trial of 63 social phobia patients followed by a double-blind relapse-prevention phase. The mean dose of tiagabine was 12.2 ± 4.0 mg/day. Twenty-seven patients completed the open-label phase but 54 were included in the ITT analyses. Of the 36 patients who withdrew from the study, 12 discontinued because of adverse events and 4 because of lack of efficacy. In the ITT analysis, significant reductions in social phobia symptoms were found as measured by the LSAS and SPIN. Significant improvements in quality of life were also found as measured by the Sheehan Disability Scale (SDS). In the ITT analysis, 40.7% (22/54) were considered to be responders (defined as a CGI ≤ 2 at end point) compared with 63.0% (17/27) of the completers. The most common adverse events were somnolence (32%) and dizziness (25%). Seventeen responders were randomized to the relapse prevention phase, where they were randomly assigned to continue on tiagabine ($N = 6$), or switch to placebo ($N = 11$). Seven patients completed this phase and the results were not reported because of the low statistical power of the small sample. (47)

Kinrys et al. (48) conducted a retrospective analysis of 14 patients treated with adjunctive tiagabine after nonresponse to an SSRI. Tiagabine was taken for a mean duration of 30.6 weeks at a mean dose of 16.4 ± 6.9 mg/day, ranging from 8 to 83 mg/day, with the SSRI and sometimes with other medications, including quetiapine, clonazepam, and bupropion. In this cohort, nine (64.2%) patients met the response criteria (defined as a CGI ≤ 2 at end point), and five (35.7%) met remission criteria (defined as a LSAS ≤ 30). Symptom response and remission were maintained in these patients at 28 weeks (48).

These two open-label reports suggest that tiagabine may be useful as a monotherapy or an augmentation therapy for treatment-resistant social phobia. However, the small sample-size, open-label design, and, in the augmentation study, the use of a variety of concomitant medications limit the generalizability of these results.

Levetiracetam

Recently, Simon et al. (49) gave levetiracetam to 20 patients with generalized social phobia for eight weeks, with doses initiated at 250 mg/day and flexibly titrated to 3000 mg/day (mean dose = 2013mg/day). Thirteen of the twenty patients completed the trial, and of those patients, three discontinued because of adverse events (drowsiness and nervousness). In the ITT analysis, there was a significant decrease in mean LSAS score from baseline to end point (20.5 points). Significant decreases in Hamilton Anxiety Scale (HAM-A) and the CGI-Severity (CGI-S) Scale scores were also found (49).

In a seven-week study of Diagnostic and Statistical Manual of Mental Disorders (DSM)-IV social anxiety disorder, 18 patients were randomly assigned (in a 2:1 ratio) to double-blind treatment with either levetiracetam (500–3000 mg/day) or placebo (50). Study medication was started at 500 mg at bedtime for four days, and increased as tolerated at the rate of 500 mg every three to four days, to 2000 mg/day by day 14, and to a maximum daily dose of 3000 mg (1500 mg b.i.d.). The mean dose of levetiracetam at the final visit was 2279 mg/day ($N = 9$), compared with 2786 mg/day for placebo ($N = 7$). The primary outcomes were the change in the BSPS from baseline and the rate of response (defined as a final CGI-I score of 1 or 2). Analyses were performed on the ITT sample using the last observation carried forward (LOCF). No statistically significant differences were observed on any measures of social anxiety, including the BSPS, LSAS, and SPIN. Response rates by CGI-I were 22% for levetiracetam and 14% for placebo ($p =$ NS). Although the differences between drug and placebo were not statistically significant, the actual magnitude of reduction was twofold greater for levetiracetam than for placebo on all three social phobia scales. The effect sizes of levetiracetam compared with placebo were 0.33 for the BSPS and 0.50 for the LSAS, representing mild-to-moderate effects. The authors noted that the low placebo response rate suggested they had a somewhat treatment-refractory group that might present a harder test for a putative treatment to demonstrate efficacy. Other limitations included the small sample size and short treatment duration. Adverse events were experienced in two of nine subjects ($N = 1$ severe headache and drowsiness, $N = 1$ disinhibition and inebriation) in the levetiracetam group, suggesting that a lower initial dose and slower titration may be preferable.

The current levetiracetam studies do not support its routine use in social phobia, but given their small sample sizes, further trials in larger samples may be warranted.

POSTTRAUMATIC STRESS DISORDER

Posttraumatic stress disorder (PTSD) is a pathological response resulting from exposure to a traumatic stressor. Three clusters of symptoms occur in PTSD: (1) persistent re-experiencing of the traumatic event (i.e., dreams and distressing recollections), (2) avoidance of stimuli associated with the trauma as well as numbing or detachment, and (3) persistent symptoms of increased arousal (31).

Evidence from placebo-controlled trials has demonstrated the efficacy of SSRIs and SNRIs in treating PTSD, making these agents first-line treatments for PTSD (51). Fluoxetine (52,53), sertraline (54–57), paroxetine, (58–60) and venlafaxine extended release (61) have all demonstrated efficacy in placebo-controlled trials. Other medications with demonstrated efficacy in PTSD include the MAOI, phenelzine (62,63), and the tricyclic antidepressants amitriptyline (64,65) and imipramine (62,63,65). Recent evidence, as described below, suggests that AEDs may be a tolerable and efficacious alternative treatment for PTSD.

Lamotrigine

A placebo-controlled trial was conducted by Hertzberg et al. (66) to evaluate the effectiveness of lamotrigine in treating PTSD. Ten patients received lamotrigine and four patients received placebo for up to 10 weeks (mean dose at end point = 380 mg/day). Improvements in avoidance or numbing and re-experiencing (i.e., flashbacks, nightmares) symptoms, as measured by the Duke Global Rating for PTSD (DGRP), were found with lamotrigine while no improvements were measured in the control group. Five (50%) patients treated with lamotrigine were classified as responders compared with one (25%) in the placebo group. Two of the ten lamotrigine patients developed a rash leading to discontinuation, while two of four placebo patients also discontinued the study due to a rash. Other side effects were judged to be mild and included sweating, drowsiness, poor concentration, thirst, restlessness, and sexual dysfunction (66). Although this study used a placebo-controlled design, the results must be interpreted with caution. The small sample size did not allow for statistical analysis of the quantifiable measures, and only one placebo patient completed the study. More studies with larger samples would allow further assessment of the potential benefits of lamotrigine in PTSD.

Topiramate

Two open-label trials of topiramate in PTSD has been reported. In the first study by Berlant et al. (67), 35 PTSD patients were given topiramate as monotherapy or as adjunctive therapy for a mean duration of treatment of 33 weeks. It was found that topiramate reduced nightmares in 79% of patients and reduced intrusions or flashbacks in 86% of patients based on self-report at end point. Fourteen of the seventeen patients who had completed the PTSD Checklist-Civilian Version (PCL-C) after four weeks of treatment had a score of 50 of less (which is below the standard cutoff score for active PTSD). Symptom improvements were reported with both topiramate monotherapy and adjunctive therapy, with a mean mono-therapy dose for full response of 43 mg/day (range 25–75 mg/day), compared with 97 mg/day (range 25–500 mg/day) for a full response with adjunctive therapy. Nine patients discontinued treatment because of side effects. These included urticaria, eating cessation, acute narrow-angle glaucoma, severe head-ache, overstimulation/panic, memory concerns, and one occurrence of emergent suicidal ideation. The topiramate doses used in this study were quite low as compared with what have been used in other psychiatric illnesses (68). Various methodological limitations make the results of this study difficult to interpret. Only half the sample completed a standardized self-report measure of PTSD, and this measure was included in the results after four weeks of treatment, which is not likely an adequate duration in order to assess response. The study also included a heterogeneous population, including different subtypes of PTSD (i.e., hallucinatory versus nonhalucinatory PTSD) and significant comorbidity (i.e., comorbid bipolar disorder), and used topiramate as both adjunctive and monotherapy.

In an effort to address some of these methodological limitation, this study was replicated in a sample of 33 consecutive civilians with PTSD, where halluci-nations were excluded, treatment lasted up to 12 weeks, and the PCL-C was used to assess all patients (69). Topiramate was administered as either monotherapy ($N = 5$) or adjunctive treatment ($N = 28$) in flexible doses and response was measured after four weeks. Results revealed a mean reduction in the PCL-C score of 49% ($p < 0.001$) and a response rate of 77% at week 4. The median time to respond was nine days, and the mean dose for those reporting a full response was 60 mg/day $\pm$ 47. By week 4, 94% of patients with nightmares and 79% of patients with intrusions at baseline reported complete cessation of their symptoms. These results are quite promising but should be interpreted with caution given the open-label design and that the monotherapy and augmentation group data are presented together (69).

Topiramate monotherapy has been evaluated in two controlled studies of PTSD. In the first, Tucker et al. (70) randomized 38 patients with noncombat-related PTSD to flexible doses of topiramate (median dose 150 mg/day, range 25–400 mg/day) or placebo for 12 weeks. No significant difference was found on the primary efficacy measure of change from baseline in the total Clinician-Administered PTSD Scale (CAPS) score (71). However, significant effects on sec-ondary outcome measures were found in favor of topiramate on the Treatment Outcome PTSD scale (TOP-8) (decrease in overall severity 68% vs. 41.6%, $p = 0.025$) and end point CGI-I scores (1.9 $\pm$ 1.2 vs. 2.6 $\pm$ 1.1, $p = 0.055$). In the second study (72), 40 veterans with PTSD were randomized to 12 weeks of topiramate or placebo. Topiramate was found to be superior on the CGI-I at weeks 6 and 8 ($p = 0.021$) as well as on the CAPS-D (hyperarousal) subscale change from baseline ($p = 0.019$).

No significant differences were found in CAPS total score, TOP 8, or other symptom severity measures.

In short, there is some evidence to indicate the helpfulness of topiramate in treating PTSD symptoms. However, available results do not show overall efficacy based on primary PTSD outcome measures. Further placebo-controlled trials that either specifically utilize monotherapy or adjunctive therapy with more homogeneous samples would allow for a better evaluation of the usefulness of topiramate in PTSD.

Gabapentin

Case reports have described the successful treatment of PTSD with gabapentin (73,74). Brannon et al. reported a reduction in nightmares and anxiety in patients suffering from PTSD and comorbid depression treated with gabapentin 1200 mg/day (73). Hamner et al. (74) conducted a retrospective chart review of 30 patients with PTSD who were treated with adjunctive gabapentin. Sixty-seven percent of patients had comorbid major depressive disorder. In nearly every case gabapentin was added to target sleep disturbance symptoms associated with PTSD. It was found that 77% of patients demonstrated "moderate" or "marked" improvements in sleep duration, as well as a decrease in the frequency of nightmares. The most common adverse events were sedation and mild dizziness (74). The results of this study should be interpreted with caution, given its retrospective nature as well as the inclusion of patients receiving multiple concomitant sedating medications. Controlled research is needed to evaluate the efficacy of gabapentin in treating the core symptoms of PTSD, as well as its usefulness as an adjunctive agent to treat nightmares and insomnia.

Valproate

Open-label data thus suggest valproate may be helpful in PTSD, but there are conflicting reports regarding its effectiveness in treating all of the core-symptom clusters of PTSD.

Symanski and Olympia (75) recorded two cases demonstrating improvements in PTSD with valproate treatment of 1000 mg/day and 1500 mg/day respectively, showing prominent reductions in irritability. In an open-trial, Fesler (76) treated 16 Vietnam veterans with valproate (mean dose = 109.3 mg/day) for one year. The majority of patients experienced significant improvements in hyperarousal and avoidant symptoms; however, little improvement was found in re-experiencing or intrusive symptoms. Gastrointestinal complaints were the most common adverse events and included abdominal cramps, indigestion, nausea, and constipation. In another study, 16 veteran outpatients with PTSD were prescribed valproate alone or adjunctively (mean dose of 1,365 mg/day) for eight weeks. Three patients dropped out because of adverse events. Of the 13 patients who completed the trial, 11 were considered responders, defined by a CGI-I less than or equal to 2. Significant improvement was also found on the CAPS total score, on the CAPS subscale scores of intrusion and hyperarousal, and on the HAM-A and Hamilton Depression Scale (HAM-D) scale scores (77). Another open-label trial of 21 patients with combat-induced PTSD treated with valproate (mean dose = 1840 mg/day) found similar results (78). Reduction was measured in all three symptom clusters using the CAPS. Six patients discontinued valproate because of intolerable side effects including rash, diarrhea, and nausea.

In a retrospective chart analysis, a sample of 325 veterans was identified through a computerized search as having both a PTSD diagnosis and having had treatment with any form of valproate (79). Fifty patients met eligibility criteria; three were treated with valproate monotherapy and 47 were treated adjunctively with a variety of psychotropic agents. The primary outcome measures were CGI-I and change in baseline CGI-S as scored by raters who were blinded to the order of visits, medication names and doses, and serum valproic acid levels. The mean valproate dose was 1070 ± 455 mg/day. Twenty-five patients (50%) were rated as very much or much improved on the CGI-I. The improved end point CGI-I differed significantly from "no change" ($p < 0.000001$). The change in CGI-S ratings differed significantly from 0, but the average change was not considered large. Patients treated in primary care had a greater improvement compared with those in the mental health setting ($p < 0.005$). Valproate dosage and serum valproic acid levels ($N = 37$) were well correlated ($r = 0.57$, $p < 0.0005$). The authors concluded that valproate treatment improves the global clinical function of veterans with PTSD.

In a more recent open-trial (80), however, valproate was not found to be effective in noncombat related PTSD. In a trial of 10 patients with PTSD related to accidents, witnessing the death of a loved one, and sexual or physical abuse, valproate monotherapy was initiated at 250 mg/day and increased up to 2000 mg/day (mean dose = 1400 ± 380 mg/day). No improvements were found in PTSD or depressive symptoms using the Posttraumatic Diagnostic Scale (PDS), the Impact of Event Scale-Revised (IES-R), and the Beck Depression Inventory (BDI), after four and eight weeks of treatment.

In a recently reported randomized controlled trial of valproate monotherapy, 86 Vietnam veterans (98% male; 95% had combat-related trauma) with a mean duration of illness of 28 years were randomized to valproate or placebo (81). No significant differences were found in the CAPS total score or in scores on the CAPS-B (re-experiencing), CAPS-D (hyperarousal), TOP-8, CGI-I, or HAM-A scales. Significant improvement was found in the reduction of CAPS-C (avoidance) and Montgomery Åsberg Depression Rating Scale (MADRS) scores as well as on symptoms of avoidance. The authors concluded that valproate was ineffective in treating PTSD in an older, male veteran population (81).

Tiagabine

Open-label studies have suggested adjunctive tiagabine may be helpful in some PTSD symptoms. An open-label case series conducted by Lara (82) examined the use of tiagabine to augment antidepressant therapy in PTSD. Six patients were included in the case series; two with comorbid bipolar depression and four with comorbid major depression. Patients started tiagabine at 2 to 4 mg/day, increasing to a maximum of 16 mg/day. Significant reduction in anxiety was found after one week of therapy, and the effect was maintained at six weeks, as measured by the change in the baseline score of the Davidson Trauma Scale (DTS) (82). Aggression levels were also significantly reduced. Similar success in treating one patient with PTSD and comorbid major depression with adjunctive tiagabine was reported by Berigan (83). In this case report, a reduction of re-experiencing symptoms was accredited to the addition of tiagabine. In addition, an open-label trial found positive results using tiagabine (mean dose = 7.3 mg/day) in six (86%) of the seven patients evaluated using the PCL-C ($p < 0.05$) (84). Of the six patients whose symptoms improved, five had an end point CGI-I score of less than or equal to 2.

Two controlled studies, however, do not support the efficacy of tiagabine monotherapy in PTSD. Davidson and et al. (85) examined the efficacy of tiagabine in PTSD utilizing a 12-week open-label phase followed by a double-blind randomization of patients who completed the open-label phase to either tiagabine continuation or switching to placebo after tapering off tiagabine for an additional 12-weeks. In the ITT sample of the open phase ($N = 26$) of tiagabine (mean dose 12.8 ± 4.3 mg/day), significant improvements were observed in all measures of PTSD, depression, general anxiety, social anxiety, resilience, and disability. After the double-blind, placebo-controlled discontinuation phase ($N = 18$), there were no significant differences between the two groups, with gains being maintained on all outcomes (85).

Davidson et al. (86) recently reported a 12-week, randomized, multicenter, double-blind study of 232 patients with PTSD who were randomly assigned to treatment with tiagabine ($N = 116$) or placebo ($N = 116$). Tiagabine was initiated at 4 mg/day (2 mg b.i.d.) and individually titrated by 4 mg/day per week to a maximum dose of 16 mg/day. The mean dose of tiagabine at end point was 11.2 mg/day (range 2.0–16.0 mg/day); for placebo equivalent the mean dose was 11.8 mg/day (range 2.0–16.0 mg/day). Efficacy was assessed using the change from baseline in the total scores on the CAPS, DTS, and TOP-8. Additional assessments included the CGI-C, Connor-Davidson Resilience Scale, SDS, and a patient-rated evaluation of sleep (sleep questionnaire). There were no significant differences between treatment groups in change from baseline in the CAPS total score or on the other efficacy outcome measures. The authors concluded that tiagabine was not significantly different from placebo in the treatment of symptoms of PTSD.

Carbamazepine

Several open-label studies have suggested that carbamazepine may be a useful treatment for PTSD. Lipper et al. (87) reported that 7 of 10 patients who met DSM-III criteria for PTSD and a comorbid personality disorder were rated as "moderately" or "very much" improved on the CGI-I scale after treatment with carbamazepine (mean dose = 780 mg/day). Patients also demonstrated a reduction in the frequency and intensity of flashbacks, nightmares, and intrusive thoughts, as measured by interview-rated and self-report scales (87). Wolf et al. (88) described improvements in the clinical condition of 10 patients with PTSD treated with carbamazepine, as assessed by staff observations and self-report, with particular improvements in violent behavior. No standardized measures, were, however, used to assess symptom improvement. The use of carbamazepine (300–1200 mg/day) in a group of 28 sexually abused children, aged 8 to 17 years with PTSD including with comorbidity [e.g., attention deficit hyperactivity disorder (ADHD), depression, oppositional defiant disorder, and polysubstance abuse), has also been reported. Of the 28 patients, 22 became free of PTSD symptoms, while 6 patients reported infrequent abuse-related nightmares (89). No standardized measures were used. These studies support the potential use of carbamazepine in PTSD, but double-blind, placebo-controlled studies are needed.

Phenytoin

In a small open-label study examining the effects of phenytoin on memory, cognition, and brain structure in PTSD, nine adult male and female patients were treated with phenytoin for a three-month period (90). Treatment was started at

300 mg/day in three divided doses and increased to 400 mg/day if plasma levels were subtherapeutic. Plasma levels of phenytoin were measured at weeks 1, 2, 3, 4, 8, and 12, and dose was adjusted to be within the therapeutic range used in the treatment of epilepsy (10–20 mg/mL). Subjects underwent magnetic resonance imaging (MRI) for measurement of whole-brain and hippocampal volume, as well as neuropsychological testing of memory and cognition, before and after treatment. Subjects showed a significant improvement in PTSD symptoms with pheytoin treatment as measured by the CAPS, showing reductions in each of the symptom clusters of intrusions, avoidance, and hyperarousal ($p < 0.05$). No significant effects were found on HAM-D or HAM-A scores.

In a subsequent publication, neuropsychological testing revealed no significant changes in memory or cognition in this sample with phenytoin treatment (91). By contrast, phenytoin administration resulted in a significant 6% increase in right whole-brain volume as measured with volumetric MRI ($p < 0.05$), as well as a 5% nonsignificant increase in right hippocampal volume. Moreover, there were significant correlations between increases in hippocampal volume and reduction of PTSD symptoms as measured with the CAPS for the intrusion cluster for both the left ($r = -0.70$, df $= 8$, $p = 0.037$) and right ($r = -0.73$, df $= 8$, $p = 0.026$) hippocampus, and for the hyperarousal cluster for right ($r = -0.70$, df $= 8$, $p = 0.048$) hippocampal volume. Correlations with total CAPS score were not significant. There was no correlation between changes in whole-brain volumes and improvements on the CAPS.

This study suggests that phenytoin may be an effective treatment for PTSD and may also be associated with changes in brain structure, particularly in right whole-brain volume. This study further indicates that medications used in the treatment of neurological and psychiatric disorders may have effects on the brain that were previously unanticipated. Of note, the mechanism by which phenytoin may affect brain structure in PTSD is not fully understood and requires further investigation.

Vigabatrin

A series of five PTSD cases augmented with vigabatrin has been reported. Vigabatrin, 250 mg to 500 mg at bedtime, was introduced to treat hypervigilance and startle which had not improved with other treatments. All five patients tolerated vigabatrin well and had a rapid amelioration of their exaggerated startle responses. No changes were found in other PTSD symptoms (92).

Oxcarbazepine

Two case reports have described improvements in PTSD symptoms with oxcarbazepine augmentation. One report describes the case of a 46-year-old man with chronic PTSD who had been unresponsive or intolerant to numerous pharmacological treatments including carbamazepine and valproate. The patient was augmented with 300 mg/day of oxcarbazepine, titrated up to 900 mg/day, along with 150 mg/day of sertraline and 0.5 mg/day of clonazepam. The patient reported experiencing less frequent and severe nightmares, as well as improvements in all areas of functioning. Gains were maintained at four-month follow-up (93). In another case report, a 38-year-old woman with PTSD and bipolar disorder who had partially responded to carbamazepine was treated with oxcarbazepine. Within a month of initiation of oxcarbazepine, she reported progressive improvement in her

PTSD symptoms. As oxcarbazepine monotherapy 750 mg b.i.d. continued, she reported significant reduction of her PTSD symptoms and stabilization of her mood without adverse effects (94).

Levetiracetam

Kinrys et al. (95) recently reported a retrospective analysis of 23 patients with DSM-IV diagnoses of PTSD who, after being deemed inadequate responders to antidepressant therapy, received adjunctive levetiracetam in a naturalistic fashion. Existing medication regimes were supplemented with a starting dose of 250 mg of levetiracetam at bedtime with a weekly dose escalation of 250 to 500 mg. The target dosage range was 1000 to 3000 mg/day given in a b.i.d. or nightly regimen, on the basis of each patient's individual response and tolerability to the drug. The primary outcome measure was the PCL-C and secondary efficacy measures included the HAM-D, CGI-S, and CGI-I. Significant improvement was found on all measures ($p < 0.001$). Thirteen (56%) patients met responder criteria at end point, as defined by PCL-C mean change $= 23.5$ and CGI-I score less than 2. Six (26%) patients met remission criteria (final CGI-S score <2). Adverse events were generally mild, and no patient stopped levetiracetam therapy because of side effects. This study indicates levetiracetam may be an effective treatment in combination with antidepressant therapy for patients with PTSD who remain symptomatic after initial intervention, but needs to be confirmed by double-blind, placebo-controlled trials.

PANIC DISORDER

Panic disorder is characterized by recurrent, unexpected panic attacks, defined as discrete periods of intense anxiety and feelings of fearfulness, terror, and often impending doom. There is persistent concern regarding future panic attacks and their consequences and the panic attacks may lead to agoraphobic avoidance. Typically avoided situations include being outside the home alone, being in a crowd, being on a bridge, or traveling in a bus, train, or automobile (31).

Tricyclic antidepressants and MAOIs were among the first pharmacological agents shown to be efficacious in the treatment of panic disorder (96–98). Currently, benzodiazepines (99–110), SSRIs (111–115), and SNRIs (116–119), either alone or in combination, are used as standard treatments for panic disorder. Among the SSRIs, fluoxetine (114,120–122), fluvoxamine (123–131) paroxetine, sertraline (132–135), citalopram (136), and escitalopram (136) have all been demonstrated efficacious in randomized clinical trials.

Gabapentin

Successful treatment of panic disorder with gabapentin has been described in case reports (17). In the only double-blind, placebo-controlled study published to date (137), Pande et al. randomly assigned 103 patients with panic disorder to gabapentin (600–3600 mg/day) or placebo for eight weeks. Although the difference in symptom severity, as measured by the Panic and Agoraphobia Scale (PAS), was insignificant between the drug and placebo groups for the entire patient sample, a significant improvement was found in an analysis of a severely ill subsample (those with a PAS baseline ≥ 20; $p = 0.04$) (137). However, no significant difference in rate of responders was found between drug and placebo in those with a baseline PAS of 20 or more (37% gabapentin versus 26.9% placebo $p = 0.437$), or between those with a baseline PAS less than 20 (45% gabapentin versus 66.7% placebo $p = 0.223$). Twelve percent of the gabapentin group discontinued the study due to adverse events compared with 4% of the placebo group (137). Common adverse events included somnolence, headache, and dizziness. Given this negative result, gabapentin should probably be reserved for use as an adjunctive therapy or for treatment nonresponders to standard therapies.

Valproate

The antipanic effects of valproate have been described in several case reports, which have included documenting the successful treatment of panic disorder with comorbid alcoholism (138), substance abuse (139), benzodiazepine withdrawal (140), and multiple sclerosis (141). A case series by Ontiveros and Fountaine (142) described the improvement of four patients with treatment-resistant panic disorder using a combination of valproate and clonazepam.

Further support for the effectiveness of valproate in treating panic disorder has come from open-label studies. Primeau et al. (143) conducted an open trial in 10 patients with panic disorder or agoraphobia with panic attacks. Patients were treated with valproate for seven weeks with an initial dose of 500 mg/day that was increased to a maximum of 2,250 mg/day. Significant improvements were noted for both panic and anxiety symptoms. Similar results were found in a six-week open-label study of valproate in 12 patients with panic disorder conducted by Woodman and Noyles (144). All 12 patients demonstrated moderate or marked improvement after the six-week trial, and the improvements gained were sustained at six-month and 18-month follow-up. Other open-trials have demonstrated the ability of valproate to block lactate-induced panic attacks (145) and to treat patients with panic disorder and mood instability resistant to conventional therapy (146).

In the only controlled study of valproate in panic disorder, Lum et al. (147) treated 12 patients in a double-blind, placebo-controlled, 2×2 crossover design with doses achieving a plasma valproic acid level between 60 and 120 mg/mL. Significant improvements in the valproate group as compared with the placebo group were noted on the CGI-S and CGI-I scales, with marked reductions in the length and intensity of panic attacks, as well as a decrease in psychic and somatic symptoms of anxiety as measured by the HAM-A scale. Five patients reported adverse events while taking valproate, which included gastrointestinal discomfort, dizziness, and somnolence (147). These preliminary results suggest that VPA may be an effective treatment for panic disorder that demonstrates a long-term effect. Larger placebo-controlled trials with long-term follow-up, however, are needed to confirm these findings.

Tiagabine

In an open-trial of five patients with panic disorder, including with comorbidity, Gruener (148) reported improvement with tiagabine (20 mg/day). Anxiety was significantly reduced in all patients at two weeks, and improvement was maintained for the entire eight-week treatment period. Similar success was found in a case series of four patients treated with tiagabine, where reductions in anxiety, agoraphobia, and panic attacks were noted (149).

Tiagabine has also been reported to reduce cholecystokinin-tetrapeptide (CCK-4)-induced panic in healthy subjects. Zwanzger et al. (150) administered

15 mg/day of tiagabine to 15 healthy volunteers for seven days. A CCK-4 challenge was given before and after the one-week treatment. A significant reduction in panic was found after the second CCK-4 challenged. A significant decrease in heart rate was also found after tiagabine treatment; however, adrenocorticotropic hormone (ACTH) and cortisol concentrations did not change.

These small studies suggest a potential antipanic effect of tiagabine. The efficacy and tolerability of this agent in panic disorder, however, must be determined with large scale double-blind, placebo-controlled trials.

Carbamazepine

The use of carbamazepine in patients with panic disorder and benzodiazepine withdrawal has suggested that carbamazepine may have antipanic effects (151). In an open trial by Tondo et al. (152), 34 patients with panic disorder with or without agoraphobia were treated with carbamazepine at a mean dose of 419 mg/day for 2 to 12 months. Patients' response was rated as "absent/scarce" or "good" on the basis of a global rating of frequency of panic attacks, degree of avoidance behavior, and adaptive functioning. Using these criteria, 20(58%) patients were rated as having a good response to medication (152).

However, in a controlled study of 14 patients with panic disorder conducted by Uhde et al. (152,153), carbamazepine was not effective. Carbamazepine treatment did not result in a significant change on any outcome measure. Forty percent of patients had a decrease in the frequency of panic attacks, 50% had an increase in panic attack frequency, and 10% demonstrated no change. Neither EEG abnormalities nor prominent psychosensory symptoms in this study predicted response to carbamazepine.

Phenytoin

McNamara and Fogel (154) described three patients who experienced a complete cessation of panic attacks with phenytoin treatment. These patients also had abnormal temporal lobe EEG patterns, comparable to interictal temporal lobe epilepsy. It is unclear whether these observations can be applied to individuals with panic disorder, as it is highly unusual for panic disorder patients to have EEG abnormalities.

Levetiracetam

A recent open-label, fixed-flexible dose study was conducted in two outpatient clinics where 18 patients with panic disorder with or without agoraphobia were treated with levetiracetam for 12 weeks (155). The mean daily dose of levetiracetam during the last two weeks of the study was 1138 mg ($\pm$627 mg; range 306 mg–2386 mg). Participants showed significant improvement on the primary efficacy measure of the CGI-S with mean scores decreasing from 4.8 ($\pm$0 0.4) to 2.7 ($\pm$1.1) ($t = 6.5$; df $= 16$; $p < 0.00$). Panic attack frequency decreased from 2.9 ($\pm$0.8) to 1.2 ($\pm$1.2) ($t = 5.9$; df $= 12$; $p < 0.00$) on the Agoraphobia, Avoidance Behavior Scale (item B of the PAS), and the mean HAM-A score decreased from 23.4 ($\pm$5.6) to 7.6 ($\pm$5.9) ($t = 8.9$; df $= 12$; $p < 0.00$). This small open-label study suggests levetiracetam may have anxiolytic effects in panic disorder, but needs to be confirmed in large double-blind, placebo-controlled studies.

Vigabatrin

Zwanzger et al. (156) reported successful vigabatrin treatment in three patients meeting DSM-IV criteria for panic disorder. After a medication-free period of at least two weeks, patients received vigabatrin at a daily dose of 2 g for six months. All patients showed a marked reduction in anxiety on the HAM-A and clear improvement in agoraphobia on the PAS after two weeks. Maximal effects of vigabatrin on anxiety as assessed by the HAM-A and PAS were observed within 4 weeks of treatment. In addition, the anxiolytic effect of vigabatrin was maintained during subsequent therapy throughout the next six months, with the occurrence of very few panic attacks.

Similar results were shown in 10 healthy volunteers who received vigabatrin 2 g per day for seven days after placebo-controlled administration of 50 μg of CCK-4 to induce panic symptoms (157). Panic symptom severity was evaluated with the Acute Panic Inventory (API) and a DSM-IV derived panic-symptom scale (PSS). Additionally, a 100-mm visual analogue scale (VAS) was used for evaluation of subjective anxiety. All subjects reported a marked reduction of CCK-4–induced panic and anxiety symptoms after one week of vigabatrin treatment. Compared with the first CCK-4 challenge, the number of reported PSS symptoms decreased by 50% from 9.4 ± 0.9 (range 5–13) to 4.7 ± 1.0 (range 0–6) after vigabatrin treatment ($F(1,9) = 45.08$, $p < 0.001$). PSS sumscores decreased by 54% from 19.7 ± 2.8 (range 3–31) to 9 ± 2.2 (range 0–25) ($F(1,9) = 9.2$, $p < 0.014$). The mean API sumscore decreased significantly by 45% from 24.0 ± 3.3 (range 10–38) to 13.2 ± 3.5 (range 0–42) ($F(1,9) = 18.96$, $p < 0.002$). Moreover, subjects reported a significant reduction of VAS-scores for anxiety from 52.0 ± 6.6 (range 30–90) to 26.5 ± 5.7 (range 0–60) ($F(1,9) = 9.56$, $p < 0.013$).

GENERALIZED ANXIETY DISORDER

Generalized anxiety disorder (GAD) is characterized by excessive and uncontrollable anxiety and worry that has been present for at least six months. The anxiety and worry is centered on a number of day to day life events, including family life, work, health and finances, and is associated with feelings of restlessness, feeling on edge, being easily tired, poor concentration, irritability, muscle tension, and sleep problems (31).

A wide spectrum of drug classes has been shown to be efficacious in the treatment of GAD. Benzodiazepines (158–167) have demonstrated safety and efficacy in more placebo-controlled trials then any other medication, but rebound and withdrawal symptoms as well as lack of efficacy in common comorbid conditions have limited their use (168). Other efficacious medications include the tricyclic imipramine (169–172), buspirone (158,164,173–176), the SSRIs, paroxetine (170,177–179), escitalopram (85,180–182), and sertraline (179,183,184), the SNRI venlafaxine (158,170,174,185–188), and the antihistamine hydroxyzine (162,176).

Gabapentin

Two case reports have described improvements in patients with GAD following the addition of gabapentin (189). Improvements in both anxiety and arousal were noted.

Pregabalin

To date, at least seven double-blind, placebo-controlled studies have demonstrated the efficacy of pregabalin in GAD. Pande et al. (190) compared the effectiveness and tolerability of pregabalin in treating GAD to that of lorazepam and a placebo. Two hundred and seventy-six patients were randomly assigned to one of four treatment groups: pregabalin 150 mg/day ($N = 69$), pregabalin 600 mg/day ($N = 70$), lorazepam 6 mg/day ($N = 68$), and placebo ($N = 69$). Significant improvements from baseline to end point were found on the HAM-A for all active treatment groups, with the high-dose pregabalin and lorazepam groups demonstrating similar anxiolytic effects. There were also significantly more responders ($\geq 50\%$ decrease in HAM-A) in patients receiving pregabalin 600 mg/day (46%) and lorazepam 6 mg/day (61%) than in those given placebo (27%). Although the side effects of pregabalin and lorazepam were similar, those in the pregabalin treatment group found the side effects more tolerable. The most common side effects for both treatments were dizziness (38.6% for 600 mg/day pregabalin and 13.2.3% for 6 mg/day lorazepam) and somnolence (35.7% for 600 mg/day pregabalin and 54.4% for 6 mg/day lorazepam). Only the lorazepam group demonstrated significantly more withdrawal effects then placebo (191).

In a double-blind, fixed-dose, placebo- and active-controlled study, Feltner et al. (163) randomized 271 patients to receive pregabalin 50 mg t.i.d. ($N = 70$), pregabalin 200 mg t.i.d. ($N = 66$), placebo ($N = 67$), or lorazepam 2 mg t.i.d. ($N = 68$) for four weeks. Adjusted mean change scores on the HAM-A (primary outcome measure) were significantly improved for pregabalin 200 mg t.i.d. [difference of 3.90 between drug and placebo; $p \leq 0.0013$ analysis of covariance (ANCOVA), df = 252] and for lorazepam [difference of 2.35; $p \leq 0.0483$ (ANCOVA), df = 252], with the significant difference between the pregabalin 200 mg t.i.d. and placebo groups seen at week 1 of treatment [$p \leq 0.0001$ (ANCOVA), df = 238].

Similar results were found in another double-blind, placebo-controlled, active comparator trial, where patients were randomized to four weeks of treatment with pregabalin 300 mg/day ($N = 91$), 450 mg/day ($N = 90$), or 600 mg/day ($N = 89$); alprazolam 1.5 mg/day ($N = 93$); or placebo ($N = 91$) (161). The end point response criterion was a 50% or greater reduction in the baseline HAM-A total score. Study drug was administered in divided doses using a t.i.d. schedule. Pregabalin and alprazolam produced a significantly greater reduction in mean $\pm$ SE HAM-A total score at LOCF end point compared with placebo: pregabalin 300 mg/day (-12.2 ± 0.8, $p < 0.001$), 450 mg/day (-11.0 ± 0.8, $p = 0.02$), and 600 mg/day (-11.8 ± 0.8, $p = 0.002$); alprazolam (-10.9 ± 0.8, $p = 0.02$); and placebo (-8.4 ± 0.8). By week 1 and at LOCF end point, the three pregabalin groups and the alprazolam group had significantly ($p < 0.01$) improved HAM-A psychic anxiety symptoms compared with the placebo group. HAM-A somatic anxiety symptoms were also significantly ($p < 0.02$) improved in the 300 and 600 mg/day pregabalin groups, but not in the 450 mg/day pregabalin (week 1, $p = 0.06$; week 4, $p = 0.32$) and the alprazolam groups (week 1, $p = 0.21$; week 4, $p = 0.15$), as compared with placebo. Of the five treatment groups, the 300 mg/day pregabalin group was the only medication group that differed statistically in global improvement at treatment end point, not only from the placebo group, but also from the alprazolam group.

Pohl et al. (191) evaluated the anxiolytic efficacy of b.i.d. versus t.i.d. dosing of pregabalin in patients with GAD. Outpatients with GAD were randomized to six weeks of double-blind treatment with pregabalin 200 mg/day (b.i.d.; $N = 78$), 400 mg/day (b.i.d.; $N = 89$), 450 mg/day (t.i.d.; $N = 88$), or placebo ($N = 86$). Mean improvement in end point HAM-A total score was significantly greater for pregabalin 200 mg/day ($p = 0.006$), 400 mg/day ($p = 0.001$), and 450 mg/day ($p = 0.005$) compared with placebo (LOCF). Pairwise comparisons of b.i.d. with t.i.d. dosing found no difference in HAM-A change score at end point. Improvement on both psychic and somatic factors of the HAM-A was rapid: significance versus placebo was achieved as early as the first assessment at week 1, with 30% or more reduction in HAM-A severity and equal or greater improvement for every subsequent visit in 38% or more patients in all three pregabalin dosage groups ($p \leq 0.001$). This study showed similar efficacy and comparable tolerability of pregabalin in GAD with b.i.d. and t.i.d. dosing.

Montgomery et al. (192) showed that pregabalin was safe, well tolerated, and rapidly efficacious across both the physical-somatic and emotional symptoms of GAD in a six-week, multicenter, randomized, double-blind, placebo-controlled comparison of pregabalin and venlafaxine. Outpatients ($N = 421$) were randomly assigned to pregabalin 400 or 600 mg/day, venlafaxine 75 mg/day, or placebo. Pregabalin at both dosages (400 mg/day, $p = 0.008$; 600 mg/day, $p = 0.03$) and venlafaxine ($p = 0.03$) produced significantly greater improvement in HAM-A total scores at LOCF end point than did placebo. Only the pregabalin 400-mg/day treatment group experienced significant improvement in all a priori primary and secondary efficacy measures. Pregabalin in both dosage treatment groups (400 mg/day, $p < 0.01$; 600 mg/day, $p < 0.001$) significantly improved HAM-A total scores at week 1, with significant improvement through LOCF end point. Statistically significant improvement began at week 2 for venlafaxine.

Khan et al. (193) evaluated the efficacy of pregabalin 150 to 600 mg/day in the elderly ($N = 277$) in an eight-week, multicenter, randomized, placebo-controlled, double-blind, parallel-group study. Patients were 65 years and older. On the primary outcome measure (change from baseline in HAM-A least squares mean total score), pregabalin-treated patients achieved a significantly greater reduction at LOCF end point than did patients who received placebo (–12.84 vs. –10.65; $p = 0.0437$). A significant reduction from baseline in mean HAM-A total score was found in favor of pregabalin at weeks 2 ($p = 0.0052$), 4 ($p = 0.0043$), 6 ($p = 0.0011$), and 8 ($p = 0.0070$). Significantly, more pregabalin-treated patients were responders at week 4 (defined as a $\geq$50% reduction in HAM-A total score) (49.3% vs. 32.9%, $p < 0.05$) and over half of pregabalin-treated patients were responders at week 8, with results approaching significance (52.6% vs. 41.1%, $p \leq 0.07$). The most common side effects among pregabalin-treated patients were dizziness (20%), somnolence (13%), headache (10%), and nausea (9%). The authors concluded that pregabalin was a safe and effective treatment of GAD in an elderly population.

Finally, the long-term efficacy of pregabalin in GAD was investigated by Smith, et al. in a treatment-discontinuation study (194). Six hundred twenty-four adult patients with DSM-IV GAD and a mean HAM-A score of 25.2 received open-label pregabalin 150 mg t.i.d. for eight weeks. Responders who had a HAM-A score of 11 or less for the weeks 7 and 8, visits were then randomized to double-blind treatment with either pregabalin ($N = 168$) or placebo ($N = 170$) for an additional 26 weeks. The primary efficacy parameter was time to relapse, defined as either: (1) a HAM-A of 20 or more and a diagnosis of GAD at two successive visits one week apart; (2) a CGI-I rated "much worse" or "very much worse" and a diagnosis of GAD at two successive visits one week apart; or (3) symptomatic worsening of anxiety which required clinical intervention. There was a significant difference between pregabalin and placebo in time to relapse ($p = 0.0001$). Significantly, more pregabalin-treated patients maintained efficacy through the double-blind period (defined as an end point CGI-I ≤ 5) as compared with placebo-treated patients (pregabalin 57.1%, placebo 36.5%; $p = 0.001$). Statistical significance in favor of pregabalin was also demonstrated on the HAM-A and the SDS (both total and individual subscale scores). Pregabalin was well tolerated, with no unexpected adverse events occurring during the eight months of the study. The results of this study clearly demonstrate the efficacy of pregabalin for the prevention of relapse of GAD during long-term treatment.

These positive, large-scale, placebo-controlled trials of pregabalin in GAD make pregabalin a new treatment alternative for GAD. Further study of its ability to treat commonly comorbid conditions, such as depressive symptoms, would allow for a better understand of its role in treating GAD, whether as a first-line agent or a strategy reserved for treatment-resistant cases, patients who cannot tolerate antidepressants, or patients for whom benzodiazepines are not indicated.

Tiagabine

There are two published case series examining tiagabine augmentation in the treatment of GAD (148,195). Five patients with GAD and comorbid major depression and/or neuropathic pain received tiagabine 6 mg/day. (148). After two weeks of tiagabine, a significant reduction in HAM-A score was found that was maintained for the eight-week treatment trial. Tiagabine was generally well tolerated. In a case series of five treatment-refractory patients (4 with GAD and 1 with major depressive and severe anxiety due to antidepressant withdrawal), tiagabine in 1-mg incremental doses was initiated either as a monotherapy or adjunctive treatment (195). Tiagabine improved anxiety and was well tolerated by all patients, including the patient with anxiety secondary to acute antidepressant withdrawal.

Similar findings were reported by Papp and Ray (196) using a mean dose of 9 mg/day of tiagabine in an eight-week treatment trial of 25 patients with GAD. Seven (37%) patients rated as much or very much improved by the CGI-I. Six (24%) patients withdrew because of adverse events, which included abnormal thinking, nausea, amnesia, anemia, asthenia, colitis, diarrhea, hallucinations, headache, migraine, and somnolence.

Rosenthal and Dolnak (197) conducted a 10-week, open-label, blind rater study of 40 patients randomized to tiagabine or paroxetine. Tiagabine and paroxetine significantly reduced measures of anxiety and depression, along with improving sleep and overall functioning. Forty percent of the tiagabine group was considered responders (defined as a ≥50% decrease in baseline HAM-A scores) compared with 60% of the paroxetine group. In both groups, 20% of patients achieved remission (defined as an end point HAM-A score ≤7). Both treatments where well tolerated, with one patient withdrawing due to adverse events while taking tiagabine and two withdrawing while taking paroxetine (197).

A recently completed double-blind, placebo-controlled trial examined tiagabine monotherapy in the treatment of GAD (198). Two hundred seventy-two patients were randomized to tiagabine ($N = 134$) (mean dose 10.5 mg/day) or placebo ($N = 132$) for eight weeks. In those who completed the trial ($N = 198$), there was a significant reduction in the primary outcome measure (HAM-A) favoring tiagabine; however, in the ITT analysis the difference did not reach statistical significance. Fifty-seven percent of patients in the tiagabine group were considered responders (much or very much improved on the CGI-I), compared with 44% of the placebo group ($p = 0.08$). Tiagabine reduced GAD symptoms according to the observed case and mixed models repeated-measures (MMRM) analyses but not the primary LOCF analysis. In a post hoc MMRM analysis, a significant difference in the mean reduction in HAM-A total score over the efficacy evaluation period was found, favoring tiagabine over placebo ($p < 0.01$). Tiagabine had an early onset of effect, as shown by significant reduction from baseline in mean HAM-A total score compared with placebo at week 1 (observed cases, $p < 0.05$). Tiagabine was generally well tolerated with dizziness, headache, and nausea as the most common adverse events. Although tiagabine did not separate from placebo in the ITT analysis, the improvements seen in the observed case and MMRM analyses suggest that tiagabine may reduce symptoms in GAD. Further placebo-controlled studies have been completed but results are not yet available. Once these results become available, we will be better able to ascertain the role of tiagabine in the treatment of GAD.

Levetiracetam

One case report has described the adjunctive use of levetiracetam in GAD. Levetiracetam 250 mg/day was added to citalopram in a 42-year-old female with GAD. Levetiracetam was associated with reduced anxiety after four days with sustained improvement at six months (199).

OBSESSIVE-COMPULSIVE DISORDER

OCD is characterized by persistent, intrusive thoughts and/or images (obsessions), and repetitive, ritualistic behaviors that the individual feels he or she must complete (compulsions) (31).

SSRIs are considered the gold standard treatment for OCD. Paroxetine (200–202), fluoxetine (203–208), citalopram (209,210), fluvoxamine (205,207,208, 211–213), sertraline (204,205,207,208,214–216) and escitalopram (217) have all demonstrated efficacy in placebo-controlled trials. Other agents shown to demonstrate efficacy are clomipramine (205,207,208,217–220) and the MAOI phenelzine (221). In treatment-resistant cases, placebo-controlled trials support the augmenting of an SSRI with haloperidol (222), pindolol (223), risperidone (224), quetiapine, (225), and olanzapine. (226) As OCD is a chronic and disabling condition, a continued search for treatment possibilities for partial responders and refractory patients is necessary.

Gabapentin

Cora-Locatelli et al. (227) described the use of gabapentin in the treatment of five patients with OCD who were partial responders to fluoxetine. Gabapentin (mean dose = 2520 mg/day) and fluoxetine (mean dose = 68 mg/day) were taken simultaneously for six weeks and the combination was relatively well tolerated. All patients demonstrated improvements in anxiety, obsessive-compulsive symptoms, sleep, and mood on the basis of clinical evaluations. However, patients experienced a rebound of psychiatric symptoms once gabapentin was discontinued (228).

Valproate

The use of valproate in treating OCD has been documented only in patients who have ceased treatment of conventional antiobsessional medication because of side effects such as anxiety, irritability, confusion, psychosis, and other cognitive impairments (229,230). Deltito (229) described the use of valproate in 10 patients with OCD who discontinued the use of medications including clomipramine, fluoxetine, sertraline, and paroxetine. Valproate was used as pretreatment, with an initial dose of 250 mg/day that was increased to a final dose of approximately 2500 mg/day. Treatment was then completed with the addition of typical anti-obsessional pharmacotherapy without the previously mentioned side effects. Successful outcomes, determined by clinical evaluation, were noted in 8 of the 10 patients. A case-report by Cora-Locatelli et al. (230) described the use of val-proate 750 mg/day in combination with 1 mg/day fluoxetine. Both treatments were started at the same time and marked changes in Yale-Brown Obsessive-Compulsive Scale (Y-BOCS), HAM-A, and HAM-D scores were found. The authors discontinued the fluoxetine as they suspected valproate to be responsible for the improvement. The patients' symptoms continued to improve with valproate monotherapy.

Carbamazepine

Three reports have described the use of carbamazepine in OCD. In a case report, a 27-year-old woman with OCD receiving inpatient treatment with a combination of carbamazepine (500 mg/day) and clomipramine (200 mg/day) displayed significant improvements in anxiety, distress, and habitual checking that allowed her to be discharged from the hospital (231). Previous psychopharmacological treatments were not effective. In an open-label trial of four patients with OCD and temporal EEG abnormalities, improvement was demonstrated in only one patient (232). In a series of nine patients treated with carbamazepine (400 to 1600 mg/day), only one of the eight who completed the trial demonstrated any improvement (233). These preliminary finding suggest that carbamazepine is likely not an effective mono-therapy for OCD; however, controlled investigations are need to adequately evaluate its efficacy.

Topiramate

To date, topiramate has been evaluated in one case report and 2 open-label trials in treatment-resistant OCD. The case report described a nine-week topiramate augmentation of paroxetine, where a significant change from baseline was found on the Y-BOCS and the CGI-I (234). In one of the open-label trials, Van Ameringen et al. (235) augmented 16 patients with topiramate (mean dose = 253.1 mg/day) for between 14 and 26 weeks. At end point, 11 (68.8%) patients were considered responders, defined as a CGI-I rating of much or very much improved. Significant improvement on the CGI-S scale was also found ($p < 0.001$). Most patients experienced one or more adverse event, which included weight loss, sedation/fatigue, paresthesia, and memory/word finding problems (235). In the other open-label trial, topiramate (mean dose of 237.5 ± 29.1 mg/day) was added to the serotonin reuptake inhibitor (SRI) of subjects with treatment-resistant OCD for 16 weeks (236). Significant changes from baseline were found in both of the primary outcome measures, the Y-BOCS ($p = 0.002$) and GAF scores ($p = 0.002$). Response, defined as an end point Y-BOCS score of less than 30% of the baseline score, was achieved by 86% of the sample. Weight loss, sedation, memory/word-finding difficulties, and paresthesias were the most common adverse events. These preliminary data may suggest a potential role for topiramate as an augmenting agent for treatment-resistant OCD, but they must be verified in double-blind, placebo-controlled trials.

Lamotrigine

There is one report of lamotrigine treatment for SRI-resistant OCD. Eight patients with an inadequate response to at least 200 mg/day of sertraline or 225 mg/day of clomipramine for a mean period of 14 weeks had lamotrigine added for at least four weeks up to a maximum dose of 100 mg/day. The SRI dose remained unchanged throughout the study period. No significant changes where found on the CGI-S or CGI-I scales. The mean baseline and end point Y-BOCS scores were 24.0 and 18.9, respectively (237). This small trial suggests that lamotrigine augmentation may not be a useful strategy for SRI-refractory OCD. However, given the potential effectiveness of topiramate, another agent with anti-glutamatergic properties, further evaluation of lamotrigine is warranted using the higher doses that are found to be effective in treating bipolar depression (238).

MIXED ANXIETY CONDITIONS

In this section, "mixed anxiety conditions" refers to studies that included patients with varying anxiety disorders.

Tiagabine

In a case series of 10 patients with an anxiety disorder or a comorbid anxiety condition considered refractory to previous antianxiety treatments, tiagabine was given as monotherapy ($N = 5$) or in combination with other medications ($N = 5$), including risperidone, citralopram, paroxetine, and clomipramine. Patients in the series had a primary diagnosis of GAD ($N = 5$), PTSD ($N = 1$), major depressive disorder ($N = 2$), bipolar disorder ($N = 1$), or schizophrenia ($N = 1$). All patients were rated as much improved or very much improved on the CGI-C scale after four weeks of tiagabine treatment, with most patients reporting marked improvement in anxiety after one week of treatment (239).

Schwartz et al. (240) conducted an eight-week open-trial of tiagabine augmentation in a sample of mixed anxiety disorders, including GAD, panic disorder, PTSD, and social phobia. Concomitant medications included SSRIs, venlafaxine, nefazodone, and alprazolam. Significant improvements from baseline in anxiety were found as measured by the HAM-A and the Beck Anxiety Inventory (BAI). At end point, 76% of patients were considered responders ($\geq$50% reduction in HAM-A), and 59% achieved remission (HAM-A total score $\leq$7).

These open trials of tiagabine in mixed anxiety disorders suggest tiagabine may have general anxiolytic effects. Conversely, the inclusion of multiple anxiety diagnoses and multiple concomitant medications significantly limits the conclusions that can be drawn from them. Moreover, placebo-controlled trials examining the efficacy of tiagabine as monotherapy and as combination therapy in individual anxiety disorders have not been robust and indicate that tiagabine may have moderate anxiolytic effects at best.

SUMMARY

A summary of the studies described in this chapter can be found in Table 1. In Table 2, we have included the level of evidence associated with each AED for each anxiety disorder. As detailed in the Canadian Clinical Practice Guidelines (241), levels of evidence are ranked from 1 to 4, which are as follows: (1) meta-analysis or

(*text continues on page 238*)

TABLE 1 Summary of Open and Controlled Trials of Anticonvulsants in Anxiety Disorders

Author(s) and yr (Ref.)	Drug	Disorder	Sample size	Design	Concomitant psychotropic medications	Outcomes	Adverse events
Van Ameringen et al., 2004 (40)	Topiramate (monotherapy)	Social phobia	23	Open trial		45.1% considered responders (CGI-I ≤ 2); 26.1% achieved remission (LSAS ≤ 30); significant decrease in LSAS	Somnolence
Pande et al., 1999 (42)	Gabapentin (monotherapy)	Social phobia	69	Double-blind, placebo-controlled trial		No significant difference in response (≥50% decrease on LSAS)	Nausea Somnolence Dizziness Fatigue
De-Paris et al., 2003 (43)	Gabapentin (monotherapy)	Social phobia	32	Open-label trial		Gabapentin at 800 mg > Gabapentin 400 mg (visual analogue mood scale item calm-excite)	Somnolence Dizziness Nausea Headaches
Pande et al., 2004 (44)	Pregabalin (monotherapy)	Social phobia	135	Double-blind, placebo-controlled trial		Significant decrease in LSAS in high-dose group (600 mg/day) Significantly more responders in high-dose group than placebo	Dizziness Somnolence Nausea Flatulence Decreased libido
Nardi et al., 1997 (44,45)	Valproic acid (monotherapy)	Social phobia	16	Open-label trial		All nonresponders	Rash, GI symptoms
Kinnys et al., 2003 (46)	Valproic acid (monotherapy)	Social phobia	17	Open-label trial		41.1% response by CGI-I	Sedation Headache Tremor GI discomfort Weight gain
Dunlop et al., 2007 (47)	Tiagabine (monotherapy)	Social phobia	54	Open-label trial		Significant reduction in LSAS and SPIN; 40.7% were responders (CGI-I ≤ 2) in the ITT sample	Somnolence Dizziness Insomnia Nausea

(Continued)

TABLE 1 Summary of Open and Controlled Trials of Anticonvulsants in Anxiety Disorders (*Continued*)

Author(s) and yr (Ref.)	Drug	Disorder	Sample size	Design	Concomitant psychotropic medications	Outcomes	Adverse events
Kinrys et al., 2004 (48)	Tiagabine (augmentation)	Treatment refractory social phobia	14	Retrospective analysis, open-label trial	SSRIs, quetiapine, clonazepam, bupropion	64.2% (9/14) met response criteria (CGI-I ≤ 2); 35.7% (5/14) met remission criteria (LSAS ≤ 30)	Sedation Tiredness Headaches
	Levetiracetam (monotherapy)	Social phobia	20	Open-label trial		Significant reduction in LSAS, CGI-S, HAM-A and HAM-D	Drowsiness Nervousness
Simon et al., 2004 (49)	Levetiracetam (monotherapy)	Social phobia	18	Double-blind, placebo-controlled pilot study		Levetiracetam = PBO Effect sizes of LEV (0.33) BSPS and 0.50 for the LSAS compared with PBO	Headaches Drowsiness Disinhibition Inebreation
Zhang et al., 2005 (50)	Lamotrigine (monotherapy)	PTSD	14	Double-blind, placebo-controlled trial		50% (5/10) of the lamotrigine group vs. 25% (1/4) of placebo group rated as "much" or "very much improved" on the DGRP	Dizziness Dry mouth Nausea Headache
Hertzberg et al., 1997 (66)	Topiramate (monotherapy and augmentation)	PTSD	33	Open-label trial	SSRIs, benzodiazepine, stimulants, atypical neuroleptics, gabapentin, lamotrigine, mirtazapine, venlafaxine, verapamil	Mean reduction in PCL-C of 49% ($p < 0.001$) and a response rate of 77% at wk 4.	Panic Nervousness Overstimulation Shakiness Clumsiness Cognitive impairment Severe headache
Berlant, 2004 (69)	Topiramate (monotherapy)	Noncombat related PTSD	38	Double-blind, placebo-controlled trial		Topiramate = PBO (CAPS—primary efficacy measure) Topiramate > PBO (TOP-8, = 0.025) Topiramate > PBO (end point CGI-I scores $p = 0.055$).	Headache Sinusitis Taste perversion Language problems Insomnia Dyspepsia Nervousness Fatigue Hypertension Difficulty with concentration/attention

Study	Drug	Disorder	N	Design	Concomitant medications	Results	Side effects
Tucker et al., 2007 (70)	Topiramate (monotherapy)	Combat-related PTSD	40	Double-blind, placebo-controlled trial		Topiramate = PBO (CAPS total, CAPS-B, CAPS-C, TOP 8, HAM-D, or HAM-A). Topiramate > PBO (wk 6 and 8 CGI-I, $p = 0.021$) Topiramate > PBO (CAPS-D, $p = 0.019$)	
Davis et al. (unpublished) (72)	Topiramate (augmentation)	PTSD	35	Open trial	Antidepressants neuroleptics anticonvulsants benzodiazepines lithium	76% had reduced nightmares; 86% had reduced flashbacks. After 4 wk 82% did not meet criteria for active PTSD	
Berlant et al., 2002 (67)	Gabapentin (augmentation)	PTSD	30	Retrospective chart review	Antidepressants antipsychotics β-blockers antiepileptics benzodiazepine	77% of patients reported moderate or marked improvements in sleep duration	
Hamner et al., 2001 (74)	Valproic acid (augmentation)	PTSD	16	Open-label trial	Antidepressants benzodiazepines neuroleptics	Decreased hyperarousal	
Fesler et al., 1991 (76)	Valproic acid (monotherapy and augmentation)	Combat-related PTSD	16	Open-label clinical trial	Fluoxetine bupropion buspirone lorazepam temazepam nefazadone	Significant improvement on CAPS total score ($p < 0.01$), on CAPS subscale scores of intrusion ($p < 0.05$) and hyperarousal ($p < .001$) and on the HAM-A and HAM-D ($p < 0.01$).	Drowziness Dizziness Irritability Headaches Vomiting Dry mouth Flushing
Clark et al., 1999 (77)	Valproic acid (augmentation)	Combat-related PTSD	21	Open-label trial	Benzodiazepines	Symptom reduction in all three clusters	
Petty et al., 2002 (78)	Valproic acid (monotherapy)	Noncombat-related PTSD	10	Open-label trial		No improvements in PTSD or depressive symptoms	Sedation Mild dizziness

(Continued)

TABLE 1 Summary of Open and Controlled Trials of Anticonvulsants in Anxiety Disorders (*Continued*)

Author(s) and yr (Ref.)	Drug	Disorder	Sample size	Design	Concomitant psychotropic medications	Outcomes	Adverse events
Otte et al., 2004 (79)	Valproic acid (augmentation and monotherapy)	PTSD	325	Retrospective chart review	Benzodiazepines Trazodone other antidepressants neuroleptics lithium buspirone other anticonvulsants methylphenidate	50% (25/50) patients were rated as "very much" or "much" improved on the CGI-I. The improved end point CGI-I differed significantly from "no change" ($p < 0.000001$)	Sedation Gastrointestinal distress
Davis et al., 2005 (80)	Divalproate (monotherapy)	PTSD	86	Randomized, placebo-controlled trial		Divalproate = PBO (CAPS total score, CAPS-B, CAPS-D, TOP-8, CGI-I or HAM-A) Divalproate > PBO (CAPS-C and MADRS)	
Davis et al. (submitted) (81)	Tiagabine (augmentation)	PTSD	6	Open-label trial	Antidepressants	Significant reduction in DTS	Urticaria Eating cessation Acute narrow-angle glaucoma Headache Memory difficulties
Lara, 2002 (82)	Tiagabine (augmentation)	PTSD with comorbidity	7	Open-label trial	Antidepressants valproic acid benzodiazepines buspirone	6/7 patients rated "markedly improved" in CGI-C	Drowsiness
Taylor, 2003 (84)	Tiagabine (monotherapy)	PTSD	26	Open-label followed by randomization to tiagabine or placebo trial		Significant reductions in open-label phase on all measures of PTSD, depression, general anxiety, social anxiety, resilience, and disability Gain, where maintained, in both tiagabine and placebo group	

Reference	Drug	Disorder	N	Study type	Comparator	Results	Side effects
Davidson et al., 2004 (85)	Tiagabine (monotherapy)	PTSD	232	Randomized, multicenter, double-blind trial		Tiagabine = PBO	Dizziness Headache Somnolence Nausea
Davidson et al., 2007 (86)	Carbamazepine (monotherapy)	PTSD	10	Open-label trial		Decrease in intensity of nightmares, flashbacks and intrusive thoughts. 7/10 responded "moderately" to "very much" on CGI-I	
Lipper et al., 1986 (87)	Carbamazepine	PTSD	10	Open-label trial		Decrease in staff observation of violent behavior and self report measures	Headache Tremor
Wolf et al., 1988 (88)	Carbamazepine (augmentation)	Childhood PTSD	28	Open-label trial	Methylphenidate clonidine sertraline fluoxetine imipramine	22/28 free of PTSD symptoms	Gastrointestinal symptoms
Looff et al., 1995 (89)	Phenytoin (monotherapy)	PTSD	9	Open-label trial		Significant improvement in PTSD (CAPS)	
Bremner et al., 2004 (90)	Phenytoin (monotherapy)	PTSD	9	Open-label trial		No significant effects were found on depression (HAM-D) or anxiety (HAM-A) scores. Significant correlation between increased hippocampal volume and reduction of PTSD symptoms. PTSD patients treated with phenytoin resulted in significant (6%) increase in right whole-brain volume ($p < 0.05$)	
	Levetiracetam (augmentation)	PTSD	23	Retrospective analysis		Significant improvement was found on all measures	Sedation Tiredness Light-headedness Dry mouth Dyspepsia
Bremner et al., 2005 (91)	Gabapentin (monotherapy)	Panic disorder	103	Double-blind, placebo-controlled trial		No significant difference in response, significant improvement in PAS for severely-ill	Headache Nausea Somnolence

(Continued)

TABLE 1 Summary of Open and Controlled Trials of Anticonvulsants in Anxiety Disorders (*Continued*)

Author(s) and yr (Ref.)	Drug	Disorder	Sample size	Design	Concomitant psychotropic medications	Outcomes	Adverse events
Kinnys et al., 2006 (95)	Valproic acid (monotherapy)	Panic disorder with/without agoraphobia	10	Open-label trial		Significant reduction in CGI-S, HAM-A, Covi Anxiety Scale, and SCL-90-Panic factor	Nausea Dizziness Drowsiness Tremor Diarrhea
Pande et al., 2000 (137)	Valproic acid (monotherapy)	Panic disorder	12	Open-label trial		Significant improvement based on CGI-S and CGI-I, HAM-A, BSI	Sedation Nausea Dry mouth
Primeau et al., 1990 (143)	Valproic acid (Monotherapy)	Panic disorder	16	Open-label trial		Significant reduction in HAM-A, 71% decrease in frequency of attacks, 43% remitted	
Woodman and Noyles, 1994 (144)	Valproic acid (monotherapy)	Panic disorder	12	Double-blind, placebo-controlled trial		Significant improvements on CGI-S, and CGI-I scales	Gastrointestinal dysfunction Dizziness Somnolence
	Valproic acid (augmentation)	Panic disorder with comorbid mood instability	13	Open-label trial	Antidepressants benzodiazepines haloperidol	Decrease in panic frequency, HAM-A, and on BAI, BDI	Nausea Increased appetite
Keck et al., 1993 (145)	Tiagabine (monotherapy)	Panic disorder	15	Open-label trial		A significant reduction in panic was found after the second CCK-4 challenge	Visual field constriction (long-term use)
Lum et al., 1990 (147)	Carbamazepine (monotherapy)	Panic disorder with/without agoraphobia	34	Open-label trial		58.8% rated as having a "good response" by at least 5 independent investigators	
Baetz and Bowen, 1998 (146)	Carbamazepine (monotherapy)	Panic disorder	14	Controlled trial		40% had a completed cessation of panic attacks, 50% had an increase, 10% had no change	Restlessness Dizziness Blurred vision Rash

Study	Drug	Disorder	N	Study design	Results	Adverse effects
Zwanzger et al., 2003 (150)	Levetiracetam (monotherapy)	Panic disorder	18	Open-label, fixed-flexible dose study trial	Significant improvement on the CGI-S (primary efficacy measure) Panic attack frequency also significantly decreased	Insomnia Irritability Headaches
Tondo et al., 1989 (152)	Viagabatrin (monotherapy)	Panic disorder	3	Open-label trial	Marked reduction in agoraphobia and anxiety (HAM-A) as early as 2 wk, and maintained during subsequent therapy throughout the next 6 mo	Dizziness Fatigue Visual field-constrictions (long-term use)
Uhde et al., 1988 (153)	Viagabatrin (monotherapy)	Panic disorder	10	Placebo-controlled (CCK-4), followed by open-label	A significant reduction in panic was found after the second CCK-4 challenge.	Visual field constrictions (long-term use)
Papp, 2006 (155)	Pregabalin (monotherapy)	GAD	276	Double-blind, placebo and active—controlled trial	Pregabalin 600 mg > PBO Lorazepam > PBO Pregabalin 600 mg = Lorazepam	Somnolence Dizziness
Zwanzger et al., 2001 (156)	Pregabalin (monotherapy)	GAD	271	Double-blind, fixed-dose, parallel-group, placebo and active-controlled trial	Pregabalin 600 mg > PBO Lorazepam > PBO	Somnolence Dizziness Weight gain
Zwanzger et al., 2001 (157)	Pregabalin (monotherapy)	GAD	454	Double-blind, placebo-controlled, active comparator trial	Pregabalin 300 mg, 450 mg and 600 mg > PBO Alprazolam > PBO	Dizziness Weight gain
Pande et al., 2003 (190)	Pregabalin (monotherapy)	GAD	341	Double-blind, placebo-controlled trial	All 3 pregabalin dosage groups > PBO	Dizziness Somnolence Dry mouth Euphoria Blurred vision Incoordination Flatulence Infection Abnormal thinking
Feltner et al., 2003 (163)	Pregabalin (monotherapy)	GAD	421	Multicenter, randomized, double blind, placebo-controlled trial	Pregabalin 400 mg/day, 600 mg/day > PBO (HAM-A total score) Venlafaxine > PBO Pregabalin 400 mg/day > PBO (all primary and secondary measures)	Dizziness Somnolence Nausea

(Continued)

TABLE 1 Summary of Open and Controlled Trials of Anticonvulsants in Anxiety Disorders (*Continued*)

Author(s) and yr (Ref.)	Drug	Disorder	Sample size	Design	Concomitant psychotropic medications	Outcomes	Adverse events
Rickels et al., 2005 (161)	Pregabalin (monotherapy)	GAD	277	Multicenter, randomized, placebo-controlled, double-blind, parallel-group study		Pregabalin > PBO	Dizziness Somnolence Headaches Nausea
Pohl et al., 2005 (191)	Pregabalin (monotherapy)	GAD	624	Open-label, double-blind trial		Pregabalin > PBO (time to relapse) Pregabalin > PBO (efficacy maintained through the double blind period as compared with double blind baseline) Pregabalin > PBO (HAM-A and the Sheehan Disability Scale)	
Montgomery et al., 2006 (192)	Tiagabine (monotherapy)	GAD	25	Open-label trial		Significant reduction in HAM-A, HADS, and LSAS; 37% responded (CGI-I $\leq$ 2)	Somnolence Asthenia Abnormal thinking
Khan et al., 2006 (193)	Tiagabine (monotherapy)	GAD	40	Open-label, blind rater, positive-controlled trial		Tiagabine and paroxetine significantly improved HAM-A scores and improved sleep quality	Headache Nausea Anorexia Dizziness
Smith et al., 2002 (194)	Tiagabine (monotherapy)	GAD	272	Double-blind, placebo-controlled trial		ITT: Tiagabine = PBO Completers: Tiagabine > PBO	Dizziness Headache Nausea
Papp and Ray, 2003 (196)	Gabapentin (augmentation)	OCD	5	Open-label trial	Fluoxetine	Significant improvement in OCD, anxiety and mood symptoms as well as sleep	
Rosenthal, 2003 (197)	Carbamazepine (monotherapy)	OCD with temporal EEG abnormalities	4	Open-label trial		1/4 demonstrated improvement	
Van Ameringen et al., 2004 (198)	Carbamazepine (monotherapy)	OCD	9	Open-label trial		1/8 who completed demonstrated improvement	Sedation

Study	Drug	Condition	N	Design	Medications	Results	Side effects
Cora-Locatelli et al., 1998 (227)	Topiramate (augmentation)	OCD	16	Retrospective, open-label case series	SSRIs fluvoxamine fluoxetine citalopram paroxetine	68.8% (11/16) of patients were rated "very much" or "much" improved on the CGI-I at end point. A significant improvement on the CGI-S score was also found ($p < 0.001$).	Weight loss Sedation/fatigue Paresthesia Memory/word-finding problems
Jenike and Brotman, 1984 (232)	Topiramate (augmentation)	OCD	12	Open-label trial	Antidepressants fluoxetine fluvoxamine citalopram paroxetine sertraline venlafaxine	Significant changes from baseline in both Y-BOCS ($p = .002$) and the GAF scores ($p = .002$).	Weight loss Sedation/fatigue Paresthesia Memory/word-finding problems
	Lamotrigine (augmentation)	OCD	8		Sertraline clomipramine	No significant changes as rated by CGI-I scale	
Joffe and Swinson, 1987 (233)	Tiagabine (monotherapy and augmentation)	Mixed conditions: GAD, PTSD, MDD, bipolar disorder, schizophrenia	10	Open-label trial	Risperidone citralopram paroxetine clomipramine	All patients rated as "much" or "very much improved" on the CGI-C after 4 wk	
Van Ameringen et al., 2006 (235)	Tiagabine (augmentation)	Mixed conditions: GAD, PTSD, panic disorder, social phobia	18	Open-label trial	SSRIs SNRI nefazodone alprazolam	Significant improvements on HAM-A and BAI; 76% of patients where responders ($\geq$50% decrease on HAM-A); 59% achieved remission HAM-A $\leq$ 7.	Cognitive slowness Somnolence Headache

Abbreviations: CGI-I, Clinical Global Impression-Improvement Score; LSAS, Liebowitz Social Anxiety Scale; SPIN, Social Phobia Inventory; SSRI, selective serotonin reuptake inhibitors; CGI-S, Clinical Global Impression-Severity Score; HAM-A, Hamilton Anxiety Rating Scale; HAM-D, Hamilton Depression Rating Scale; PBO, placebo; BSPS, Brief Social Phobia Scale; PTSD, posttraumatic traumatic stress disorder; DGRP, Duke Global Rating Scale for PTSD; PCL-C, TPSD Checklist—Civilian Version; CAPS, Clinician-Administered PTSD Scale; TOP-8, Treatment Outcome PTSD; DTS, Davidson Trauma Scale; CGI-C, Clinical Global Impression-Change score; PAS, Panic and Agoraphobia Scale; SCL-90, Symptom Checklist-90; BSI, Brief Symptom Inventory; BAI, Beck Anxiety Inventory; BDI, Beck Depression Inventory; CCK-4, cholecystokinin-tetrapeptide; GAD, generalized anxiety disorder; OCD, obsessive-compulsive disorder; EEG, electroencephalogram; Y-BOCS, Yale-Brown Obsessive-Compulsive Scale; GAF, Global Assessment of Functioning; HADS, Hospital Anxiety and Depression Scale.

TABLE 2 Levels of Evidence for Epileptic Use in Anxiety Disorders

Drug	Panic disorder	OCD	PTSD	Social phobia	GAD
Lamotrigine		Level 4	Level 2		
Topiramate		Level 3	Level 1(–ve)[a]	Level 3	
Gabapentin	Level 2 (–ve)[a]	Level 4	Level 3	Level 2	Level 4
Pregabalin				Level 2	Level 1
Valproic acid	Level 2	Level 4	Level 2 (–ve)[a]	Level 3	
Tiagabine	Level 3		Level 3	Level 3	Level 2
Carbamazepine	Level 3	Level 4	Level 3		
Levetiracetam	Level 3		Level 4	Level 2	Level 4
Phenytoin	Level 4		Level 4		
Vigabatrin	Level 3		Level 4		
Oxcarbazepine			Level 4		

Note: Level of evidence criteria (241) are as follows:
Level 1: Meta-analysis or replicated randomized controlled trial (RCT) that includes a placebo condition.
Level 2: At least 1 RCT with placebo or active comparison condition.
Level 3: Uncontrolled trial with 10 or more subjects.
Level 4: Anecdotal case reports.
[a]Negative results of RCT.

replicated, randomized controlled trial that includes a placebo condition (the highest level of evidence); (2) at least one randomized controlled trial with placebo or active comparison condition; (3) uncontrolled trial with at least 10 or more subjects; and (4) anecdotal reports or expert opinions.

The psychotropic use of AEDs is an active area of research, with a number of case reports, case series, and open trials suggesting the potential efficacy of these treatments in a variety of anxiety disorders (Table 1). The strongest evidence, level 1, can be found for pregabalin in GAD (Table 2). Level 2 evidence suggests efficacy of lamotrigine in PTSD, gabapentin in social phobia, pregabalin in social phobia and generalized anxiety with comorbidity, and valproate in panic disorder (Table 2). Of note, despite level 1 evidence criteria being met for lamotrigine in PTSD and valproate in panic disorder, these results need to be viewed with caution, given the very small sample sizes used in the supporting studies.

The remainder of the evidence for AEDs in the treatment of anxiety disorders remains at level 3 or 4. Although there have been numerous studies and reports describing the use of AEDS in anxiety disorders, they have suffered from a number of methodological problems. These include inadequate sample size, lack of placebo controls, heterogeneous patients samples, use of inadequate doses of medication, lack of controlling for patient variables such as comorbidity, disorder subtype and use of concomitant medications, as well as the reliance on impressionistic outcome measures such as the CGI-scale.

Although AEDS seem to be promising treatments for anxiety disorders, it is not yet clear where their place will be in the spectrum of treatments available for these conditions. Given the very preliminary data on the efficacy of AEDs in anxiety disorders, their current clinical use should be reserved for treatment-refractory individuals, as augmentation strategies for partial responders, and as alternative treatments for those individuals who cannot tolerate first-line treatments, such as SSRIs, or those who are not appropriate candidates for benzodiazepines. There is currently no evidence to support the use of AEDs as first-line treatments with the exception of pregabalin in GAD. In addition, for AEDs that have thus far shown some evidence of benefit in the treatment of anxiety disorders, their potential use in combination with mood stabilizers in bipolar disorder patients who suffer from a comorbid anxiety disorder should be considered.

Future research examining the potential use of AEDs in anxiety disorders will require large-scale controlled trials in a number of these disorders, including head-to-head comparisons with first-line treatments and examinations of clinical subgroups that may preferentially respond to AEDs. In addition, it may be warranted to evaluate the potential use of AEDs in youth with anxiety disorders given the current concerns about the safety and efficacy of SSRIs in this age group.

REFERENCES

1. van Steveninck AL, Wallnofer AE, Schoemaker RC, et al. A study of the effects of long-term use on individual sensitivity to temazepam and lorazepam in a clinical population. Br J Clin Pharmacol 1997; 44:267–275.
2. Cowley DS, Roy-Byrne PP, Radant A, et al. Benzodiazepine sensitivity in panic disorder: Effects of chronic alprazolam treatment. Neuropsychopharmacology 1995; 12: 147–157.
3. Rapport DJ, Calabrese JR. Tolerance to fluoxetine. J Clin Psychopharmacol 1993; 13: 361–361.
4. Pope HG, Mcelroy SL, Keck PE, et al. Valproate in the treatment of acute mania: a placebo-controlled study. Arch Gen Psychiatry 1991; 48:62–68.
5. Lerer B, Moore N, Meyendorff E, et al. Carbamazepine versus lithium in mania: a double-blind study. J Clin Psychiatry 1987; 48:89–93.
6. Quirk GJ, Gehlert DR. Inhibition of the amygdala: key to pathological states? Ann N Y Acad Sci 2003; 985:263–272.
7. LeDoux JE. The Emotional Brain. New York, NY: Simon & Schuster, 1996.
8. Lydiard RB. The role of GABA in anxiety disorders. J Clin Psychiatry 2003; 64(suppl 3): 21–27.
9. Goddard AW, Mason GF, Almai A, et al. Reductions in occipital cortex GABA levels in panic disorder detected with 1h-magnetic resonance spectroscopy. Arch Gen Psychiatry 2001; 58:556–561.
10. Smith TA. Type A gamma-aminobutryric acid (GABAA) receptors subunits and benzodiazepines binding site sensitivity. Nature 1978; 274:383–385.
11. Rosenberg DR, MacMaster FP, Keshavan MS, et al. Decrease in caudate glutamatergic concentrations in pediatric obsessive-compulsive disorder patients taking paroxetine. J Am Acad Child Adolesc Psychiatry 2000; 39:1096–1103.
12. Mathew SJ, Coplan JD, Gorman JM. Neurobiological mechanisms of social anxiety disorder. Am J Psychiatry 2001; 158:1558–1567.
13. Satoh M, Foong FW. A mechanism of carbamazepine-analgesia as shown by bradykinin-induced trigeminal pain. Brain Res Bull 1983; 10:407–409.
14. Burchiel KJ. Carbamazepine inhibits spontaneous activity in experimental neuromas. Exp Neurol 1988; 102:249–253.
15. Chapman V, Suzuki R, Chamarette HL, et al. Effects of systemic carbamazepine and gabapentin on spinal neuronal responses in spinal nerve ligated rats. Pain 1998; 75: 261–272.
16. Tanelian DL, Cousins MJ. Combined neurogenic and nociceptive pain in a patient with pancoast tumor managed by epidural hydromorphone and oral carbamazepine. Pain 1989; 36:85–88.
17. Pollack MH, Matthews J, Scott EL. Gabapentin as a potential treatment for anxiety disorders. Am J Psychiatry 1998; 155:992–993.
18. Calabrese JR, Bowden CL, Sachs GS, et al. A double-blind placebo-controlled study of lamotrigine monotherapy in outpatients with bipolar I depression. lamictal 602 study group. J Clin Psychiatry 1999; 60:79–88.
19. Rigo JM, Hans G, Nguyen L, et al. The anti-epileptic drug levetiracetam reverses the inhibition by negative allosteric modulators of neuronal GABA- and glycine-gated currents. Br J Pharmacol 2002; 136:659–672.

20. Grant SM, Faulds D. Oxcarbazepine. A review of its pharmacology and therapeutic potential in epilepsy, trigeminal neuralgia and affective disorders. Drugs 1992; 43: 873–888.
21. McAuley JW, Biederman TS, Smith JC, et al. Newer therapies in the drug treatment of epilepsy. Ann Pharmacother 2002; 36:119–129.
22. Tecoma ES. Oxcarbazepine. Epilepsia 1999; 40:S37–S46.
23. Wamil AW, McLean MJ. Phenytoin blocks N-methyl-D-aspartate responses of mouse central neurons. J Pharmacol Exp Ther 1993; 267:218–227.
24. Kawano H, Sashihara S, Mita T, et al. Phenytoin, an antiepileptic drug, competitively blocked non-NMDA receptors produced by xenopus oocytes. Neurosci Lett 1994; 166: 183–186.
25. Frampton JE, Foster RH. Pregabalin: in the treatment of generalised anxiety disorder. CNS Drugs 2006; 20:685–693 (discussion 694–695).
26. Fink-Jensen A, Suzdak PD, Swedberg MD, et al. The gamma-aminobutyric acid (GABA) uptake inhibitor, tiagabine, increases extracellular brain levels of GABA in awake rats. Eur J Pharmacol 1992; 220:197–201.
27. Borden LA, Murali Dhar TG, Smith KE, et al. Tiagabine, SK&F 89976-A, CI-966, and NNC-711 are selective for the cloned GABA transporter GAT-1. Eur J Pharmacol 1994; 269:219–224.
28. Biton V, Edwards KR, Montouris GD, et al. Topiramate titration and tolerability. Ann Pharmacother 2001; 35:173–179.
29. Harden CL. New antiepileptic drugs. Neurology 1994; 44:787–795.
30. Ben-Menachem E. Pharmacokinetic effects of vigabatrin on cerebrospinal fluid amino acids in humans. Epilepsia 1989; 30(suppl 3):S12–S14.
31. American Psychiatric Association. Diagnostic and Statistical Manual of Mental Disorders. 4th ed. Washington, DC: American Psychiatric Association, 1994.
32. Stein MB, Fyer AJ, Davidson JRT, et al. Fluvoxamine treatment of social phobia (social anxiety disorder): a double-blind, placebo-controlled study. Am J Psychiatry 1999; 156: 756–760.
33. Van Ameringen MA, Lane RM, Walker JR, et al. Sertraline treatment of generalized social phobia: a 20-week, double-blind, placebo-controlled study. Am J Psychiatry 2001; 158: 275–281.
34. Liebowitz MR, Mangano R. Comparison of venlafaxine extended-release (ER) and paroxetine in the short-term treatment of SAD. Arch Gen Psychiatry 2005; 62: 190–198.
35. Gelernter CS, Uhde TW, Cimbolic P, et al. Cognitive-behavioral and pharmacological treatments of social phobia: a controlled-study. Arch Gen Psychiatry 1991; 48:938–945.
36. Liebowitz MR, Schneier F, Campeas R, et al. Phenelzine vs atenolol in social phobia. A placebo-controlled comparison. Arch Gen Psychiatry 1992; 49:290–300.
37. Heimberg RG, Liebowitz MR, Hope DA, et al. Cognitive behavioral group therapy vs phenelzine therapy for social phobia: 12-week outcome. Arch Gen Psychiatry 1998; 55: 1133–1141.
38. Fahlen T, Nilsson HL, Borg K, et al. Social phobia: the clinical efficacy and tolerability of the monoamine oxidase -A and serotonin uptake inhibitor brofaromine. A double-blind placebo-controlled study. Acta Psychiatr Scand 1995; 92:351–358.
39. Schneier FR, Goetz D, Campeas R, et al. Placebo-controlled trial of moclobemide in social phobia. Br J Psychiatry 1998; 172:70–77.
40. Van Ameringen M, Mancini C, Pipe B, et al. An open trial of topiramate in the treatment of generalized social phobia. J Clin Psychiatry 2004; 65:1674–1678.
41. Stein MB, Pollack MH, Mangano R. Long-term treatment of generalized SAD with venlafaxine extended release. Poster presented at: The 23rd Annual Conference of the Anxiety Disorders Association of America; March 27–30, 2003; Toronto, Canada.
42. Pande AC, Davidson JR, Jefferson JW, et al. Treatment of social phobia with gabapentin: a placebo-controlled study. J Clin Psychopharmacol 1999; 19:341–348.
43. de-Paris F, Sant'Anna MK, Vianna MR, et al. Effects of gabapentin on anxiety induced by simulated public speaking. J Psychopharmacol 2003; 17:184–188.

44. Pande AC, Feltner DE, Jefferson JW, et al. Efficacy of the novel anxiolytic pregabalin in social anxiety disorder: a placebo-controlled, multicenter study. J Clin Psychopharmacol 2004; 24:141–149.
45. Nardi AE, Mendolwicz M, Versiani FM. Valproic acid in social phobia: an open trial. Biol Psychiatry 1997; 42:S118.
46. Kinrys G, Pollack MH, Simon NM, et al. Valproic acid for the treatment of social anxiety disorder. Int Clin Psychopharmacol 2003; 18:169–172.
47. Dunlap BW, Papp L, Garlow SJ, et al. Tiagabine for social anxiety disorder. Human Psychopharmacol 2007; 22:241–244.
48. Kinrys G, Soldani F, Hsu D, et al. Adjunctive tiagabine for treatment refractory social anxiety disorder. Poster presented at: The 157th Annual Meeting of the American Psychiatric Association; May 1–6, 2004; New York, NY.
49. Simon NM, Worthington JJ, Doyle AC, et al. An open-label study of levetiracetam for the treatment of social anxiety disorder. J Clin Psychiatry 2004; 65:1219–1222.
50. Zhang W, Connor KM, Davidson JR. Levetiracetam in social phobia: a placebo controlled pilot study. J Psychopharmacol 2005; 19:551–553.
51. Ballenger JA, Davidson JRT, Lecrubier Y, et al. Consensus statement on posttraumatic stress disorder from the international consensus group on depression and anxiety. J Clin Psychiatry 2000; 61:60–66.
52. Connor KM, Sutherland SM, Tupler LA, et al. Fluoxetine in post-traumatic stress disorder. Randomised, double-blind study. Br J Psychiatry 1999; 175:17–22.
53. van der Kolk BA, Dreyfuss D, Michaels M, et al. Fluoxetine in posttraumatic stress disorder. J Clin Psychiatry 1994; 55:517–522.
54. Davidson JR, Rothbaum BO, van der Kolk BA, et al. Multicenter, double-blind comparison of sertraline and placebo in the treatment of posttraumatic stress disorder. Arch Gen Psychiatry 2001; 58:485–492.
55. Brady K, Pearlstein T, Asnis GM, et al. Efficacy and safety of sertraline treatment of posttraumatic stress disorder: a randomized controlled trial. JAMA 2000; 283:1837–1844.
56. Zohar J, Amital D, Miodownik C, et al. Double-blind placebo-controlled pilot study of sertraline in military veterans with posttraumatic stress disorder. J Clin Psychopharmacol 2002; 22:190–195.
57. Tucker P, Potter-Kimball R, Wyatt DB, et al. Can physiologic assessment and side effects tease out differences in PTSD trials? A double-blind comparison of citalopram, sertraline, and placebo. Psychopharmacol Bull 2003; 37:135–149.
58. Tucker P, Zaninelli R, Yehuda R, et al. Paroxetine in the treatment of chronic posttraumatic stress disorder: results of a placebo-controlled, flexible-dosage trial. J Clin Psychiatry 2001; 62:860–868.
59. Marshall RD, Beebe KL, Oldham M, et al. Efficacy and safety of paroxetine treatment for chronic PTSD: a fixed-dose, placebo-controlled study. Am J Psychiatry 2001; 158: 1982–1988.
60. Stein DJ, Davidson J, Seedat S, et al. Paroxetine in the treatment of post-traumatic stress disorder: pooled analysis of placebo-controlled studies. Expert Opin Pharmacother 2003; 4:1829–1838.
61. Davidson J, Lipschitz A, Musgnung J. Venlafaxinw XR and sertraline in PTSD: a placebo-controlled study. Eur Neuropsychopharmacol 2003; 13:S380.
62. Kosten TR, Frank JB, Dan E, et al. Pharmacotherapy for posttraumatic stress disorder using phenelzine or imipramine. J Nerv Ment Dis 1991; 179:366–370.
63. Frank JB, Kosten TR, Giller EL Jr., et al. A randomized clinical trial of phenelzine and imipramine for posttraumatic stress disorder. Am J Psychiatry 1988; 145:1289–1291.
64. Davidson J, Kudler H, Smith R, et al. Treatment of posttraumatic-stress-disorder with amitriptyline and placebo. Arch Gen Psychiatry 1990; 47:259–266.
65. Davidson JR, Kudler HS, Saunders WB, et al. Predicting response to amitriptyline in posttraumatic stress disorder. Am J Psychiatry 1993; 150:1024–1029.
66. Hertzberg MA, Butterfield MI, Feldman ME, et al. A preliminary study of lamotrigine for the treatment of posttraumatic stress disorder. Biol Psychiatry 1999; 45:1226–1229.

67. Berlant J, van Kammen DP. Open-label topiramate as primary or adjunctive therapy in chronic civilian posttraumatic stress disorder: a preliminary report. J Clin Psychiatry 2002; 63:15–20.
68. Chengappa KN, Rathore D, Levine J, et al. Topiramate as add-on treatment for patients with bipolar mania. Bipolar Disord 1999; 1:42–53.
69. Berlant JL. Prospective open-label study of add-on and monotherapy topiramate in civilians with chronic nonhallucinatory posttraumatic stress disorder. BMC Psychiatry 2004; 4:24.
70. Tucker P, Trautman RP, Wyatt DB, et al. Efficacy and safety of topiramate monotherapy in civilian posttraumatic stress disorder: a randomized, double-blind, placebo-controlled study. J Clin Psychiatry 2007; 68:201–206.
71. Blake DD, Weathers FW, Nagy LM, et al. The development of a clinician-administered PTSD scale. J Trauma Stress 1995; 8:75–90.
72. Davis EA. Topiramate for PTSD. Presented at: The 160th Annual Meeting of the American Psychiatric Association; May 19–24, 2007; San Diego, California.
73. Brannon N, Labbate L, Huber M. Gabapentin treatment for posttraumatic stress disorder. Can J Psychiatry 2000; 45:84.
74. Hamner MB, Brodrick PS, Labbate LA. Gabapentin in PTSD: A retrospective, clinical series of adjunctive therapy. Ann Clin Psychiatry 2001; 13:141–146.
75. Szymanski HV, Olympia J. Divalproex in posttraumatic stress disorder. Am J Psychiatry 1991; 148:1086–1087.
76. Fesler FA. Valproate in combat-related posttraumatic stress disorder. J Clin Psychiatry 1991; 52:361–364.
77. Clark RD, Canive JM, Calais LA, et al. Divalproex in posttraumatic stress disorder: an open-label clinical trial. J Trauma Stress 1999; 12:395–401.
78. Petty F, Davis LL, Nugent AL, et al. Valproate therapy for chronic, combat-induced posttraumatic stress disorder. J Clin Psychopharmacol 2002; 22:100–101.
79. Davis LL, Ambrose SM, Newell JM, et al. Divalproex for the treatment of posttraumatic stress disorder: a retrospective chart review. Int J Psychiatry Clin Pract 2005; 9:278–283.
80. Otte C, Wiedemann K, Yassouridis A, et al. Valproate monotherapy in the treatment of civilian patients with non-combat-related posttraumatic stress disorder: An open-label study. J Clin Psychopharmacol 2004; 24:106–108.
81. Davis EA. Divalporex for PTSD. Presented at: The 160th Annual Meeting of the American Psychiatric Association; May 19–24, 2007; San Diego, California.
82. Lara ME. Tiagabine for augmentation of antidepressant treatment of post-traumatic stress disorder. Presented at: The 22nd National Conference of the Anxiety Disorders Association of America; March 21–24, 2002; Austin, TX.
83. Berigan T. Treatment of posttraumatic stress disorder with tiagabine. Can J Psychiatry 2002; 47:788.
84. Taylor FB. Tiagabine for posttraumatic stress disorder: a case series of 7 women. J Clin Psychiatry 2003; 64:1421–1425.
85. Connor KM, Davidson JR, WEisler RH, et al. Tiagabine for posttraumatic stress disorder: effects of open-label and double-blind discontinuation treatment. Psychopharmacology (Berl) 2006; 184:21–26.
86. Davidson JR, Brady K, Mellman TA, et al. The efficacy and tolerability of tiagabine in adult patients with post-traumatic stress disorder. J Clin Psychopharmacol 2007; 27: 85–88.
87. Lipper S, Davidson JR, Grady TA, et al. Preliminary study of carbamazepine in post-traumatic stress disorder. Psychosomatics 1986; 27:849–854.
88. Wolf ME, Alavi A, Mosnaim AD. Posttraumatic stress disorder in vietnam veterans clinical and EEG findings; possible therapeutic effects of carbamazepine. Biol Psychiatry 1988; 23:642–644.
89. Looff D, Grimley P, Kuller F, et al. Carbamazepine for PTSD. J Am Acad Child Adolesc Psychiatry 1995; 34:703–704.
90. Bremner JD, Mletzko T, Welter S, et al. Treatment of posttraumatic stress disorder with phenytoin: an open-label pilot study. J Clin Psychiatry 2004; 65:1559–1564.

91. Bremner JD, Mletzko T, Welter S, et al. Effects of phenytoin on memory, cognition and brain structure in post-traumatic stress disorder: a pilot study. J Psychopharmacol 2005; 19:159–165.
92. Macleod AD. Vigabatrin and posttraumatic stress disorder. J Clin Psychopharmacol 1996; 16:190–191.
93. Berigan T. Oxcarbazepine treatment of posttraumatic stress disorder. Can J Psychiatry 2002; 47:973–974.
94. Malek-Ahmadi P, Hanretta AT. Possible reduction in posttraumatic stress disorder symptoms with oxcarbazepine in a patient with bipolar disorder. Ann Pharmacother 2004; 38:1852–1854.
95. Kinrys G, Wygat LE, Pardo TB, et al. Levetiracetam for treatment-refactory PTSD. J Clin Psychiatry 2006; 67:211–214.
96. Andersch S, Rosenberg NK, Kullingsjo H, et al. Efficacy and safety of alprazolam, imipramine and placebo in treating panic disorder. A Scandinavian multicenter study. Acta Psychiatr Scand Suppl 1991; 365:18–27.
97. Modigh K, Westberg P, Eriksson E. Superiority of clomipramine over imipramine in the treatment of panic disorder: a placebo-controlled trial. J Clin Psychopharmacol 1992; 12: 251–261.
98. Sheehan DV, Ballenger J, Jacobsen G. Treatment of endogenous anxiety with phobic, hysterical, and hypochondriacal symptoms. Arch Gen Psychiatry 1980; 37:51–59.
99. Tesar GE, Rosenbaum JF, Pollack MH, et al. Double-blind, placebo-controlled comparison of clonazepam and alprazolam for panic disorder. J Clin Psychiatry 1991; 52:69–76.
100. Boyer W. Serotonin uptake inhibitors are superior to imipramine and alprazolam in alleviating panic attacks: a meta-analysis. Int Clin Psychopharmacol 1995; 10:45–49.
101. Schweizer E, Pohl R, Balon R, et al. Lorazepam vs. alprazolam in the treatment of panic disorder. Pharmacopsychiatry 1990; 23:90–93.
102. Beauclair L, Fontaine R, Annable L, et al. Clonazepam in the treatment of panic disorder: a double-blind, placebo-controlled trial investigating the correlation between clonazepam concentrations in plasma and clinical response. J Clin Psychopharmacol 1994; 14:111–118.
103. Moroz G, Rosenbaum JF. Efficacy, safety, and gradual discontinuation of clonazepam in panic disorder: a placebo-controlled, multicenter study using optimized dosages. J Clin Psychiatry 1999; 60:604–612.
104. Rosenbaum JF, Moroz G, Bowden CL. Clonazepam in the treatment of panic disorder with or without agoraphobia: a dose-response study of efficacy, safety, and discontinuance. Clonazepam panic disorder dose-response study group. J Clin Psychopharmacol 1997; 17:390–400.
105. Valenca AM, Nardi AE, Nascimento I, et al. Double-blind clonazepam vs placebo in panic disorder treatment. Arq Neuropsiquiatr 2000; 58:1025–1029.
106. Charney DS, Woods SW. Benzodiazepine treatment of panic disorder: a comparison of alprazolam and lorazepam. J Clin Psychiatry 1989; 50:418–423.
107. de Jonghe F, Swinkels J, Tuynman-Qua H, et al. A comparative study of suriclone, lorazepam and placebo in anxiety disorder. Pharmacopsychiatry 1989; 22:266–271.
108. Dunner DL, Ishiki D, Avery DH, et al. Effect of alprazolam and diazepam on anxiety and panic attacks in panic disorder: a controlled study. J Clin Psychiatry 1986; 47:458–460.
109. Noyes R Jr., Anderson DJ, Clancy J, et al. Diazepam and propranolol in panic disorder and agoraphobia. Arch Gen Psychiatry 1984; 41:287–292.
110. Noyes R Jr., Burrows GD, Reich JH, et al. Diazepam versus alprazolam for the treatment of panic disorder. J Clin Psychiatry 1996; 57:349–355.
111. Ballenger JC, Wheadon DE, Steiner M, et al. Double-blind, fixed-dose, placebo-controlled study of paroxetine in the treatment of panic disorder. Am J Psychiatry 1998; 155:36–42.
112. Londborg PD, Wolkow R, Smith WT, et al. Sertraline in the treatment of panic disorder. A multi-site, double-blind, placebo-controlled, fixed-dose investigation. Br J Psychiatry 1998; 173:54–60.
113. Asnis GM, Hameedi FA, Goddard AW, et al. Fluvoxamine in the treatment of panic disorder: a multi-center, double-blind, placebo-controlled study in outpatients. Psychiatry Res 2001; 103:1–14.

114. Michelson D, Allgulander C, Dantendorfer K, et al. Efficacy of usual antidepressant dosing regimens of fluoxetine in panic disorder: randomised, placebo-controlled trial. Br J Psychiatry 2001; 179:514–518.

115. Pollack M, Mangano R, Entsuah R, et al. A randomized controlled trial of venlafaxine ER and paroxetine in the treatment of outpatients with panic disorder. Psychopharmacology (Berl) 2007; 194(2):233–242.

116. Liebowitz M, Asnis G, Tzanis E, et al. Venlafaxine extended release versus placebo in the short-term treatment of panic disorders [abstract NR194] In: American Psychiatric Association. New Research Abstracts, Annual Meeting of the American Psychiatric Association; May 1–6; Washington (DC): American Psychiatric Association; 2004.

117. Pollack MH, Worthington JJ III, Otto MW, et al. Venlafaxine for panic disorder: results from a double-blind, placebo-controlled study. Psychopharmacol Bull 1996; 32:667–670.

118. Bradwejn J, Ahokas A, Stein DJ, et al. Venlafaxine extended-release capsules in panic disorder: flexible-dose, double-blind, placebo-controlled study. Br J Psychiatry 2005; 187: 352–359.

119. Michelson D, Lydiard RB, Pollack MH, et al. Outcome assessment and clinical improvement in panic disorder: evidence from a randomized controlled trial of fluoxetine and placebo. The fluoxetine panic disorder study group. Am J Psychiatry 1998; 155:1570–1577.

120. Ribeiro L, Busnello JV, Kauer-Sant'Anna M, et al. Mirtazapine versus fluoxetine in the treatment of panic disorder. Braz J Med Biol Res 2001; 34:1303–1307.

121. Tiller JWG, Bouwer C, Behnke K. Moclobemide and fluoxetine for panic disorder. International Panic Disorder Study Group. Eur Arch Psychiatry Clin Neurosci 1999; 249: S7–S10.

122. Sharp DM, Power KG, Simpson RJ, et al. Global measures of outcome in a controlled comparison of pharmacological and psychological treatment of panic disorder and agoraphobia in primary care. Br J Gen Pract 1997; 47:150–155.

123. Black DW, Wesner R, Bowers W, et al. A comparison of fluvoxamine, cognitive therapy, and placebo in the treatment of panic disorder. Arch Gen Psychiatry 1993; 50:44–50.

124. Bakish D, Hooper CL, Filteau MJ, et al. A double-blind placebo-controlled trial comparing fluvoxamine and imipramine in the treatment of panic disorder with or without agoraphobia. Psychopharmacol Bull 1996; 32:135–141.

125. Den Boer JA, Westenberg HG. Serotonin function in panic disorder: a double blind placebo controlled study with fluvoxamine and ritanserin. Psychopharmacology (Berl) 1990; 102:85–94.

126. Hoehn-Saric R, McLeod DR, Hipsley PA. Effect of fluvoxamine on panic disorder. J Clin Psychopharmacol 1993; 13:321–326.

127. Bakker A, van Balkom AJ, Spinhoven P. SSRIs vs. TCAs in the treatment of panic disorder: a meta-analysis. Acta Psychiatr Scand 2002; 106:163–167.

128. Oehrberg S, Christiansen PE, Behnke K, et al. Paroxetine in the treatment of panic disorder. A randomised, double-blind, placebo-controlled study. Br J Psychiatry 1995; 167:374–379.

129. Bakker A, van Dyck R, Spinhoven P, et al. Paroxetine, clomipramine, and cognitive therapy in the treatment of panic disorder. J Clin Psychiatry 1999; 60:831–838.

130. Lecrubier Y, Bakker A, Dunbar G, et al. A comparison of paroxetine, clomipramine and placebo in the treatment of panic disorder. Collaborative paroxetine panic study investigators. Acta Psychiatr Scand 1997; 95:145–152.

131. Sheehan DV, Burnham DB, Iyengar MK, et al. Efficacy and tolerability of controlled-release paroxetine in the treatment of panic disorder. Panic Disorder Study Group. J Clin Psychiatry 2005; 66:34–40.

132. Pohl RB, Wolkow RM, Clary CM. Sertraline in the treatment of panic disorder: a double-blind multicenter trial. Am J Psychiatry 1998; 155:1189–1195.

133. Pollack MH, Otto MW, Worthington JJ, et al. Sertraline in the treatment of panic disorder: a flexible-dose multicenter trial. Arch Gen Psychiatry 1998; 55:1010–1016.

134. Pollack MH, Rapaport MH, Clary CM, et al. Sertraline treatment of panic disorder: response in patients at risk for poor outcome. J Clin Psychiatry 2000; 61:922–927.

135. Lepola U, Arato M, Zhu Y, et al. Sertraline versus imipramine treatment of comorbid panic disorder and major depressive disorder. J Clin Psychiatry 2003; 64:654–662.

136. Stahl SM, Gergel I, Li D. Escitalopram in the treatment of panic disorder: a randomized, double-blind, placebo-controlled trial. J Clin Psychiatry 2003; 64:1322–1327.
137. Pande AC, Pollack MH, Crockatt J, et al. Placebo-controlled study of gabapentin treatment of panic disorder. J Clin Psychopharmacol 2000; 20:467–471.
138. Brady KT, Sonne S, Lydiard RB. Valproate treatment of comorbid panic disorder and affective disorders in two alcoholic patients. J Clin Psychopharmacol 1994; 14:81–82.
139. Roberts JM, Malcolm R, Santos AB. Treatment of panic disorder and comorbid substance abuse with divalproex sodium. Am J Psychiatry 1994; 151:1521.
140. McElroy SL, Keck PE Jr., Lawrence JM. Treatment of panic disorder and benzodiazepine withdrawal with valproate. J Neuropsychiatry Clin Neurosci 1991; 3:232–233.
141. Marazziti D, Cassano GB. Valproic acid for panic disorder associated with multiple sclerosis. Am J Psychiatry 1996; 153:842–843.
142. Ontiveros A, Fontaine R. Sodium valproate and clonazepam for treatment-resistant panic disorder. J Psychiatry Neurosci 1992; 17:78–80.
143. Primeau F, Fontaine R, Beauclair L. Valproic acid and panic disorder. Can J Psychiatry 1990; 35:248–250.
144. Woodman CL, Noyes R Jr. Panic disorder: treatment with valproate. J Clin Psychiatry 1994; 55:134–136.
145. Keck PE Jr., Taylor VE, Tugrul KC, et al. Valproate treatment of panic disorder and lactate-induced panic attacks. Biol Psychiatry 1993; 33:542–546.
146. Baetz M, Bowen RC. Efficacy of divalproex sodium in patients with panic disorder and mood instability who have not responded to conventional therapy. Can J Psychiatry 1998; 43:73–77.
147. Lum M, Fontaine R, Elie R, et al. Divalproex sodium's antipanic effect in panic disorder: a placebo-controlled study. Biol Psychiatry 1990; 27:164A.
148. Gruener D. Tiagabine as an augmenting agent for the treatment of anxiety. Presented at: The 22nd National Conference of the Anxiety Disorders Association of America; 2002; Austin, TX.
149. Zwanzger P, Baghai TC, Schule C, et al. Tiagabine improves panic and agoraphobia in panic disorder patients. J Clin Psychiatry 2001; 62:656–657.
150. Zwanzger P, Eser D, Padberg F, et al. Effects of tiagabine on cholecystokinin-tetrapeptide (CCK-4)-induced anxiety in healthy volunteers. Depress Anxiety 2003; 18:140–143.
151. Lawlor BA. Carbamazepine, alprazolam withdrawal, and panic disorder. Am J Psychiatry 1987; 144:265–266.
152. Tondo L, Burrai C, Scamonatti L, et al. Carbamazepine in panic disorder. Am J Psychiatry 1989; 146:558–559.
153. Uhde TW, Stein MB, Post RM. Lack of efficacy of carbamazepine in the treatment of panic disorder. Am J Psychiatry 1988; 145:1104–1109.
154. McNamara ME, Fogel BS. Anticonvulsant-responsive panic attacks with temporal lobe EEG abnormalities. J Neuropsychiatry Clin Neurosci 1990; 2:193–196.
155. Papp LA. Safety and efficacy of levetiracetam for patients with panic disorder: results of an open-label, fixed-flexible dose study. J Clin Psychiatry 2006; 67:1573–1576.
156. Zwanzger P, Baghai T, Boerner RJ, et al. Anxiolytic effects of vigabatrin in panic disorder. J Clin Psychopharmacol 2001; 21:539–540.
157. Zwanzger P, Baghai TC, Schuele C, et al. Vigabatrin decreases cholecystokinin-tetrapeptide (CCK-4) induced panic in healthy volunteers. Neuropsychopharmacology 2001; 25:699–703.
158. Mitte K, Noack P, Steil R, et al. A meta-analytic review of the efficacy of drug treatment in generalized anxiety disorder. J Clin Psychopharmacol 2005; 25:141–150.
159. Lydiard RB, Ballenger JC, Rickels K. A double-blind evaluation of the safety and efficacy of abecarnil, alprazolam, and placebo in outpatients with generalized anxiety disorder. Abecarnil Work Group. J Clin Psychiatry 1997; 58(suppl 11):11–18.
160. Moller HJ, Volz HP, Reimann IW, et al. Opipramol for the treatment of generalized anxiety disorder: a placebo-controlled trial including an alprazolam-treated group. J Clin Psychopharmacol 2001; 21:59–65.

161. Rickels K, Pollack MH, Feltner DE, et al. Pregabalin for treatment of generalized anxiety disorder: a 4-week, multicenter, double-blind, placebo-controlled trial of pregabalin and alprazolam. Arch Gen Psychiatry 2005; 62:1022–1030.

162. Llorca PM, Spadone C, Sol O, et al. Efficacy and safety of hydroxyzine in the treatment of generalized anxiety disorder: a 3-month double-blind study. J Clin Psychiatry 2002; 63: 1020–1027.

163. Feltner DE, Crockatt JG, Dubovsky SJ, et al. A randomized, double-blind, placebo-controlled, fixed-dose, multicenter study of pregabalin in patients with generalized anxiety disorder. J Clin Psychopharmacol 2003; 23:240–249.

164. Laakmann G, Schule C, Lorkowski G, et al. Buspirone and lorazepam in the treatment of generalized anxiety disorder in outpatients. Psychopharmacology (Berl) 1998; 136: 357–366.

165. Fresquet A, Sust M, Lloret A, et al. Efficacy and safety of lesopitron in outpatients with generalized anxiety disorder. Ann Pharmacother 2000; 34:147–153.

166. Rickels K, Schweizer E, DeMartinis N, et al. Gepirone and diazepam in generalized anxiety disorder: a placebo-controlled trial. J Clin Psychopharmacol 1997; 17:272–277.

167. Rickels K, DeMartinis N, Aufdembrinke B. A double-blind, placebo-controlled trial of abecarnil and diazepam in the treatment of patients with generalized anxiety disorder. J Clin Psychopharmacol 2000; 20:12–18.

168. Rickels K, Rynn M. Pharmacotherapy of generalized anxiety disorder. J Clin Psychiatry 2002; 63:9–16.

169. Rickels K, Downing R, Schweizer E, et al. Antidepressants for the treatment of generalized anxiety disorder. A placebo-controlled comparison of imipramine, trazodone, and diazepam. Arch Gen Psychiatry 1993; 50:884–895.

170. Kanczinski F, Lima MS, Souza JS, et al. Antidepressants for generalized anxiety disorder. Cochrane Database Syst Rev 2003; 2:CD003592.

171. Hoehn-Saric R, McLeod DR, Zimmerli WD. Differential effects of alprazolam and imipramine in generalized anxiety disorder: somatic versus psychic symptoms. J Clin Psychiatry 1988; 49:293–301.

172. Rocca P, Fonzo V, Scotta M, et al. Paroxetine efficacy in the treatment of generalized anxiety disorder. Acta Psychiatr Scand 1997; 95:444–450.

173. Strand M, Hetta J, Rosen A, et al. A double-blind, controlled trial in primary care patients with generalized anxiety: a comparison between buspirone and oxazepam. J Clin Psychiatry 1990; 51(suppl):40–45.

174. Davidson JR, DuPont RL, Hedges D, et al. Efficacy, safety, and tolerability of venlafaxine extended release and buspirone in outpatients with generalized anxiety disorder. J Clin Psychiatry 1999; 60:528–535.

175. Pollack MH, Worthington JJ, Manfro GG, et al. Abecarnil for the treatment of generalized anxiety disorder: a placebo-controlled comparison of two dosage ranges of abecarnil and buspirone. J Clin Psychiatry 1997; 58(suppl 11):19–23.

176. Lader M, Scotto JC. A multicentre double-blind comparison of hydroxyzine, buspirone and placebo in patients with generalized anxiety disorder. Psychopharmacology (Berl) 1998; 139:402–406.

177. Pollack MH, Zaninelli R, Goddard A, et al. Paroxetine in the treatment of generalized anxiety disorder: results of a placebo-controlled, flexible-dosage trial. J Clin Psychiatry 2001; 62:350–357.

178. Rickels K, Zaninelli R, McCafferty J, et al. Paroxetine treatment of generalized anxiety disorder: a double-blind, placebo-controlled study. Am J Psychiatry 2003; 160: 749–756.

179. Ball SG, Kuhn A, Wall D, et al. Selective serotonin reuptake inhibitor treatment for generalized anxiety disorder: a double-blind, prospective comparison between paroxetine and sertraline. J Clin Psychiatry 2005; 66:94–99.

180. Goodman WK, Bose A, Wang Q. Treatment of generalized anxiety disorder with escitalopram: pooled results from double-blind, placebo-controlled trials. J Affect Disord 2005; 87:161–167.

181. Baldwin DS, Huusom AK, Maehlum E. Escitalopram and paroxetine in the treatment of generalised anxiety disorder: randomised, placebo-controlled, double-blind study. Br J Psychiatry 2006; 189:264–272.
182. Goodman WK, Bose A, Wang Q. Treatment of generalized anxiety disorder with Escitalopram: pooled results from double-blind, placebo-controlled trials. J Affect Disord 2005; 87:161–167.
183. Rynn MA, Siqueland L, Rickels K. Placebo-controlled trial of sertraline in the treatment of children with generalized anxiety disorder. Am J Psychiatry 2001; 158:2008–2014.
184. Allgulander C, Dahl AA, Austin C, et al. Efficacy of sertraline in a 12-week trial for generalized anxiety disorder. Am J Psychiatry 2004; 161:1642–1649.
185. Sheehan DV. Venlafaxine extended release (XR) in the treatment of generalized anxiety disorder. J Clin Psychiatry 1999; 60(suppl 22):23–28.
186. Rickels K, Pollack MH, Sheehan DV, et al. Efficacy of extended-release venlafaxine in nondepressed outpatients with generalized anxiety disorder. Am J Psychiatry 2000; 157: 968–974.
187. Nimatoudis I, Zissis NP, Kogeorgos J, et al. Remission rates with venlafaxine extended release in Greek outpatients with generalized anxiety disorder: a double-blind, randomized, placebo controlled study. Int Clin Psychopharmacol 2004; 19:331–336.
188. Katz IR, Reynolds CF III, Alexopoulos GS, et al. Venlafaxine ER as a treatment for generalized anxiety disorder in older adults: pooled analysis of five randomized placebo-controlled clinical trials. J Am Geriatr Soc 2002; 50:18–25.
189. Pollack MH, Matthews J, Scott EL. Gabapentin as a potential treatment for anxiety disorders. Am J Psychiatry 1998; 155:992–993.
190. Pande AC, Crockatt JG, Feltner DE, et al. Pregabalin in generalized anxiety disorder: a placebo-controlled trial. Am J Psychiatry 2003; 160:533–540.
191. Pohl RB, Feltner DE, Fieve RR, et al. Efficacy of pregabalin in the treatment of generalized anxiety disorder: double-blind, placebo-controlled comparison of BID versus TID dosing. J Clin Psychopharmacol 2005; 25:151–158.
192. Montgomery SA, Tobias K, Zornberg GL, et al. Efficacy and safety of pregabalin in the treatment of generalized anxiety disorder: a 6-week, multicenter, randomized, double-blind, placebo-controlled comparison of pregabalin and venlafaxine. J Clin Psychiatry 2006; 67:771–782.
193. Khan A, Farfel GM, Brock JD, et al. Efficacy and safety of pregabalin in the treatment of generalized anxiety disorder in elderly patients. 2006.
194. Smith W, Feltner D, Kavoussi R. Pregabalin in generalized anxiety disorder: long term efficacy and relapse prevention. Eur Neuropsychopharmacol 2002; 12:S350–S350.
195. Schaller JL, Thomas J, Rawlings D. Low-dose tiagabine effectiveness in anxiety disorders. MedGenMed 2004; 6:8.
196. Papp LA, Ray S. Tiagabine treatment of generalized anxiety disorder. Presented at: The 156th Annual Meeting of the American Psychiatric Association; 2003; San Francisco, CA.
197. Rosenthal M. Tiagabine for the treatment of generalized anxiety disorder: a randomized, open-label, clinical trial with paroxetine as a positive control. J Clin Psychiatry 2003; 64:1245–1249.
198. Van Ameringen M, Pollack MH, Roy-Byrne. A randomized, double-blind, placebo-controlled study of tiagabine in patients with generalized anxiety disorder. 2004.
199. Pollack M. Levetiractam (keppra) for anxiety. Curbside Consultant 2002; 1(4):468–474.
200. Zohar J, Judge R. Paroxetine versus clomipramine in the treatment of obsessive-compulsive disorder. OCD paroxetine study investigators. Br J Psychiatry 1996; 169: 468–474.
201. Denys D, van der Wee N, van Megen HJ, et al. A double blind comparison of venlafaxine and paroxetine in obsessive-compulsive disorder. J Clin Psychopharmacol 2003; 23:568–575.
202. Hollander E, Allen A, Steiner M, et al. Acute and long-term treatment and prevention of relapse of obsessive-compulsive disorder with paroxetine. J Clin Psychiatry 2003; 64: 1113–1121.

203. Tollefson GD, Rampey AH Jr., Potvin JH, et al. A multicenter investigation of fixed-dose fluoxetine in the treatment of obsessive-compulsive disorder. Arch Gen Psychiatry 1994; 51:559–567.

204. Bergeron R, Ravindran AV, Chaput Y, et al. Sertraline and fluoxetine treatment of obsessive-compulsive disorder: results of a double-blind, 6-month treatment study. J Clin Psychopharmacol 2002; 22:148–154.

205. Piccinelli M, Pini S, Bellantuono C, et al. Efficacy of drug treatment in obsessive-compulsive disorder. A meta-analytic review. Br J Psychiatry 1995; 166:424–443.

206. Zitterl W, Meszaros K, Hornik K, et al. Efficacy of fluoxetine in Austrian patients with obsessive-compulsive disorder. Wien Klin Wochenschr 1999; 111:439–442.

207. Greist JH, Jefferson JW, Kobak KA, et al. Efficacy and tolerability of serotonin transport inhibitors in obsessive-compulsive disorder: a meta-analysis. Arch Gen Psychiatry 1995; 52:53–60.

208. Ackerman DL, Greenland S. Multivariate meta-analysis of controlled drug studies for obsessive-compulsive disorder. J Clin Psychopharmacol 2002; 22:309–317.

209. Montgomery SA, Kasper S, Stein DJ, et al. Citalopram 20 mg, 40 mg and 60 mg are all effective and well tolerated compared with placebo in obsessive-compulsive disorder. Int Clin Psychopharmacol 2001; 16:75–86.

210. Pallanti S, Quercioli L, Bruscoli M. Response acceleration with mirtazapine augmentation of citalopram in obsessive-compulsive disorder patients without comorbid depression: a pilot study. J Clin Psychiatry 2004; 65:1394–1399.

211. Goodman WK, Kozak MJ, Liebowitz M, et al. Treatment of obsessive-compulsive disorder with fluvoxamine: a multicentre, double-blind, placebo-controlled trial. Int Clin Psychopharmacol 1996; 11:21–29.

212. Mundo E, Maina G, Uslenghi C. Multicentre, double-blind, comparison of fluvoxamine and clomipramine in the treatment of obsessive-compulsive disorder. Int Clin Psychopharmacol 2000; 15:69–76.

213. Mundo E, Rouillon F, Figuera ML, et al. Fluvoxamine in obsessive-compulsive disorder: similar efficacy but superior tolerability in comparison with clomipramine. Hum Psychopharmacol 2001; 16:461–468.

214. Kronig MH, Apter J, Asnis G, et al. Placebo-controlled, multicenter study of sertraline treatment for obsessive-compulsive disorder. J Clin Psychopharmacol 1999; 19:172–176.

215. Hoehn-Saric R, Ninan P, Black DW, et al. Multicenter double-blind comparison of sertraline and desipramine for concurrent obsessive-compulsive and major depressive disorders. Arch Gen Psychiatry 2000; 57:76–82.

216. Bisserbe J, Lane R, Flament M. A double-blind comparison of sertraline and clomipramine in outpatients with obsessive compulsive disorder. Eur Psychiatry 1997; 12:82–93.

217. Fineberg NA, Pampaloni I, Pallanti S, et al. Escitalopram in obsessive-compulsive disorder: a randomized, placebo-controlled, paroxetine-referenced, fixed-dose, 24-week study. Curr Med Res Opin. 2007; Apr; 23(4):701–711.

218. Kobak KA, Greist JH, Jefferson JW, et al. Behavioral versus pharmacological treatments of obsessive compulsive disorder: a meta-analysis. Psychopharmacology (Berl) 1998; 136: 205–216.

219. The Clomipramine Collaborative Study Group. Clomipramine in the treatment of patients with obsessive-compulsive disorder. Arch Gen Psychiatry 1991; 48:730–738.

220. Vallejo J, Olivares J, Marcos T, et al. Clomipramine versus phenelzine in obsessive-compulsive disorder. A controlled clinical trial. Br J Psychiatry 1992; 161:665–670.

221. Jenike MA, Baer L, Minichiello WE, et al. Placebo-controlled trial of fluoxetine and phenelzine for obsessive-compulsive disorder. Am J Psychiatry 1997; 154:1261–1264.

222. McDougle CJ, Goodman WK, Leckman JF, et al. Haloperidol addition in fluvoxamine-refractory obsessive-compulsive disorder: a double-blind, placebo-controlled study in patients with and without tics. Arch Gen Psychiatry 1994; 51:302–308.

223. Dannon PN, Sasson Y, Hirschmann S, et al. Pindolol augmentation in treatment-resistant obsessive compulsive disorder: a double-blind placebo controlled trial. Eur Neuropsychopharmacol 2000; 10:165–169.

224. McDougle CJ, Epperson CN, Pelton GH, et al. A double-blind, placebo-controlled study of risperidone addition in serotonin reuptake inhibitor-refractory obsessive-compulsive disorder. Arch Gen Psychiatry 2000; 57:794–801.
225. Denys D, de Geus F, van Megen HJ, et al. A double-blind, randomized, placebo-controlled trial of quetiapine addition in patients with obsessive-compulsive disorder refractory to serotonin reuptake inhibitors. J Clin Psychiatry 2004; 65:1040–1048.
226. Bystritsky A, Ackerman DL, Rosen RM, et al. Augmentation of serotonin reuptake inhibitors in refractory obsessive-compulsive disorder using adjunctive olanzapine: a placebo-controlled trial. J Clin Psychiatry 2004; 65:565–568.
227. Cora-Locatelli G, Greenberg BD, Martin J, et al. Gabapentin augmentation for fluoxetine-treated patients with obsessive-compulsive disorder. J Clin Psychiatry 1998; 59:480–481.
228. Cora-Locatelli G, Greenberg BD, Martin JD, et al. Rebound psychiatric and physical symptoms after gabapentin discontinuation. J Clin Psychiatry 1998; 59:131.
229. Deltito JA. Valproate pretreatment for the difficult-to-treat patient with OCD. J Clin Psychiatry 1994; 55:500.
230. Cora-Locatelli G, Greenberg BD, Martin JD, et al. Valproate monotherapy in an SRI-intolerant OCD patient. J Clin Psychiatry 1998; 59:82.
231. Iwata Y, Kotani Y, Hoshino R, et al. Carbamazepine augmentation of clomipramine in the treatment of refractory obsessive-compulsive disorder. J Clin Psychiatry 2000; 61: 528–529.
232. Jenike MA, Brotman AW. The EEG in obsessive-compulsive disorder. J Clin Psychiatry 1984; 45:122–124.
233. Joffe RT, Swinson RP. Carbamazepine in obsessive-compulsive disorder. Biol Psychiatry 1987; 22:1169–1171.
234. Hollander E, Dell'Osso B. Topiramate plus paroxetine in treatment-resistant obsessive-compulsive disorder. Int Clin Psychopharmacol 2006; 21:189–191.
235. Van Ameringen M, Mancini C, Patterson B, et al. Topiramate augmentation in treatment-resistant obsessive-compulsive disorder: a retrospective, open-label case series. Depress Anxiety 2006; 23:1–5.
236. Rubio G, Jimenez-Arriero MA, Martinez-Gras I, et al. The effects of topiramate adjunctive treatment added to antidepressants in patients with resistant obsessive-compulsive disorder. J Clin Psychopharmacol 2006; 26:341–344.
237. Kumar TC, Khanna S. Lamotrigine augmentation of serotonin re-uptake inhibitors in obsessive-compulsive disorder. Aust N Z J Psychiatry 2000; 34:527–528.
238. Bowden CL, Calabrese JR, Sachs G, et al. A placebo-controlled 18-month trial of lamotrigine and lithium maintenance treatment in recently manic or hypomanic patients with bipolar I disorder. Arch Gen Psychiatry 2003; 60:392–400.
239. Crane D. Tiagabine for the treatment of anxiety. Depress Anxiety 2003; 18:51–52.
240. Schwartz TL, Azhar N, Husain J, et al. An open-label study of tiagabine as augmentation therapy for anxiety. Ann Clin Psychiatry 2005; 17:167–172.
241. Canadian Psychiatric Association. Clinical practice guidelines management of anxiety disorders. Can J Psychiatry 2006; 51(suppl 2):7S.

Antiepileptics in the Treatment of Alcohol Withdrawal and Alcohol Use Relapse Prevention

Mark A. Frye, Victor M. Karpyak, and Daniel Hall-Flavin
Department of Psychiatry and Psychology, Mayo Clinic, Rochester, Minnesota, U.S.A.

Ihsan M. Salloum
Department of Psychiatry, University of Miami, Miller School of Medicine, Miami, Florida, U.S.A.

Andrew McKeon
Department of Neurology, Mayo Clinic, Rochester, Minnesota, U.S.A.

Doo-Sup Choi
Departments of Psychiatry and Psychology and Molecular Pharmacology, Mayo Clinic, Rochester, Minnesota, U.S.A.

INTRODUCTION

In the World Health Organization's Global Burden of Disease Study (1), alcohol use disorders (abuse and dependence) ranked fifth in the undeveloped world and second in the developed world (ages 15–44 years) in disability-adjusted life years (DALYs); this measure is a composite of time lost because of premature mortality and time lived with a disability. In the United States alone, approximately 18 million people, or 7% of the population, suffer from alcohol abuse or dependence. The direct and indirect economic burden ascribed to alcohol use is estimated to be $185 billion (2). Clearly, more effective prevention and treatment of this major public health problem is needed.

For years, treatment for alcohol dependence predominantly focused on behavioral approaches or negative-reinforcement drug therapy such as disulfiram. Novel drug development over the last 10 to 15 years, as noted by the U.S. Food and Drug Administration (FDA) indications of naltrexone (1995), acamprosate (2004), and naltrexone extended-release injectable suspension (2006), has resulted in an increasing pharmacopoeia for the treatment of alcohol use disorders.

Over the course of the last 50 years, the language of an FDA alcoholism indication has evolved substantially from the 1951 indication of disulfiram ("management of selected chronic alcohol patients who want to remain in a state of enforced sobriety so that supportive and psychotherapeutic treatment may be applied to best advantage") to the 1995 naltrexone label ("an adjunct to other measures, including psychological and social counseling, in the treatment of alcohol dependence") and finally to the acamprosate 2004 label ("for the maintenance of sobriety in patients with alcohol dependence who are abstinent at treatment initiation as a part of a comprehensive management program, including psychosocial support") (3,4). This evolution in labeling not only reflects an increased understanding of the neurobiological underpinnings of addiction but also a conceptual change on how to integrate psychosocial, psychotherapeutic, and biologic treatments to maximize outcome measures such as complete abstinence and, more recently, reduction of hazardous drinking. Despite these advances, many alcoholics do not optimally respond to these current treatments. There remains an unmet need for pharmacological treatment options for both alcohol withdrawal and relapse prevention.

As recently reviewed by Mckeon et al. (5), the neurobiology of alcohol withdrawal is a complex set of voltage-dependent calcium channel, neuro-transmitter, and receptor-mediated interactions. Several neuromodulatory changes are potentially relevant when reviewing the mechanism of action of antiepileptic drugs (AEDs) and their potential utility in the treatment of alcohol withdrawal and relapse prevention. Acute alcohol ingestion has an inhibitory effect at N-methyl-D-aspartate (NMDA) receptors, reducing excitatory glutamatergic transmission (6,7), and an agonistic effect at gamma-aminobutyric acid type-A (GABA$_A$) receptors, which promotes inhibitory transmission. There is a subsequent NMDA receptor upregulation and GABA$_A$ receptor downregulation associated with chronic exposure to alcohol leading to tolerance (8). The roles are reversed during early abstinence, with enhanced NMDA receptor function, reduced GABAergic trans-mission, and dysregulation of the noradrenergic and dopaminergic systems, leading to many of the symptoms and signs of the alcohol withdrawal syndrome (9,10). Also, voltage-dependent calcium influx modulates neurotransmitter release and expression of genes that regulate production of NMDA and GABA receptor proteins; the continued presence of alcohol increases voltage-operated calcium channel expression and contributes to alcohol tolerance and the alcohol withdrawal syndrome (11).

The alcohol withdrawal syndrome is defined by two or more of the following after cessation or reduction of heavy or prolonged alcohol use: autonomic hyperactivity (sweating, tachycardia); psychomotor activation; anxiety/agitation; increased hand tremor; insomnia; nausea or vomiting; transient visual, tactile, or auditory illusions or hallucinations; and tonic-clonic seizures. While some alcohol withdrawal syndromes are mild and do not require treatment, if severe, it may be complicated by alcohol withdrawal seizures and delirium tremens (12). The chronic heavy user of alcohol is the typical patient who develops alcohol with-drawal seizures and is thought to occur secondary to a kindling effect of recurrent detoxifications (13).

Relapse prevention is the treatment intervention employed when a patient has been safely detoxified from alcohol and is now sober. This is often a time of great psychiatric instability as patients will commonly suffer from insomnia and have symptoms of anxiety, depression, or mania/hypomania at a subsyndromal or syndromal level. There may also be continued cravings for alcohol and anticipatory anxiety regarding psychosocial adjustments that need to be established in a new sober environment. By the *Diagnostic and Statistical Manual of Mental Disorders* (DSM-IV) criteria, most patients who start relapse prevention treatment have yet to meet or have just met criteria for abuse or dependence in early partial or full remission (14).

The AEDs have increasingly been identified as efficacious and effective compounds for treatment of both alcohol withdrawal and relapse prevention (15–17). The kindling model, well known in epilepsy and preclinical testing of AEDs, has also been proposed to be the neurophysiological mechanism by which alcohol withdrawal symptoms become more progressive with repeated episodes (18). This has been confirmed in retrospective and prospective clinical studies.

Brown et al. (19) studied male alcoholics with ($N = 25$) and without ($N = 25$) alcohol withdrawal–related seizures at the time of index admission for alcohol detoxification. In this study, 48% of the seizure group and only 12% of the non-seizure group had a history of greater than five prior detoxification admissions. Booth and Blow (20) reported that men with delirium tremens, alcoholic halluci-nations, and withdrawal seizures at index detoxification were more likely than men without these symptoms to have subsequent readmissions for alcoholism, with-drawal symptoms, and withdrawal seizures.

Although the intermediate (oxazepam, lorazepam) and longer-acting benzodiazepines (diazepam, clonazepam) are the established agents for treating alcohol detoxification, there has been interest in developing other compounds with less addiction potential and a reduced sedative side-effect burden. In fact, com-parative studies in alcohol withdrawal have shown that the AED carbamazepine decreases global distress and anxiety more than the benzodiazepines oxazepam and lorazepam, respectively. As anxiety and depressive symptoms can increase the likelihood of relapse, these limitations to the standard of benzodiazepine treatment are relevant. Other possible advantages of AEDs over benzodiazepines include the absence of potentiation of alcohol intoxication and their long-term use for seizure prevention in epilepsy. With this background, the AEDs carbamazepine, dival-proex, topiramate, lamotrigine, and gabapentin would appear to be promising treatments for alcohol withdrawal or relapse prevention.

CARBAMAZEPINE/OXCARBAZEPINE

Carbamazepine (Tegretol®) is approved for use in the United States for the treat-ment of trigeminal neuralgia and for temporal lobe epilepsy (complex partial seizures). Carbamazepine was synthesized as a potential antidepressant, but its atypical profile in a number of animal models led to its initial development for pain control and seizure disorders. It is now recognized in most guidelines as a second-line mood stabilizer useful in the treatment and prevention of both phases of bipolar disorder. A long-acting sustained-release formulation (Carbatrol®) has been approved by the FDA for partial seizures, generalized seizures, and trige-minal neuralgia. Under an alternate name (Equetro®), the long-acting formulation has been FDA approved for the treatment of acute mania. The structure and chemistry of carbamazepine are closely related to the more recently introduced anticonvulsant oxcarbazepine (Trileptal®).

Carbamazepine inhibits voltage-dependent sodium channels, activates voltage-dependent potassium channels, and suppresses withdrawal-induced kindling in limbic structures (21). Animal studies have shown that carbamazepine is able to prevent alcohol withdrawal seizures and reduce withdrawal symptoms (22,23). A recent retrospective pooled analysis (24) encompassing 540 patients with alcohol withdrawal reported that carbamazepine (mean dose 540 mg/day) in combination with tiapride, a benzamide D2/D3-receptor antagonist, was safe and effective in reducing quantified signs and symptoms of alcohol withdrawal. In total, 103 (19%) had a history of alcohol withdrawal delirium and 151 (28%) of an epileptic seizure during withdrawal; these rates were reduced to 0.9% and 1.5%, respectively, while on carbamazepine-tiapride treatment. Keck et al. (25) reviewed six studies that evaluated carbamazepine's efficacy for treatment of withdrawal symptoms. In a seven-day trial comparing carbamazepine ($N = 32$; 800 mg/day) to oxazepam ($N = 34$; 120 mg/day) in the treatment of acute alcohol withdrawal, both drugs were effective; however, carbamazepine was more effective than oxazepam in decreasing global distress as measured by the Clinical Institute Withdrawal Assessment for Alcohol-Revised (CIWA-Ar) score (26). More recently, Malcolm et al. compared the effects of carbamazepine (600–800 mg/day) and lorazepam (6–8 mg/day) in divided doses in a randomized double-blind controlled trial (27). The CIWA-Ar was used to assess alcohol withdrawal symptoms on days 1 through 5 and then post medication on days 7 and 12. Both drugs were equally efficacious at treating the symptoms of alcohol withdrawal, but carbamazepine had greater efficacy than lorazepam in preventing posttreatment relapses to drinking over the 12 days of follow-up in those with multiple alcohol withdrawals. Furthermore, carbamazepine was associated with a greater reduction in anxiety symptoms, as measured by the Zung Anxiety Scale.

A Cochrane database systematic review (28) demonstrated that carbamazepine had a small but statistically significant protective effect over benzodiazepines. There was also a nonsignificant reduction in seizures and side effects favoring patients treated with AEDs over patients treated with other drugs in that review.

More direct evidence for the use of carbamazepine in the treatment of alcohol dependence comes from a placebo-controlled pilot study of 29 alcohol-dependent patients. Carbamazepine increased time to first drink and time to first heavy drinking within the first 120 days of the study. There was no difference between carbamazepine and placebo after one year, but low patient compliance complicates this finding (29). Complimentary to this work is the study of Bjorkqvist et al. (30), where alcohol-dependent patients randomized to carbamazepine returned to vocational functioning faster than alcohol-dependent patients randomized to placebo.

Oxcarbazepine (Trileptal®) is currently FDA approved for the treatment of partial seizures in children and adults. It is the 10-keto-analog of carbamazepine with no epoxide metabolite, less hepatic metabolism, and fewer drug-drug interactions. These advantages may explain the overall greater tolerability of oxcarbazepine over carbamazepine (31–33). Oxcarbazepine is a prodrug and is rapidly metabolized to a pharmacologically active monohydroxyderivative, which has been shown to reduce high voltage-dependent calcium channels and subsequent NMDA glutamatergic transmission (34).

Oxcarbazepine has shown comparable effects to carbamazepine in the treatment of the alcohol withdrawal syndrome in one randomized, single-blind study (35). However, a recent multisite, six-day, double-blind, detoxification trial of 50 inpatients reported that oxcarbazepine was no different than placebo in the primary outcome measure of clomethiazole (a GABA-mediated sedative hypnotic) rescue medication use (36). The authors highlighted that the study was underpowered and that the protocol-driven threshold for trigger-based clomethiazole use may have been lower than what is done clinically, thereby reducing the potential to demonstrate a drug-placebo difference.

The data for oxcarbazepine in relapse prevention are more promising, as there are two small proof-of-concept studies comparing the AED to two standard antidipsotropic drugs (37,38). In a 24-week randomized, parallel-group, open-label clinical trial of 30 acutely detoxified alcohol-dependent patients, oxcarbazepine (1200 mg/day) was compared with acamprosate (1998 mg/day) by survival analysis with time to first severe relapse (defined as ethanol consumptions of greater than 60 g/day for males and 48 g/day for females) as the primary outcome measure (37). While the effect size for survival analysis favored oxcarbazepine, the primary outcome measure was not significantly different between groups. In a

12-week randomized, open-label, comparison study of naltrexone 50 mg/day ($N = 27$), oxcarbazepine 1500 to 1800 mg/day ($N = 29$), and oxcarbazepine 600 to 900 mg/day ($N = 28$), a significantly larger number of subjects remained completely abstinent with high-dose oxcarbazepine (59%) compared with low-dose oxcarbazepine (43%) or naltrexone (41%). High-dose oxcarbazepine was also associated with a greater reduction in hostility-aggression subscores of the SCL-90-R and an overall better response rate in dual-diagnosis patients compared with the other two treatments (38).

DIVALPROEX

Valproic acid (*N*-dipropylacetic acid) is a simple branched chain carboxylic acid with a number of formulation derivatives, including divalproex sodium (Depakote®), divalproex sodium extended release (Depakote ER®), and valproate sodium injection (Depacon®). Divalproex is approved by the FDA for (*i*) monotherapy or adjunctive therapy of complex partial seizures that occur in isolation or in conjunction with other types of seizures, (*ii*) monotherapy and adjunctive therapy of simple and complex absence seizures, (*iii*) adjunctive therapy for patients with multiple seizures that include absence seizures, (*iv*) acute manic and mixed episodes associated with bipolar disorder with or without psychosis, and (*v*) prophylaxis of migraine. Intravenous valproate sodium is currently FDA approved as an alternative in patients for whom oral administration is temporarily not feasible [i.e., those who are unresponsive or otherwise on nothing-by-mouth (NPO) status]. The drug has been shown to enhance GABA activity and suppress glutamate function via NDMA receptors (39,40).

Divalproex has been studied in the treatment of alcohol withdrawal in both open and randomized trials. In a one-week open-label study, inpatients with alcohol dependence were randomized to valproate (1200 mg/day) or control treatment with chlormethiazole or other tranquilizers, multivitamins, and fluid replacements. Five seizures occurred during the study (all in the control group) and withdrawal symptoms resolved more quickly with valproate, even though fewer valproate-treated patients received chlormethiazole (41). In a second study of 23 inpatients hospitalized for dysphoric mania, complicated by substance use (primarily alcohol), treatment with divalproex resulted not only in dysphoric symptom reduction [as measured by the Young Mania Rating Scale (YMRS) and the Hamilton Rating Scale for Depression (HAM-D)], but also in effective alcohol withdrawal symptom reduction and abstinence over the subsequent 20-week prospective follow-up (42). Mild hepatocellular enzyme elevation (not >3 times normal) at the time of admission, presumably related to alcohol ingestion, decreased over the study period. In a one-week double-blind, placebo-controlled study of nonbipolar subjects ($N = 36$) with alcohol withdrawal, subjects randomized to divalproex (1500 mg/day) required less rescue oxazepam than the placebo group (43). Furthermore, only 6% of patients in the divalproex group had an increase in withdrawal symptoms (as measured by CIWA-Ar) over time, whereas 40% of patients in the placebo group experienced an increase in CIWA-Ar scores. The ability to reduce benzodiazepine use in patients undergoing detoxification with divalproex without further significant hepatocellular risk (i.e., liver function tests decreased during detoxification) is a benefit clinically.

An open randomized trial pilot study by Longo et al. (44) evaluated divalproex in the treatment of both alcohol withdrawal and sustained abstinence in patients with alcohol dependence. Divalproex (mean dose 1500 mg/day) was as effective as standard chlordiazepoxide treatment in reducing alcohol withdrawal symptoms. Further benefit (i.e., increasing rate of abstinence) was observed at six weeks follow-up in those subjects who were maintained on divalproex compared with subjects who received either the benzodiazepine or divalproex only in the acute detoxification phase.

Alcohol relapse prevention has also been evaluated with divalproex (45). Twenty-nine outpatients with alcohol dependence participated in a 12-week, double-blind, placebo-controlled, pilot trial of divalproex. Mean valproic acid level at week 12 was 88.2 µg/mL. All patients received weekly cognitive behavioral therapy during the trial. There was a greater reduction in irritability in the divalproex treatment group, and a smaller percentage of divalproex-treated patients relapsed to heavy drinking (37%) compared with placebo-treated patients (63%; $p \leq 0.05$). There were no significant differences in reported side effects or abnormal laboratory values; in both treatment groups, a reduction in hepatocellular enzymes [alanine aminotransferase (ALT), aspartate aminotransferase (AST), and gamma-glutamyltransferase (GGT)] was observed during the course of the study. Given the extensive comorbidity of alcoholism with other Axis I disorders, particularly bipolar disorders, treatment with divalproex may stabilize mood and help treat components of alcoholism (withdrawal and relapse prevention). These results have now been replicated and extended.

In a 24-week, double-blind, placebo-controlled study of bipolar patients with comorbid active alcoholism maintained on lithium and psychosocial treatment as usual, divalproex showed greater effects than placebo on several measures of drinking (46). Of the 25 patients randomized to placebo, 68% returned to heavy drinking (defined as ≥ 4 drinks/day in women; ≥ 5 drinks/day in men) compared with 44% of the 27 randomized to divalproex ($p = 0.02$). Liver function tests ALT and AST did not differ between treatment groups, but gamma-glutamyltranspeptidase (GTP) was higher in those on placebo and was correlated with the amount of alcohol consumed per week. Of patients who did return to heavy drinking, time to relapse was significantly delayed for those on divalproex (93 days) compared with those on placebo (62 days; $p = 0.02$). Of note, this was one of the first studies to address the treatment of both drinking behavior and acute mood symptoms, which is an important situation regularly encountered in clinical practice.

TOPIRAMATE

Topiramate (Topomax®) is a sulfamate fructopyranose derivative that is FDA approved for the treatment of complex partial epilepsy, primary generalized epilepsy, seizures associated with Lennox-Gastaut syndrome, and prevention of migraine headache. Although five placebo-controlled studies of topiramate monotherapy in acute mania failed to show any demonstrable difference compared with placebo, topiramate shows promise as a treatment for alcohol dependence (47). First, topiramate has several mechanisms of action that theoretically are important in relation to treating alcoholism. Topiramate facilitates GABAergic neurotransmission through a nonbenzodiazepine site on the $GABA_A$ receptor; this action decreases extracellular release of midbrain dopamine, which is thought to mediate the craving and reward related to alcohol. In addition, topiramate antagonizes glutamate activity at AMPA and kainate receptors (48).

Second, mounting clinical trial data indicate topiramate is an effective treatment for alcohol dependence. In a prospective, open-label, 70-day study of 24 patients with alcohol dependence, adjunctive topiramate (mean dose 261 mg/day) significantly reduced alcohol consumption and craving as measured by a visual analog scale (49). A subsequent placebo-controlled study reported similar results. In addition to a brief weekly behavioral therapy to enhance medication compliance, 150 subjects with alcohol dependence were randomized to placebo or topiramate (50). The groups were matched on age, baseline drinking, and age of onset of problem drinking. The Timeline Follow Back (TLFB) method was the primary drinking outcome measure. There were no baseline differences between groups in TLFB measures of drinking outcome. At study endpoint, there were no group differences in dropout or completion rates or attrition from adverse events. However, topiramate (mean daily dose 120 ±38 mg/day) was statistically superior to placebo on all drinking and craving measures. This study was recently replicated in a 14-week, double-blind, randomized, placebo-controlled trial in 371 patients with alcohol dependence who also received a weekly compliance enhancement intervention (51). Subjects randomized to topiramate (mean dose 170 mg/day), compared with those receiving placebo, had a significantly reduced percentage of heavy drinking days. The percentage of heavy drinking days for the topiramate group was reduced from 82% at baseline to 44% at study endpoint; the placebo group's drinking was reduced from 82% at baseline to 52% at study endpoint. Topiramate was also associated with significant reductions in plasma GGT, AST, ALT, and body mass index (BMI). There was no correlation between topiramate dose and percent reduction of heavy drinking days.

GABAPENTIN

Gabapentin (Neurontin®) is approved for the adjunctive treatment of complex partial epilepsy with and without secondary generalization and postherpetic neuralgia. Calcium channel blockade and enhanced synthesis of brain GABA have been suggested as the potential antiepileptic mechanisms of action of this agent (52). Gabapentin has been shown to decrease excitability and convulsions in animal models of alcohol withdrawal (53). The lack of hepatic metabolism, cytochrome P450 enzyme induction, protein-binding, and addictive properties make gabapentin a potentially useful compound in this patient population.

Interest in gabapentin for treating the alcohol withdrawal syndrome grew after several positive reports emerged, using various doses of the drug, including starting at 400 mg three times daily and tapering over five days (54). One study demonstrated an efficacy similar to phenobarbital in treating the alcohol withdrawal syndrome (55). Another controlled trial, however, did not substantiate a benefit over placebo (56). This latter study included 61 inpatients admitted for a one-week alcohol detoxification who were randomized to gabapentin (400 mg q.i.d.) versus placebo with a protocol-driven trigger for the rescue medication clomethiazole (1 capsule = 192 mg). The primary outcome was the amount of rescue medication received in the first 24 hours, which was 6.2 capsules for the gabapentin group and 6.1 capsules for the placebo group. During the withdrawal study, there was a significant increase in the Profile of Mood State (POMS) vigor subscore in the gabapentin compared with the placebo group; this finding was particularly robust in the group with comorbid depression.

Despite the conflicting results for gabapentin in alcohol withdrawal, there is increasing recognition of its therapeutic benefit for the sleep disturbance component of the alcohol withdrawal syndrome. In an open-label pilot study, low-dose gabapentin (mean dose 900 mg/day) in the treatment of alcohol withdrawal, in comparison with trazodone, was associated with greater improvement in sleep problems, as assessed with the Sleep Problems Questionnaire (57). In a controlled trial in patients with a history of multiple previous alcohol withdrawals, gabapentin, in comparison with lorazepam, was associated with significant reductions in self-report sleep disturbances and sleepiness (58).

There is one four-week placebo-controlled, randomized, double-blind study evaluating gabapentin in alcohol abuse relapse prevention (59). After detoxification, 60 male alcohol-dependent subjects who had been drinking on average 17 drinks/day for the preceding three months were randomized to gabapentin (300 mg b.i.d.) versus placebo. The gabapentin group showed a significant reduction in the number of drinks per day, the percent heavy drinking days, and in craving for alcohol, specifically automaticity of drinking. In addition, gabapentin-treated patients showed an increase in percentage of abstinent days.

LAMOTRIGINE

Lamotrigine (Lamictal®) is currently FDA approved for simple and complex partial seizures, primary generalized tonic clonic seizures, the difficult-to-treat generalized seizures of Lennox-Gastaut syndrome, and the maintenance phase of bipolar I disorder. Lamotrigine inhibits presynaptic glutamate release through inhibition of sodium and calcium channels (60,61). Additionally, lamotrigine has been shown to modulate basal extracellular levels of serotonin and dopamine (62). Recent animal work has shown that pretreatment with lamotrigine was associated with significant reductions in both cue-induced reinstatement of alcohol-seeking behavior and voluntary alcohol intake after alcohol deprivation (63); both of these animal models have become widely used in examining the efficacy of drug therapy in preventing alcohol seeking and relapse.

Like other antiglutamatergic AEDs, lamotrigine may have some effectiveness in alcohol withdrawal. A recent double-blind study found lamotrigine 25 mg q.i.d. superior to placebo and equivalent to diazepam in the treatment of alcohol withdrawal in individuals with alcohol dependence (64).

While there are no clinical trials of lamotrigine in alcohol relapse prevention, lamotrigine has been reported to reduce drinking in alcoholics with bipolar disorder (65). In this open-label study, alcohol-dependent subjects with bipolar disorder received lamotrigine either as monotherapy or add-on therapy to other mood stabilizing medications for 12 weeks. Significant reductions in drinks per week, craving for alcohol, and carbohydrate-deficient transferrin were reported. Improved alcohol outcomes were paralleled by reductions in both mania and depression ratings. This study has a number of limitations, including small sample size and no control group for comparison. Moreover, it is unclear whether improved drinking outcomes were a cause or consequence of improved mood stability.

CONCLUSION

Studies completed to date suggest that nonbenzodiazepine, GABAergic, or antiglutamatergic AEDs may be effective treatments for the alcohol withdrawal syndrome and for preventing alcohol abuse relapse. Carbamazepine has the largest amount of evidence-based data for short-term efficacy for alcohol withdrawal followed by divalproex, with single studies providing support for topiramate and lamotrigine. For alcohol abuse relapse prevention or reduction in hazardous drinking, topiramate, divalproex, and to a lesser degree (because of sample size or study design), carbamazepine, oxcarbazepine, and gabapentin appear to be promising. Further controlled study is encouraged.

Generally, in studies of alcohol withdrawal and relapse prevention, AEDs were well tolerated with few serious adverse events. However, these agents are not without serious side effects (15,17,25,31). Carbamazepine, in addition to the difficulty of establishing stable blood levels due to its cytochrome P450 autoinduction properties, may produce significant hyponatremia and rare severe skin reactions. The hyponatremia risk is greater with oxcarbazepine (32,33). There are black box warning labels for serious dermatological conditions for carbamazepine, oxcarbazepine, and lamotrigine. One of the major concerns with the use of valproate in actively drinking or recovering alcoholics is the potential for hepatic and/or pancreatic compromise. Valproate has black box warnings for the rare but serious side effects, hepatic failure and pancreatitis. Thus far, most studies of divalproex in patients with alcohol abuse or dependence have reported a decrease, rather than increase, in liver function tests, presumably because of a decrease in alcohol use. Topiramate may produce cognitive deficits such as word-finding difficulties with prevalence rates varying from 7% in patients with epilepsy (66) to 27% in patients with migraine (67). Another concern with AEDs is their reproductive and teratogenic effects. Thus, careful reproductive history taking and education are essential before initiating treatment, as are ongoing monitoring and counseling, when using these medications in women of childbearing potential (68).

Many of the reviewed AEDs are conventional mood stabilizers (carbamazepine, divalproex, lamotrigine), and thus, in comparison with disulfiram, acamprosate, or naltrexone, may be preferred treatments in active dually diagnosed bipolar patients. Clinically, this is not an insignificant group as women and men with bipolar disorder are 7.4 and 2.8 times more likely than their counterparts in the general population to meet criteria for alcohol abuse or dependence (69). In one study, greater amounts of depression and anxiety were correlates in bipolar women with abuse alcohol, suggesting that alcohol abuse was a form of self-medication and that earlier and more effective intervention of these target symptoms could lessen the incidence of alcohol comorbidity (70).

The use of combined medications to decrease alcohol use among these patients may also be a viable option (71). In a randomized, open-label, pilot study, the combined pharmacotherapy of valproate plus naltrexone was compared with valproate alone in acutely ill, actively drinking bipolar alcoholics over an eight-week period. Those receiving the combination of valproate plus naltrexone versus valproate alone had a better outcome on avoiding relapse to alcohol use and on improvement in alcohol craving and mood symptoms. As always, careful consideration of the risk-benefit ratio of using adjunctive medications must be undertaken as polypharmacy, while prevalent, does pose some clinical challenges in the treatment of bipolar disorder (72).

It is very encouraging that interest and efforts at evaluating pharmacotherapeutic compounds for alcohol use disorders has substantially increased over the past few years. Antiepileptic mood stabilizers such as carbamazepine, divalproex, and lamotrigine, as well as the AEDs oxcarbazepine, gabapentin, and topiramate, appear to be promising agents for the treatment of alcohol withdrawal and relapse prevention. With such a diverse group of treatments potentially available (AEDs and antidipsotropics), it will be valuable to better understand how both withdrawal symptom management and relapse prevention management are achieved.

REFERENCES

1. Murray CJ, Lopez AD. Global mortality, disability, and the contribution of risk factors. Global Burden of Disease Study. Lancet 1997; 349(9063):1436–1442.
2. Li T, Hewitt B, Grant B. Alcohol use disorders and mood disorders: a National Institute on Alcohol Abuse and Alcoholism perspective. Biol Psychiatry 2004; 56:718–720.
3. USP DI® Drug Information for the Health Care Professional and PDR, 2006.
4. Physicians Desk Reference. 60th ed. Montvale, NJ: Thomson PDR, 2006.
5. McKeon A, Frye MA, Delanty N. The alcohol withdrawal syndrome. J Neurol Neurosurg Psychiatry 2008 (In press).
6. Tsai G, Gastfriend DR, Coyle JT. The glutamatergic basis of human alcoholism. Am J Psychiatry 1995; 152:332–340.
7. Tsai G, Coyle JT. The role of glutamatergic neurotransmission in the pathophysiology of alcoholism. Annu Rev Med 1998; 49:173–184.
8. Sanna E, Mostallino MC, Busonero F, et al. Changes in GABA(A) receptor gene expression associated with selective alterations in receptor function and pharmacology after ethanol withdrawal. J Neurosci 2003; 23:11711–11724.
9. Nutt D. Alcohol and the brain. Pharmacological insights for psychiatrists. Br J Psychiatry 1999; 175:114–119.
10. Lingford-Hughes A, Nutt D. Neurobiology of addiction and implications for treatment. Br J Psychiatry 2003; 182:97–100.
11. Kovacs GL. Natriuretic peptides in alcohol withdrawal: central and peripheral mechanisms. Curr Med Chem 2003; 10:2559–2576.
12. Seitz PF. The sensorium in delirium tremens and alcoholic hallucinosis. Am J Psychiatry 1951; 108:145.
13. Lechtenberg R, Worner TM. Total ethanol consumption as a seizure risk factor in alcoholics. Acta Neurol Scand 1992; 85:90–94
14. American Psychiatric Association, American Psychiatric Association Task Force on DSM-IV, Teton Data Systems (firm). Diagnostic and Statistical Manual of Mental Disorders DSM-IV-TR. 4th ed. Washington, DC: American Psychiatric Association, 2000.
15. Ait-Saoud N, Malcolm RJ, Johnson BA. An overview of medications for the treatment of alcohol withdrawal and alcohol dependence with an emphasis on the use of older and newer anticonvulsants. Addict Behav 2006; 31:1628–1649.
16. Leggio L, Kenna GA, Swift RM. New developments for the pharmacological treatment of alcohol withdrawal syndrome. A focus on non-benzodiazepine GABAergic medications. Prog Neuro-Psychopharmacol Biol Psychiatry 2008 (In press).
17. Malcolm R, Myrick H, Brady KT, et al. Update on anticonvulsants for the treatment of alcohol withdrawal. Am J Addict 2001; 10(S):16–23.
18. Ballenger JC, Post RM. Kindling as a model for alcohol withdrawal syndromes. Br J Psychiatry 1978; 133:1–14.
19. Brown ME, Anton RE, Malcom R, et al. Alcohol detoxification and withdrawal seizures clinical support for a kindling hypothesis. Biol Psychiatry 1988; 23:507–514.
20. Booth BM, Blow FC. The kindling hypothesis: further evidence from a U.S. national study of alcoholic men. Alcohol Alcohol 1993; 28:593–598.
21. Armijo JA, Shushtarian M, Valdizan EM, et al. Ion channels and epilepsy. Curr Pharm Des 2005; 11:1975–2003.
22. Chu NS. Carbamazepine: prevention of alcohol withdrawal seizures. Neurology 1979; 29:1397–1401.
23. Strzelec JS, Czarnecka E. Influence of clonazepam and carbamazepine on alcohol withdrawal syndrome, preference and development of tolerance to ethanol in rats. Pol J Pharmacol 2001; 53:117–124.
24. Soyka M, Schmidt P, Franz M, et al. Treatment of alcohol withdrawal syndrome with a combination of tiapride/carbamazepine: results of a pooled analysis in 540 patients. Eur Arch Psychiatry Clin Neurosci 2006; 256:395–401.

25. Keck PE Jr., McElroy SL, Friedman LM. Valproate and carbamazepine in the treatment of panic and posttraumatic stress disorders, withdrawal states, and behavioral dyscontrol syndromes. J Clin Psychopharmacol 1992; 12:36S–41S.
26. Malcolm R, Ballenger JC, Sturgis ET, et al. Double-blind controlled trial comparing carbamazepine to oxazepam treatment of alcohol withdrawal. Am J Psychiatry 1989; 146:617–621.
27. Malcolm R, Myrick H, Roberts J, et al. The effects of carbamazepine and lorazepam on single versus multiple previous alcohol withdrawals in an outpatient randomized trial. J Gen Intern Med 2002; 17:349–355.
28. Polycarpou A, Papanikolaou P, Ioannidis JP, et al. Anticonvulsants for alcohol withdrawal. Cochrane Database Syst Rev 2005; 3:CD005064.
29. Mueller TI, Stout RL, Rudden S, et al. A double-blind, placebo-controlled pilot study of carbamazepine for the treatment of alcohol dependence. Alcohol Clin Exp Res 1997; 21:86–92.
30. Bjorkqvist SE, Isohanni M, Makela R, et al. Ambulant treatment of alcohol withdrawal symptoms with carbamazepine: a formal multicentre double-blind comparison with placebo. Acta Psychiatr Scand 1976; 53:333–342.
31. Keck PE, McElroy SL. Clinical pharmacodynamics and pharmacokinetics of antimanic and mood stabilizing medications. J Clin Psychiatry 2002; 63:(suppl 4):3–122.
32. Glauser TA. Oxcarbazepine in the treatment of epilepsy. Pharmacotherapy 2001; 21: 904–919.
33. Beydoun A, Kutluay E. Oxcarbazepine. Expert Opin Pharmacother 2002; 3:59–71.
34. Wellington K, Goa KL. Oxcarbazepine: an update on its efficacy in the management of epilepsy. CNS Drugs 2001; 15:137–163.
35. Schik G, Wedegaertner FR, Liersch J, et al. Oxcarbazepine versus carbamazepine in the treatment of alcohol withdrawal. Addict Biol 2005; 10:283–288.
36. Koethe D, Juelicher A, Nolden BM, et al. Oxcarbazepine: efficacy and tolerability during treatment of alcohol withdrawal: a double-blind, randomized, placebo-controlled multicenter pilot study. Alcohol Clin Exp Res 2007; 31:1188–1194.
37. Croissant B, Diehl A, Klein O, et al. A pilot study of oxcarbazepine versus acamprosate in alcohol-dependent patients. Alcohol Clin Exp Res 2006; 4:630–635.
38. Martinotti G, Di Nicola M, Romanelli R, et al. High and low dosage oxcarbazepine versus naltrexone for the prevention of relapse in alcohol dependent patients. Hum Psychopharmacol 2007; 22:149–156.
39. Keck PE, McElroy SL, Friedman LM. Valproate and carbamazepine in the treatment of panic and posttraumatic stress disorders, withdrawal states, and behavioural dyscontrol syndromes. J Clin Pscyhopharmacol 1992; 12(1 suppl):36S–41S.
40. Loscher W. Basic pharmacology of valproate: a review after 35 years of clinical use for the treatment of epilepsy CNS Drug 2002; 16:669–694.
41. Lambie D, Johnson RH, Vijayasenan ME, et al. Sodium valproate in the treatment of the alcohol withdrawal syndrome. Aust NZ J Psychiatry 1980; 14:213–215.
42. Brady KT, Sonne SC, Anton R, et al. Valproate in the treatment of acute bipolar affective episodes complicated by substance abuse: a pilot study. J Clin Psychiatry 1995; 56:118–121.
43. Reoux JP, Saxon AJ, Malte CA, et al. Divalproex sodium in alcohol withdrawal: a randomized double-blind placebo-controlled clinical trial. Alcohol Clin Exp Res 2001; 25: 1324–1329.
44. Longo LP, Campbell T, Hubatch S. Divalproex sodium (Depakote) for alcohol withdrawal and relapse prevention. J Addict Dis 2002; 21(2):55–64.
45. Brady KT, Myrick H, Henderson S, et al. The use of divalproex in alcohol relapse prevention: a pilot study. Drug Alcohol Depend 2002; 67(3):323–330.
46. Salloum IM, Cornelius JR, Daley DC, et al. Efficacy of valproate maintenance in patients with bipolar disorder and alcoholism: a double-blind placebo controlled study. Arch Gen Psychiatry 2005; 62(1):37–45.
47. Kushner SF, Khan A, Olson WH. Topiramate monotherapy in the management of acute mania: results of four double-blind placebo controlled trials. Bipolar Disord 2006; 8:15–27.
48. Moghaddam B, Bolinao ML. Glutamatergic antagonists attenuate ability of dopamine uptake blockers to increase extracellular levels of dopamine: implications for tonic influence of glutamate on dopamine release. Synapse 1994; 18:337–342.

49. Rubio G, Ponce G, Jimenez-Arriero MA, et al. Effectiveness of topiramate in control of alcohol craving. Eur Neuropsychoparmacol 2002; 12(suppl 3):S367.
50. Johnson BA, Ait-Daoud N, Bowden CL, et al. Oral topiramate for treatment of alcohol dependence: a randomised controlled trial. Lancet 2003; 361(9370):1677–1685.
51. Johnson BA, Rosenthal N, Capece JA, et al. Topiramate for treating alcohol depndence: a randomized controlled trial. JAMA 2007; 298:1641–1651.
52. McLean M. Clinical pharmacokinetics of gabapentin. Neurology 1994; 44:S17–S22.
53. Watson WP, Robinson E, Little HJ. The novel anticonsultant gabapentin protects against both convulsant and anxiogenic aspects of the ethanol withdrawal syndrome. Neuropharmacology 1997; 36:1369–1375.
54. Bozikas V, Petrikis P, Gamvrula K, et al. Treatment of alcohol withdrawal with gabapentin. Prog Neuropsychopharmacol Biol Psychiatry 2002; 26:197–199.
55. Mariani JJ, Rosenthal RN, Tross S, et al. A randomized, open-label, controlled trial of gabapentin and phenobarbital in the treatment of alcohol withdrawal. Am J Addict 2006; 15:76–84.
56. Bonnet U, Banger M, Leweke FM, et al. Treatment of acute alcohol withdrawal with gabapentin: results from a controlled two-center trial. J Clin Psychopharmacol 2003; 23:514–519.
57. Karam-Hage M, Brower KJ. Open pilot study of gabapentin versus trazodone to treatment insomnia in alcoholic outpatients. Psychiatry Clin Neurosci 2003; 57:542–544.
58. Malcolm R, Myrick LH, Veatch LM, et al. Self-reported sleep, sleepiness, and repeated alcohol withdrawals: a randomized, double blind, controlled comparison vs. lorazepam vs. gabapentin. J Clin Sleep Med 2007; 15:24–32.
59. Furieri FA, Nakamura-Palacios EM. Gabapentin reduces alcohol consumption and craving: a randomized, double-blind, placebo-controlled trial. J Clin Psychiatry 2007; 11:1691–1700.
60. Lees G, Leach MJ. Studies on the mechanism of action of the novel anticonvulsant lamotrigine using primary neurological cultures from rat cortex. Brain Res 1993; 612:190–199.
61. Wang SJ, Sibra TS, Gean PW. Lamotrigine inhibition of glutamate release from isolated cerebrocortical nerve terminals by suppression of voltage activated calcium channel activity. Neuroreport 2001; 12:2255–2258.
62. Ahmad S, Fowler LJ, Whitton PS. Effects of acute and chronic lamotrigine treatment on basal and stimulated extracellular amino acids in the hippocampus of freely moving rats. Brain Res 2004; 1029:41–47.
63. Vengelien V, Heidbreder CA, Spanagel R. The effects of lamotrigine on alcohol seeking and relapse. Neuropharmacology 2007; 53:951–957.
64. Krupitsky EM, Rudenko AA, Burakov AM, et al. Antiglutamatergic strategies for ethanol detoxification: comparison with placebo and diazepam. Alcohol Clin Exp Res 2007; 31:604–611.
65. Rubio G, Lopez-Munoz F, Alamo C. Effects of lamotrigine in patients with bipolar disorder. Bipolar Disord 2006; 8:289–293.
66. Mula M, Trimble MR, Thompson P, et al. Topiramate and word-finding difficulties in patients with epilepsy. Neurology 2003; 60(7):1104–1107
67. Coppola F, Rossi C, Mancini ML, et al. Language disturbances as a side effect of prophylactic treatment of migraine. Headache 2008; 48(1):86–94.
68. Altshuler LL, Cohen L, Szuba MP, et al. Pharmacologic management of psychiatric illness during pregnancy: dilemmas and guidelines. Am J Psychiatry 1996; 154(5):592–606.
69. Frye MA, Altshuler LL, McElroy SL, et al. Gender differences in prevalence, risk, and clinical correlates of alcoholism comorbidity in bipolar disorder. Am J Psychiatry 2003; 160:883–889.
70. Salloum IM, Cornelius JR, Mezzich JE, et al. Characterizing female bipolar alcoholic patients presenting for initial evaluation. Addict Behav 2001; 26:341–348.
71. Salloum IM, Cornelius JR, Daley DC, et al. Efficacy of valproate in bipolar alcoholics: a double blind, placebo-controlled study. Presented at: the Fifth International Conference on Bipolar Disorder; June 12–14, 2003; Pittsburgh, PA.
72. Frye MA, Ketter TA, Leverich GS, et al. The increasing use of polypharmacotherapy for refractory mood disorders: 22 years of study. J Clin Psychiatry 2000; 61(1):9–15.

14 Antiepileptic Drugs in the Treatment of Drug Use Disorders

Kyle M. Kampman
University of Pennsylvania School of Medicine, Philadelphia, Pennsylvania, U.S.A.

INTRODUCTION

Antiepileptic drugs (AEDs) such as phenobarbital have been traditionally used in the treatment of sedative-hypnotic dependence to help patients withdraw safely from sedatives, including benzodiazepines. More recently, newer AEDs, including carbamazepine and valproate, have also shown some potential in treating benzodiazepine withdrawal. AEDs such as GVG [gamma-vinyl gamma-aminobutyric acid (GABA)], topiramate, and tiagabine may be promising for the treatment of stimulant dependence, primarily as relapse-prevention medications. Finally, AEDs such as carbamazepine and lamotrigine may be particularly beneficial in helping drug-addicted patients with comorbid mood disorders achieve and maintain abstinence from drugs of abuse, including from stimulants.

ANTIEPILEPTIC DRUGS FOR THE TREATMENT OF SEDATIVE-HYPNOTIC WITHDRAWAL

For many years, phenobarbital has been used to facilitate withdrawal from sedative hypnotics (1). Its usefulness as a detoxification medication is related to its cross-tolerance with other sedatives including benzodiazepines (2). Phenobarbital acts primarily by facilitating transmission at the $GABA_A$ receptor, as do sedatives, including benzodiazepines (3). Although patients addicted to benzodiazepines could be treated by gradually tapering the dose of the benzodiazepine or other sedative to which they are already addicted, phenobarbital is favored by many clinicians because of its long half-life and because many clinicians believe that it is better not to administer the drug of abuse during treatment.

Withdrawal from high doses of benzodiazepines (doses much higher than recommended therapeutic doses) is usually done in a hospital setting. The starting dose of phenobarbital can be calculated on the basis of the patient's history of benzodiazepine use over the past month. A dose of 30 mg of phenobarbital is roughly equivalent to 10 mg of diazepam, 25 mg of chlordiazepoxide, 1 mg of alprazolam, or 2 mg of clonazepam (4). The calculated phenobarbital-equivalent dose is given in three divided doses each day. Because patients often cannot give an accurate estimate of the type or dose of sedative they have been abusing, they need to be closely observed after the first few doses of phenobarbital and the dose adjusted on the basis of clinical response. The maximum starting dose of phenobarbital is 500 mg daily. After two days of stabilization, the dose is decreased by 30 mg daily (4). Patients addicted to lower doses of benzodiazepines (i.e., those within the therapeutic range) can also be detoxified using phenobarbital replacement, but the rate of the taper is usually much longer, i.e., many weeks to months in an outpatient setting.

More recently, other AEDs such as carbamazepine and valproate have been tested with some success for the treatment of benzodiazepine withdrawal. Carbamazepine's mechanism of action is unique. It has no effect on benzodiazepine receptors or on the GABA receptor complex in general. Carbamazepine limits the repetitive firing of action potentials by slowing the rate of recovery of voltage-activated sodium channels from inactivation (2). Its ability to inhibit electrical activation in the limbic system is thought to be a possible mechanism of action for the treatment of sedative withdrawal. It has been hypothesized that repeated withdrawal from alcohol or other sedatives induces long-lasting neuronal changes that alter the organism's response to sedatives, resulting in more severe withdrawal symptoms (5). Carbamazepine has been shown to be effective in blocking the progression of disorders on the basis of the kindling model, such as bipolar disorder, alcohol withdrawal, and electrically induced kindling in rats (6–8). Thus, it was hypothesized that carbamazepine would be effective as a treatment for sedative-hypnotic withdrawal based on its effects on kindling (5).

There have been several case series and open trials reported in the literature, supporting the use of carbamazepine for the treatment of benzodiazepine withdrawal (9–14). In most cases, carbamazepine was added to a tapering dose of benzodiazepine, although in at least one open trial, the benzodiazepines were abruptly stopped when carbamazepine was started (11).

There has been only one double-blind, controlled trial of carbamazepine as an adjunct to a tapering dose of benzodiazepine to treat benzodiazepine withdrawal (15). In this trial, 40 benzodiazepine-dependent patients were randomized to carbamazepine 200 to 800 mg daily or placebo. After starting study medication, patients' benzodiazepine doses were tapered 25% per week. Patients assigned to carbamazepine were significantly more likely to be abstinent from benzodiazepines five weeks after the taper was complete compared with placebo-treated patients (15). However, the difference between carbamazepine- and placebo-treated patients was no longer statistically significant at 12 weeks after taper completion. Carbamazepine-treated patients reported less severe withdrawal symptoms compared with placebo-treated patients, but this effect was significant only at a trend level. Carbamazepine was reasonably well tolerated. The most commonly experienced side effects included headache, nausea, and mental impairment (15).

Valproate has also been used for benzodiazepine withdrawal. Its anticonvulsant effects appear to be mediated by a prolonged recovery of voltage-activated sodium ion channels from inactivation (2). In addition, valproate may increase brain GABA levels. It stimulates the activity of the GABA synthetic enzyme glutamic acid decarboxylase and inhibits the GABA degradative enzymes GABA transaminase and succinic semialdehyde dehydrogenase (2). Valproate's usefulness in the treatment of benzodiazepine withdrawal is thought to be related to its ability to increase GABAergic neurotransmission.

The evidence supporting the usefulness of valproate for the treatment of benzodiazepine withdrawal consists of two small case studies and one double-blind trial. In one case, valproate treatment appeared to facilitate benzodiazepine tapering (16). In the other, therapy with valproate appeared to reduce protracted abstinence symptoms in four patients recently detoxified from benzodiazepines (17). In the only double-blind, controlled trial of valproate for benzodiazepine withdrawal, Rickels and colleagues compared the serotonergic antidepressant trazodone with valproate and to placebo in 78 benzodiazepine-dependent patients (18). Patients were stabilized on a dose of benzodiazepine and then pretreated for two weeks with either trazodone 100 to 500 mg daily, valproate 500 to 2500 mg daily, or placebo. After two weeks, patients' benzodiazepines were tapered 25% each week. All treatments were continued for five weeks post taper. Follow-up evaluations were conducted 5 and 12 weeks after completion of the taper. At the five-week follow-up, both the trazodone- and valproate-treated patients were significantly more likely to be free from benzodiazepines than the placebo-treated patients. At the 12-week follow-up, however, there were no statistically significant differences in benzodiazepine use between the three groups. Additionally, neither trazodone nor valproate was effective in reducing benzodiazepine withdrawal symptom severity (18).

In sum, the evidence supporting the usefulness of carbamazepine and valproate for the treatment of benzodiazepine withdrawal is not overwhelming. While several open trials and case series suggest carbamazepine may be useful, the one double-blind trial did not completely support carbamazepine's efficacy. Carbamazepine was associated with a higher rate of abstinence from benzodiazepines five weeks after completing a benzodiazepine taper, but this effect was not seen at 12-week follow-up. In addition, carbamazepine had no effect on benzodiazepine withdrawal symptom severity. The data supporting the efficacy of valproate for benzodiazepine detoxification are even weaker, with only two very small case series suggesting the drug's utility in this area. No open trials have been published, and the results of the one double-blind trial of valproate for benzodiazepine detoxification are similar to those obtained for carbamazepine. Valproate was associated with a higher rate of benzodiazepine abstinence five weeks after completing a benzodiazepine taper compared with placebo, but this effect was not seen at 12-week follow-up.

ANTIEPILEPTIC DRUGS FOR THE TREATMENT OF STIMULANT DEPENDENCE

AEDs have received a great deal of study for the treatment of cocaine dependence where they have been mainly viewed as potentially helpful for the prevention of relapse. None are FDA approved for the treatment of cocaine dependence, and most of the data supporting their usefulness in this area come from small, pilot clinical trials that have not yet been replicated in large well-controlled trials. Initially, it was believed that AEDs that were useful in the control of kindled seizures, such as carbamazepine, would be useful for the treatment of cocaine dependence. However, in three separate double-blind, placebo-controlled trials, carbamazepine was not found to be better than placebo for the treatment of cocaine dependence (19–21). More recently, attention has shifted to AEDs that have GABAergic properties, and these medications appear to hold more promise. These GABAergic AEDs may be able to affect the mesocortical dopaminergic reward center in a way that reduces craving and prevents relapse in cocaine-dependent patients.

The mesocortical dopamine system plays a central role in the reinforcing effects of cocaine (22–25). Mesocortical dopaminergic neurons receive modulatory inputs from both GABergic and glutamatergic neurons. GABA is primarily an inhibitory neurotransmitter in the central nervous system, and activation of GABAergic neurons tends to decrease activity in the dopaminergic reward system. Preclinical trials of AEDs that enhance GABAergic neurotransmission have suggested that these compounds reduce the dopamine response to both cocaine administration and to conditioned reminders of prior cocaine use (26–28).

GABAergic medications also reduce self-administration of cocaine in animal models (29,30). Therefore, GABAergic medications could prevent relapse either by blocking cocaine-induced euphoria or by reducing craving caused by exposure to conditioned reminders of prior cocaine use. Some promising GABAergic AEDs include GVG, tiagabine, and topiramate.

GVG is an AED that has been in use in many countries throughout the world for a number of years, but not the United States. It is an irreversible inhibitor of GABA transaminase and thus elevates brain GABA concentrations. Preclinical trials of GVG have been promising. GVG has been shown to block cocaine- and cocaine cue–induced increases in nucleus accumbens dopamine (27,31). It has also been shown to block cocaine self-administration in rodents (29). Similar results have been shown for GVG with both amphetamine and methamphetamine (28).

There has been only one clinical trial of GVG for the treatment of stimulant dependence. This was a small open-label trial involving 20 patients with either cocaine or amphetamine dependence. In this trial, GVG treatment was well tolerated and was associated with significant reductions in stimulant use in 40% of patients (32).

GVG has not been approved for use in the United States because of an association with visual field defects. However, available data suggest that such visual field defects occur after relatively long-term exposure to GVG and that brief treatment with GVG may be safely conducted (33,34). Large-scale, well-controlled trials of GVG for both cocaine and amphetamine dependence have, therefore, been planned.

Tiagabine is another GABAergic AED that may be promising for the treatment of cocaine dependence. Currently approved for the treatment of seizures, it is a selective blocker of the presynaptic GABA reuptake transporter type 1 (35). Tiagabine was found to be well tolerated and moderately effective for improving abstinence in a pilot study that included 45 cocaine- and opiate-dependent patients participating in a methadone maintenance program. In this 10-week trial, the number of cocaine metabolite–free urine samples increased by 33% in the group treated with tiagabine (24 mg/day) and decreased by 14% in the placebo-treated group (36). The results of this trial were recently replicated in another 10-week trial also conducted in cocaine- and opiate-dependent patients stabilized on methadone. Patients treated with tiagabine (24 mg/day; $N = 25$) significantly reduced their cocaine use compared with placebo-treated patients ($N = 25$). At the end of the trial, tiagabine-treated patients submitted 48% cocaine-free urine samples compared with 24% cocaine-free samples for the placebo group (37).

Topiramate may be an excellent medication for relapse prevention based on its effects on both GABA and glutamate neurotransmission. Topiramate facilitates GABA neurotransmission and increases cerebral levels of GABA (38,39). It also inhibits glutamate neurotransmission through blockade of α-amino-3 hydroxy-5-methyl-4-isoxazole propionic acid (AMPA)/kainate receptors (40). In animal models of cocaine relapse, blockade of AMPA receptors in the nucleus accumbens has been shown to prevent reinstatement of cocaine self-administration (41).

In a 13-week, double-blind, placebo-controlled pilot trial of topiramate involving 40 cocaine-dependent patients, topiramate-treated patients were significantly more likely to be abstinent during the last five weeks of treatment compared with placebo-treated patients (42). In addition, among patients who returned for at least one visit after receiving medication, topiramate-treated patients were significantly more likely to achieve at least three weeks of continuous abstinence from cocaine compared with placebo-treated patients (59% vs. 26%). Topiramate-treated patients were also significantly more likely than placebo-treated patients to be rated very much improved on their last visit (71% vs. 32%) (42). Topiramate is currently undergoing large-scale confirmatory trials for the treatment of cocaine dependence as well as for the treatment of combined cocaine and alcohol dependence.

AEDs are among the most promising medications for the treatment of cocaine dependence. Medications such as GVG and topiramate may be efficacious for many drugs of abuse in addition to cocaine, including nicotine and alcohol. However, at this time there are no large-scale, well-controlled trials that have shown any AED to be efficacious for the treatment of cocaine or amphetamine dependence. More research is needed before any AED can be recommended for the treatment of cocaine or amphetamine dependence.

ANTIEPILEPTIC DRUGS FOR THE TREATMENT OF DRUG DEPENDENCE AND COMORBID MOOD DISORDERS

AEDs have been shown to be effective for the treatment of bipolar disorder (43). Mood disorders, in general, and bipolar disorder, in particular, are commonly seen in patients with substance use disorders (44). For the treatment of drug-dependent patients with comorbid mood disorders, at least two AEDs have shown some promise: carbamazepine and lamotrigine.

Carbamazepine was not found to be effective for the treatment of cocaine dependence in three separate double-blind, placebo-controlled trials (19–21). However, it is an effective medication for the treatment of bipolar disorder and its mood-stabilizing properties may help cocaine-dependent patients with comorbid mood disorders reduce their cocaine use. In one double-blind, placebo-controlled trial, Brady and colleagues found that, among cocaine-dependent patients with comorbid mood disorders, those treated with carbamazepine were less likely to relapse to cocaine use (45). This trial involved 139 cocaine-dependent patients, 57 with a comorbid mood disorder. Of those with mood disorders, 33 had major depression or dysthymia and 24 had bipolar disorder or cyclothymia. Patients were treated with carbamazepine 800 mg daily or placebo. Among patients with a comorbid mood disorder, carbamazepine treatment was associated with a significantly longer time to relapse to cocaine use. By contrast, among patients without a comorbid mood disorder, carbamazepine had no effect on cocaine use.

There is some evidence from two open trials that lamotrigine may be effective for the treatment of cocaine dependence in patients with bipolar disorder. Brown and colleagues conducted two open trials of lamotrigine that included a total of 62 cocaine-dependent patients with comorbid bipolar disorder (bipolar I, II, or bipolar disorder NOS) (46,47). In the most recent trial, lamotrigine was added to the patient's ongoing regimen and titrated up to a maximum dose of 300 mg/day (average dose 155 mg/day). Over the 36-week trial, mood symptoms declined, as did cocaine craving and dollars spent for cocaine. In addition, there was a significant correlation between improvement in mood symptoms and reductions in cocaine craving and cocaine use (47).

In sum, among bipolar patients with comorbid cocaine dependence, there is preliminary evidence that AEDs may be effective for the treatment of both mood and drug dependence symptoms. In a double-blind trial, carbamazepine reduced relapse to cocaine in patients with co-occurring bipolar and unipolar mood disorders. In two open trials in bipolar patients, lamotrigine treatment was associated with less cocaine craving and less cocaine use. These data need to be replicated in larger, well-controlled clinical trials before either medication can be recommended for the treatment of cocaine dependent patients with comorbid mood disorders.

REFERENCES

1. Smith DE, Wesson DR. Phenobarbital technique for treatment of barbiturate dependence. Arch Gen Psychiatry 1971; 24(1):56–60.
2. McNamara JO. Drugs effective in the therapy of the epilepsies. In: Hardman JG, Limbard LE, eds. Goodman and Gillman's The Pharmacological Basis of Therapeutics. 10th ed. New York, NY: McGraw Hill, 2001:521–547.
3. Charney D, Mihic S, Harris R. Hypnotics and sedatives. In: Hardman J, Limbird L, Goodman Gilman A, eds. Goodman and Gillman's The Pharmacological Basis of Therapeutics. 10th ed. New York, NY: McGraw Hill, 2001:399–427.
4. Wesson D, Smith D, Seymore M. Sedative-hypnotics and tricyclics. In: Lowinson J, Ruiz P, Millman R, et al. eds. Substance Abuse, A Comprehensive Textbook. 2nd ed. Philadelphia, PA: Williams and Wilkins, 1992:217–279.
5. Mueller TI, Stout RL, Rudden S, et al. A double-blind, placebo-controlled pilot study of carbamazepine for the treatment of alcohol dependence. Alcohol Clin Exp Res 1997; 21(1): 86–92.
6. Post RM, Weiss SR, Chuang DM. Mechanisms of action of anticonvulsants in affective disorders: comparisons with lithium. J Clin Psychopharmacol 1992; 12(suppl 1):S23–S35.
7. Ballenger JC, Post RM. Kindling as a model for alcohol withdrawal syndromes. Br J Psychiatry 1978; 133:1–14.
8. Silver JM, Shin C, McNamara JO. Antiepileptogenic effects of conventional anticonvulsants in the kindling model of epilespy. Ann Neurol 1991; 29(4):356–363.
9. Klein E, Uhde TW, Post RM. Preliminary evidence for the utility of carbamazepine in alprazolam withdrawal. Am J Psychiatry 1986; 143(2):235–236.
10. Ries RK, Roy-Byrne PP, Ward NG, et al. Carbamazepine treatment for benzodiazepine withdrawal. Am J Psychiatry 1989; 146(4):536–537.
11. Ries R, Cullison S, Horn R, et al. Benzodiazepine withdrawal: clinicians' ratings of carbamazepine treatment versus traditional taper methods. J Psychoactive Drugs 1991; 23(1):73–76.
12. Swantek SS, Grossberg GT, Neppe VM, et al. The use of carbamazepine to treat benzodiazepine withdrawal in a geriatric population. J Geriatr Psychiatry Neurol 1991; 4(2): 106–109.
13. Garcia-Borreguero D, Bronisch T, Apelt S, et al. Treatment of benzodiazepine withdrawal symptoms with carbamazepine. Eur Arch Psychiatry ClinNeurosci 1991; 241(3): 145–150.
14. Klein E, Colin V, Stolk J, et al. Alprazolam withdrawal in patients with panic disorder and generalized anxiety disorder: vulnerability and effect of carbamazepine. Am J Psychiatry 1994; 151(12):1760–1766.
15. Schweizer E, Rickels K, Case WG, et al. Carbamazepine treatment in patients discontinuing long-term benzodiazepine therapy. Effects on withdrawal severity and outcome. Arch Gen Psychiatry 1991; 48(5):448–452.
16. McElroy SL, Keck PE Jr., Lawrence JM. Treatment of panic disorder and benzodiazepine withdrawal with valproate. J Neuropsychiatry Clin Neurosci 1991; 3(2):232–233.
17. Apelt S, Emrich HM. Sodium valproate in benzodiazepine withdrawal. Am J Psychiatry 1990; 147(7):950–951.
18. Rickels K, Schweizer E, Garcia Espana F, et al. Trazodone and valproate in patients discontinuing long-term benzodiazepine therapy: effects on withdrawal symptoms and taper outcome. Psychopharmacology 1999; 141(1):1–5.

19. Montoya ID, Levin FR, Fudala PJ, et al. Double-blind comparison of carbamazepine and placebo for treatment of cocaine dependence. Drug Alcohol Depend 1995; 38(3):213–219 (comment).
20. Cornish JW, Maany I, Fudala PJ, et al. Carbamazepine treatment for cocaine dependence. Drug Alcohol Depend 1995; 38(3):221–227 (comment).
21. Kranzler HR, Bauer LO, Hersh D, et al. Carbamazepine treatment of cocaine dependence: a placebo-controlled trial. Drug Alcohol Depend 1995; 38(3):203–211 (comment).
22. Roberts DCS, Koob GF, Klonoff P, et al. Extinction and recovery of cocaine self-administration following 6-hydroxydopamine lesions of the nucleus accumbens. Pharmacol Biochem Behav 1980; 12:781–787.
23. Koob G, Vaccarino F, Amalric M, et al. Positive reinforcement properties of drugs: search for neural substrates. In: Engel J, Oreland L, eds. Brain Reward Systems and Abuse. New York, NY: Raven Press, 1987:35–50.
24. Goeders NE, Dworkin SI, Smith JE. Neuropharmacological assessment of cocaine self-administration into the medial prefrontal cortex. Pharmacol Biochem Behav 1986; 24: 1429–1440.
25. Dworkin SI, Smith JE. Neurobehavioral pharmacology of cocaine. In: Clouet D, Ashgar K, Brown R, eds. Mechanisms of Cocaine Abuse and Toxicity. National Institute on Drug Abuse Research Monograph Number 88. Washington, DC: U.S. Government Printing Office, 1988:185–198.
26. Dewey S, Smith G, Logan J, et al. GABAergic inhibition of endogenous dopamine release measured in vivo with 11c- raclopride and positron emission tomography. J Neurosci 1992; 12(10):3773–3780.
27. Dewey SL, Chaurasia CS, Chen CE, et al. GABAergic attenuation of cocaine-induced dopamine release and locomotor activity. Synapse 1997; 25(4):393–398.
28. Gerasimov MR, Ashby CR Jr., Gardner EL, et al. Gamma-vinyl GABA inhibits methamphetamine, heroin, or ethanol-induced increases in nucleus accumbens dopamine. Synapse 1999; 34(1):11–19.
29. Kushner SA, Dewey SL, Kornetsky C. The irreversible gamma-aminobutyric acid (GABA) transaminase inhibitor gamma-vinyl-GABA blocks cocaine self-administration in rats. J Pharmacol Exp Ther 1999; 290(2):797–802.
30. Roberts DC, Andrews MM, Vickers GJ. Baclofen attenuates the reinforcing effects of cocaine in rats. Neuropsychopharmacology 1996; 15(4):417–423.
31. Morgan AE, Dewey SL. Effects of pharmacologic increases in brain GABA levels on cocaine-induced changes in extracellular dopamine. Synapse 1998; 28(1):60–65.
32. Brodie JD, Figueroa E, Laska EM, et al. Safety and efficacy of gamma-vinyl GABA (GVG) for the treatment of methamphetamine and/or cocaine addiction. Synapse 2005; 55(2):122–125.
33. Manuchehri K, Goodman S, Siviter L, et al. A controlled study of vigabatrin and visual abnormalities. Br J Ophthalmol 2000; 84(5):499–505.
34. Schmitz B, Schmidt T, Jokiel B, et al. Visual field constriction in epilepsy patients treated with vigabatrin and other antiepileptic drugs: a prospective study. J Neurol 2002; 249 (4):469–475.
35. Schachter S. Tiagabine. Epilepsia 1999; 40:S17–S22.
36. Gonzalez G, Sevarino K, Sofuoglu M, et al. Tiagabine increases cocaine-free urines in cocaine-dependent methadone-treated patients: results of a randomized pilot study. Addiction 2003; 98(11):1625–1632.
37. Gonzalez G, Desai R, Sofuoglu M, et al. Clinical efficacy of gabapentin versus tiagabine for reducing cocaine use among cocaine dependent methadone-treated patients. Drug Alcohol Depend 2007; 87:1–9.
38. Kuzniecky R, Hetherington H, Ho S, et al. Topiramate increases cerebral GABA in healthy humans. Neurology 1998; 51(2):627–629.
39. Petroff OA, Hyder F, Mattson RH, et al. Topiramate increases brain GABA, homocarnosine, and pyrrolidinone in patients with epilepsy. Neurology 1999; 52(3):473–478.
40. Gibbs J, Sombati S, DeLorenzo R, et al. Cellular actions of topiramate: blockade of kainate-evoked inward currents in cultured hippocampal neurons. Epilepsia 2000; (suppl 1):S10–S16.

41. Cornish JL, Kalivas PW. Glutamate transmission in the nucleus accumbens mediates relapse in cocaine addiction. J Neurosci 2000; 20(RC89):1–5 (rapid communication).
42. Kampman KM, Pettinati H, Lynch KG, et al. A pilot trial of topiramate for the treatment of cocaine dependence. Drug Alcohol Depend 2004; 75(3):233–240.
43. McElroy SL, Keck PE Jr. Pharmacologic agents for the treatment of acute bipolar mania. Biol Psychiatry 2000; 48(6):539–557.
44. Regier DA, Farmer ME, Rae DS, et al. Comorbidity of mental disorders with alcohol and other drug abuse. Results from the Epidemiologic Catchment Area (ECA) Study. JAMA 1990; 264(19):2511–2518 (comment).
45. Brady KT, Sonne SC, Malcolm RJ, et al. Carbamazepine in the treatment of cocaine dependence: subtyping by affective disorder. Exp Clin Psychopharmacol 2002; 10(3): 276–285.
46. Brown ES, Nejtek VA, Perantie DC, et al. Lamotrigine in patients with bipolar disorder and cocaine dependence. J Clin Psychiatry 2003; 64(2):197–201.
47. Brown ES, Perantie DC, Dhanani N, et al. Lamotrigine for bipolar disorder and comorbid cocaine dependence: a replication and extension study. J Affect Disord 2006; 93(1–3):219–222.

15 Antiepileptics as Potential Aids to Smoking Cessation

Robert M. Anthenelli
Tri-State Tobacco and Alcohol Research Center, Department of Psychiatry, University of Cincinnati College of Medicine and Cincinnati Veterans Affairs Medical Center, Cincinnati, Ohio, U.S.A.

Jaimee L. Heffner and Candace S. Johnson
Tri-State Tobacco and Alcohol Research Center, Department of Psychiatry, University of Cincinnati College of Medicine, Cincinnati, Ohio, U.S.A.

INTRODUCTION

Cigarette smoking is endemic among individuals with psychiatric disorders, and it is estimated that such persons smoke approximately 45% of the cigarettes sold in the United States (1). Smoking prevalence rates and how heavily a person smokes are positively correlated with the number of psychiatric diagnoses an individual reports (1). Thus, patients with serious mental illnesses (i.e., bipolar disorder and schizophrenia) comorbid with substance use disorders represent one of the most deeply entrenched subpopulations of smokers that mental health professionals and tobacco specialists will treat.

As evidenced by the breadth of diagnoses covered in this book, psychiatrists have grown comfortable using antiepileptic drugs (AEDs) to treat many different psychiatric disorders. However, the notion of using anticonvulsants as potential aids to smoking cessation has received relatively less consideration. The purpose of this chapter is to provide the reader with a pharmacological rationale as to why AEDs may have use in treating nicotine dependence and to review the few pilot studies that have been conducted to date, which show promise for this new strategy.

PHARMACOLOGICAL RATIONALE

GABA/Glutamate Modulation of Nicotine-Induced Dopamine Release

Like other drugs of abuse, nicotine stimulates the mesocorticolimbic dopamine reinforcement circuit (2). This circuitry, which has been conserved throughout evolution in all higher animals, seems primarily involved with reinforcing life's natural rewards such as motivating feeding and sexual behaviors to enhance the species' chances for survival (3). At its core are dopamine neurons located in the ventral tegmental area (VTA), which send their projections rostrally to areas of the cortex [e.g., medial prefrontal cortex (PFC)] and limbic system [e.g., nucleus accumbens (Nacc)] (Fig. 1). These dopamine neurons receive inputs from a variety of neurotransmitters and neuromodulators, but, as depicted in the figure, of central importance to one's understanding of how AEDs affect this circuitry are stimulatory inputs from glutamatergic and cholinergic afferents and inhibitory signals from GABAergic interneurons and more remote sites.

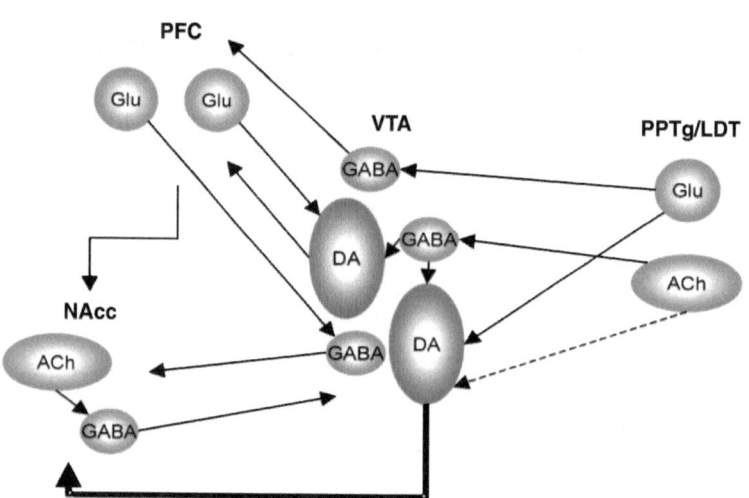

FIGURE 1   Nicotine's stimulatory effects on the brain's reward circuitry. In this simplified schematic of brain reward center connectivity, dopamine (DA), acetylcholine (ACh), GABA, and glutamate (Glu) neurons are illustrated in select brain nuclei involved in drug reward. Nicotinic acetylcholine receptors (nAChRs) that usually bind ACh from cholinergic projections originating in the pedunculopontine tegmental and laterodorsal tegmental nuclei (PPTg/LDT) are commandeered by exogenous nicotine in tobacco smoke to reinforce nicotine intake and smoking-related behaviors. Antiepileptic drugs such as topiramate may counterbalance some of nicotine's effects. *Abbreviations*: VTA, ventral tegmental area; Nacc, nucleus accumbens; PFC, prefrontal cortex. *Source*: From Ref. 4.

Electrophysiological studies have demonstrated that nicotine stimulates dopamine release in the Nacc in at least three ways (4). First, nicotine from exogenous cigarette smoke binds to nicotinic acetylcholine receptors (nAChRs) located on the VTA dopamine cell bodies to directly promote dopamine release (4). Second, nAChRs located on the terminals of excitatory glutamatergic projections synapsing on VTA dopamine neurons are stimulated by nicotine, leading to the efflux of glutamate and its subsequent stimulation of dopamine release. Third, in what appears to be a two-step process that most likely involves the release of endocannabinoids (5), long-loop and interneuronal GABAergic inputs on VTA dopamine neurons are desensitized. This desensitization of inhibitory GABAergic signaling, combined with the additive stimulatory effects of the glutamatergic and cholinergic systems, summate to favor excitation of dopamine neurons in response to nicotine. The net result of these neurochemical events is the reinforcement of nicotine intake and those smoking behaviors that caused it.

In addition to these mechanisms through which nicotine produces its rewarding effects, the deficits in brain reward function found during nicotine withdrawal have been proposed as another important factor that contributes to nicotine addiction (6). Here again, glutamatergic and, possibly, GABAergic modulation of the mesocorticolimbic system is believed to play a prominent role. Regarding the former, Markou and colleagues have found that presynaptic group II metabotropic glutamate (mGluII) receptors and postsynaptic ionotropic α-amino-3-hydroxy-5-methyl-4-isoxazoleproprionate (AMPA)/kainate receptors play important roles in modulating reward deficits in an animal model simulating aspects of nicotine withdrawal (6,7). Blocking excitatory glutamatergic and enhancing GABAergic neurotransmission appear to also dampen nicotine and other drug (alcohol and opiates) withdrawal states, and this may involve effects on norepinephrinergic activity in the locus coeruleus (8).

In summary, while other neurotransmitters and modulators are clearly involved (9), it is the confluence of GABAergic, glutamatergic, and cholinergic inputs on the mesocorticolimbic dopamine system, which plays an important role in mediating nicotine's reinforcing properties. These same systems appear to be involved in the aversive withdrawal syndrome that accompanies nicotine abstinence. Thus, in the next section, it should become clear why certain AEDs, which affect the balance of excitatory glutamatergic and inhibitory GABAergic neurotransmission, may play a role in the treatment of nicotine dependence.

Anticonvulsants' Effects on GABA/Glutamate Balance

The traditional (i.e., phenobarbital, primidone, phenytoin, carbamazepine, and valproate) and "new" AEDs (i.e., felbamate, gabapentin, lamotrigine, topiramate, tiagabine, levetiracetam, oxcarbazepine, and zonisamide) share some overlapping features in mechanisms of action, but the second generation of anticonvulsants is most relevant to this discussion. Among these newer agents, a MEDLINE search of these drugs with the keywords nicotine, tobacco, smoking cessation, and cigarettes revealed 34 articles, from which two of the new AEDs became the focus of our investigation.

Gabapentin (Neurontin™)

First approved by the U.S. Food and Drug Administration (FDA) as an AED in 1993, gabapentin is primarily used off-label for a variety of pain and psychiatric syndromes discussed elsewhere in this textbook (10). Structurally analogous to gamma-aminobutryic acid (GABA), its precise mechanism of action in humans is not known. However, preclinical studies provide evidence that it inhibits glutamate release and enhances GABA concentrations in the brain (11).

In 2001, two case reports from different groups hypothesized that gabapentin might have use as an aid to smoking cessation. Crockford et al., in a report on gabapentin's use in the treatment of benzodiazepine withdrawal, noticed that in addition to blunting cravings for benzodiazepines, this AED also blocked urges to smoke cigarettes in a woman with a combination of benzodiazepine dependence and anxiety (12). In a similar vein, Myrick and colleagues reported that gabapentin decreased nicotine withdrawal symptoms and craving in a man who abused homemade nicotine nasal spray (13). These anecdotal clinical observations, along with the hypothesis that GABAergic facilitators should have benefit in nicotine addiction (14), have led to two small pilot studies of gabapentin for smoking cessation described below.

Following up on their clinical observations, the Canadian group mentioned above conducted a single-site, six-week, randomized, open-label pilot study of gabapentin (1800 mg/day) versus bupropion slow release (SR) (150 mg b.i.d.) in 36 women (61%) and men (39%) motivated to quit smoking. The purpose of the trial was to determine an effect size for gabapentin in a subsequent, more definitive comparison study (15). Although the study was not adequately powered to detect significant differences between gabapentin- and bupropion SR-treated participants, more patients treated with the FDA-approved smoking cessation aid quit smoking

(5 of 19 or 26.3%) compared with those smokers treated with the investigational medication (1 of 17 or 5.9%). Reductions in withdrawal severity also favored bupropion SR; however, gabapentin was associated with fewer dropouts due to adverse events (12%) than the first-line agent (26%). Although the study lacked a placebo control group, the authors characterized the cessation rate with gabapentin as "disappointing[ly]" low.

Sood and colleagues were more optimistic when interpreting the results of their eight-week, single-arm, open-label trial of gabapentin (up to 1800 mg/day) as an aid to smoking cessation in 50 female (56%) and male (44%) chronic smokers. Like the previous study, the trial was designed to estimate the effect size of this AED in initiating smoking abstinence, but the authors also explored the drug's effects on tobacco withdrawal, including urges to smoke. They found an end-of-treatment, seven-day point prevalence abstinence rate of 28%, and that 24% of smokers were able to achieve at least four weeks of carbon monoxide (CO)-confirmed continuous abstinence. At six months, the weekly point prevalence and prolonged smoking abstinence rates were 20% and 16%, respectively. Although the overall nicotine withdrawal score post treatment did not significantly differ from baseline, self-reported desire to smoke was significantly lower. Of interest to our own work presented later in this chapter, the Mayo group also found a modestly robust [odds ratio (OR) = 2.1] but nonsignificant association between gender and the likelihood of achieving abstinence with male gabapentin-treated participants faring better than women. Impressed with the medication's tolerability and compliance, the authors concluded that gabapentin may promote smoking abstinence and that further placebo-controlled, randomized clinical trials were warranted (11).

In summary, anecdotal case reports and at least one small pilot study in smokers motivated to quit indicate that gabapentin may have some potential to promote smoking abstinence, but the results are mixed. While the unimpressive results observed in the White et al. study compared with the Sood et al. report might be explained by methodological differences and that first study's choice to compare the anticonvulsant with a first-line approved medication in an open-label fashion, the small sample sizes and the lack of placebo-controlled groups limit the interpretability of both trials.

Topiramate (Topamax™)

Topiramate is a broad-spectrum AED first approved for use as an anticonvulsant in 1996. It was subsequently approved by the FDA for use in migraine prophylaxis, and its appetite-suppressing and weight loss effects have led to randomized clinical trials in obesity as well. More recently, this medication has been considered as a novel treatment for a variety of substance use disorders including alcohol (16,17), cocaine (18), and opiate dependence (19).

Topiramate has multiple mechanisms of action that include: (*i*) sodium and calcium channel blockade, (*ii*) glutamate receptor antagonism, (*iii*) GABA potentiation, and (*iv*) carbonic anhydrase (CA-II and CA-IV) inhibition (10,20). However, for purposes of this discussion on nicotine dependence, it is topiramate's effects as an AMPA/kainate receptor antagonist (21) and allosteric modulator of the GABA$_A$ receptor (22) that appear to underlie its glutamate inhibitory and GABA facilitatory effects, respectively. The medication also has compelling weight loss properties (23). While the precise molecular mechanisms underlying these effects on body weight remain unknown, central effects on hypothalamic neuropeptide-Y Y1 and

Y5 receptors, corticotropin-releasing hormone (24), and lateral hypothalamic AMPA/kainate-mediated feeding behaviors (25) may play a role. Moreover, topiramate appears to have clear-cut peripheral effects on energy balance, perhaps by regulating hepatic expression of genes involved in lipid metabolism (26).

Preclinical evidence for topiramate as a potential pharmacotherapy for nicotine dependence. Dewey and colleagues were the first group to speculate that topiramate may have a role in treating tobacco dependence (27). Following up on work they had performed using gamma-vinyl GABA, which blocks GABA degradation (14), these investigators used microdialysis techniques to measure nicotine-induced increases in monoamine release in the Nacc region of rats following pretreatment with topiramate. They found that topiramate pretreatment significantly inhibited nicotine-induced increases in dopamine and norepinephrine, but not serotonin activity (27). Furthermore, these effects were maintained even in sensitized animals. However, as we will see below, it was not until several years later that clinical researchers picked up on this preclinical speculation and tested it in human laboratory paradigms and clinical trials.

Human laboratory studies of topiramate and nicotine. Sofuoglu et al. conducted a double-blind, placebo-controlled, crossover laboratory study of topiramate's effects on hemodynamic and subjective drug effects in 12 smokers who came to the laboratory after an overnight smoking abstinence period (8). On each of the three experimental days, participants received either placebo, topiramate 25 mg, or topiramate 50 mg in a noncounterbalanced order (i.e., the 50-mg topiramate dose always followed the 25-mg dose). Two hours later, participants received a saline injection followed by 0.5 and 1.0 mg/70 kg IV nicotine. They found that topiramate at a dose of 50 mg significantly attenuated heart rate increases induced by nicotine as compared with 25 mg or placebo. Compared with placebo, topiramate also enhanced several ratings of subjective effects of nicotine that included "drug strength" and "drug liking" (8). They interpreted the dose-dependent cardiovascular effects as possibly due to topiramate's blockade of AMPA/kainate receptors in the locus coeruleus decreasing norepinephrinergic tone. Interestingly, citing preclinical work that topiramate enhances dopamine release in the prefrontal cortexes of rats (28), these authors speculated that topiramate might work to counterbalance the deficits in reward threshold associated with nicotine withdrawal (8). While the extent to which the results from this small, preliminary human laboratory study apply to topiramate as an aid to smoking cessation are debatable, the speculation that topiramate might work primarily to attenuate nicotine withdrawal warrants further consideration.

A larger study of 25 male and 15 female smokers who underwent laboratory testing following a subacute administration of topiramate over a nine-day treatment period (up to a maximum dosage of 75 mg/day) found little evidence to support the hypothesis that topiramate may be effective for smoking cessation. In this randomized, placebo-controlled study, participants were rapidly titrated up to 75 mg of topiramate achieving a final dose of 75 mg for the last two days. On the testing day, and after a three-hour period of smoking abstinence, participants underwent cue reactivity and cigarette smoking test paradigms with brief 30-minute breaks between the neutral and active cigarette cue sessions and cigarette smoking session, respectively (29). The investigators found that topiramate-treated participants ($N = 19$) endorsed more withdrawal symptoms following a three-hour abstinence period compared with the self-reports of withdrawal symptomatology obtained nine days previously and evaluated 30 minutes after ad lib smoking [i.e., 2 (nonabstinent vs. abstinent) by 2 (topiramate vs. placebo) analysis of variance (ANOVA) results were positive at $p < 0.05$] (29). Furthermore, topiramate-treated participants endorsed higher levels of "reward" on the five-item Cigarette Evaluation Questionnaire that assessed the subject's response to a smoked cigarette. The authors concluded that their findings call into "question the utility of topiramate treatment for smoking cessation."

In summary, the results of two small, laboratory-based studies evaluating acute and subacute effects of low-dose topiramate on intravenous nicotine cue reactivity and controlled smoking, respectively, do not provide much evidence to support topiramate's use as an aid to smoking cessation. However, as the reader will observe in the next section, the findings from these laboratory studies run counter to the more promising results observed in clinical trials. We think that several factors influence the predictive validity of these laboratory studies. First, the dosages of topiramate used were likely subtherapeutic to adequately test its effects. Second, the acute and subacute topiramate administration schemes do not come close to approximating the six- or eight-week dosage titration schedules followed by our group (30–32) or that of Johnson et al. (33), respectively, in the preliminary clinical trials. Third, it is possible that the increase in withdrawal symptoms observed in the study by Reid et al. (29) represents acute or subacute drug effects rather than frank nicotine withdrawal phenomena. Finally, neither of the laboratory studies considered potential gender differences in the interpretation of their results, which, as we hope to demonstrate below, may have profound effects on topiramate's efficacy in smoking.

Clinical trials of topiramate as a potential aid to smoking cessation.   Johnson and colleagues were the first group to report that topiramate (up to a maximal dosage of 300 mg daily) promoted spontaneous smoking abstinence in alcohol-dependent individuals who had taken the drug to help them quit drinking (33). Specifically, these investigators performed a secondary data analysis on the 94 smokers who participated in the larger ($N = 150$) alcoholism clinical trial. The topiramate-treated smokers ($N = 45, 76\%$ men) and placebo group ($N = 45, 73\%$ men) were similar on baseline cotinine concentrations and self-reported number of days on which cigarettes were smoked in the three months prior to randomization; however, the topiramate group reported significantly greater daily drinking rates at baseline than participants receiving placebo. Two outcome measures were used to determine smoking abstinence: (*i*) weekly self-reports of any smoking using the Timeline Follow-back technique and (*ii*) serum cotinine levels at weeks 0, 3, 6, 9, and 12. Using the former outcome measure in a main effects repeated-measures analysis, the investigators reported that topiramate-treated alcoholic smokers were greater than four times more likely to "achieve self-reported abstinence" than those individuals receiving placebo (OR = 4.46, 95% CI = 1.08–18.39, $p = 0.04$). On the basis of a dichotomized serum cotinine concentration cut-off score to distinguish smokers versus nonsmokers, the advantage of topiramate over placebo appeared even larger (OR = 4.97, 95% CI = 1.1–23.4, $p = 0.04$).

These results are noteworthy because the study was not designed to enroll participants who were motivated to quit smoking; but rather, only recruited individuals who sought to reduce or abstain from drinking. Moreover, while all study participants received a weekly, 20-minute compliance enhancement therapy intended to enhance medication adherence, no formal advice to quit smoking or concomitant psychosocial intervention to aid quitting was delivered. Furthermore, while topiramate-associated reductions in alcohol drinking were related to the odds of smoking abstinence (OR = 1.04, 95% CI = 1.01–1.06, $p = 0.02$), the authors made a compelling argument that decreased drinking alone could not explain the strength of the results (33). While the ORs obtained are most likely inflated because of the unorthodox outcome measures utilized (e.g., defining nonsmoking using a cutoff serum cotinine concentration of 28 ng/mL, not assessing daily smoking or measuring expired CO levels at each weekly visit), this naturalistic change in smoking behavior observed in alcoholic patients treated with topiramate is consistent with observations made by other investigators who have used this drug in other patient groups (Susan L. McElroy and Paul E. Keck Jr., personal communication).

Khazaal et al. reported results from a nonrandomized, uncontrolled flexible dose study of 13 smokers (10 of whom expressed a desire to quit smoking) who were prescribed topiramate for a variety of reasons (34). Although further limited by the lack of any biochemical verification of abstinence, these investigators reported that 46% of topiramate-treated patients were abstinent at 60 days and that an additional two subjects had reduced their smoking by greater than 50%. Although severely hampered by the obvious design and methodological issues, when combined with the provocative findings of Johnson et al. (33), it seems reasonable to conclude, as these authors did, that controlled randomized trials were needed to confirm their preliminary observations.

The first controlled clinical trial of topiramate to aid smoking cessation. On the basis of an idea proposed by Drs. McElroy and Keck and in collaboration with these investigators, Anthenelli et al. conducted the first randomized, double-blind, placebo-controlled trial of topiramate (up to 200 mg daily) in nonalcoholic smokers who were motivated to quit smoking. The purpose of this preliminary study was to determine the feasibility, efficacy, and safety of this AED in initiating short-term smoking abstinence.

As described in detail elsewhere (30–32), 49 female and 38 male smokers ($N = 87$) who smoked an average of 10 or more cigarettes a day in the past 60 days were randomized 1:1 to either topiramate or placebo. Study medication was gradually titrated up to a maximal target dosage of 200 mg daily taken in divided doses using the titration schedule described in Table 1.

TABLE 1 Double Blind Topiramate/Placebo Dosing-Titration Schedule

Study day	Study medication		Total daily dose	
	25 mg tablets	100 mg tablets	Topiramate	Placebo
1–7	1 tablet h.s.		25 mg	Matching tablet(s)
8–14	1 tablet b.i.d. (a.m./p.m.)		50 mg	
15–21	2 tablets a.m./1 tablet p.m.		75 mg	
22–28	2 tablets b.i.d. (a.m./p.m.)		100 mg	
29–35	3 tablets b.i.d. (a.m./p.m.)		150 mg	
36–42		1 tablet b.i.d. (a.m./p.m.)	200 mg	

In this 11-week, single-site trial, a five-week maintenance period followed the six-week titration period. The target quit date was set for day 42, allowing one week of steady state concentrations of topiramate at the maximal dosage to be reached. To be similar with recommendations issued by the Society for Research on Nicotine and Tobacco Workgroup on Abstinence Measures (35), a one-week grace period was allowed, with the primary efficacy end point defined as a minimum of four weeks of prolonged abstinence during weeks 8 to 11 of the trial. Self-reported continuous abstinence was assessed at each weekly visit and verified by expired CO breath levels of less than or equal to 10 ppm. In addition to study medication, all participants received a weekly, brief (~10 minutes), manual-guided smoking cessation intervention on the basis of the principles outlined in *Clearing the Air*, the National Cancer Institute's self-help booklet (36).

Demographics and baseline characteristics of the study participants as a function of gender and treatment group are summarized in Table 2. Overall, the groups were similar on these measures, with two exceptions: (*i*) men in the placebo group smoked more heavily than placebo-treated women and (*ii*) topiramate-treated men had made significantly more prior quit attempts than women in the topiramate group. Given our interest in gender differences, these variables were included as covariates in the logistic regression results that follow.

Figure 2 depicts our main study findings. Topiramate produced gender-specific effects on smoking cessation; men on topiramate were nearly 16 times more likely to quit than women taking the mediation (38% vs. 4%, OR = 15.6, 95% CI = 1.7–146.4, $p = 0.016$). A significant overall effect on cessation was not observed at this 200 mg/day b.i.d. dosing range, however.

We also examined the effects of topiramate on nicotine withdrawal and post-smoking cessation weight change as secondary end points. Regarding the former, repeated measures ANOVA-assessing changes in weekly mean total Minnesota Nicotine Withdrawal Scale scores revealed further gender-specific effects: topiramate-treated men reported decreased withdrawal symptoms compared with topiramate-treated women [mean difference = 4.8 ± 2.2, standard error (SE), $p < 0.04$] and men taking placebo [mean difference = 4.8 ± 2.3 (SE), $p < 0.04$]. In contrast, there were no significant gender-by-treatment-interaction effects on body weight change. However, topiramate-treated individuals had an adjusted mean weight loss of 1.51 kg, while women and men taking placebo had essentially no weight change (-0.01 kg, $p < 0.0001$). On average, male cessators on placebo gained 3.30 kg, whereas topiramate led to a 0.72 kg weight loss ($p = 0.03$).

Study discontinuation rates due to adverse events were significantly higher in the topiramate group (23%) versus placebo (2%). The most commonly reported treatment-emergent adverse events in the topiramate arm were paraesthesias, fatigue, difficulty with concentration/attention, and nervousness, each of which had incidence rates greater than or equal to 10% higher than on placebo.

Taken together, we found potential gender-specific effects of topiramate as an aid to smoking cessation. Male smokers had markedly greater quit rates than female smokers, and these gender differences extended to tobacco withdrawal as well. Topiramate significantly reduced postcessation weight gain regardless of gender and the medication was generally well tolerated despite higher discontinuation rates than placebo.

In summary, preclinical findings (27), an uncontrolled open-label trial (34), and a study measuring spontaneous smoking remissions in alcohol-dependent patients (33) provided preliminary evidence that topiramate may be a potential

TABLE 2 Descriptive and Baseline Smoking and Clinical Characteristics

| | Overall (N = 87) | | Placebo (N = 44) | | | | Topiramate (N = 43) | | | | P-value[b] |
			Male (1) (N = 22)		Female (2) (N = 22)		Male (3) (N = 16)		Female (4) (N = 27)		
Age	43.7	± 9.0	45.8	± 9.1	40.9	± 9.8	44.8	± 7.7	43.7	± 8.7	0.31
BMI (kg/m²)	29.1	± 6.9	29.1	± 4.2	26.6	± 6.1	31.0	± 6.3	30.0	± 9.0	0.21
Cigarettes/day	23.8	± 9.5	28.5	± 11.7	20.2	± 7.9	25.1	± 7.9	22.3	± 8.1	0.02 (1>2)
FTND score	6.1	± 2.0	6.6	± 2.4	5.6	± 1.8	5.7	± 1.5	6.4	± 2.2	0.26
No. of previous quit attempts	2.8	± 2.6	3.5	± 3.2	2.9	± 2.0	3.8	± 3.5	1.6	± 1.3	0.02 (3>4)
Withdrawal symptoms[a] (0–40)	3.9	± 5.9	4.6	± 6.0	4.6	± 7.7	2.4	± 2.0	3.7	± 5.9	0.66
No. of Caucasians(%)	69 (79%)		20 (91%)		16 (73%)		15 (94%)		18 (67%)		0.09

Mean ± standard deviation shown except as noted.
[a] Mean total score for days −7 to −1.
[b] ANOVA F-test w/Tukey adjustment.
Abbreviations: BMI, body mass index; FTND, Fagerström Test for Nicotine Dependence; ANOVA, analysis of variance.

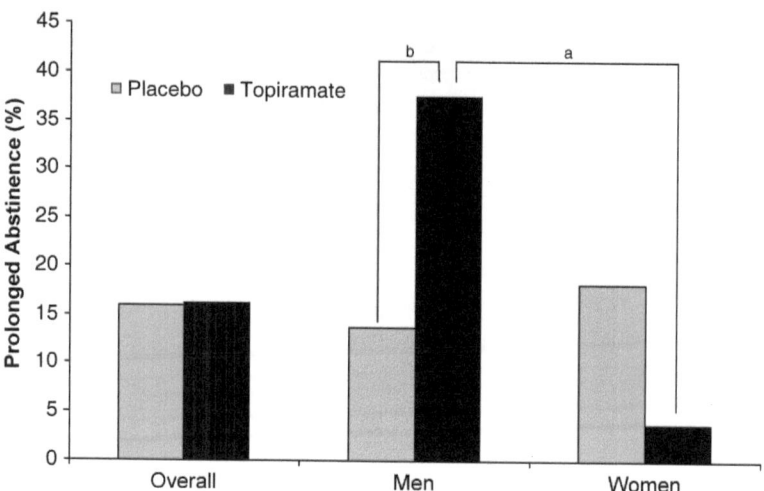

FIGURE 2 Four-week prolonged abstinence rates in smokers treated with topiramate vs. placebo. [a]Topiramate-treated men vs. topiramate-treated women, $p = 0.016$. [b]Topiramate-treated men vs. placebo-treated men, $p = 0.098$.

pharmacotherapy for tobacco dependence. In the first formal test of this hypothesis, we found that topiramate's triad of effects aiding smoking abstinence, mitigating nicotine withdrawal, and preventing postcessation weight gain make it a promising agent for treating tobacco addiction, at least in men. Further research is warranted because the causes of this gender-by-treatment-interaction effect remain to be determined and need to be interpreted cautiously, given the small sample sizes.

CONCLUSIONS

In this chapter, we have attempted to summarize findings from a growing body of studies exploring the potential utility of AEDs as aids to smoking cessation. We contend that the pharmacological rationale behind this approach is strong, but that more preclinical and clinical studies need to be performed to determine whether these medications can be used to effectively treat tobacco addiction. Clearly, there remains a need to develop alternative pharmacotherapies for nicotine dependence, and medications that have the potential to attenuate nicotine withdrawal and curb postcessation weight gain are highly desirable.

As others have suggested (8,37), we believe that AEDs for smoking cessation might have special use in dually dependent smokers—patients with nicotine as well as alcohol, cocaine, or possibly opiate dependence. Furthermore, should our preliminary findings of a gender-specific effect of topiramate as an aid to smoking cessation be substantiated, this may usher in an era of personalized treatment for tobacco addiction. Finally, as new agents with improved side-effect profiles are developed, these medications may have broader use in our battle against this pernicious disorder that plagues so many psychiatric patients.

REFERENCES

1. Lasser K, Boyd JW, Woolhandler S, et al. Smoking and mental illness: a population-based prevalence study. JAMA 2000; 284(20):2606–2610.
2. Pontieri FE, Tanda G, Orzi F, et al. Effects of nicotine on the nucleus accumbens and similarity to those of addictive drugs. Nature 1996; 382(6588):255–257.
3. Kelley AE. Memory and addiction: shared neural circuitry and molecular mechanisms. Neuron 2004; 44(1):161–179.
4. Fagen ZM, Mansvelder HD, Keath JR, et al. Short- and long-term modulation of synaptic inputs to brain reward areas by nicotine. Ann N Y Acad Sci 2003; 1003:185–195.
5. Anthenelli RM. Cannabinoid antagonists: CB1 receptors as a therapeutic target for nicotine dependence. In: George TP, ed. Medication Treatments for Nicotine Dependence. 1st ed [chap. 13]. Boca Raton, FL: Taylor & Francis, 2006:187–198.
6. Kenny PJ, Gasparini F, Markou A. Group II metabotropic and alpha-amino-3-hydroxy-5-methyl-4-isoxazole propionate (AMPA)/kainate glutamate receptors regulate the deficit in brain reward function associated with nicotine withdrawal in rats. J Pharmacol Exp Ther 2003; 306(3):1068–1076.
7. Liechti ME, Markou A. Interactive effects of the mGlu5 receptor antagonist MPEP and the mGlu2/3 receptor antagonist LY341495 on nicotine self-administration and reward deficits associated with nicotine withdrawal in rats. Eur J Pharmacol 2007; 554(2–3):164–174.
8. Sofuoglu M, Poling J, Mouratidis M, et al. Effects of topiramate in combination with intravenous nicotine in overnight abstinent smokers. Psychopharmacology (Berl) 2006; 184(3–4):645–651.
9. Watkins SS, Koob GF, Markou A. Neural mechanisms underlying nicotine addiction: acute positive reinforcement and withdrawal. Nicotine Tob Res 2000; 2(1):19–37.
10. LaRoche SM, Helmers SL. The new antiepileptic drugs: scientific review. JAMA 2004; 291(5):605–614.
11. Sood A, Ebbert JO, Schroeder DR, et al. Gabapentin for smoking cessation: a preliminary investigation of efficacy. Nicotine Tob Res 2007; 9(2):291–298.
12. Crockford D, White WD, Campbell B. Gabapentin use in benzodiazepine dependence and detoxification. Can J Psychiatry 2001; 46(3):287.
13. Myrick H, Malcolm R, Henderson S, et al. Gabapentin for misuse of homemade nicotine nasal spray. Am J Psychiatry 2001; 158(3):498.
14. Dewey SL, Brodie JD, Gerasimov M, et al. A pharmacologic strategy for the treatment of nicotine addiction. Synapse 1999; 31(1):76–86.
15. White WD, Crockford D, Patten S, et al. A randomized, open-label pilot comparison of gabapentin and bupropion SR for smoking cessation. Nicotine Tob Res 2005; 7(5):809–813.
16. Rubio G, Ponce G, Jimenez-Arriero MA, et al. Effectiveness of topiramate in control of alcohol craving. Eur Psypharmacol, 2002:S63.
17. Johnson BA, Ait-Daoud N, Bowden CL, et al. Oral topiramate for treatment of alcohol dependence: a randomised controlled trial. Lancet 2003; 361(9370):1677–1685.
18. Kampman KM, Pettinati H, Lynch KG, et al. A pilot trial of topiramate for the treatment of cocaine dependence. Drug Alcohol Depend 2004; 75(3):233–240.
19. Zullino DF, Cottier AC, Besson J. Topiramate in opiate withdrawal. Prog Neuropsychopharmacol Biol Psychiatry 2002; 26(6):1221–1223.
20. Ait-Daoud N, Malcolm RJ Jr., Johnson BA. An overview of medications for the treatment of alcohol withdrawal and alcohol dependence with an emphasis on the use of older and newer anticonvulsants. Addict Behav 2006; 31(9):1628–1649.
21. Angehagen M, Ben Menachem E, Ronnback L, et al. Topiramate protects against glutamate- and kainate-induced neurotoxicity in primary neuronal-astroglial cultures. Epilepsy Res 2003; 54(1):63–71.
22. White HS, Brown SD, Woodhead JH, et al. Topiramate modulates GABA-evoked currents in murine cortical neurons by a nonbenzodiazepine mechanism. Epilepsia 2000; 41 (suppl 1):S17–S20.

23. Wilding J, Van Gaal L, Rissanen A, et al. A randomized double-blind placebo-controlled study of the long-term efficacy and safety of topiramate in the treatment of obese subjects. Int J Obes Relat Metab Disord 2004; 28(11):1399–1410.

24. York DA, Singer L, Thomas S, et al. Effect of topiramate on body weight and body composition of Osborne-Mendel rats fed a high-fat diet: alterations in hormones, neuropeptide, and uncoupling-protein mRNAs. Nutrition 2000; 16(10):967–975.

25. Stanley BG, Ha LH, Spears LC, et al. Lateral hypothalamic injections of glutamate, kainic acid, D,L-alpha-amino-3-hydroxy-5-methyl-isoxazole propionic acid or N-methyl-D-aspartic acid rapidly elicit intense transient eating in rats. Brain Res 1993; 613(1): 88–95.

26. Liang Y, She P, Wang X, et al. The messenger RNA profiles in liver, hypothalamus, white adipose tissue, and skeletal muscle of female Zucker diabetic fatty rats after topiramate treatment. Metabolism 2006; 55(10):1411–1419.

27. Schiffer WK, Gerasimov MR, Marsteller DA, et al. Topiramate selectively attenuates nicotine-induced increases in monoamine release. Synapse 2001; 42(3):196–198.

28. Okada M, Yoshida S, Zhu G, et al. Biphasic actions of topiramate on monoamine exocytosis associated with both soluble N-ethylmaleimide-sensitive factor attachment protein receptors and Ca(2+)-induced Ca(2+)-releasing systems. Neuroscience 2005; 134(1): 233–246.

29. Reid MS, Palamar J, Raghavan S, et al. Effects of topiramate on cue-induced cigarette craving and the response to a smoked cigarette in briefly abstinent smokers. Psychopharmacology (Berl) 2007; 192(1):147–158.

30. Anthenelli RM, Blom TJ, McElroy SL, et al. A double-blind, placebo-controlled trial of topiramate as an aid to smoking cessation. Poster presented at: The 12th Annual Meeting of the Society for Research on Nicotine and Tobacco (SRNT); February, 2006; Orlando, FL.

31. Anthenelli RM, Blom TJ, Heffner JL, et al. Preliminary evidence for gender-specific effects of topiramate in smoking cessation. Poster presented at: The 13th Annual Meeting of the Society for Research on Nicotine and Tobacco (SRNT); February, 2007; Austin, TX.

32. Anthenelli RM, Blom TJ, McElroy SL, et al. Preliminary evidence for gender-specific effects of topiramate as a potential aid to smoking cessation: gender effects of topiramate in smoking cessation. Addiction 2008; 103:687–694.

33. Johnson BA, Ait-Daoud N, Akhtar FZ, et al. Use of oral topiramate to promote smoking abstinence among alcohol-dependent smokers: a randomized controlled trial. Arch Intern Med 2005; 165(14):1600–1605.

34. Khazaal Y, Cornuz J, Bilancioni R, et al. Topiramate for smoking cessation. Psychiatry Clin Neurosci 2006; 60(3):384–388.

35. Hughes JR, Keely JP, Niaura RS, et al. Measures of abstinence in clinical trials: issues and recommendations. Nicotine Tob Res 2003; 5(1):13–25.

36. US Department of Health and Human Services. Clearing the Air (NIH Publication No. 03-1647). Bethesda, MD: National Cancer Institute, 2003.

37. Johnson BA. Topiramate-induced neuromodulation of cortico-mesolimbic dopamine function: a new vista for the treatment of comorbid alcohol and nicotine dependence? Addict Behav 2004; 29(7):1465–1479.

16 Antiepileptic Drugs in Obesity, Psychotropic-Associated Weight Gain, and Eating Disorders

Susan L. McElroy, Anna I. Guerdjikova, and Paul E. Keck, Jr.
Lindner Center of HOPE, Mason, and Department of Psychiatry, University of Cincinnati College of Medicine, Cincinnati, Ohio, U.S.A.

Harrison G. Pope, Jr. and James I. Hudson
Department of Psychiatry, Harvard Medical School, Boston, and McLean Hospital, Belmont, Massachusetts, U.S.A.

INTRODUCTION

Obesity, psychotropic-associated weight gain, and eating disorders are each important public health problems that overlap, especially in clinical populations. Although the degree, nature, and causes of this overlap are not well understood, antiepileptic drugs (AEDs) are increasingly being used in the treatment of these three conditions. In this chapter, we review the data supporting the effectiveness of various AEDs in the treatment of patients with obesity, psychotropic-associated weight gain, and eating disorders. We then discuss some of the theoretic implications of the usefulness of these agents for these three conditions.

OBESITY

Obesity, an excess of body fat, is most often clinically defined by the body mass index (BMI), which is calculated by dividing weight (in kilograms) by the square of height (in meters) (1–4). According to most medical guidelines, obesity in adults is a BMI greater than or equal to 30 kg/m^2 and extreme (morbid) obesity is a BMI greater than or equal to 40 kg/m^2. Overweight is a BMI of 25 to less than 30 kg/m^2, normal weight is a BMI 18.5 to less than 25 kg/m^2, and underweight is a BMI less than or equal to 18.5 kg/m^2. In children and adolescents, overweight is often defined as a BMI for age more than or equal to the sex-specific 95th percentile (5).

The prevalence of obesity has substantially increased worldwide over the past 30 years. The most recent prevalence estimates based on national height and weight measurements in 2003–2004 found that 32.2% of United States (U.S.) adults were obese and 17.1% of children and adolescents were overweight (5). Importantly, the prevalence of extreme obesity may be increasing at a much faster rate among adults in the U.S. than is the prevalence of moderate obesity (4,6).

Obesity is presently viewed as a chronic heterogeneous metabolic disease that, in most cases, is due to genetic factors adversely interacting with a sedentary, overly caloric environment (4,7,8). It is associated with numerous medical conditions (including cardiovascular disease, hypertension, dyslipidemias, type 2 diabetes, and many cancers), disability, and an increased risk for premature death (1–4,9).

Although obesity is currently viewed primarily as a medical illness and is not listed in the Diagnostic and Statistical Manual of Mental Disorders, 4th edition (DSM-IV) (10), it has also been conceptualized as a stress-sensitive psychosomatic disorder that may be related to some forms of mental illness (11,12). Thus, clinical studies have repeatedly shown that obesity patients seeking weight loss treatment have elevated rates of psychopathologic symptoms and mental disorders, especially mood, eating, and anxiety disorders (11–14). Recent methodologically rigorous epidemiologic studies have confirmed that obesity is associated with mood, anxiety, and binge eating disorders (15–19). Data from the National Comorbidity Survey-Replication (NCS-R) finding associations between obesity and mood disorders with odds ratios in the range of 1.2 to 1.5 lead the authors to conclude that nearly 25% of cases of obesity in the general population were attributable to the association with mood disorders (16). In addition, because most people with obesity are unable to stop overeating despite its deleterious consequences, obesity has also been conceptualized as an addiction to food (20). It has therefore been suggested that obesity, or at least some of its aspects, be included in the DSM-V as a brain disorder (20,21).

Pharmacotherapy of Obesity

Currently available antiobesity drugs can be broadly categorized into agents that reduce food intake by acting on the central nervous system (CNS) (appetite suppressants) and those that modify fat absorption or otherwise alter metabolism (metabolic agents) (22–27). The former includes the noradrenergic agents phentermine, mazindol, and diethylpropion, the monoamine reuptake inhibitor sibutramine, and the selective cannabinoid-1 receptor antagonist rimonabant. The latter includes the lipase inhibitor orlistat. Phetermine, mazindol, and diethylpropion are approved by the U.S. Food and Drug Administration (FDA) for short-term use in obesity (e.g., for acute weight loss only), whereas sibutramine and orlistat are also approved for long-term use (e.g., for both acute weight loss and maintenance of weight loss). Rimonabant is currently available in more than 30 countries in Europe, America, and Asia, but an FDA advisory panel of outside experts unanimously recommended in June, 2007, that the drug not be approved for sale in the United States because of safety concerns related to psychiatric and neurologic side effects, especially depression and suicidality (26,28).

Most guidelines recommend that weight loss drugs be used for patients with a BMI greater than or equal to 30, and for patients with a BMI greater than or equal to 27 who have concomitant obesity-related risk factors or diseases (1,2). It is also recommended that these drugs be used in combination with behavioral weight management.

The amount of weight loss attributed to available antiobesity drugs is modest—typically less than 5 kg at one year (22,25–27). This weight loss is often associated with metabolic benefits but may also be associated with problematic side effects. Sibutramine is associated with small improvements in glycemic control but with modest increases in heart rate and blood pressure (22–26). Orlistat is associated with small improvements in blood pressure, lipid profiles, and fasting blood glucose but with an increase in adverse gastrointestinal events (22–26). Rimonabant is associated with improvement in waist circumference, HDL-cholesterol, triglycerides, blood pressure, and insulin resistance, but an increase in gastrointestinal, neurologic, and psychiatric side effects (26–28). The latter include depressive and suicidal events, anxiety, psychomotor agitation, and sleep disorders.

Various psychotropics (e.g., fluoxetine, bupropion) have also been evaluated for weight loss and metabolic benefits in obesity (29,30). Although some agents show promise, none have clear advantages over available antiobesity medications, at least for obese patients without psychopathology. Thus, there is a great need for novel pharmacologic agents in the treatment of obesity (22).

Antiepileptics in Obesity

Antiepileptics studied in obesity to date in placebo-controlled trials include topiramate (31–39), zonisamide (40,41), and lamotrigine (42). Of these AEDs, topiramate has received the most systematic attention (see Table 1). Most of these studies were stimulated in part by findings that these agents were associated with weight loss in controlled clinical trials in patients with epilepsy (43).

Topiramate

Nine controlled trials have evaluated topiramate ($N = 8$) or a controlled-release formulation of topiramate ($N = 1$) for weight loss in subjects with obesity (see Table 1). In one study, subjects were required to have comorbid essential hypertension (34); in four studies, subjects were required to have concurrent type 2 diabetes (36–39). In all nine studies, topiramate was superior to placebo for weight loss at all doses (range 64–400 mg/day) and at all end points (range 28 weeks–1 year) evaluated. A meta-analysis of six of these studies reported that mean weight loss for topiramate at six months was 6.5% above placebo (CI, 4.8% to 8.3%) ($I^2 = 87\%$; $p < 0.001$ for heterogeneity) (22,31–35,39). The four long-term studies (durations 40 weeks–1 year) showed that topiramate was associated with weight loss that increased for up to one year without plateauing (32,33,37,39). If replicated in future studies, this finding is notable because it would distinguish topiramate from other currently available antiobesity medications, the weight loss effects of which usually plateau after six months of treatment.

In the study of topiramate in obese subjects with comorbid hypertension, there were significant decreases in diastolic, but not systolic, blood pressure in the two groups receiving topiramate compared with the placebo group (34). In all four studies of topiramate in obese subjects with comorbid type 2 diabetes, topiramate-treated patients showed significant decreases in glycosylated hemoglobin (HbA1$_c$) compared with placebo-treated patients (36–39). In two of these studies, topiramate also significantly decreased urinary albumin excretion (38,39).

Several studies assessed correlates of weight reduction associated with topiramate. Topiramate-associated weight loss was found to be associated with decreased energy intake (35), decreases in measures of adiposity, such as total body fat mass and total abdominal adipose tissue (35), and improvements in some metabolic variables in healthy populations (32). The latter included significant reductions in systolic and diastolic blood pressure in normotensive subjects (32) and decreases in plasma glucose or insulin in nondiabetic subjects (32). On the other hand, in a study of 68 sedentary men with abdominal obesity, topiramate did not alter 24-hour daily energy expenditure, as evaluated by whole-body indirect calorimetry (35).

Adverse events related to the central or peripheral nervous systems or to psychiatric disorders were most commonly reported. These included paresthesias, fatigue, difficulty with attention, concentration and/or memory, taste perversion, and anorexia. In the adverse event analysis of the meta-analysis of six studies, paresthesias and changes in taste were the two events reported much more commonly in topiramate-treated patients than in placebo-treated patients (pooled odds ratio, 20.18 and 11.14, respectively; relative risk 4.92 and 9.19, respectively) (22).

In several studies, depression and/or mood problems were reported to be more common with topiramate than placebo, usually with the highest topiramate

TABLE 1 Randomized, Placebo-Controlled Trials of Topiramate for Weight Loss in Obesity

Study	N[a]	TPM dose(s) (mg/day)	Duration	Findings
Bray et al., 2003	385 healthy obese subject (BMI 30–49.9) or overweight/obese subjects with controlled hypertension or dyslipidemia (BMI 27–49.9)[a,b]	64, 96, 192, 384	6 mo	Mean baseline weight loss at 24 wk was 5.0%, 4.8%, 6.3%, and 6.3% in the 64, 96, 192, and 384 mg/day TPM groups, respectively, compared with 2.6% in the PBO group ($p < 0.05$ from wk 4)
Wilding et al., 2004	1289 healthy obese subjects (BMI 30–49.9) or overweight/obese subjects with controlled hypertension or dyslipidemia (BMI 27–49.9)	96, 192, 256	1 yr	Mean baseline weight loss was 7.0%, 9.1%, and 9.7% in the 96, 192, and 256 mg/day TPM groups, respectively, compared with 1.7% in the PBO group ($p < 0.001$). TPM was also associated with improvement in blood pressure and glucose tolerance
Astrup et al., 2004	561 obese subjects (BMI 30–49.9) who lost ≥ 8% of their enrollment weight on an 8-wk low-calorie run-in phase; 293 analyzed for efficacy[a,b]	96, 192	44 wk	Subjects receiving TPM lost 15.4% (96 mg/day) and 16.5% (192 mg/day) of their enrollment weight at wk 44 compared with 8.9% in the PBO group ($p < 0.001$). Also, significantly more TPM subjects lost 5%, 10%, and 15% of their randomization weight than PBO patients
Tonstad et al., 2005	531 overweight/obese subjects (BMI 27–50) with hypertension	96, 192	28 wk	Mean weight loss from baseline for the PBO, 96, and 192 mg/day groups were 1.9%, 5.9%, 6.5%, respectively ($p < 0.0001$ for both comparisons with PBO). Decreases in diastolic, but not systolic, blood pressure were significant for both TPM doses
Tremblay et al., 2007	68 abdominally obese men (BMI 27–40)	400	6 mo	Mean weight loss from baseline at 6 mo was 3.2 kg in the TPM group compared with a mean weight gain of 1.1 kg in the PBO group ($p < 0.01$)
Eliasson et al., 2007	38 obese patients with T2DM (BMI 27–50); 22 completers analyzed for efficacy[c]	96 mg b.i.d.	11 mo	Mean weight loss from baseline in TPM patients ($N = 9$) at 5,8, and 11 months was 6.0 ± 3.5, 6.8 ± 4.4, respectively, and 7.2 ± 4.3 kg compared with 0.01 ± 2.5 kg at 11 mo in PBO patients ($N = 13$) ($p < 0.0001$). TPM-treated patients also had significant decreases in HbA1$_c$ and FBG compared with PBO-treated patients

Study	Subjects	Dose (mg/day)	Duration	Results
Toplak et al., 2007	646 overweight/obese subjects (BMI 27–50) with T2DM controlled by metformin randomized; 307 analyzed for efficacy[a,b]	96,192	24 wk	Mean weight loss from baseline for the PBO, 96, and 192 mg/day groups were 1.7%, 4.5%, and 6.5%, respectively ($p < 0.001$ for both comparisons with PBO). TPM-treated patients also had significant decreases in HbA1c and systolic blood pressure.
Rosenstock et al., 2007	111 overweight/obese subjects (BMI $\geq$ 27) with T2DM treated with diet and exercise alone or with metformin[a]	175	16 wk	Mean weight loss from baseline for the PBO and TPM groups was 2.3% (2.5 kg) and 5.8% (6.0 kg), respectively ($p < 0.001$). HbA1c improved 0.4% and 0.9% for the PBO and TPM groups, respectively ($p < 0.001$). TPM also significantly reduced blood pressure and urinary albumin excretion.
Stenlof et al., 2007	535 overweight/obese subjects (BMI 27–50) with drug-naïve T2DM (HbA1c < 10.5%) who completed a 6-wk placebo run-in; 229 analyzed for efficacy[b]	96,192	40 wk	Mean weight loss from baseline at end of week 40 for the PBO, 96, and 192 mg/day groups were 2.5%, 6.6%, and 9.1%, respectively ($p < 0.001$ for both comparisons with PBO). Mean decrease in HbA1c was 0.2%, 0.6%, and 0.7%, respectively ($p < 0.001$ vs. PBO). TPM also significantly reduced blood pressure and urinary albumin excretion

[a] Subjects with psychiatric disorders specifically excluded.
[b] Subjects participated in an ancillary nonpharmacologic weight loss program.
[c] Subjects were receiving treatment of their type 2 diabetes with diet or sulfonylurea.
Abbreviations: BMI, body mass index; FBG, fasting blood glucose; HbA1c, glycosylated hemoglobin; PBO, placebo; T2DM, type 2 diabetes; TPM, topiramate.

doses used (31–33,36,38). One of these studies reported suicidal-related events, with eight (6.2%) such events occurring in topiramate-treated patients versus none in placebo-treated patients (32).

Zonisamide

To date, two controlled studies have evaluated zonisamide in obesity—one as monotherapy (40) and the other as a combination therapy with bupropion sustained release (SR) (41). A randomized, open-label study of zonisamide combined with bupropion SR in obese women has also been reported (44).

In the monotherapy study, 60 obese subjects were treated for 16 weeks with double-blind zonisamide ($N = 30$) or placebo ($N = 30$) in combination with a hypocaloric diet (40). The double-blind 16-week treatment phase was followed by an optional single-blind 16-week extension trial. Subjects' mean age was 37 years, 92% were women, and their mean BMI at baseline was 36 kg/m². Zonisamide was begun at 100 mg/day and doses were subsequently increased to a maximum of 600 mg/day on the basis of tolerability and response. Fifty-one subjects completed the 16-week acute phase; 36 completed the entire 32 weeks of treatment. The mean highest daily dose of zonisamide was 426 mg.

During the double-blind 16-week phase, subjects receiving zonisamide lost an average of 5.9 kg (6.0% of baseline body weight) compared with 0.9 kg (1.0% of baseline body weight) for subjects receiving placebo ($p < 0.001$). Seventeen (57%) of the zonisamide group and three (10%) of the placebo group lost $\geq$5% of body weight ($p < .001$) by week 16.

At week 32, the mean (SD) weight loss for the zonisamide group ($N = 19$) was 9.2 (1.7) kg (9.4% loss) compared with 1.5 (0.7) kg (1.8% loss) for the placebo group ($N = 17$). Ten (53%) of nineteen zonisamide subjects and none of the placebo subjects lost greater than or equal to 10% of body weight at week 32 ($p < 0.001$). There were also significantly greater reductions in mean waist circumference, systolic blood pressure, diastolic blood pressure, and fat mass for zonisamide-treated subjects compared with placebo-treated subjects. There were no changes in heart rate or lipid levels.

Zonisamide was well tolerated, with fatigue being the only side effect more common with zonisamide than placebo. Only one subject receiving zonisamide withdrew for an adverse effect. Mean serum creatinine levels were significantly increased with zonisamide versus placebo.

In the combination therapy study, Orexigen Therapeutics evaluated fixed dosages of zonisamide with bupropion SR in a phase II clinical trial. It was reported on the corporation's Web site that, on an intent-to-treat (ITT) basis, the combination demonstrated a mean weight loss of 5.8% at 24 weeks; on a completer basis, mean weight loss was 9.2% at 24 weeks (41). Details about dosages and adverse events were not provided.

In the open-label study, 18 obese women (mean BMI 36.8 kg/m²) were randomly assigned to receive the combination of zonisamide (increased to 400 mg/day over 4 weeks) and bupropion SR (increased to 200 mg/day after 2 weeks) ($N = 9$) or zonisamide alone ($N = 9$) for 12 weeks (44). All subjects were also prescribed a balanced hypocaloric diet. The combination group lost more body weight than the zonisamide group [mean (SE) = 7.2 (1.2) kg (7.5%) vs. 2.9 (0.7) kg (3.1%); $p = 0.003$]. Six subjects in the combination group and two in the zonisamide group lost at least 5% of body weight. Twelve subjects ($N = 7$ combination, $N = 5$ zonisamide) completed the 12-week trial; two subjects (both receiving the combination) withdrew because of neuropsychiatric side effects. There were no serious adverse events. The authors concluded that combination treatment with zonisamide in combination with bupropion SR resulted in more weight loss than treatment with zonisamide alone (44).

Lamotrigine

In the one controlled lamotrigine study, 40 obese subjects (BMI of 30 to <40) were randomly assigned to receive lamotrigine 200 mg/day or placebo for up to 26 weeks (42). There was a trend toward a decrease in body weight and a statistically significant difference in mean change in BMI from baseline to endpoint with lamotrigine compared with placebo. Mean change in body weight from baseline to endpoint was -6.4 lb $\pm$ 10.26 lbs for lamotrigine and -1.2 ± 7.09 lbs for placebo ($p = 0.062$). Mean change in BMI was -1.5 ± 2.8 for lamotrigine and -0.1 ± 1.1 for placebo ($p = 0.04$). Subjects were significantly more satisfied with lamotrigine treatment than with placebo ($p = 0.0065$). There were no differences in other secondary measures, which included change from baseline to endpoint in percent body fat, serum lipid and HbAl$_c$ values, and scores on the Impact of Weight Quality of Life scale.

Other AEDs

At least two other AEDs, felbamate and levetiracetam, have been associated with anorexia and/or weight loss in patients with epilepsy (43,45,46). However, we were unable to locate any reports of these drugs in the treatment of obesity. For felbamate, this may be due to its association with serious idiosyncratic adverse effects, including aplastic anemia and liver failure (45). For levetiracetam, this may be due to weight loss being a relatively uncommon side effect (46).

No other currently available AEDs are regularly associated with weight loss. Indeed, several agents are associated with weight gain. These include valproate, pregablin, gabapentin, vigabatrin, and, to a lesser extent, carbamazepine (43,47,48). Importantly, valproate has been associated with obesity, insulin resistance, and polycystic ovarian syndrome (PCOS), the latter especially in girls with epilepsy (43,47,49).

PSYCHOTROPIC-INDUCED WEIGHT GAIN

Many of the medications used to treat patients with mental disorders are associated with weight gain (43,47,50–56). These include most antipsychotics, many mood stabilizers, and some antidepressants. Importantly, medications associated with weight gain may also be associated with the medical complications associated with obesity, including dyslipidemias, hyperglycemia and type 2 diabetes, and hypertension (53,57,58).

There is no widely accepted operational definition of psychotropic-associated weight gain. Common definitions have been a greater than or equal to 5% or greater than or equal to 7% increase of basal body weight since medication initiation. In the emerging *Guidance for Industry Developing Products for Weight Management*, the FDA states that "patients eligible for participation in trials examining the efficacy and safety of products for the treatment of medication-induced weight gain should have a documented increase in body weight of at least 5% within 6 months of starting a drug known to cause weight gain" (59; p. 10).

    The pathogenesis of psychotropic-associated weight gain is unknown. Some factors are medication-related, as weight gain is far more likely to occur with certain medications than others. Thus, weight gain is more common with clozapine and olanzapine than other antipsychotics, and with valproate than other AEDs and lithium. However, since not all patients gain weight with a particular drug, factors related to the individual and the environment are also thought to be involved in psychotropic-associated weight gain. For example, individual factors associated with antipsychotic-induced weight gain in patients with psychotic disorders may include variations in the 5-hydroxytryptamine 2C and adrenergic α *2a* receptor genes (60) and the development of binge eating and binge eating disorder (BED) (61). For lithium-associated weight gain, such a factor in patients with bipolar disorder may be pre-existing obesity (62).

Pharmacotherapy of Psychotropic-Associated Weight Gain

Although no medication is currently approved by the FDA for the treatment of psychotropic-induced weight gain, preliminary data from double-blind, placebo-controlled trials suggest sibutramine, reboxetine, and amantadine may be helpful in reducing antipsychotic-associated weight gain, at least over the short term (56,63). Metformin may be effective for antipsychotic-associated weight gain in children and adolescents (64), but studies on its effectiveness in adults have produced mixed results (63,65). Medications that have not been efficacious in controlled trials include fluoxetine and phenylpropanolamine (56,63).

    As noted earlier, the FDA has proposed preliminary guidelines for the development of medications for drug-induced weight gain (59). The current document states these guidelines will be similar to those for developing a drug for weight loss in general. Thus, in addition to having medication-induced weight gain defined as a greater than or equal to 5% increase in body weight within six months of starting a drug known to cause weight gain, the guidelines stipulate that potential subjects have "BMIs greater than or equal to 27 kg/m^2 with comorbidities or greater than or equal to 30 kg/m^2 with or without comorbidities at the time of screening" (59; p. 10). In addition to having drug-induced weight gain, subjects must also be obese or overweight with comorbid conditions.

Antiepileptics in Psychotropic-Associated Weight Gain

Two placebo-controlled studies and one randomized, open-label trial suggest topiramate may reduce antipsychotic-induced weight gain in schizophrenia (66–68). In one controlled study, 66 inpatients with schizophrenia receiving antipsychotic medication and "carrying excess weight" (mean BMI 28.1 kg/m^2) were given topiramate 100 mg/day, topiramate 200 mg/day, or placebo for 12 weeks (66). In the topiramate 200-mg/day group, body weight, BMI, and waist and hip circumference decreased significantly compared with the topiramate 100-mg/day and placebo groups. Scores on the Clinical Global Impression-Severity (CGI-S) and the Brief Psychiatric Rating Scale (BPRS) also significantly decreased over the 12-week period, but the decreases were not thought to be clinically meaningful. The waist-to-hip ratio (WHR) did not change in any group. In the other controlled study, 43 women with mood or psychotic disorders who had gained weight while receiving olanzapine therapy were randomized to topiramate ($N = 25$) or placebo ($N = 18$) for 10 weeks (67). Weight loss was significantly greater in the topiramate-treatment group by 5.6 kg. Patients receiving topiramate also experienced significantly greater improvement in measures of health-related quality of life and psychologic impairments. In the open-label trial, 60 male outpatients with schizophrenia were randomized to receive treatment with olanzapine plus topiramate (maximum dose 50 mg b.i.d.) or olanzapine alone for 12 weeks (68). Both groups gained weight during the 12-week treatment period, but the topiramate-treated group gained significantly less weight (at weeks 4, 8, and 12).

One placebo-controlled study (69) and two comparison trials (70,71) suggest topiramate may be superior to placebo and at least as effective as bupropion and sibutramine in psychotropic-associated weight gain in patients with bipolar disorder. In the controlled study, adjunctive topiramate was ineffective for manic symptoms after 12 weeks in 287 bipolar I manic or mixed patients receiving lithium or valproate, but was associated with significantly greater reductions in body weight (-2.5 vs. 0.2 kg, $p < 0.001$) and BMI (-0.84 vs. 0.07 kg/m^2, $p < 0.001$) (69). In a single-blind comparator trial in 36 outpatients with bipolar I depression, adjunctive bupropion and topiramate each decreased both depressive symptoms and body weight after eight weeks of treatment (70). Specifically, bupropion and topiramate-treated patients showed similar rates of antidepressant responses (59% vs. 56%), but topiramate was associated with greater mean weight loss (5.8 kg vs. 1.2 kg).

In a 24-week, open-label, flexible-dose, comparison trial, 46 euthymic outpatients with a bipolar disorder (types I, II, or NOS) who had a BMI ≥ 30kg/m^2, or ≥ 27 with obesity-related comorbid medical conditions, and psychotropic-associated weight gain [defined as a weight gain of 10 lbs (4.5 kg) since initiation of their current psychotropic regimen] received topiramate ($N = 28$; 25–600 mg/day) or sibutramine ($N = 18$; 5–15 mg/day) for 24 weeks (71). Patients receiving either drug lost comparable amounts of weight (2.8 $\pm$ 3.5 kg for topiramate and 4.1 $\pm$ 5.7 kg, sibutramine) and displayed similar rates of weight loss (0.82 kg/week and 0.85 kg/week, respectively). However, only four (22%) patients receiving sibutramine and six (21%) receiving topiramate completed the trial. In addition, the attrition patterns for the two drugs were different, with patients discontinuing topiramate doing so early in treatment and patients discontinuing sibutramine doing so throughout treatment. Analyses showed that higher ratings of manic and depressive symptoms significantly increased risk for early topiramate discontinuation as compared with that for sibutramine. It was concluded that adjunctive sibutramine and topiramate may have comparable weight loss effects in overweight or obese bipolar patients with psychotropic-associated weight gain, but each were associated with similarly high discontinuation rates with different attrition profiles. Specifically, it was suggested that compared with sibutramine, topiramate discontinuation might be more likely to occur early in treatment and be more dependent upon manic and depressive symptoms.

Other data suggest topiramate may be effective in psychotropic-associated weight gain. Three open-label, prospective trials suggest that initiating treatment with the combination of topiramate with either risperidone or olanzapine may successfully stabilize mood in patients with bipolar disorder while preventing weight gain (72–74). Open-label reports also suggest the weight loss associated with adjunctive topiramate in bipolar patients may be long term and associated with improvement in metabolic variables (75,76). Finally, topiramate has been used to treat weight gain in patients with treatment-resistant major depression receiving antidepressants, patients with anxiety disorders receiving SSRIs, and patients with autism receiving antipsychotics (77–81).

To date, there are no controlled studies of other AEDs in patients with psychotropic-induced weight gain. Adjunctive treatment with zonisamide, however, was associated with weight loss in the three open-label studies of the drug in bipolar patients receiving mood stabilizers and antipsychotics that reported effects on weight (82–84). In addition, lamotrigine monotherapy has been associated with weight loss in obese patients with bipolar disorder who responded to the drug (62,85). Bowden et al. conducted a post hoc analysis to assess the weight changes in obese ($N = 155$) and nonobese ($N = 399$) bipolar I patients from two placebo-controlled, 18-month studies comparing lamotrigine with lithium (62). Among obese patients, mean changes in weight at week 52 were −4.2, +6.1, and −0.6 kg with lamotrigine, lithium, and placebo, respectively. Decreases in weight with lamotrigine were significant ($p < 0.05$) compared with placebo at weeks 20, 36, and 44; they were significant compared with lithium at weeks 12, 20, 28, 36, 44, and 52. Among nonobese patients, mean changes in weight at week 52 were −0.5, +1.1, and +0.7 with lamotrigine, lithium and placebo, respectively, with no significant differences between groups. It was concluded that obese patients with bipolar I disorder lost weight while taking lamotrigine and gained weight while taking lithium, whereas nonobese patients did not change weight with either drug. In another analysis of these same data, in which the effect of 52 weeks of lamotrigine maintenance therapy was assessed retrospectively in the entire patient group regardless of baseline weight status, mean weight remained stable with lamotrigine and placebo, but increased with lithium as compared to lamotrigine (85).

EATING DISORDERS

Two eating disorders, anorexia nervosa (anorexia) and bulimia nervosa (bulimia), are recognized as diagnostic entities in the DSM-IV, and a third, BED, is proposed in DSM-IV as a possible new diagnostic entity [and given as an example of eating disorder not otherwise specified (NOS)] (10). Pica, rumination disorder, and feeding disorders of infancy or early childhood are listed in the DSM-IV under Disorders of Feeding and Eating that are usually first diagnosed in infancy or early childhood. Night eating syndrome (NES) has been proposed to be a distinct eating disorder, but it is not mentioned in DSM-IV (86). Although there are a variety of operational definitions for NES in the literature and most include the features of morning anorexia, evening hyperphagia, and sleep disturbance, its status as a distinct diagnostic entity is controversial. Finally, sleep-related eating disorders, characterized by nocturnal eating after awakening from sleep, have been described (87). These disorders may meet DSM-IV criteria for parasomnia NOS. Some authorities have proposed that NES and sleep-related eating disorders are related and exist on a continuum (87).

Growing epidemiologic data indicate that BED may be more common than bulimia and anorexia combined. For example, the lifetime prevalence estimates of DSM-IV BED, bulimia, and anorexia from the National Comorbidity Survey Replication (NCS-R) were 2.8%, 1.0%, and 0.6%, respectively (19). In addition, 4.5% of the population had any lifetime binge eating, defined as binge eating episodes occurring at least twice a week for at least three months. Less is known about the epidemiology of pica, rumination disorder, feeding disorders of infancy or early childhood, NES, or sleep-related eating disorders (86–90). While available data suggest some of these disorders are rare, others may be more common than once thought, especially pica, rumination, and NES.

It is unknown if the prevalence of eating disorders are changing over time, but data from the NCS-R suggests that the incidence of bulimia and BED has increased with successive birth cohorts (19). Anorexia, bulimia, and BED are associated with medical morbidity, other psychiatric disorders (especially mood, anxiety, and substance use disorders), and impairment (19,91,92). Pica is similarly associated with medical complications and other psychiatric disorders (88,89). Anorexia, by definition, is associated with low body weight, whereas BED is associated with obesity, including severe obesity (18,19,91). Both genetic and environmental factors are thought to contribute to the pathophysiology of anorexia, bulimia, and BED (18,93–96).

There is a growing literature on the pharmacotherapy of eating disorders, and many patients with eating disorders receive psychotropic medications, particularly antidepressants. Several guidelines (91,97) and reviews (98–103) suggest that SSRIs are reasonable first- or second-line treatments for bulimia or BED on the basis of controlled studies showing that these drugs are superior to placebo in reducing binge eating, at least over the short term. Indeed, the only medication approved by the FDA for the treatment of an eating disorder is fluoxetine for bulimia. Several other types of antidepressants have also been shown effective for bulimia, including tricyclics, monoamine oxidase inhibitors, trazodone, and bupropion (104). All of these agents reduce purging as well as binge eating behavior. Bupropion, however, is contraindicated for bulimia, because of an elevated risk of seizures (105). Although several types of antidepressants have also been shown effective for the binge eating of BED (98–101,103), these medications are less satisfactory in inducing weight loss. By contrast, two placebo-controlled studies, including one large multicenter trial with 304 subjects, suggest sibutramine reduces both binge eating and excessive body weight in BED (106,107).

Overall, then, the available pharmacotherapeutic armamentarium for eating disorders is still less than adequate. Many patients with bulimia or BED have inadequate responses to antidepressants and other agents, and these medications have proven even less effective for anorexia (101,108,109). New medical treatments for eating disorders are therefore needed.

Antiepileptics in Eating Disorders

Topiramate, zonisamide, and carbamazepine are the AEDs that have been studied to date in randomized, placebo-controlled trials in subjects with DSM-defined eating disorders. Topiramate has been studied in two studies of bulimia (110–112) and three studies of BED (113–115); zonisamide in one study of BED (116); and carbamazepine in one study of bulimia (117–119). Phenytoin has been studied in two controlled trials of patients of various weights with compulsive or binge eating (119–121).

Topiramate

The AED that has received the most study thus far in eating disorders is topiramate. Four positive-controlled studies have shown that topiramate monotherapy reduces binge eating, other aspects of eating disorder psychopathology, and excessive body weight in 567 subjects with bulimia ($N = 2$ studies, 99 subjects) or BED ($N = 2$ studies, 468 subjects) (110–114). A fifth placebo-controlled study found topiramate added to cognitive behavior therapy (CBT) improved the effectiveness of the later, increasing remission of binge eating and weight loss, in 73 subjects with BED (115).

In the first study in bulimia, a 10-week trial in 69 subjects, topiramate (median dose 100 mg/day; range 25–400 mg/day) was superior to placebo in reducing the frequency of binge and purge days (days during which at least one binge eating or purging episode occurred; $p = 0.004$); the bulimia/uncontrollable overeating ($p = 0.005$), body dissatisfaction ($p = 0.007$), and drive for thinness ($p = 0.002$) subscales on the Eating Disorder Inventory; the bulimia/food preoccupation ($p = 0.019$) and dieting ($p = 0.031$) subscales of the Eating Attitudes Test; and body weight (mean decrease of 1.8 kg for topiramate vs. 0.2 kg increase for placebo; $p = 0.004$) (110,111). Remission rates from binge eating and/or purging were 23% for topiramate and 6% for placebo ($p = .08$). The topiramate group had a significantly greater reduction in mean Hamilton Rating scale for Anxiety (HAM-A) score then the placebo group ($p = 0.046$). The reduction in mean HAM-D score was also greater in the topiramate group but did not reach statistical significance ($p = 0.069$). Significantly more topiramate-treated subjects compared with placebo-treated subjects reported improvement on the Patient Global Improvement scale ($p = 0.004$). Dropout rates were 34% for topiramate and 47% for placebo. In the second study, 60 subjects with DSM-IV bulimia for at least 12 months received topiramate ($N = 30$) or placebo ($N = 30$) for 10 weeks (112). Topiramate was begun at 25 mg/day, titrated to 250 mg/day in the sixth week, and the dosage then held constant. Topiramate was associated with significant decreases in the frequency of binging/purging (defined as a >50% reduction; 37% for topiramate and 3% for placebo); body weight (difference in weight loss between the 2 groups = 3.8 kg); and all SF 36 Health Survey scales (all $ps < 0.001$). Five (17%) subjects on topiramate and six (20%) subjects on placebo were considered dropouts. All subjects tolerated topiramate well.

In the first controlled study in BED, 61 subjects with DSM-IV BED and obesity (defined as a BMI $\geq$ 30) received topiramate ($N = 30$) or placebo ($N = 31$) for 14 weeks (113). Topiramate was significantly superior to placebo in reducing binge frequency, as well as global severity of illness, obsessive-compulsive features of binge eating symptoms, body weight, and BMI. Topiramate-treated subjects experienced a 94% reduction in binge frequency and a mean weight loss of 5.9 kg, whereas placebo-treated subjects experienced a 46% reduction in binge frequency and a mean weight loss of 1.2 kg. Dropout rate, however, was high: 14 (47%) of subjects receiving topiramate and 12 (39%) subjects receiving placebo failed to complete the trial. The most common side effects associated with topiramate were paresthesias, dry mouth, headache, and dyspepsia.

Completers ($N = 35$) were offered participation in a 42-week open-label extension trial of topiramate (122). Forty-four patients (31 who received topiramate in the open-label trial plus 13 who received topiramate in the double-blind study only) received at least one dose of topiramate; 43 patients provided outcome measures at a median final dose of 250 mg/day. Mean weekly binge frequency declined significantly from baseline to final visit for all 43 patients (-3.2; $p < 0.001$), for the 15 patients who received topiramate during the controlled and open-label studies (-4.0; $p < 0.001$), and for the 15 patients who received topiramate only during the open-label trial (-2.5; $p = .044$). Patients also exhibited a statistically significant reduction in body weight. The most common reasons for topiramate discontinuation were protocol nonadherence ($N = 17$) and adverse events ($N = 14$).

The second controlled study of topiramate in BED was a multicenter trial in which subjects with DSM-IV BED with three or more binge eating days/week, a BMI between 30 and 52 kg/m^2, and no current psychiatric disorders or substance abuse were randomized 1:1 to topiramate or placebo for 16 weeks (114). A total of

407 subjects enrolled; 13 failed to meet inclusion criteria, resulting in 195 top-iramate and 199 placebo subjects who were evaluated for efficacy. Topiramate significantly reduced binge eating days/week (-3.5 ± 1.9 vs.-2.5 ± 2.1), binge episodes/week (-5.0 ± 4.3 vs. -3.4 ± 3.8), weight (-4.5 ± 5.1 kg vs. 0.2 ± 3.2 kg), and BMI (-1.6 ± 1.8 kg/m^2 vs. 0.1 ± 1.2 kg/m^2) compared with placebo (all $ps < 0.001$). Topiramate also significantly decreased obsessive-compulsive symptoms as assessed with the Yale Brown Obsessive-Compulsive Scale Modified for Binge Eating (YBOCS-BE); overall, motor, and nonplanning impulsiveness scores of the Barratt Impulsiveness Scale, Version II; cognitive restraint, disinhibition, and hunger subscores of the Three Fractor Eating Questionnaire (TFEQ), and overall, social, and family life disability scores of the Sheehan Disability Scale. Fifty eight percent of topiramate-treated subjects achieved remission compared with 29% of placebo-treated subjects ($p < 0.001$). Discontinuation rates were 30% in each group; adverse events were the most common reason for topiramate discontinuation (16%; placebo, 8%). Paresthesias, upper respiratory tract infection, somnolence, and nausea were the most common side effects with topiramate.

The third controlled study of topiramate in BED was another multicenter trial in which 73 subjects with DSM-IV BED and obesity (defined as a BMI ≥ 30) were randomized to CBT (19 sessions) and topiramate ($N = 37$) or placebo ($N = 36$) for 21 weeks (115). The primary outcome measure was weight change. Topiramate was associated with a significantly greater rate of weight reduction over the course of treatment ($p < 0.001$), with subjects taking topiramate attaining a clinically significant weight loss (-6.8 kg) compared with those taking placebo (-0.9 kg). Although rates of reduction of binge frequencies, Binge Eating Scale scores, and BDI scores did not differ between groups during treatment, a greater number of subjects in the topiramate group (31/37) attained remission of binge eating as compared to subjects in the placebo group (22/36; $p = 0.03$). No difference between groups was found in completion rates; one subject (topiramate group) withdrew for an adverse effect. Paresthesias and taste perversion were more frequent with topiramate, and insomnia was more frequent with placebo ($p < 0.05$).

Topiramate has also been reported in case descriptions and open-label studies to reduce binge eating, purging and/or overweight in eating disorder patients with comorbid mood disorders—either as monotherapy or when given with anti-depressants and/ or mood stabilizers (123–126). The drug has been successfully used to reduce binge eating and weight loss difficulties after adjustable gastric banding or gastric bypass surgery (127,128). It has been reported to reduce nighttime eating and decrease body weight in patients with NES, and to reduce nocturnal eating in patients with sleep-related eating disorders (129,130). There is also a description of topiramate reducing binge eating in a woman with epilepsy (131).

However, two case reports of therapeutic topiramate use in anorexia are mixed. In one, topiramate significantly improved the concurrent anorexia of a patient with bipolar disorder (132); in the other, topiramate possibly "triggered" a recurrent episode of anorexia in a woman with an extensive psychiatric history receiving the drug for epilepsy (133). There are also isolated reports of abuse of topiramate by eating disorder patients to lose weight (134,135).

Zonisamide

One controlled study suggests zonisamide reduces binge eating and induces weight loss in patients with BED and obesity. In this single-center, flexible-dose

(100–600 mg/day) trial, 60 outpatients with DSM-IV BED and obesity (BMI ≥ 30) received zonisamide ($N = 30$) or placebo ($N = 30$) for 16 weeks (116). Compared with placebo, zonisamide was associated with a significantly greater rate of reduction in binge-eating episode frequency ($p = 0.021$), body weight ($p < 0.0001$), BMI ($p = 0.0001$), and scores on the Clinical Global Impression-Severity (CGI-S) ($p < 0.0001$), YBOCS-BE ($p < 0.0001$), and TFEQ Disinhibition ($p < 0.0001$) scales. The mean (SD) zonisamide daily dose at endpoint evaluation was 436 (159) mg/day. Of note, plasma leptin levels did not change with weight loss. However, plasma ghrelin concentrations (which are thought to be decreased in obesity and BED) increased with zonisamide but decreased with placebo ($p = 0.0001$).

This controlled trial was stimulated by an open-label study in which 15 outpatients with BED and obesity [mean (SD) BMI = 40.0 (6.8) kg/m^2] received flexible-dose zonisamide (100–600 mg/day) over a 12-week period (136). Eight patients completed the trial; the seven patients who discontinued zonisamide prematurely did so because of lack of response ($N = 1$), protocol nonadherence ($N = 2$), and adverse events ($N = 4$). Nonetheless, both random regression and endpoint analyses found a highly significant decrease in binge-eating episode frequency, binge day frequency, BMI, body weight, and scores on the CGI-S, YBOCS-BE total, and TFEQ hunger and disinhibition scales ($p < 0.0001$ for all measures in both analyses except $p = 0.001$ for endpoint analysis of binge eating frequency, $p = 0.0001$ for endpoint analysis of TFEQ disinhibition, and $p = 0.0008$ for endpoint analysis of TFEQ hunger).

Carbamazepine and Related AEDs

In the only double-blind, placebo-controlled study of carbamazepine in an eating disorder, 16 patients with DSM-III bulimia and at least one binge per week and no binge-free intervals of longer than three weeks during the previous year received the drug in a crossover design (117–119). The first six patients were treated at six-week intervals over 18 weeks in a placebo-carbamazepine placebo or a carbamazepine-placebo-carbamazepine sequence. The next 10 patients were treated over 12 weeks in two six-week intervals of placebo-carbamazepine or carbamazepine-placebo. Overall, there was no significant difference in response between carbamazepine and placebo. One patient had a complete remission of binge eating, one patient had a marked response, and three additional patients improved on carbamazepine compared with baseline but did not show a difference on drug compared with placebo. Of note, the patient who had a remission had a comorbid cyclothymic disorder; she showed marked improvement in her mood as well as her bulimic symptoms while receiving carbamazepine.

There are few other reports of carbamazepine or related AEDs in eating disorders. There is a description of a patient with anorexia and cyclothymia who experienced a remission of binge eating and mood symptoms on the combination of carbamazepine with lithium (119,137). There is also a report of two patients with bulimia whose co-occurring self-mutilating behavior responded to oxcarbazepine, a keto analog of carbamazepine (138). The one patient whose eating disorder was not in remission when oxcarbazepine was added, however, continued to vomit. There are also two cases of the use of carbamazepine in pica. One report describes the successful treatment of coprophagia (a form of pica) due to a glioblastoma with carbamazepine (139). In the other report, the pica of a severely mentally handicapped man with depression failed to respond to carbamazepine but responded to the antidepressant lofepramine (140).

Finally, a case of fulminant hepatic failure from acetaminophen in an anorexic patient treated with carbamazepine has been described (141).

Phenytoin

Early positive open-label reports of phenytoin in patients with binge eating (142–144) were followed by two placebo-controlled trials, one of which was negative (121) and the other modestly positive (120). In the negative trial, four obese patients with bulimia were treated with phenytoin in a crossover design (121). There were no significant differences between phenytoin and placebo on any outcome measure and none of the subjects showed a marked response to drug.

In the modestly positive study, 19 of 20 subjects with severe binge eating completed a 12-week crossover trial comparing phenytoin with placebo (120). Subjects received phenytoin or placebo for six weeks each. Twelve subjects had final serum phenytoin levels of 10 to 20 mg/mL; five had levels of 5 to 10 mg/mL. Subjects treated first with phenytoin experienced a 37% decrease in binge frequency ($p < 0.01$), but when administered placebo, they experienced no change in binge frequency. Subjects treated first with placebo experienced no change in binge frequency, and they did experience a 39% decrease after switching to phenytoin ($p < 0.01$). When the two groups were compared, there were significantly fewer binges in the phenytoin-placebo group than in the placebo-phenytoin group ($p < 0.02$), indicating a carryover effect for the phenytoin-first sequence. Of the 19 completers, 8 (42%) showed a moderate or better response ($\geq 50\%$ reduction in binge episode frequency) on phenytoin. One subject experienced a remission of binge eating and five others had a marked response (defined as $\geq 75\%$ reduction in binge episode frequency).

As noted, these two controlled studies were preceded by descriptions of phenytoin reducing compulsive eating in patients of various weights. In the first report, Green and Rau presented 9 of 10 patients with compulsive eating binges who were successfully treated with phenytoin (142). Four patients were underweight and diagnosed as having anorexia, two were of normal weight, and four were obese. Green and Rau noted that nine of the patients had EEG abnormalities, hypothesized that binge eating might be related to epilepsy, and ultimately expanded their investigation to a series of 47 patients (144). Of these, 27 (57%) showed a "good" response and 20 (43%) showed an "uncertain" or "poor" response. They found that patients with abnormal EEGs [21(70%) of 30] were significantly more likely to have good responses than those with normal EEGs [6 (35%) of 17; $p < 0.001$].

Other AEDs

Valproate has been reported to be effective in three hospitalized patients with bulimia and comorbid rapid-cycling bipolar disorder (119,145,146). All three patients were young women (two were 17 and one 20 years of age), had mildly abnormal EEG's, and were previously unresponsive or only partially responsive to lithium and antipsychotics. Two patients were treated with valproate alone, and one was treated with valproate in combination with lithium. All patients had an excellent clinical response to valproate, with marked improvement of both binge eating and mood symptoms. In one case, bulimic and mood symptoms recurred on two occasions when plasma valproic acid levels fell below 50 μg/mL.

The combination of valproate and clonazepam has been reported effective for both eating symptoms and seizures in a 13-year-old girl with anorexia and epilepsy (147).

However, valproate has been reported to worsen binge eating and enhance weight gain in patients with BED and comorbid bipolar disorder (123). There also has been one report of a patient with epilepsy who developed pica and weight loss when treated with levetiracetam (46).

SUMMARY

The effectiveness of AEDs in obesity, psychotropic-induced weight gain, and eating disorders is summarized in Table 2. At this time, available data suggest that topiramate, zonisamide, and possibly lamotrigine may have beneficial effects in at least one of these conditions. Of these AEDs, topiramate appears to have the broadest spectrum of action as a weight loss and anti-binge eating agent, with efficacy (at least over the short term) in obesity, antipsychotic-induced weight gain, bulimia, and BED. Zonisamide may have efficacy in obesity and BED; preliminary open-label data suggest it might also be effective in psychotropic-associated weight gain. Lamotrigine may have some efficacy in obesity and might be associated with weight loss in obese bipolar patients responding to the drug. Phenytoin might be effective in some patients with compulsive binge eating, but available data are too mixed to make definitive conclusions. Carbamazepine and valproate may be effective in patients with bulimia or anorexia when they treat an associated psychiatric (e.g., mood) or neurologic (e.g., seizure) disorder; otherwise, both agents, especially valproate, are associated with weight gain. Moreover, valproate has been associated with worsening of binge eating and weight gain in BED with comorbid bipolar disorder.

The role of AEDs in the treatment of obesity, psychotropic-associated weight gain, and eating disorders is presently unclear. Despite the large amount of empiric data supporting topiramate's efficacy for weight loss in obesity, an FDA indication for this use was not pursued because of the drug's side effect profile. Indeed, Rosenstock et al. concluded that the CNS and psychiatric adverse events of topiramate made it unsuitable for the treatment of obesity and diabetes (38). However, the drug may be useful in cases of treatment-resistant obesity, including in patients who have failed to respond to antiobesity medication or bariatric surgery (127,128).

TABLE 2 Summary of AEDs Studied in Obesity, Psychotropic-Associated Weight Gain, or Eating Disorders

| AED | Obesity | Condition | | | |
		Psychotropic-associated weight Gain	Anorexia nervosa	Bulimia nervosa	Binge eating disorder
Topiramate	++++	+++	NT	+++	+++
Zonisamide	++	+	NT	NT	++
Lamotrigine	++	NT	NT	NT	NT
Phenytoin	NT	NT	NT	NT	NT
Carbamazepine	NT	NT	NT	−	NT

++++Efficacy in ≥ 3 randomized, double-blind, placebo-controlled trials.
+++Efficacy in ≥2 randomized, double-blind, placebo-controlled trials.
++Efficacy in ≥ 1 randomized, double-blind, placebo-controlled trials.
+Efficacy in open trials.
−At least 1 negative controlled trial.
NT Not tested.

In contrast, topiramate appears to be used with more acceptance in treating psychotropic-induced weight gain, perhaps because there are so few options for this condition and psychiatrists are generally comfortable managing the drug's neurologic and psychiatric side effects. For bulimia, topiramate is presently considered an option for patients resistant to other treatments (91). By contrast, our group considers topiramate a viable first-line choice for BED associated with obesity (114). We consider using zonisamide in BED patients seeking or requiring pharmacotherapy who have failed or are unable to tolerate SSRIs, sibutramine or other serotonin norepinephrine-reuptake inhibitors, or topiramate, and in patients with treatment-resistant bulimia who have failed SSRIs and topiramate.

The potential mechanisms of action of AEDs in these conditions are unknown. One type of mechanism by which topiramate, zonisamide, or lamotrigine might reduce body weight in obesity, psychotropic-induced weight gain, and/or BED is by decreasing ingestive behavior, including pathologic forms of over-ingestion such as binge eating (113,114,116). Topiramate has in fact been shown to induce weight loss and decrease weight gain in rodent models of obesity in part by reducing caloric intake, although the mechanism by which it does this is unknown (148–152). Topiramate, zonisamide, and lamotrigine each have potential sites of action that might contribute to effects on eating behavior. All three AEDs affect glutamate transmission, albeit in different ways (153–157), and growing evidence suggests glutamate plays a key role in regulating feeding behavior and body weight (158–160). Topiramate was shown to upregulate neuropeptide Y (NPY), galanin, and corticotropin-releasing hormone (CRH) immunoreactivities in the hypothalamus and to increase serum leptin in Flinders rats (161); NPY and leptin reduce feeding behavior, and galanin and CRH are also thought to modulate appetite (161,162). Additionally, zonisamide affects central serotonin and dopamine function, which are also known to regulate feeding behavior (40,162–164). Alternatively, topiramate and zonisamide might reduce ingestion via their side effects of dyspepsia, nausea, and taste perversion. The latter mechanisms, however, would not likely account for the weight loss seen in obese patients receiving lamotrigine.

A second possible mechanism is that topiramate, zonisamide, and/or lamotrigine reduce forms of overeating motivated by the rewarding properties of food (20,21,165). These forms of overeating could include binge eating as well as compulsive eating, grazing, subjective overeating, emotional eating, night eating, and eating induced by craving. A reduction in "reward-induced" overeating might lead to weight loss. This view would be consistent with the notion that obesity, psychotropic-induced weight gain, and eating disorders with binge eating might represent food addictions (20,165). Supporting this possibility are controlled trials showing topiramate superior to placebo in reducing alcohol and cocaine use in subjects with alcohol and cocaine dependence (166–168), and the finding that topiramate inhibits nicotine-induced elevation of dopamine in rodent brain (169).

A third possible mechanism is that topiramate, zonisamide, and possibly lamotrigine reduce overeating, and hence body weight, via a general effect on pathologic impulsivity, rather than having specific effects on ingestive behavior or reward. Supporting this mechanism are findings that these AEDs may decrease other pathologic impulsive behaviors. Thus, in addition to decreasing alcohol and cocaine use in patients with substance use disorders (166–168), topiramate has been shown superior to placebo in reducing aggression and/or anger in men and women with borderline personality disorder (170,171) and women with major depression (172). Lamotrigine has similarly been shown superior to placebo in reducing aggression in women with borderline personality disorder (173). Growing research has shown that, like addictive, cluster B personality, and mood disorders, both eating disorders and obesity are characterized by features of pathologic impulsivity (174–177). Topiramate, zonisamide, and possibly lamotrigine might therefore benefit these conditions via an anti-impulsivity effect that spans diagnostic categories

A fourth possible mechanism is that these AEDs induce weight loss via direct metabolic effects. For patients with BED or bulimia, direct weight loss might secondarily lead to reductions in binge eating. Support for this mechanism comes from rodent models of obesity showing that topiramate induces weight loss or prevents weight gain in part by stimulation of energy expenditure (149–152) and from other rodent models showing that topiramate has direct effects on glucose and lipid metabolism (178–181). It has also been hypothesized that carbonic anhydrase inhibitors, including topiramate and zonisamide, induce weight loss by inhibiting carbonic anhydrase–mediated de novo lipogenesis (182). It should be noted, however, that Eliasson et al. (37) cultured explants of human adipose tissue with topiramate and found no effects on lipolysis or the antilipolytic effect of insulin.

Yet another possible mechanism is that AEDs may sometimes reduce overeating or binge eating through their anticonvulsant or thymoleptic properties. Although a clear link between obesity or eating disorders and epilepsy has not been demonstrated, several lines of evidence suggest there might sometimes be neurologic contributions to their etiologies. First, population-based, case-control studies have suggested that anorexia and bulimia are associated with specific obstetric and perinatal complications (95,96). Second, some women with bulimia may have a reduced seizure threshold (105,119,183). Third, a number of neurologic conditions are characterized by eating and/or weight dysregulation, including Prader-Willi syndrome, Klein-Levin syndrome, and damage to the hypothalamus and temporal lobes (184–188). These conditions sometimes benefit from AEDs (184,187,189–191). In short, AEDs may be effective in obesity and eating disorders when there are neurologic, epileptogenic, or neurodevelopmental contributions to the etiology, but this possibility needs to be systematically explored.

Regarding AEDs and their thymoleptic properties, as noted earlier, growing research indicates a relationship between eating disorders and mood disorders, eating disorders and obesity, and obesity and mood disorders. Despite being associated with weight gain, valproate and carbamazepine may exert anti–binge eating effects in bulimia when they effectively treat a comorbid bipolar disorder (117–119,146,147). Conversely, valproate may worsen BED—even when stabilizing an associated bipolar disorder (123)—just as it can exacerbate obesity when treating comorbid bipolar disorder (51,52). Indeed, since many other mood stabilizers cause appetite stimulation and weight gain, it has been hypothesized that the weight gain of these compounds may be related to their therapeutic properties and that, analogous to individuals with bipolar disorder and comorbid substance use disorders, those with comorbid obesity or BED may be overeating or binge eating to "self medicate" their affective symptoms (71). The relationship among mood, eating, and weight dysregulation clearly needs further investigation, as does the role AEDs may play in treating patients who have dysfunction in each of these three domains.

In conclusion, this review suggests that certain AEDs, especially topiramate and zonisamide, may have a role in the treatment of obesity, psychotropic-induced weight gain, BED, and bulimia. Lamotrigine may be an important treatment consideration for the bipolar patient with obesity. Further study is needed to clarify for which patient subgroups these agents might be most useful. In addition, future AEDs associated with anorexia or weight loss might also be considered as potential therapeutic agents for these conditions.

REFERENCES

1. National Institutes of Health (National Heart, Lung, and Blood Institute): Clinical Guidelines on the Identification, Evaluation and Treatment of Overweight and Obesity in Adults. The Evidence Report. Bethesda, MD: National Institutes of Health, 1998.
2. Bray GA, Bouchard C, eds. Handbook of Obesity. Etiology and Pathophysiology, 2nd ed. New York, NY: Marcel Dekker, 2004.
3. Bray GA. Obesity: the disease. J Med Chem 2006; 49:4001–4007.
4. Hensrud DD, Klein S. Extreme obesity: a new medical crisis in the United States. Mayo Clin Proc 2006; 81(10 suppl):S5–S10.
5. Ogden CL, Carroll MD, Curtin LR, et al. Prevalence of overweight and obesity in the United States, 1999–2004. JAMA 2006; 295:1549–1555.
6. Sturm R. Increases in morbid obesity in the USA: 2000–2005. Public Health 2007; 121: 492–496.
7. Friedman JM. A war on obesity, not the obese. Science 2003; 299:856–858.
8. Friedman JM. Modern science versus the stigma of obesity. Nat Med 2004;10:563–569.
9. Van Gaal LF, Mertens IL, DeBlock CE. Mechanisms linking obesity with cardiovascular disease. Nature 2006; 444:875–880.
10. American Psychiatric Association. Diagnostic and Statistical Manual of Mental Disorders. 4th ed. Washington, DC: American Psychiatric Association, 1994.
11. McElroy SL, Kotwal R, Malhotra S, et al. Are mood disorders and obesity related? A review for the mental health professional. J Clin Psychiatry 2004; 65:634–651.
12. Bornstein SR, Schuppenies A, Wong M-L, et al. Approaching the shared biology of obesity and depression: the stress axis as the locus of gene-environment interactions. Mol Psychiatry 2006; 11:892–902.
13. Black DW, Goldstein RB, Mason EE. Prevalence of mental disorders in 88 morbidly obese bariatric clinic patients. Am J Psychiatry 1992; 149:227–234.
14. McElroy SL, Allison DA, Bray GA, eds. Obesity and Mental Disorders. New York, NY: Taylor & Francis Group, 2006.
15. Onyike CU, Crum RM, Lee HB, et al. Is obesity associated with major depression? Results from the Third National Health and Nutrition Examination Survey. Am J Epidemiol 2003; 158:1139–1147.
16. Simon GE, Von Korff M, Saunders K, et al. Association between obesity and psychiatric disorders in the US adult population. Arch Gen Psychiatry 2006; 63:824–830.
17. McIntyre RS, Konarski JZ, Wilkins K, et al. Obesity in bipolar disorder and major depressive disorder: results from a national community health survey on mental health and well-being. Can J Psychiatry 2006; 51:274–280.
18. Hudson JI, Lalonde JK, Berry JM, et al. Binge eating disorder as a distinct familial phenotype in obese individuals. Arch Gen Psychiatry 2006; 63:313–319.
19. Hudson JI, Hiripi E, Pope HG Jr., et al. The prevalence and correlates of eating disorders in the national comorbidity survey replication. Biol Psychiatry 2006, 61, 348–358.
20. Volkow ND, O'Brien CP. Issues for DSM-V: should obesity be included as a brain disorder? Am J Psychiatry 2007; 164:708–710.
21. Devlin MJ. Is there a place for obesity in DSM-V? Int J Eat Disord 2007; 40(suppl): S83–S88 (comment in Int J Eat Disord 2007; 40 (suppl):S104-S106; Int J Eat Disord 2007; 40(suppl):S107–S110).
22. Li Z, Maglione M, Tu W, et al. Meta-analysis: pharmacologic treatment of obesity. Ann Intern Med 2005; 142:532–546.
23. Ioannides-Demos LL, Proietto J, McNeil JJ. Pharmacotherapy for obesity. Drugs 2005; 65: 1391–1418.
24. Hofbauer KG, Nicholson JR, Boss O. The obesity epidemic: current and future pharmacological treatments. Ann Rev Pharmacol Toxicol 2007; 47:565–592.

25. Haddock CK, Poston WS, Dill PL, et al. Pharmacotherapy for obesity: a quantitative analysis of four decades of published randomized clinical trials. Int J Obes Relat Metab Disord 2002; 26:262–273.
26. Padwal RS, Majumdar SR. Drug treatments for obesity: orlistat, sibutramine, and rimonobant. Lancet 2007; 369:71–77.
27. Curioni C, André C. Rimonabant for overweight or obesity. Cochrane Database Syst Rev 2006; (4):CD006162.
28. http://www.fda.gov/ohrms/dockets/ac/07/briefing/2007-4306b1-fda-backgrounder.pdf. Accessed June 25, 2007.
29. Appolinario JC, Bueno JR, Coutinho W. Psychotropic drugs in the treatment of obesity: what promise? CNS Drugs 2004; 18:629–651.
30. Gadde KM, Xiong GL. Buproprion for weight reduction. Expert Rev Neurother 2007; 7:17–24.
31. Bray GA, Hollander P, Klein S, et al. A 6-month randomized, placebo-controlled, dose-ranging trial of topiramate for weight loss in obesity. Obes Res 2003; 11:722–733.
32. Wilding J, Gaal L, Rissanen A, et al. A randomized double-blind placebo-controlled study of the long-term efficacy and safety of topiramate in the treatment of obese subjects. Int J Obes Relat Metab Disord 2004; 28:1399–1410.
33. Astrup A, Caterson I, Zelissen P, et al. Topiramate: long-term maintenance of weight loss induced by a low-calorie diet in obese subjects. Obes Res 2004; 12:1658–1669.
34. Tonstad S, Tykarski A, Weissgarten J, et al. Efficacy and safety of topiramate in the treatment of obese subjects with essential hypertension. Am J Cardiol 2005; 96:243–251.
35. Tremblay A, Chaput J-P, Bérubé S, et al. The effect of topiramate on energy balance in obese men: a 6-month double-blind randomized placebo-controlled study with a 6-month open-label extension. Eur J Clin Pharmacol 2007; 63:123–134.
36. Toplak H, Hamann A, Moore R, et al. Efficacy and safety of topiramate in combination with metformin in the treatment of obese subjects with type 2 diabetes: a randomized, double-blind, placebo-controlled study. Int J Obesity 2007; 31:138–146.
37. Elisasson B, Gudbjörnsdottir S, Cederholm J, et al. Weight loss and metabolic effects of topiramate in overweight and obese type 2 diabetic patients: randomized double-blind placebo-controlled trial. Int J Obes 2007; 31:1140–1147.
38. Rosenstock J, Hollander P, Gadde KM, et al. A randomized, double-blind, placebo-controlled multicenter study to assess the efficacy and safety of topiramate controlled-release in the treatment of obese, type 2 diabetic patients. Diabetes Care 2007; 30:1480–1486.
39. Stenlöf K, Rössner S, Vercruysse F, et al. Topiramate in the treatment of obese subjects with drug-naive type 2 diabetes. Diabetes Obes Metab 2007; 9:360–368.
40. Gadde KM, Franciscy DM, Wagner HR II, et al. Zonisamide for weight loss in obese adults: a randomized controlled trial. JAMA 2003; 289:1820–1825.
41. Orexigen. Products. Available at: http://www.orexigen.com/products/products14/. Accessed June 22, 2007.
42. Meredith CH. A single-center, double-blind, placebo-controlled evaluation of lamotrigine in the treatment of obesity in adults. J Clin Psychiatry 2006; 67(2):258–262.
43. Biton V. Effect of antiepileptic drugs on bodyweight: overview and clinical implications for the treatment of epilepsy. CNS Drugs 2003; 17:781–791.
44. Gadde KM, Yonish GM, Foust MS, et al. Combination therapy of zonisamide and bupropion for weight reduction in obese women: a preliminary, randomized, open-label study. J Clin Psychiatry 2007; 68:1226–1229.
45. Pellock JM, Faught E, Leppik IE, et al. Felbamate: consensus of current clinical experience. Epilepsy Res 2006; 71:89–101.
46. Hadjikoutis S, Pickersgill TP, Smith PE. Drug points: weight loss associated with levetiracetam. BMJ 2003; 327:905.
47. Jallon P, Picard F. Bodyweight gain and anticonvulsants: a comparative review. Drug Saf 2001; 24:969–978.
48. Hamandi K, Sander JW. Pregbalin: a new antiepileptic drug for refractory epilepsy. Seizure 2006; 15:73–78.

49. Prabhakar S, Sahota P, Kharbanda PS, et al. Sodium valproate, hyperandrogenism and altered ovarian function in Indian women with epilepsy: a prospective study. Epilepsia 2007; 48:1371–1377.
50. Allison DB, Mentore JL, Heo M, et al. Antipsychotic-induced weight gain: a comprehensive research synthesis. Am J Psychiatry 1999; 156:1686–1696.
51. Aronne LJ, Segal KR. Weight gain in the treatment of mood disorders. J Clin Psychiatry 2003; 64(suppl 8):22–29.
52. Keck PE Jr., McElroy SL. Bipolar disorder, obesity, and pharmacotherapy-associated weight gain. J Clin Psychiatry 2003; 64:1426–1435.
53. American Diabetes Association; American Psychiatric Association; American Association of Clinical Endocrinologists; North American Association for the Study of Obesity. Consensus development conference on antipsychotic drugs and obesity and diabetes. J Clin Psychiatry 2004; 65:267–272.
54. Baptista T, Zarate J, Joober R, et al. Drug-induced weight gain, an impediment to successful pharmacotherapy: focus on antipsychotics. Curr Drug Targets 2004; 5:279–299.
55. Gentile S. Long-term treatment with atypical antipsychotics and the risk of weight gain. A literature analysis. Drug Safety 2006; 29:303–319.
56. McIntyre RS, Soczynska JK, Bordbar K, et al. Antipsychotic-associated weight gain. In: Bermudes RA, Keck PE Jr., McElroy SL, eds. Managing Metabolic Abnormalities in the Psychiatrically Ill. A Clinical Guide for Psychiatrists. Washington, DC: American Psychiatric Publishing, 2007,165–201.
57. Marder SR, Essock SM, Miller AL, et al. Physical health monitoring of patients with schizophrenia. Am J Psychiatry 2004; 161:1334–1349.
58. Bermudes RA, Keck PE Jr., McElroy SL. Metabolic risk assessment, monitoring, and interventions. Translating what we have learned into practice. In: Bermudes RA, Keck PE Jr., McElroy SL, eds. Managing Metabolic Abnormalities in the Psychiatrically Ill. A Clinical Guide for Psychiatrists. Washington, DC: American Psychiatric Publishing, 2007, 277–302.
59. U.S. Department of Health and Human Services Food and Drug Administration Center for Drug Evaluation and Research (CDER). Guidance for industry developing products for weight management. Revised February 2007. Available at: http://www.fda.gov/cder/guidance/index.htm.
60. Muller DJ, Kennedy JL. Genetics of antipsychotic treatment emergent weight gain in schizophrenia. Pharmacogenomics 2006; 7:863–887.
61. Thiesen FM, Linden A, Geller F, et al. Spectrum of binge eating symptomatology in patients treated with clozapine and olanzapine. J Neural Trans 2003; 110:111–121.
62. Bowden CL, Calabrese JR, Ketter TA, et al. Impact of lamotrigine and lithium on weight in obese and nonobese patients with bipolar I disorder. Am J Psychiatry 2006; 163:1199–1201.
63. Faulkner G, Cohn T, Remington G. Interventions to reduce weight gain in schizophrenia. Cochrane Database Syst Rev 2007; (1):CD 005148.
64. Klein DJ, Cottingham EM, Sorter M, et al. A randomized, double-blind, placebo-controlled trial of metformin treatment of weight gain associated with initiation of atypical antipsychotic therapy in children and adolescents. Am J Psychiatry 2006; 153:2072–2079.
65. Baptista T, Rangel N, Fernandez V, et al. Metformin as an adjunctive treatment to control body weight and metabolic dysfunction during olanzapine administration: a multicentric, double-blind, placebo-controlled trial. Schizophr Res 2007; 93:99–108.
66. Ko YH, Joe SH, Jung IK, et al. Topiramate as an adjuvant treatment with atypical antipsychotics in schizophrenic patients experiencing weight gain. Clin Neuropharmacol 2005; 28:169–175.
67. Nickel MK, Nickel CN, Muehlbacher M, et al. Influence of topiramate on olanzapine-related adiposity in women. A random, double-blind, placebo-controlled study. J Clin Psychopharmacol 2005; 25:211–217.
68. Kim JH, Yim SJ, Nam JH. A 12-week, randomized, open-label, parallel-group trial of topiramate in limiting weight gain during olanzapine treatment in patients with schizophrenia. Schizophr Res 2006; 82:115–117.

69. Roy Chengappa KN, Schwarzman LK, Hulihan JF, et al. Adjunctive topiramate therapy in patients receiving a mood stabilizer for bipolar I disorder: a randomized, placebo-controlled trial. J Clin Psychiatry 2006; 67:1698–1706.

70. McIntyre RS, Mancini DA, McCann S, et al. Topiramate versus bupropion SR when added to mood stabilizer therapy for the depressive phase of bipolar disorder: a preliminary single-blind study. Bipolar Disord 2002; 4:207–213.

71. McElroy SL, Frye MA, Altshuler LL, et al. A 24-week, randomized, controlled trial of adjunctive sibutramine versus topiramate in the treatment of weight gain in overweight or obese patients with bipolar disorders. Bipolar Disord 2007; 9:426–434.

72. Vieta E, Goikolea JM, Olivares JM, et al. 1-year follow-up of patients treated with risperidone and topiramate for a manic episode. J Clin Psychiatry 2003; 64:834–839.

73. Vieta E, Sanchez-Moreno J, Goikolea JM, et al. Effects on weight and outcome of long-term olanzapine-topiramate combination treatment in bipolar disorder. J Clin Psychopharmacol 2004; 24:374–378.

74. Bahk WM, Shin YC, Woo J, et al. Topiramate and divalproex in combination with risperidone for acute mania: a randomized open-label study. Prog Neuropsychopharmacol Biol Psychiatry 2005; 29:115–121.

75. McElroy SL, Suppes T, Keck PE, et al. Open-label adjunctive topiramate in the treatment of bipolar disorders. Biol Psychiatry 2000; 47:1025–1033.

76. Chengappa KN, Levine J, Rathore D, et al: Long-term effects of topiramate on bipolar mood instability, weight change and glycemic control: a case series. Eur Psychiatry 2001; 16:186–190.

77. Dursun SM, Devarajan S. Accelerated weight loss after treating refractory depression with fluoxetine plus topiramate: possible mechanisms of action? Can J Psychiatry 2001; 46:287–288.

78. Carpenter LL, Leon Z, Yasmin S, et al. Do obese depressed patients respond to topiramate? A retrospective chart review. J Affect Disord 2002; 69:251–255.

79. Woods TM, Eichner SF, Franks AS. Weight gain mitigation with topiramate in mood disorders. Ann Pharmacother 2004; 38:887–891.

80. Van Ameringen M, Mancini C, Pipe B, et al. Topiramate treatment for SSRI-induced weight gain in anxiety disorders. J Clin Psychiatry 2002; 63:981–984.

81. Canitano R. Clinical experience with topiramate to counteract neuroleptic induced weight gain in 10 individuals with autistic spectrum disorders. Brain Dev 2005; 27: 228–232.

82. McElroy SL, Suppes T, Keck PE Jr., et al. Open-label adjunctive zonisamide in the treatment of bipolar disorders: a prospective trial. J Clin Psychiatry 2005; 66:617–624.

83. Ghaemi SN, Zablotsky B, Filkowski MM, et al. An open prospective study of zonisamide in acute bipolar depression. J Clin Psychopharmacol 2006; 26:385–388.

84. Wang PW, Yang YS, Chandler RA, et al. Adjunctive zonisamide for weight loss in euthymic bipolar disorder patients: a pilot study. J Psychiatr Res 2008; 42:451–457.

85. Sachs G, Bowden C, Calabrese JR, et al. Effects of lamotrigine and lithium on body weight during maintenance treatment of bipolar I disorder. Bipolar Disord 2006; 8: 175–181.

86. Streigel-Moore RH, Franko DL, May A, et al. Should night eating syndrome be included in the DSM? Int J Eat Disord 2006; 39:544–549.

87. Winkelman JW. Sleep-related eating disorder and night eating syndrome: sleep disorders, eating disorders, or both? Sleep 2006; 29:876–877.

88. Parry-Jones B, Parry-Jones WL. Pica: symptom or eating disorders? A historical assessment. Br J Psychiatry 1992; 160:341–354.

89. Rose EA, Porcerelli JH, Neale AV. Pica: common but commonly missed. J Am Board Fam Pract 2000; 13:353–358.

90. Birmingham CL, Firoz T. Rumination in eating disorders: literature review. Eat Weight Disord 2006; 11:e85–e89.

91. American Psychiatric Association. Practice Guideline for the Treatment of Patients with Eating Disorders. 3rd. ed. Am J Psychiatry 2006; 163(July suppl):4–54.

92. Javaras KN, Pope HG Jr., Lalonde JK, et al. Co-occurance of binge eating disorder with psychiatric and medical disorders. J Clin Psychiatry 2008 (E-pub ahead of print).

93. Slof-Op't Landt MC, van Furth EF, Meulenbelt I, et al. Eating disorders: from twin studies to candidate genes and beyond. Twin Res Hum Genet 2005; 8:467–482.
94. Jarvaris KN, Laird NM, Reichborn-Kjennerud T, et al. Familiality and heritability of binge eating disorder: results of a case-control family study and a twin study. Int J Eating Disord 2008; 41:174–179.
95. Cnattingius S, Hultman CM, Dahl M, et al. Very preterm birth, birth trauma, and the risk of anorexia nervosa among girls. Arch Gen Psychiatry 1999; 56:634–638.
96. Favaro A, Tenconi E, Santonastaso P. Perinatal factors and the risk of developing anorexia nervosa and bulimia nervosa. Arch Gen Psychiatry 2006; 63:82–88.
97. National Institute for Clinical Excellence (NICE). Eating disorders. Core interventions in the treatment and management of anorexia nervosa, bulimia nervosa and related eating disorders. Clinical guideline no 9. London, UK: British Psychological Society, 2004.
98. Carter WP, Hudson JI, Lalonde JK, et al. Pharmacologic treatment of binge eating disorder. Int J Eat Disord 2003; 34(suppl):S74–S88.
99. Appolinario JC, McElroy SL. Pharmacological approaches in the treatment of binge eating disorder. Curr Drug Targets 2004; 5:301–307.
100. Steffen KJ, Roerig JL, Mitchell JE, et al. Emerging drugs for eating disorder treatment. Expert Opin Emerg Drugs 2006; 11:315–336.
101. Berkman ND, Bulik CM, Brownley KA, et al. Management of eating disorders. Evidence Report/Technology Assessment No. 135. (Prepared by the RTI International-University of North Carolina Evidence-Based Practice Center under Contract no 290-02-0016.) AHRQ Publication No. 06-E010. Rockville, MD: Agency for Healthcare Research and Quality, 2006.
102. Shapiro JR, Berkman ND, Brownley KA, et al. Bulimia nervosa treatment: a systematic review of randomized controlled trials. Int J Eat Disord 2007; 40:321–336.
103. Brownley KA, Berkman ND, Sedway JA, et al. Binge eating disorder treatment: a systematic review of randomized controlled trials. Int J Eat Disord 2007; 40:337–348.
104. Hudson JI, Pope HG Jr., Carter WP. Pharmacologic therapy of bulimia nervosa. In: Goldstein E, ed. The Management of Eating Disorders and Obesity. Totowa, NJ: Humana Press, 1999: 19–32.
105. Horne RL, Ferguson JM, Pope HG Jr., et al. Treatment of bulimia with bupropion: a multicenter controlled trial. J Clin Psychiatry 1988; 49:262–266.
106. Appolinario JC, Bacaltchuk J, Sichieri R, et al. A randomized, double-blind, placebo-controlled study of sibutramine in the treatment of binge-eating disorder. Arch Gen Psychiatry 2003; 60:1109–1116.
107. Wilfley DE, Crow SJ, Hudson JI, et al. Efficacy of sibutramine for the treatment of binge eating disorder: a randomized multi-center placebo-controlled double-blind study. Am J Psychiatry 2008; 165:51–58.
108. Walsh BT, Kaplan AS, Attia E, et al. Fluoxetine after weight restoration in anorexia nervosa: a randomized controlled trial. JAMA 2006; 296:934.
109. Bulik CM, Berkman ND, Brownley KA, et al. Anorexia nervosa treatment: a systematic review of randomized controlled trials. Int J Eat Disord 2007; 40:310–320.
110. Hoopes SP, Reimherr FW, Hedges DW, et al. Treatment of bulimia nervosa with topiramate in a randomized, double-blind, placebo-controlled trial, part 1: improvement in binge and purge measures. J Clin Psychiatry 2003; 64:1335–1341.
111. Hedges DW, Reimherr FW, Hoopes SP, et al. Treatment of bulimia nervosa with topiramate in a randomized, double-blind, placebo-controlled trial, part 2: improvement in psychiatric measures. J Clin Psychiatry 2003; 64:1449–1454.
112. Nickel C, Tritt K, Muehlbacher M, et al. Topiramate treatment in bulimia nervosa patients: a randomized, double-blind, placebo-controlled trial. Int J Eat Disord 2005; 38:295–300.
113. McElroy SL, Arnold LM, Shapira NA, et al: Topiramate in the treatment of binge eating disorder associated with obesity: a randomized, placebo-controlled trial. Am J Psychiatry 2003; 160:255–261.

114. McElroy SL, Hudson JI, Capece JA, et al. Topiramate for the treatment of binge eating disorder associated with obesity: a placebo-controlled study. Biol Psychiatry 2007; 61:1039–1048.

115. Claudino AM, de Oliveira IR, Appolinario JC, et al. Double-blind, randomized, placebo-controlled trial of topiramate plus cognitive-behavior therapy in binge-eating disorder. J Clin Psychiatry 2007; 68:1324–1332.

116. McElroy SL, Kotwal R, Guerdjikova AI, et al. Zonisamide in the treatment of binge eating disorder with obesity: a randomized controlled trial. J Clin Psychiatry 2006; 67: 1897–1906.

117. Kaplan AS, Garfinkel PE, Darby PL, et al. Carbamazepine in the treatment of bulimia. Am J Psychiatry 1983; 140:1225–1226.

118. Kaplan AS. Anticonvulsant treatment of eating disorders. In: Garfinkel PE, Garner DM, eds. The Role of Drug Treatments for Eating Disorders. New York: Brunner/Mazel, 1987: 96–123.

119. Hudson JI, Pope HG Jr. The role of anticonvulsants in the treatment of bulimia. In: McElroy SL, Pope HG Jr., eds. Use of Anticonvulsants in Psychiatry. New York, NY: Oxford Univ Press, 1988: 141–153.

120. Wermuth BM, Davis KL, Hollister LE, et al. Phenytoin treatment of binge eating syndrome. Am J Psychiatry 1977; 134:1249–1253.

121. Greenway FL, Dahms WT, Bray GA. Phenytoin as a treatment of obesity associated with compulsive eating. Curr Ther Res 1977; 21: 338–42.

122. McElroy SL, Shapira NA, Arnold LM, et al. Topiramate in the long-term treatment of binge-eating disorder associated with obesity. J Clin Psychiatry 2004; 65:1463–1469.

123. Shapira NA, Goldsmith TD, McElroy SL. Treatment of binge-eating disorder with topiramate: a clinical case series. J Clin Psychiatry 2000; 61:368–372.

124. Schmidt do Prado-Lima PA, Bacaltchuck J. Topiramate in treatment-resistant depression and binge eating disorder. Bipolar Disord 2002; 4:271–273.

125. Felstrom A, Blackshaw S. Topiramate for bulimia nervosa with bipolar II disorders. Am J Psychiatry 2002; 159:1246–1247.

126. Barbee JG. Topiramate in the treatment of severe bulimia nervosa with comorbid mood disorders: a case series. Int J Eat Disord 2003; 33:456–472.

127. Zilberstein B, Pajecki D, Garcia de Brito AC, et al. Topiramate after adjustable gastric banding in patients with binge eating and difficulty losing weight. Obes Surg 2004; 14:802–805.

128. Guerdjikova AI, Kotwal R., McElroy SL. Response of recurrent binge eating and weight gain to topiramate in patients with binge eating disorder after bariatric surgery. Obes Surg 2005; 15:273–277.

129. Winkelman JW. Treatment of nocturnal eating syndrome and sleep-related eating disorder with topiramate. Sleep Med 2003; 4:243–246.

130. Tucker P, Masters B, Nawar O. Topiramate in the treatment of comorbid night eating syndrome and PTSD: a case study. Eat Disord 2004; 12:75–78.

131. Knable M. Topiramate for bulimia nervosa in epilepsy. Am J Psychiatry 2001; 158: 322–323.

132. Guille C, Sachs G. Clinical outcome of adjunctive topiramate treatment in a sample of refractory bipolar patients with comorbid conditions. Prog Neuropsychopharmacol Biol Psychiatry 2002; 26:1035–1039.

133. Rosenow F, Knake S, Hebebrand J. Topiramate and anorexia nervosa. Am J Psychiatry 2002; 159:2112–2113.

134. Colom F, Vieta E, Benabarre H, et al. Topiramate abuse in a bipolar patient with an eating disorder. J Clin Psychiatry 2001; 62:475–476.

135. Chung AM, Reed MD. Intentional topiramate ingestion in an adolescent female. Ann Pharmacother 2004; 38:1439–1442.

136. McElroy SL, Kotwal R, Hudson JI, et al. Zonisamide in the treatment of binge-eating disorder: an open-label, prospective trial. J Clin Psychiatry 2004; 65:50–56.

137. Hudson JI, Pope HG Jr., Jonas JM, et al. Treatment of anorexia nervosa with anti-depressants. J Clin Psychopharmacol 1985; 5:17–23.

138. Cordas TA, Tavares H, Calderoni DM, et al. Oxcarbazepine for self-mutilating bulimic patients. Int J Neuropsychopharmacol 2006; 9:769–771.
139. Stewart JT. Treatment of coprophagia with carbamazepine. Am J Psychiatry 1995; 152:295.
140. Jawed SH, Krishnan VH, Prasher VP, et al. Worsening of pica as a symptom of depressive illness in a person with severe mental handicap. Br J Psychiatry 1993; 162: 835–837.
141. Young CR, Mazure CM. Fulminant hepatic failure from acetaminophen in an anorexic patient treated with carbamazepine. J Clin Psychiatry 1998; 59:622.
142. Green RS, Rau JH. Treatment of compulsive eating disturbances with anticonvulsant medication. Am J Psychiatry 1974; 131:428–432.
143. Rau JH, Green RS. Compulsive eating: a neuropsychologic approach to certain eating disorders. Compr Psychiatry 1975; 16:223–231.
144. Rau JH, Struve FA, Green RS. Electroencephalographic correlates of compulsive eating. Clin Electroencephalogr 1979; 10:180–189.
145. Herridge PL, Pope HG Jr. Treatment of bulimia and rapid-cycling bipolar disorder with sodium valproate: a case report. J Clin Psychopharmacol 1985; 5:229–230.
146. McElroy SL, Keck PE Jr., Pope HG Jr. Sodium valproate: its use in primary psychiatric disorders. J Clin Psychopharmacol 1987; 7: 16–24.
147. Tachibana N, Sugita Y, Teshima Y, et al. A case of anorexia nervosa associated with epileptic seizures showing favorable responses to sodium valproate and clonazepam. Jpn J Psychiatry Neurol 1989; 43:77–84.
148. York DA, Singer L, Thomas S, et al. Effect of topiramate on body weight and body composition of Osborne-mendel rats fed a high-fat diet: alterations in hormones, neuropeptide, and uncoupling-protein mRNAs. Nutrition 2000; 16:967–975.
149. Picard F, Deshaies Y, Lalonde J, et al. Topiramate reduces energy and fat gains in (Fa/?) and obese (fa/fa) Zucker rats. Obes Res 2000; 8:656–663.
150. Richard D, Ferland J, Lalonde J, et al. Influence of topiramate in the regulation of energy balance. Nutrition 2000; 16:961–966.
151. Richard D, Picard F, Lemieux C, et al. The effects of topiramate and sex hormones on energy balance of male and female rats. Int J Obes Relat Metab Disord 2002; 26:344–353.
152. Lalonde J, Samson P, Poulin S, et al. Additive effects of leptin and topiramate in reducing fat deposition in lean and obese ob/ob mice. Physiol Behav 2004; 80:415–420.
153. Shank RP, Gardocki JF, Streeter AJ, et al. An overview of the preclinical aspects of topiramate: pharmacology, pharmacokinetics, and mechanism of action. Epilepsia 2000; 41(suppl 1):S3–S9.
154. Kaminski RM, Banerjee M, Rogawski MA. Topiranate selectively protects against seizures induced by ATPA, a GluR5 kainate receptor agonist. Neuropharmacology 2004; 46:1097–1104.
155. Okada M, Kawata Y, Mizuno K, et al. Interaction between Ca2+, K+, carbamazepine and zonisamide on hippocampal extracellular glutamate monitored with a microdialysis electrode. Br J Pharmacol 1998; 124:1277–1285.
156. Ueda Y, Doi T, Tokumaru J, et al. Effect of zonisamide on molecular regulation of glutamate and GABA trasporter proteins during epileptogenesis in rats with hippocampal seizures. Brain Res Mol Brain Re 2003; 116:1–6.
157. White HS, Smith MD, Wilcox KS. Mechanisms of action of antiepileptic drugs Int Rev Neurobiol 2007; 81:85–110.
158. Stanley BG, Ha LH, Spears LC, et al. Lateral hypothalamic injections of glutamate, kainic acid, D,L-alpha-amino-3 hydroxy-5-methyl-isoxazole propionic acid or N-methyl-D-aspartic acid rapidly elicit intense transient eating in rats. Brain Res 1993; 613:88–95.
159. Zeni, LAZR, Seidler HBK, De Carvalho NAS, et al. Glutamatergic control of food intake in pigeons: Effects of central injections of glutamate, NMDA, and AMPA receptor agonists and antagonists. Pharmacol Biochem Behav 2000; 65:67–74.
160. Zheng H, Patterson C, Berthoud HR. Behavioral analysis of anorexia produced by hindbrain injections of AMPA receptor antagonist NBQX in rats. Am J Physiol Regul Integr Comp Physiol 2002; 282:R147–R155.

161. Husum H, Van Kammen D, Termeer E, et al. Topiramate normalizes hippocampal NPY-LI in flinders sensitive line 'depressed' rats and upregulates NPY, galanin, and CRH-LI in the hypothalamus: implications for mood-stabilizing and weight loss-inducing effects. Neuropsychopharmacol 2003; 28 :1292–1299.
162. Meister B. Neurotransmitters in key neurons of the hypothalamus that regulate feeding behavior and body weight. Physiol Behav 2007; 92:263–271.
163. Okada M, Hirano T, Kawata Y, et al. Biphasic effects of zonisamide on serotonergic system in rat hippocampus. Epilepsy Res 1999; 34:187–197.
164. Okada M, Kaneko S, Hirano T, et al. Effects of zonisamide on dopaminergic system. Epilepsy Res 1995; 22:193–205.
165. Gold MS, Star J. Eating disorders. In: Lowinson JH, Ruiz P, Millman RB, eds. Substance Abuse A Comprehensive Textbook, 2nd ed. York, Pennsylvania: Williams and Wilkins, 2004: 469–488.
166. Johnson BA, Ait-Daoud N, Bowden CL, et al. Oral topiramate for treatment of alcohol dependence: a randomized controlled trial. Lancet 2003; 361:1677–1685.
167. Johnson BA, Rosenthal N, Capece J, et al. Topiramate for treating alcohol dependence: a randomized controlled trial. JAMA 2007; 298:1641–1651.
168. Kampman KM, Pettinati H, Lynch KG, et al. A pilot trial of topiramate for the treatment of cocaine dependence. 2004; 75:233–240.
169. Schiffer WK, Gerasimov MR, Marsteller DA, et al. Topiramate selectively attenuates nicotine-induced increases in monoamine release. Synapse 2001; 42:196–198.
170. Nickel MK, Nickel C, Kaplan P, et al. Treatment of aggression with topiramate in male borderline patients: A double-blind, placebo controlled study. Biol Psychiatry 2005; 57:495–499.
171. Nickel MK, Nickel C, Mitterlehner FO, et al. Topiramate treatment of aggression in female borderline personality disorder patients: A double-blind placebo-controlled study. J Clin Psychiatry 2004; 65:1515–1519.
172. Nickel C, Lahman C, Tritt K, et al. Topiramate in treatment of depressive and anger symptoms in female depressive patients: a randomized double-blind, placebo-controlled study. J Affect Disord 2005; 87: 243–252.
173. Tritt K, Nickel C, Lahmann C, et al. Lamotrigine treatment of aggression in female borderline-patients: a randomized, double-blind, placebo-controlled study. J Psychopharmacol 2005; 19:287–291.
174. Nasser JA, Gluck ME, Geliebter A. Impulsivity and test meal intake in obese binge eating women. Appetite 2004; 43:303–307.
175. McElroy S, Kotwal R. Binge eating. In: Hollander E, Stein DJ, eds. Clinical Manual of Impulse-Control Disorders. Washington, DC: American Psychiatric Publishing, 2006: 115–148.
176. Nederkoorn C, Smulders FT, Havermans RC, et al. Impulsivity in obese women. Appetite 2006; 47:253–256
177. McElroy SL, Kotwal R, Keck PE Jr, et al. Comorbidity of bipolar and eating disorders: distinct or related disorders with shared dysregulations? J Affect Disord 2005; 86: 107–127.
178. Wilkes JJ, Nguyen MT, Bandyopadhyay GK, et al. Topiramate treatment causes skeletal muscle insulin sensitization and increased Acrp30 secretion in high-fat-fed male Wistar rats. Am J Physiol Endocrinol Metab 2005; 289:E1015–E1022.
179. Liang Y, Chen X, Osborne M, et al. Topiramate ameliorates hyperglycaemia and improves glucose-stimulated insulin release in ZDF rats and db/db mice. Diabetes Obes Metab 2005; 7:360–369.
180. Wilkes JJ, Nelson E, Osborne M, et al. Topiramate is an insulin-sensitizing compound in vivo with direct effects on adipocytes in female ZDF rats. Am J Physiol Endocrinol Metab 2005; 288:E617–E624.
181. Ha E, Yim SV, Jung KH, et al. Topiramate stimulates glucose transport through AMP-activated protein kinase-mediated pathway in L6 skeletal muscle cells. Pharmacogenomics J 2006; 6:327–332.
182. De Simone G, Supuran CT. Antiobesity carbonic anhydrase inhibitors. Curr Top Med Chem 2007; 7:879–884.

183. Alper K, Schwartz KA, Kolts RL, et al. Seizure incidence in psychopharmacological clinical trials: an analysis of food and drug administration (FDA) summary basis of approval reports. Biol Psychiatry 2007; 62:345–354.
184. Jobe A, Lewis D, Wainwright M, et al. Three children with a syndrome of obesity and overgrowth, atypical psychosis, and seizures: a problem in neuropsychopharmacology. J Child Neurol 2000; 15:518–528.
185. Gilmour J, Skuse D, Pembrey M. Hyperphagic short stature and Prader-Willi syndrome: a comparison of behavioral phenotypes, genotypes and indices of stress. Br J Psychiatry 2001; 179:250–254.
186. Arnulf I, Zeitzer JM, File J, et al. Kleine-Levin syndrome: a systematic review of 186 cases in the literature. Brain 2005; 128:2763–2776.
187. Goscinski I, Kwiatkowski S, Polak J, et al. The Kluver-Bucy syndrome. J Neurosurg Sci 1997; 41:269–272.
188. Daousi C, Dunn AJ, Foy PM, et al. Endocrine and neuroanatomic features associated with weight gain and obesity in adult patients with hypothalamic damage. Am J Med 2005; 118:45–50.
189. Tu JB, Hartridge C, Izawa J. Psychopharmacological aspects of Prader-Willi Syndrome. J Am Acad Child Adolesc Psychiatry 1992; 31:1137–1140.
190. Smathers SA, Wilson JG, Nigro MA. Topiramate effectiveness in Prader-Willi syndrome. Pediatr Neurol 2003; 28:130–133.
191. Mukaddes NM, Kora ME, Bilge S. Carbamazepine for Kleine-Levin Syndrome. J Am Acad Child Adolesc Psychiatry 1999; 38:791–792.

17 Antiepileptic Drugs in the Treatment of Impulsivity and Aggression and Impulse Control and Cluster B Personality Disorders

Heather A. Berlin and Eric Hollander
*Department of Psychiatry, Mount Sinai School of Medicine,
New York, New York, U.S.A.*

INTRODUCTION

We review here evidence that suggest that antiepileptic drugs (AEDs) (a.k.a. anti-convulsants) may be effective for the treatment of impulsivity and aggression across a range of psychiatric disorders. AEDs are increasingly used as primary or adjunctive treatments for impulse control disorders (ICDs) and cluster B personality disorders [in particular borderline personality disorder (BPD)]. Thus, in addition to the reviewing the effects of AEDS on the symptoms of impulsivity and aggression across a variety of diagnoses, we will focus on ICDs and BPD. The AEDs valproate (e.g., divalproex sodium), carbamazepine, and lamotrigine have U.S. Food and Drug Administration (FDA) indications for the treatment of bipolar disorder. Other AEDs, like oxcarbazepine, gabapentin, topiramate, levetiracetam, phenytoin, and tiagabine, are often used as mood stabilizers but do not have FDA indication for bipolar disorder. Use of off-label AEDs requires careful monitoring and publication of all significant results, including adverse effects. The choice of specific AED is often dependent on drug-drug interactions and side-effect profile (1). Side effects from AEDs are typically mild to moderate. Although data regarding longer-term safety of the newer AEDs are limited, they may have more desirable side-effect profiles.

Impulsivity and Aggression

Impulsivity and aggression are natural behaviors controlled by brain mechanisms, which are essential for survival in all species. Understanding those mechanisms may lead to targeted treatment strategies for this symptom domain when these behaviors become dysfunctional. The concept of impulsivity covers a wide range of "actions that are poorly conceived, prematurely expressed, unduly risky, or inappropriate to the situation and that often result in undesirable outcomes" (2). Moeller et al. (3) defined impulsivity as: "a predisposition toward rapid, unplanned reactions to internal or external stimuli without regard to the negative consequences of these reactions to the impulsive individual or to others." Aggressive behavior has been defined as a verbal or physical act directed against a person or object that can potentially cause physical or emotional harm that occurs in a premeditated or impulsive manner (3,4). The symptoms of impulsivity and aggression are a significant public health problem and can be manifested by self-injurious behavior (SIB), suicide, suicide attempts, substance abuse, accidents (e.g., motor vehicle), domestic violence, assault, and destruction of property (5–10). Intervention can occur at the symptom, syndrome, or behavioral level.

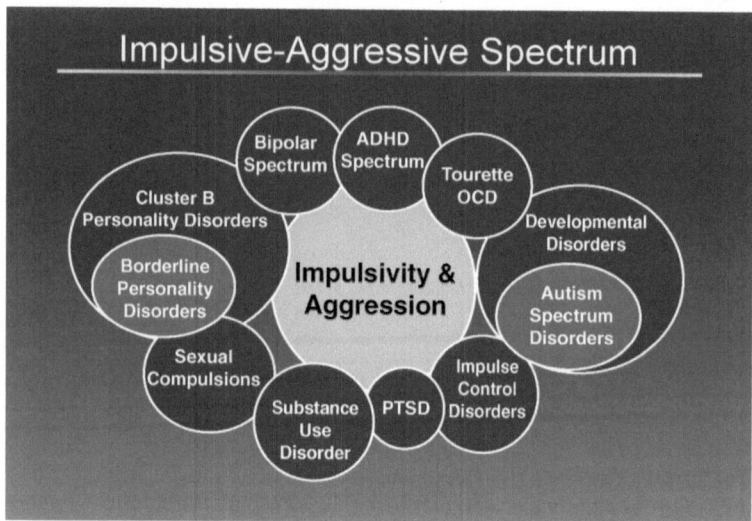

FIGURE 1 Impulsive-aggressive spectrum. *Abbreviations*: ADHD, attention deficit hyperactivity disorder; OCD, obsessive-compulsive disorder; PTSD, posttraumatic stress disorder.

Impulsive and aggressive behaviors can be conceptualized as existing on a spectrum where they are the core symptoms of a broad range of psychiatric disorders that are often comorbid with one another, like cluster B personality disorders, ICDs, autism spectrum disorders, and bipolar disorder (Fig. 1). This is based on similarities in associated clinical features (e.g., age of onset, clinical course, comorbidity) and response to pharmacological treatment [e.g., selective serotonin reuptake inhibitors (SSRIs)], suggesting a high degree of overlap among disorders (11). Further, impulsivity can be thought of as part of a compulsive-impulsive dimensional model, where impulsivity and compulsivity represent polar opposite complexes that can be viewed along a continuum of compulsive and impulsive disorders (Fig. 2). One endpoint marks compulsive or risk-aversive behaviors characterized by overestimation of the probability of future harm, exemplified by obsessive-compulsive disorder (OCD). The other endpoint designates impulsive action characterized by the lack of complete consideration of the negative results of such behavior, exemplified by borderline disorder and antisocial personality disorder (ASPD). Anti-impulsive medication classes include SSRIs, serotonin (5-HT)1A agonists, 5-HT2 antagonists (Table 1), lithium, AEDs, atypical and typical antipsychotics, β blockers, α2-agonists (e.g., clonidine, guanfacine), opiate antagonists (e.g., naltrexone), and dopamine agonists (e.g., stimulants, bupropion).

There are many contributing factors to impulsivity and aggression such as genes, gender, environment, psychiatric disorders, and substance abuse. Early environment can alter a person's neurochemistry related to impulsivity and aggression (12). The neurochemistry of aggression and impulsivity may involve serotonin, gamma-aminobutyric acid (GABA), glutamate, norepinephrine, dopamine, androgens, vasopressin, and nitric oxide.

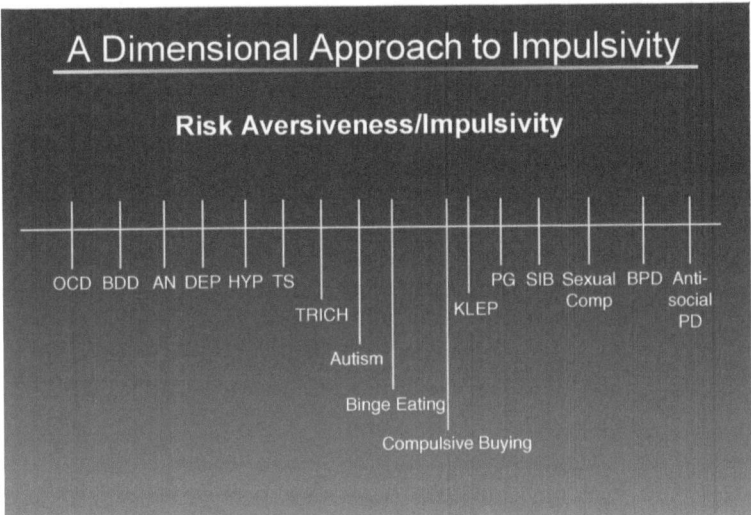

FIGURE 2 A dimensional approach to impulsivity. *Abbreviations*: OCD, obsessive-compulsive disorder; BDD, body dysmorphic disorder; AN, anorexia; DEP, depression; HYP, hypochondriasis; TS, Tourette's syndrome; TRICH, trichotillomania; KLEP, kleptomania; PG, pathological gambling; SIB, self-injurious behavior; Comp, compulsion; BPD, borderline personality disorder; PD, personality disorder.

TABLE 1 Mechanisms of Impulsive Behavioral Disturbances

Serotonin-sensitive	Serotonin-resistant
Low serotonin	Severe arousal
Impulsive aggression	Multiple disturbances
Trait dependent	Mixed-state trait
Increased serotonin function would ameliorate disturbance	Decreased arousal would ameliorate disturbance

Neural Substrates

The orbitofrontal cortex (OFC), with its extensive reciprocal connections with the amygdala (which is implicated in emotional behavior) (13,14), may play a role in correcting or regulating emotional and behavioral responses (15–19). Limbic-orbitofrontal circuit dysfunction may be involved in impulsivity and aggression, at least in a subgroup of patients (20). Impulsivity and aggression may conceivably involve increased limbic discharge, decreased OFC function, and/or hypoactive frontolimbic circuitry (21). Studies suggest that the amygdala and OFC act as part of an integrated neural system, as well as alone, in guiding decision making and adaptive response selection on the basis of stimulus-reinforcement associations (13,22–25). Thus, underactivation of prefrontal areas involved in inhibiting behavior, overstimulation of the limbic regions involved in drive, or a combination of both may result in disinhibited and aggressive behaviors.

For example, in 15 healthy subjects, Pietrini et al. (26) found that compared with imagined scenarios involving emotionally neutral behavior, imagined scenarios involving aggressive behavior were associated with significant emotional reactivity and reductions in reginal cerebral blood flow (rCBF) in the ventromedial prefrontal cortex (PFC). These results in healthy subjects support previous animal and human studies, which suggest the involvement of the OFC in the expression of aggressive behavior. Reduced serotonergic activity has been associated with impulsive aggression in personality-disordered patients in metabolite, pharmacological challenge, and position emission tomography (PET) studies. In an [^{18}F] fluorodeoxyglucose PET study (27), six impulsive-aggressive patients with intermittent explosive disorder (IED) and five healthy volunteers were evaluated for changes in regional glucose metabolism after administration of d,l-fenfluramine (a serotonergic releasing agent) or placebo. Healthy controls showed increases in glucose metabolism in the orbitofrontal, ventral medial frontal, cingulate, and inferior parietal cortices, while impulsive-aggressive patients had no significant increases in glucose metabolism in any region after fenfluramine. Compared with controls, impulsive-aggressive patients also had significantly blunted metabolic responses in orbitofrontal, ventral medial, and cingulate cortices but not in inferior parietal lobe. These results suggest that impulsive-aggressive personality disorder patients have reduced serotonergic modulation of orbital frontal, ventral medial frontal, and cingulate cortices.

OFC [Brodmann area (BA) 10] and ventrolateral PFC (BA 47) activation are thought to exhibit top-down control over limbic pathways (28,29). The amygdala is known to receive major visual input from sensory areas of the cortex, which provide fast responses to simple perceptual and associative aspects of external stimuli (30). Thus, in addition to subcortical pathways of emotional processing, which are thought to act automatically even without awareness of stimuli (31), the OFC and ventrolateral PFC, with their strong interconnections with subcortical areas implicated in emotional behavior, may play a role in correcting emotional responses (15,18,19). In fact, using functional magnetic resonance imaging (FMRI), an abnormal elevation of CBF in the ventrolateral PFC in response to aversive emotional stimuli was found in four of six BPD subjects, but not in controls (29), and was also reported during induced aversive emotional states in patients with anxiety disorders or depression (28). This part of the PFC is directly connected with the basal nucleus of the amygdala, and has been regarded as a gateway for distinctive sensory information, and may modulate or inhibit amygdala-driven emotional responses and thus provide top-down control of the amygdala (28,32,33).

ANTIEPILEPTIC DRUGS AND IMPULSE CONTROL DISORDERS

IED, kleptomania, pyromania, pathological gambling, trichotillomania, and ICDs not otherwise specified (NOS) are the classic disorders of impulse control listed under "impulse-control disorders not elsewhere classified" in the Diagnostic and Statistical Manual of Mental Disorders IV-Text Revision (DSM-IV-TR) (34), in which impulsivity is a core and defining symptom. Further, currently categorized under ICDs-NOS, but proposed to be included as individual ICDs in the DSM-V, are impulsive-compulsive sexual behaviors, shopping, Internet addiction, and excoriation (skin picking). The essential feature of an ICD is the failure to resist an impulse, drive, or temptation to perform an act that is harmful to the person or to others. Additional features include increasing tension or arousal before the act; pleasure, gratification, or relief at the time of the act; and self-reproach or guilt following the act. Impulsivity also plays a significant role in a wide range of other psychiatric disorders, including mood disorders (particularly mania), personality disorders (borderline and antisocial), eating disorders [e.g., binge eating disorder (BED), bulimia nervosa], substance use disorders, schizophrenia, attention deficit hyperactivity disorder (ADHD), paraphilias, conduct disorder, and neurological disorders with disinhibition.

There is gender predominance for most of the ICDs. Pathological gambling, IED, pyromania, and sexual compulsions are more prevalent in males, whereas kleptomania, trichotillomania, SIB, compulsive shopping, and BED are more prevalent in females. This differential gender distribution indicates that both men and women express impulsivity but do so in different ways. The reasons for this differential gender distribution are unclear but may be related to genetic factors, differences in serotonin turnover, hormonal differences, or social/environmental pressures.

We review here treatment studies of ICDs with AEDs, focusing on pathological gambling as an ICD that may be successfully treated with AEDs.

Pathological Gambling

Pathological gambling has traits in common with many different psychiatric disorders (Fig. 3). The link between pathological gambling and antisocial disorders, including ASPD, conduct disorder, and adult antisocial behavior, is largely determined by genetic propensity. Slutske et al. (35) found that genetic factors account for 61% to 86% of the overlap between antisocial behaviors and pathological gambling and 16% to 22% of the variance for pathological gambling overall. Nonfamilial environmental factors also significantly contribute to pathological gambling and to ASPD and adult antisocial behavior. Antisocial behavior is not just a consequence of pathological gambling but also an independent psychiatric symptom. Further, the risk of alcohol abuse/dependence and adult antisocial behavior overlap, suggesting that impulsivity is a mediator in these conditions. In

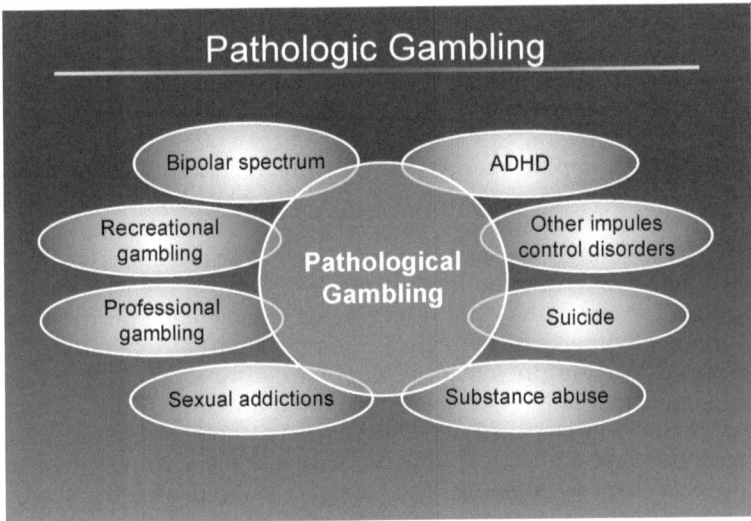

FIGURE 3 Pathological gambling. *Abbreviation*: ADHD, attention deficit hyperactivity disorder.

other words, impulsivity can be thought of as a common endophenotype, or nonobvious underlying trait, in these and related psychiatric disorders.

In FMRI studies, researchers observed that, compared with healthy subjects, pathological gamblers have decreased activity in their ventromedial PFC during presentation of gambling cues (36) and during a cognitive inhibition task (e.g., Stroop color-word) (37). The ventromedial PFC is associated with decision making (38), and the OFC plays a role in the processing of rewards during the expectancy and experiencing of monetary gains or losses (17,39–41). In a recent imaging study of pathological gamblers ($N = 7$), Hollander et al. (41) found that during a gambling task, monetary reward, as opposed to game points, was associated with significantly higher metabolic activity in the primary visual cortex (BA 17), cingulate gryus (BA 24), putamen, and OFC (BAs 47 and 10).

An understanding of the neurobiology of pathological gambling is beginning to emerge. Serotonin (5-HT) is linked to behavioral initiation and disinhibition, which are important in the onset of the gambling cycle and the difficulty in ceasing gambling behavior. Norepinephrine is associated with the arousal and risk taking in patients with pathological gambling. Dopamine is linked to positive and negative reward and the addictive component of pathological gambling (42). Studies suggest that potentially useful treatments for pathological gambling include the SSRIs clomipramine (43) and fluvoxamine (44–46), the opioid antagonist naltrexone (which may reduce the "high" associated with gambling) (47), the mood stabilizer lithium (48–50), and the AEDs carbamazepine (51), valproate (49), and topiramate (46).

While SSRIs may be effective for some patients with pathological gambling (43–46), those with comorbid conditions, like bipolar spectrum disorders, may relapse during such treatment. Thus treatment with AEDs for pathological gambling has been suggested, especially when bipolar mood symptoms are present. In the first controlled trial of mood stabilizers in pathological gambling, Pallanti et al. (49) compared the efficacy and safety of lithium and valproate in nonbipolar pathological gamblers. At the end of the 14-week trial, both the lithium and valproate groups showed comparable significant improvement in mean score on the Yale-Brown Obsessive-Compulsive Scale Modified for Pathological Gambling (YBOCS-PG). Thirteen (68.4%) of the nineteen patients taking valproate and 14 (60.9%) of the 23 patients taking lithium were responders based on a Clinical Global Impressions-Improvement Scale (CGI-I) score of much or very much improved.

Dannon et al. (46) compared the effectiveness of randomly assigned topiramate versus fluvoxamine in the treatment of male pathological gamblers. After 12 weeks, 9 of the 12 topiramate completers reported full remission of gambling behavior, and three completers had a partial remission. The CGI-I score was significantly better for the topiramate group at the 12-week visit as compared with baseline. Six of the eight fluvoxamine completers reported a full remission and the remaining two completers reported a partial remission. The fluvoxamine group showed improvement in the CGI-I score at week 12 but the change was not significant. Hollander (personal communication, 2007) recently completed a randomized, 14-week, double-blind, placebo-controlled, multicenter trial of topiramate (flexibly dosed to 300 mg or the maximum tolerated dose) in 50 subjects with pathological gambling. The primary endpoint was the change from baseline in the obsession component of the YBOCS-PG. Data analysis is presently ongoing.

Other ICDs

Topiramate has been reported to be effective in the treatment of a number of ICDs other than pathological gambling (46), including kleptomania (52), skin picking (53,54), trichtillomania (55), and IED (56,57). For example, topiramate augmentation of clomipramine/fluvoxamine was reported useful in a case of trichotillomania (58). In an open-label pilot study, Lochner et al. (55) evaluated topiramate mono-therapy in 14 adults with trichotillomania. Patients received 16 weeks of flexible-dose treatment (50–250 mg/day), followed by a flexible-dose taper over two to four weeks. Severity of hair pulling in those who completed the 16-week trial ($N = 9$) decreased significantly from baseline to endpoint according to the Massachusetts General Hospital Hair Pulling Scale. Although CGI-I scores (a secondary outcome measure) suggested that hair pulling was not significantly reduced, six of nine completers were classified as responders. Five patients dropped out because of adverse effects. These results suggest that topiramate may be useful in the treatment of some patients with trichtillomania.

Prader-Willi syndrome (PWS) is a multisystem neurogenetic obesity disorder with behavioral manifestations, including hyperphagia, compulsive behaviors, mild to moderate mental retardation, and SIBs in the form of skin picking, nail biting, and rectal gouging. In the first published study of topiramate for the treatment of PWS or SIB, Shapira et al. (53) reported attenuation of SIBs resulting in lesion healing in three PWS adults treated with topiramate in an eight-week open-label trial. In another eight-week open-label study, Shapira et al. (54) evaluated adjunctive therapy with topiramate in eight adults with PWS. Topiramate did not significantly change compulsions, calories consumed, body mass index (BMI), or increased self-reported appetite. However, there was a clinically significant improvement in the self-injury characteristics (i.e., skin picking) of this syndrome. Double-blind or crossover studies are needed to establish the role of topiramate in attenuating SIB in PWS and other disorders involving SIB.

Regarding other ICDs, Dannon (52) reported three kleptomaniac patients who responded well to topiramate given either alone or in combination with SSRIs. Kaufman et al. (59) described two patients with ICDs with aggressive features and postencephalitic epilepsy where adjunctive tiagabine, a novel GABA reuptake inhibitor AED, was effective in the management of both epilepsy and severe impulsive and aggressive behaviors. This is consistent with observations that GABAergic modulation is important in impulsive aggression. De Dios Perrino et al. (56) reported three IED patients in whom good control of aggressive behavior was achieved using SSRIs in combination with carbamazepine. Indeed, in a survey completed by 2543 psychiatrists in the United States in 1988, carbamazepine was reported to be moderately to markedly effective in 65.2% of IED patients and 43.0% of BPD patients (57). In sum, AEDs may be effective treatments for ICDs, but more appropriately powered randomized, double-blind, placebo-controlled trials are needed.

ANTIEPILEPTIC DRUGS AND CLUSTER B PERSONALITY DISORDERS

Borderline Personality Disorder

We review here AED treatment studies across cluster B personality disorders. Since the majority of studies focus specifically on BPD, we will also discuss BPD in this section.

Personality disorders are characterized by interpersonal styles that are rigid and constant over time with onset before adulthood. BPD has been the most extensively studied among the current personality disorders. The DSM-IV-TR (34) classifies BPD as an axis II cluster B personality disorder with criteria that include affective instability, impulsive risk-taking behavior, inappropriate and intense anger, fear of abandonment, unstable relationships that rapidly shift between idealization and devaluation, unstable self-image, feelings of emptiness, dissociative experiences, SIB like superficial skin cutting or burning, and multiple suicide attempts. The designation of BPD as an axis II disorder reflects the historical conceptualization that personality disorders are psychologically and developmentally rooted, rather than biologically based and genetically determined like axis I disorders. Recently, alternative conceptualizations of BPD in particular and personality disorders in general have arisen, providing a theoretical rationale for the investigation into their neurobiology.

BPD is characterized by the core features of affective instability (possibly related to increased responsivity of the cholinergic system) and impulsivity and aggression (both thought to be related to reduced serotonergic brain activity). A typical symptom for BPD is the tendency to have outbursts of aggressive impulsivity (60). BPD is associated with high levels of functional impairment, treatment utilization, and mortality by suicide (61,62). Approximately 10% of patients with BPD commit suicide (63). BPD has an estimated prevalence of 1% to 2% of the U.S. population (34,64–67), with men constituting only about 25% of patients (67). The disorder accounts for approximately 10% of all psychiatric outpatients and 20% of acute inpatient hospitalizations (34,68,69). There are several psychotherapies for the treatment of BPD, like dialectic behavior therapy, but they are very time consuming, therapists must be specially trained, and patients must be highly motivated, as many are resistant to treatment. Thus, pharmacotherapy may serve as a useful adjunct to psychotherapeutic interventions in BPD, and a combination of these approaches may be most effective (70,71).

In evaluating the use of medications for treating personality disorders, one can (i) treat the disorder itself, (ii) treat associated axis I disorders, or (iii) treat symptom clusters/psychobiological dimensions within and across disorders (72). Three symptom clusters that can be targeted in BPD are impulsivity and aggression, mood symptomatology, and psychotic-like symptoms. No single medication is thought to be effective for all three of these symptom clusters (73). New and old antipsychotics, monoamine oxidase inhibitors (MAOIs), SSRIs, and AEDs are all currently used for BPD (74). Tricyclics are used to decrease irritability and aggression, but are lethal in overdose; MAOIs are used for affective instability, but risks include hypertensive crisis; SSRIs are used to decrease anger, irritability, and aggression, but comorbid bipolar spectrum patients may develop rapid cycling; antipsychotics are used to improve psychosis, but side effects are common and controlled data are lacking; and benzodiazepines are used to decrease episodes of behavioral dyscontrol. In a review of the treatment of rapid-cycling bipolar disorder, which overlaps with BPD, Coryell (75) stated that placebo-controlled studies so far provided the most support for the use of lithium and lamotrigine as prophylactic agents. The combination of lithium and carbamazepine, valproate, or lamotrigine for maintenance has some support from controlled studies, as does the adjunctive use of olanzapine. However, it appears that AEDs are used more widely than lithium in treating BPD.

Valproate

Recently, AED trials have focused on valproate, a widely used mood stabilizer, and to a lesser extent on the newer anticonvulsants, for efficacy in BPD. Valproate has been shown to improve symptoms of irritability, agitation, aggression, and anxiety in patients with BPD (76–81). In an open-label study, eight BPD patients completed an eight-week trial of valproate (76). Half of the patients were rated as overall responders, with significant to modest decreases in depression, anxiety, anger, impulsivity, rejection sensitivity, and irritability, as measured by Overt Aggression Scale-Modified (OAS-M) and Symptom Checklist-90 (SCL-90) scores. Wilcox (77) treated 30 BPD inpatients in a naturalistic open study of valproate. Brief Psychiatric Rating Scale (BPRS) scores (particularly the anxiety subcomponents), aggressive outbursts, and time in seclusion significantly decreased during the six-week trial. In addition to treating the aggressive and impulsive symptoms of BPD patients, valproate may also be helpful in treating BPD patients who report changeable mood (i.e., those who have mood instability but who are subsyndromal for major depression or hypomania) (82). In one valproate treatment study, six of nine BPD patients with mood instability (defined by the BPD DSM-III-R diagnostic criterion "affective instability due to marked reactivity of mood"), without bipolar or current major depression, were responders in that their CGI score on their last visit was "much improved" or better (82). Responders showed a greater reduction in Hamilton Rating Scale for Depression (HAM-D) scores than nonresponders.

In a preliminary, double-blind trial, BPD outpatients were treated for 10 weeks with valproate ($N = 12$) or placebo ($N = 4$) (80). There was significant improvement from baseline in measures of global symptom severity (as assessed by the CGI-I) and functioning [as assessed by the Global Assessment of Function (GAF) scale], following treatment. A high dropout rate precluded finding significant differences between the treatment groups in the intent-to-treat (ITT) analyses. However, all results were in the predicted direction so that patients in the treatment group had decreases in scores on the Aggression Questionnaire and the Beck Depression Inventory (BDI) compared with placebo. In another controlled, double-blind study of valproate, efficacy was examined in 30 women with comorbid BPD and bipolar II disorder over six months of treatment (81). Valproate, at an average dose of 850 mg/day (blood levels between 50 and 100 mg/L), was well tolerated and superior to placebo in diminishing interpersonal sensitivity and anger/hostility as measured by the SCL-90 and overall aggression as measured by the OAS-M. Taken together, these studies suggest valproate may be more effective than placebo for global symptomatology, level of functioning, aggression, and depression in BPD.

Since valproate may improve impulsive aggression, irritability, and global severity in patients with cluster B personality disorders (9), Hollander et al. (83) examined clinical characteristics of BPD outpatients that might predict response of impulsive aggression to valproate. In this randomized, double-blind, 12-week study, valproate ($N = 20$) was superior to placebo ($N = 32$) in reducing impulsive aggression in BPD patients. Both pretreatment trait impulsivity and state aggression symptoms, independently of one another, predicted a favorable response to valproate relative to placebo. However, baseline affective instability did not affect differential treatment response. These may help identify BPD patient subgroups or baseline characteristics (e.g., those with high levels of trait impulsivity or state aggression) that could guide future trials of AEDs. These data also suggest that BPD may be characterized by independent symptom domains that are amenable to treatment (40,84).

Carbamazepine and Oxcarbazepine

Carbamazepine, an anticonvulsant with effects on subcortical limbic structures, is effective in the treatment of several psychiatric disorders, including bipolar mania. Because patients with BPD show prominent affective symptomatology and symptoms suggestive of an epileptoid disorder, carbamazepine might be useful in treating BPD. In fact, in a double-blind, crossover trial, carbamazepine decreased the severity of behavioral dyscontrol in 11 women with BPD significantly more than placebo (85). In another double-blind, placebo-controlled, crossover study, carbamazepine led to a dramatic, highly significant decrease in clinician-rated behavioral dyscontrol and had a modest effect on mood in female BPD outpatients with prominent behavioral dyscontrol and without current major depression (86). However, one carbamazepine study of 20 BPD inpatients without concurrent depression or concomitant medications yielded negative results (87). After four weeks of treatment at standard doses, carbamazepine was no better than placebo in treating depression, behavioral dyscontrol, or global symptomatology. In another study, 3 (18%) of 17 BPD patients developed melancholia during carbamazepine treatment, which remitted upon discontinuation of carbamazepine (88). Thus, while carbamazepine may be an effective medication for some BPD patients, clinicians should be alert for any worsening in depressive symptoms.

More recently, Bellino et al. (89) tested 17 DSM-IV-TR-diagnosed BPD outpatients with oxcarbazepine, an AED that is structurally related to carbamazepine and sometimes used for treating patients with bipolar disorders, substance abuse, schizoaffective disorder, and treatment-resistant psychosis. Patients were administered oxcarbazepine 1200 to 1500 mg/day and evaluated at baseline, and after 4 and 12 weeks of treatment. A statistically significant response to oxcarbazepine was observed according to change in mean scores on the CGI-S, BPRS, and Hamilton Rating Scale for Anxiety (HAM-A); in interpersonal relationships, impulsivity, affective instability, and outbursts of anger items; and in total score of the Borderline Personality Disorder Severity Index. Oxcarbazepine was well tolerated with no severe adverse effects; four patients discontinued treatment due to noncompliance. Thus, oxcarbazepine may be an effective and safe treatment for some BPD patients. However, controlled studies are needed.

Topiramate

In an eight-week, double-blind, placebo-controlled trial of topiramate to treat aggression in females with DSM-IV-diagnosed BPD, the topiramate group ($N = 19$) showed significantly more efficacy than the placebo group ($N = 10$) (90) as measured by four subscales (i.e., the state-anger, trait-anger, anger-out, and anger-control subscales) of the State Trate Anger Expression Inventory (STAXI) scale. Significant changes on the same four STAXI subscales were also observed in males with DSM-IV-diagnosed BPD treated with topiramate ($N = 22$) in a similarly designed eight-week, double-blind, placebo ($N = 20$) controlled study (91). In both studies, topiramate was well tolerated and significant weight loss was observed. These findings suggest topiramate may be a safe and effective treatment of anger in both men and women with BPD and correspond with other studies where topiramate therapy resulted in significantly decreased symptoms of aggression (92,93).

Recently, Loew et al. explored whether topiramate could influence BPD patients' borderline psychopathology, health-related quality of life, and interpersonal problems (94,95). DSM-IV SCID-II–diagnosed BPD women were randomly assigned in a 1:1 ratio to topiramate titrated from 25 to 200 mg/day ($N = 28$) or placebo ($N = 28$) for 10 weeks. Significant changes were observed on the somatization, interpersonal sensitivity, anxiety, hostility, phobic anxiety, and Global Severity Index scales of the SCL-90 in the topiramate-treated subjects after 10 weeks. In addition, significant differences were found on all eight scales of the SF-36 Health Survey and in the overly autocratic, competitive, introverted, and expressive scales of the Inventory of Interpersonal Problems. Significant weight loss was also observed.

Finally, do Prado-Lima et al. (96) reported a woman with BPD and a history of childhood trauma who showed a significant clinical response with a low dosage of topiramate. The authors suggested that topiramate might decrease emotional and behavioral reactivity by facilitating memory extinction.

Lamotrigine

In a small, open trial of lamotrigine in eight BPD patients without concurrent major depression, two subjects discontinued because of adverse events or noncompliance and three did not respond (97). However, the remaining three were robust responders with a marked increase in their overall level of functioning, a cessation of impulsive behaviors like promiscuity, substance abuse, and suicidality, and maintenance of response at one-year follow-up. In a retrospective study of borderline symptoms in bipolar patients, it was estimated that 43% of this subgroup experienced a reduction in such symptoms during lamotrigine treatment (98).

Tritt et al. (99) investigated the efficacy of lamotrigine in the treatment of aggression in 24 women meeting Structured Clinical Interview for DSM-IV (SCID) criteria for BPD. In this double-blind, placebo-controlled study, subjects were randomly assigned in a 2:1 ratio to lamotrigine ($N = 18$) or placebo ($N = 9$) for eight weeks. Compared with the placebo group, highly significant changes on four STAXI scales (e.g., state-anger, trait-anger, anger-out, anger-control) were observed in subjects treated with lamotrigine after eight weeks. All the patients tolerated lamotrigine relatively well, and it had no clinically significant effect on body weight.

Weinstein and Jamison (100) assessed lamotrigine treatment for affective instability symptoms of BPD patients. Charts of patients treated with lamotrigine in a private practice during 2003–2004 were reviewed. Patients were included in the analysis if they had been given a DSM-IV-R diagnosis of BPD; had continued to display affective instability while taking their previous medications before lamotrigine initiation; had received a CGI-S score before and after lamotrigine therapy; had been treated with lamotrigine, as monotherapy or adjunctive therapy, at a dose ranging from 50 to 200 mg/day; and continued to take lamotrigine for at least three months. The charts of 13 patients met inclusion criteria. All patients were female, 19 to 43 years of age, and had reported continuing symptoms of affective instability despite treatment with two to seven psychotropic drugs, including, but not limited to, fluoxetine, paroxetine, escitalopram, buproprion, and clonazepan. The duration of lamotrigine treatment ranged from 3 to 15 months. The patients had initial CGI-S scores of 5 or 6 and final scores of 1 or 2, except one patient with an initial score of 3 and a final score of 1 and another patient with an initial score of 6 and a final score of 7.

In sum, there is preliminary evidence that lamotrigine may have efficacy in treating BPD symptomatology, especially symptoms of anger, affective instability, and impulsivity.

Cluster B Personality Disorders

Many researchers have recommended AEDs for the treatment of the affective, impulsive, and aggressive symptoms of cluster B personality disorders in general. Stein (101) has suggested that carbamazepine and lithium may help some personality-disordered people with episodic behavioral dyscontrol and aggression, even in the absence of affective, organic, or epileptic features. Stone (63) has suggested that BPD patients with bipolar II may benefit from lithium or from carbamazepine if irritability is prominent. In a review of double-blind, placebo-controlled drug trials for personality disorders, Hori (102) concluded that patients with BPD and behavioral dyscontrol respond to carbamazepine, which reduces episodes of dyscontrol, and that patients with personality disorders with aggressive behavior respond to lithium. Coccaro and Kavoussi (103) concluded that affective instability in BPD, which may be related to abnormalities in the brain's adrenergic and cholinergic systems, appears to respond to lithium and carbamazepine. In another review, Pelissolo and Lepine (104) argued that for cluster B personality disorders, especially antisocial and BPD, positive results have been obtained using lithium, carbamazepine, and valproate for aggressive and impulsive behaviors.

In an eight-week open trial of valproate in patients with at least one personality disorder who had failed one SSRI trial, six of eight completers showed a significant decline in irritability and impulsive aggression on the OAS-M score (78). Hollander et al. (9) conducted a large, placebo-controlled, multicenter trial of valproate for the treatment of impulsive aggression in cluster B personality disorders, IED, or posttraumatic stress disorder (PTSD). These different diagnoses were included in the same study, as they have the symptom dimension of impulsivity and aggression, which could benefit from the same treatment. Entry criteria required evidence of current impulsive-aggressive behavior (e.g., two or more impulsive-aggressive outbursts per week on average for the previous month) and an OAS-M score of 15 or greater. Ninety-one (43 valproate; 48 placebo) of the 96 randomized cluster B personality disorder patients were included in the ITT data set (defined as subjects who received at least one dose of the study drug and had at least one postbaseline OAS-M rating). The most common primary diagnosis was BPD (55% of patients), followed by cluster B personality disorder NOS (21%), narcissistic (13%), antisocial (10%), and histrionic (1%) personality disorders. Subjects were randomized to 12 weeks of valproate or placebo, and OAS-M (aggression and irritability) and CGI scores were obtained weekly (except for weeks 5 and 7).

A treatment effect was not observed when all three diagnostic groups were combined, but valproate was superior to placebo in the treatment of impulsive aggression, irritability, and global severity in the subgroup of patients with cluster B personality disorders. A treatment effect was observed in both ITT and evaluable (defined as receiving at least 21 days of treatment with study drug) data sets for cluster B personality disorder patients in terms of average OAS-M Aggression scores over the last four weeks of treatment. In the cluster B evaluable data set, statistically significant treatment differences favoring valproate were also observed for component items of the OAS-M Aggression scale (including verbal assault and assault against objects), OAS-M Irritability scale, and CGI-S at multiple time points throughout the study. Across psychiatric diagnoses, 21 (17%) patients in the valproate group prematurely discontinued because of an adverse event, compared with four (3%) patients in the placebo group.

These results support previous findings of decreased impulsive-aggressive behavior and irritability in BPD patients treated with valproate (80), including in those who failed to respond to other agents with antiaggressive properties (i.e., SSRIs) (78). Unlike a previous pilot study where valproate was superior to placebo for the treatment of irritability and hostility in women with bipolar II and BPD (81), patients in the study by Hollander et al. (9) were excluded if they had bipolar disorder I or II with recent (i.e., past year) hypomania. This suggests that the effect of valproate in impulsive aggression may be unrelated to its effect in mania. However, the possibility that the impulsive aggression of cluster B personality disorders has an affective component or that valproate is treating a subclinical mood disorder in cluster B personality disorders cannot be excluded.

Gabapentin is an AED structurally similar to GABA, with unclear mechanisms of action and a good safety profile. Biancosino et al. (105) reported a case of successful gabapentin treatment of chronic impulsive-aggressive behavior in a patient with severe BPD. Morana et al. (106) treated 29 cluster B personality disorder outpatients (8 antisocial, 13 impulsive, 7 histrionic, and 1 narcissistic type) with gabapentin (1200 mg/day), alone or with other drugs (antipsychotics, mood stabilizers, and benzodiazepines). After six weeks of treatment, there was an improvement in 23 (79.9%) patients, with a decrease in aggressiveness, impulsivity, antisocial behavior, and drug abuse and an improvement in their concentration, introspection capabilities, and interest in productive activities, as reported by patients and their caregivers. Morana and Camara (107) found that after more than four years of study of personality disorder patients from the Personality Disorder Ambulatory of the Department of Psychiatry of Sao Paulo University Medical School, about 79.3% of the patients treated with gabapentin had reduced their antisocial behaviors, as reported by patient informers. The authors observed a decrease in aggressiveness, impulsiveness, offender behavior, and drug abuse, and a general improvement in tolerance, concentration, and introspective capacity, with a greater interest in productive activities. It has been suggested that gabapentin reduces reactivity and turbulent behavior perhaps because of its inhibitory effect in central neurotransmission (108). The authors concluded that, in their clinical experience, gabapentin was the most effective mood stabilizer for the treatment of personality disorders.

Summary

A symptom-specific method using current empirical evidence for drug efficacy in each symptom domain of BPD is proposed for treatment. Drugs in each medication class have some potential utility against specific symptoms of BPD (109). As there is no "drug of choice" to treat BPD, a more rational clinical approach might be to treat different symptom clusters (e.g., cognitive, affective, impulsive, and aggressive) rather than the disorder itself. On the basis of the above evidence, we suggest that selective AEDs may be effective in treating the affective, impulsive, and aggressive symptoms of BPD and other cluster B personality disorders.

ANTIEPILEPTIC DRUGS AND IMPULSIVITY AND AGGRESSION ACROSS DIAGNOSES

The antiaggressive effects of AEDs in patients with neurological disorders make them good candidates for the treatment of aggression in the context of psychopathology. AEDs are generally considered the treatment of choice for patients with abnormal EEG findings and outbursts of rage (110). In a retrospective chart review, Salpekar et al. (111) identified 38 children with bipolar spectrum disorders and epilepsy comorbidity. Common bipolar symptoms included impulsivity, psycho-motor agitation, and explosive rage. Forty-two medication trials with 11 different AEDs were identified. Of the 30 cases in which AED monotherapy was attempted, carbamazepine, valproate, lamotrigine, and oxcarbazepine were associated with better CGI-I ratings than were other AEDs. In many cases, selected AEDs appeared to simultaneously treat both epilepsy and mood disorder. However, with the exception of cluster B personality disorders, AEDs have received only preliminary exploration in the treatment of impulse control and aggression in psychiatric disorders, without an associated seizure disorder.

Nonetheless, there is some evidence for the efficacy of valproate and carba-mazepine for the treatment of pathological aggression in patients with organic brain syndromes, dementia, psychosis, and, as discussed, personality disorders (109,110). Firm evidence for the efficacy of valproate or carbamazepine in man-aging aggression and/or agitation following traumatic brain injury (TBI) is lacking (112). In a literature review of AEDs for migraine, neuropathic pain, movement disorders, pervasive developmental disorders, bipolar disorder, and aggressive behavior in children and adolescents, Golden et al. (113) concluded that valproate is "probably effective" in decreasing aggressive behavior, carbamazepine is "probably ineffective" in treating aggression, and lamotrigine is "possibly inef-fective" for the core symptoms of pervasive developmental disorders. They also concluded that the data are insufficient to make recommendations about the efficacy of AEDs in these conditions in children and adolescents.

The likelihood of aggression may increase from stress or environmental overstimulation, problems related to impulsivity, or neurotransmitter balances, favoring dopamine and excitatory amino acid transmission over serotonin and inhibitory amino acid (GABA) transmission (114). AEDs may work by altering the inhibitory excitatory amino acid balance in favor of GABA, thereby protecting against overstimulation and raising the convulsive threshold when aggression is associated with a seizure disorder. Useful AEDs might also be those that combine dopaminergic and serotonergic actions (114).

Treatments for aggression should be based on the underlying causes. Barratt (115) proposed that aggression could be divided into three general categories: (*i*) medically related, where aggression is a symptom secondary to a neurological, psychiatric, or other medical disorder; (*ii*) premeditated, predatory, or planned, where the aggressive behavior is an instrumental response; and (*iii*) impulsive, where aggression is a trigger response in that information is not processed in an adap-tive way during the temper outburst. Barratt hypothesized that certain anticonvul-sants (e.g., phenytoin, carbamazepine) would be effective for treating impulsive aggression.

Valproate

Valproate, which enhances GABA neurotransmission, was first introduced as an AED in 1967. Its use in the treatment of aggressive and violent behaviors has been reported in the literature as far back as 1988. This literature, which includes several double-blind, placebo-controlled studies (9,80,81,83,116), supports the use of val-proate in the treatment of hostility/aggression, impulsive aggression, and affective instability in patients in a variety of psychiatric and neuropsychiatric disorders.

Thus, valproate has been reported to be effective against impulsive aggression and/or hostility in subjects with bipolar disorder (9,74,77,80–83,117) and adolescents with aggression and labile mood (118,119). Improved behavioral dyscontrol and aggression with valproate treatment has also been noted in patients with PTSD (120–122), temper outbursts (118,119,123), TBI (124,125), dementia (116,126–129), and autism (130).

In a review of studies of nonbipolar subjects with aggressive and violent behaviors (the most frequent diagnoses were dementia, organic brain syndromes, and mental retardation), valproate was found to be effective in 77% of 164 subjects in 17 studies, though these were open studies that often included more than one treatment (131). Wroblewski et al. (125) described the effectiveness of VPA in reducing and improving destructive and aggressive behaviors in five patients with TBI. In all cases, valproate was effective after other pharmacological interventions had failed, and neurobehavioral improvement was fairly rapid, often within one to two weeks. Although AEDs may be best suited for subacute or chronic treatment (114), rapid stabilization of severe agitation has been reported with intravenous valproate (132). Buchalter and Lantz (127) described a patient with vascular dementia in whom valproate led to reduced overt aggression, diminished impulsivity, and improved functional status. In a retrospective study of a long-term care database of elderly nursing home residents with a history of dementia-related behavior problems, Meinhold et al. (133) found that valproate therapy had beneficial effects on various behavioral, mood, and cognitive indicators, as monotherapy with benzodiazepines, and with antipsychotics, and at both higher and lower doses. In general, the higher-dose valproate group had more favorable results.

In a retrospective study (130), 14 patients with DSM-IV-diagnosed autism, Asperger's disorder, or pervasive developmental disorder NOS, with or without a history of seizure disorders or EEG abnormalities, received open-label treatment with valproate. Ten (71%) patients had a sustained response to valproate, as assessed by the CGI-I scale. Improvement was noted in the core autistic symptoms of social interaction, speech/communication skills, and repetitive behaviors as well as the associated features of affective instability, impulsivity, and aggression. Valproate was generally well tolerated. By contrast, no treatment difference was observed between groups in a prospective, eight-week, randomized, double-blind, placebo-controlled study of 30 outpatient subjects ($N = 20$ boys) with pervasive developmental disorders (ages 6–20 years) with significant aggression (134). However, these negative findings should not be considered conclusive, partly because of the large placebo response, subject heterogeneity, and small sample size.

Evidence supporting the use of valproate in the treatment of juvenile bipolar disorder with reactive aggression has grown (135,136). In one study, three boys with ADHD associated with giant somatosensory evoked potentials (SEP) responded well to valproate extended-release (ER) in particular, showing reduced hyperactivity and impulsivity (137). In two patients, previous methylphenidate treatment had worsened symptoms, suggesting that they may have had bipolar spectrum conditions. Valproate was also effective in a randomized, controlled trial of adolescent males with conduct disorder openly treated with high-dose or low-dose VPA (138). There was significant improvement in the high-dose group on a number of outcome measures, including self-reported weekly impulse control. Donovan et al. (119) sought to replicate open-label findings where 10 adolescents with a disruptive behavior disorder, who met operationalized criteria for explosive temper and mood lability, showed improvement with valproate for five weeks (118).

In the double-blind, placebo-controlled crossover study (119,120), outpatient children and adolescents (ages 10–18 years) with a disruptive behavior disorder (oppositional defiant disorder or conduct disorder), who met the specific criteria for explosive temper and mood lability, were randomly assigned to receive six weeks of valproate or placebo. At the end of phase one, 8 of 10 subjects responded to valproate and 0 of 10 responded to placebo. Twelve of the 15 subjects who completed both phases had a superior response to valproate.

In a randomized, double-blind, 28-day study, valproate and quetiapine showed similar efficacy for the treatment of impulsivity and reactive aggression related to co-occurring bipolar and disruptive behavior disorders in adolescents ($N = 33$) (139). In a retrospective, case-controlled study, Gobbi et al. (140) compared the effects of topiramate, valproate, and their combination in 45 psychiatric inpatients with schizophrenia, schizoaffective, or bipolar disorder with marked aggression and agitation. Topiramate-treated patients showed a decrease in mean OAS scores, episodes of agitation, and strict surveillance interventions. The effect was similar in the valproate-alone and combination valproate-topiramate treatment groups. However, valproate alone, but not topiramate alone, decreased the intensity of agitation episodes; and valproate alone and the valproate-topiramate combination decreased the number of psychotic disorganization episodes. MacMillan et al. (141) reviewed medical records of 31 pediatric bipolar disorder patients (age < 18 years) with severe aggression who received valproate ($N = 20$) or oxcarbazepine ($N = 11$). Overall CGI-S scores and CGI-S scores specific to aggression significantly improved from baseline to the four-month time point with valproate but not oxcarbazepine. Discontinuation rates from adverse events were similar. However, more discontinuations due to worsening aggression occurred with oxcarbazepine (27.3% vs. none for valproate). In a medical records review of 42 patients (ages 12–19 years) hospitalized for acute mania and discharged with a diagnosis of DSM-III-R or DSM-IV bipolar disorder, a history of ADHD was associated with a significantly diminished acute response to both valproate and lithium as a treatment for their bipolar manic phase (142). Response rates for lithium versus valproate in subjects with and without ADHD did not differ.

Barzman et al. (143) retrospectively reviewed the charts of 46 children and adolescents admitted to a crisis stabilization center with prominent impulsive aggression and irritability who met criteria for a potential pediatric bipolar phenotype and who responded to valproate. Significant improvements were obtained on the Children's Global Assessment Scale, with significant decreases on the OAS and the Anger-Hostility Subscale of the SCL-90 at discharge, following a maximal 14-day stay. No severe side effects were reported. The above data are in line with valproate response in children and adolescents with explosive temper and mood instability (118,119) and suggest that such symptoms, together with impulsive aggression, irritability, and other manic symptoms, may constitute a pediatric valproate-responsive bipolar spectrum disorder. In a 12-week, open-label trial of valproate in 24 bipolar offspring, ages 6 to 18 years (17 boys), with mixed diagnoses of major depression, cyclothymia, ADHD, and oppositional defiant disorder, 71% of subjects were considered valproate responders by the OAS (144). Thus, youths who were at high risk for bipolar disorder experienced an overall decrease in aggressive behavior in response to valproate.

Prospective, randomized, double-blind, placebo-controlled trials are needed to further assess valproate's optimal usage for the treatment of aggression and impulsivity across psychiatric disorders.

Carbamazepine and Oxcarbazepine

In the 1980s, carbamazepine became an AED of primary interest in treating impulsive aggression because it was the drug of choice for treating temporal lobe epilepsy patients with aggressive outbursts and irritability (145). Several reviews have since then concluded that carbamazepine reduces aggressive and associated behaviors across a wide range of diagnoses (146–149). Carbamazepine has been reported effective in treating pathological aggression in dementia (150) and in decreasing combativeness, agitated behavior, irritability, and disinhibition in subjects with head injuries (151,152). Freymann et al. (153) described the successful use of carbamazepine in a 78-year-old Alzheimer's disease patient with hypersexual behavior. The efficacy of carbamazepine in this case is in parallel to its effects on aggression and agitation in dementia (150). One open-label study of inpatient children with conduct disorder found statistically and clinically significant declines of explosiveness and aggression (154). A double-blind, placebo-controlled trial, however, found no difference between carbamazepine and placebo, and side effects were common (146). Indeed, the few placebo-controlled trials with carbamazepine have been small and in diverse patient populations (147,148). For example, Mattes (155) randomly assigned propranolol or carbamazepine treatment for temper outbursts to 80 patients with diverse diagnoses. Both medications were beneficial, but a diagnosis of ADHD predicted better response to propranolol, and a diagnosis of IED predicted better response to carbamazepine.

The ICD-10 diagnosis "Organic Personality Disorder," listed under "Personality Change Due to a General Medical Condition" in the DSM-IV, may involve aggression and impulsivity. Many different treatments have been proposed for this condition, including carbamazepine. Munoz and Gonzalez Torres (156) described a 28-year-old male who had aggressive episodes along with an intensification of previous personality traits, sexual exhibitionism, promiscuity, suspiciousness, and low impulse control after a severe brain injury sustained in a car accident. Antipsychotics, benzodiazepines, and antidepressants had no effect. After two months of carbamazepine treatment, the patient had marked improvement with the absence of aggressive episodes and exhibitionistic behavior, a tendency toward normalization of mood and anxiety, stabilization of his social and family relationships, and employment. Morikawa et al. (157) reported a 19-year-old male who had a personality change, marked by irritability, aggression, labile mood, childishness, irresponsibility, and lack of motivation, six months after a mild injury to his left frontotemporal cortex from a motorbike accident. He was diagnosed with posttraumatic personality disorder and treated with clonazepam, which moderately improved his symptoms but caused drowsiness. Within a few days of the addition of carbamazepine, he improved to his preinjury personality. After clonazepam was discontinued, he maintained good mental status and at two-year follow-up continued to be well. Lewin and Sumners (158) described an 18-year-old man who, following a traffic accident, developed episodic dyscontrol. Two years post injury, carbamazepine treatment was started and his aggressive outbursts subsided.

Oxcarbazepine, like carbamazepine, is effective for complex partial seizures and may have mood-stabilizing effects (159). In a double-blind, placebo-controlled, 10-week study, adult outpatients with clinically significant impulsive aggression were randomized to placebo (N = 24) or oxcarbazepine (N = 24) (160). Nine patients dropped out because of adverse events, but 45 completed at least four weeks of treatment. Results showed a benefit from oxcarbazepine compared with placebo on OAS-M scores and patient-rated global improvement. Guadino et al. (161) described an adolescent with treatment-resistant aggression (and a mood disorder and ADHD), which improved with oxcarbazepine, the only side effect being sedation. Cordas et al. (162) presented two cases of severe bulimia and BPD, in which self-mutilating behavior was successfully controlled with oxcarbazepine treatment.

Topiramate

Topiramate, a newer AED, which acts on voltage-activated sodium channels and glutamate and GABA receptors, has also been reported to be effective in a variety of aggressive patients (92). In a retrospective chart review study, Janowsky et al. (93) examined topiramate treatment in 22 severely or profoundly intellectually disabled, institutionalized adults, most with a concurrent mood disorder. Patients were treated for aggression, SIBs, destructive/disruptive behaviors, and/or other challenging and maladaptive behaviors. Significant decreases in global severity scores, cumulative aggression, and worst behavior rates occurred, especially when comparing the three months before and the three to six months after starting topiramate. In a randomized, double-blind, placebo-controlled, 10-week study of topiramate in 64 females diagnosed with recurrent major depressive disorder, topiramate significantly reduced anger and depressive symptoms compared with placebo (163). There was also significant weight loss in the topiramate group and topiramate was relatively well tolerated. In seven patients with PWS, topiramate reduced aggressive and SIB, improved mood, and stabilized weight (164). These reports correspond with other studies in which topiramate resulted in significantly decreased aggressive symptoms (90,91).

Impulsivity plays a significant role in a wide range of psychiatric disorders including eating disorders like BED. Topiramate has also shown efficacy in the treatment of a number of disorders involving impulsivity including BED (165,166). BED is characterized by recurrent episodes of binge eating that are not followed by the regular use of inappropriate compensatory weight loss behaviors. It is often associated with overweight or obesity and psychopathology. The literature offers support, including from double-blind, placebo-controlled trials, for the use of antidepressants, appetite suppressants (e.g., sibutramine), and AEDs in the treatment of BED (167–169). Topiramate, in particular, appears to be promising for the treatment of BED because of its beneficial effects on body weight as well as impulsivity.

In a preliminary naturalistic, open-label study with topiramate, 9 of 13 BED outpatients showed a moderate or better response of binge eating symptoms after beginning treatment that was maintained for 3 to 30 months (165). Two other patients had moderate or marked responses that subsequently diminished and the remaining two patients had a mild or no response. In another preliminary study, treatment with topiramate (150 mg daily) was administered over 16 weeks to eight obese patients with BED and no medical or psychiatric comorbidity (170). All six of the trial completers showed reduced binge eating. Four patients had a complete remission, and two had a marked reduction in binge eating frequency. Patients also had significant weight loss. In a 14-week, double-blind, flexible-dose topiramate trial, 61 BED outpatients with obesity were randomly assigned to receive topiramate ($N = 30$) or placebo ($N = 31$) (166). Compared with placebo, topiramate resulted in a significantly greater rate of reduction in binge frequency, binge day frequency, BMI, weight, and scores on the CGI-S and the Y-BOCS modified for binge eating (Y-BOCS-BE) (166). Topiramate was also found to have positive effects for the long-term treatment of BED in a 42-week, open-label extension trial (171) of the acute study (166). For all patients ($N = 43$) receiving topiramate during either the double-blind or open-label extension study, there was a significant decline from baseline to final visit in weekly binge frequency, CGI-Score, Y-BOCS-BE total, and compulsion, and obsession subscale scores, weight, and BMI.

Zilberstein et al. (172) analyzed 16 patients with binge eating and inadequate weight loss after adjustable gastric banding while receiving topiramate for three months (12.5–50 mg/day). There was a mean increase in excess weight loss from 20.4% to 34.1% without the need for band readjustment. Two patients, however, could not tolerate topiramate. Dolberg et al. (173) reported the effects of adjunctive topiramate on eating patterns and weight in 17 patients with TBI, posttraumatic epilepsy, and weight gain of various etiologies. The six patients with BED had the most pronounced effects, with marked decreases in binges and a normalization of BMI. In another study, three obese BED patients, who had recurrent binge eating and weight gain after initially successful bariatric surgery, reported complete improvement of their binge eating and displayed weight loss after receiving top-iramate for 10 months on average (174). De Bernardi et al. (175) reported a BED patient who was unresponsive to several treatments but was successfully treated with topiramate. In a 10-week double-blind, placebo-controlled study, topiramate was also effective in reducing the frequency of binging/purging and body weight in bulimic patients (176).

Topiramate may also be effective in treating self-mutilating behavior. Top-iramate improved self-mutilation and manic symptoms in two patients with bipolar disorder and BPD (177). Further, topiramate (200 mg/day) administered in an on-off-on design to a 24-year-old woman with bipolar II depression and BPD led to long-term remission of self-mutilation despite the persistence of depression (178). No self-injurious acts occurred over nine months, and mood was sufficiently stabilized.

Dolengevich et al. (179) evaluated 11 child and adolescent outpatients with impulsive behavioral disorders by DSM-IV criteria at one and three months after starting topiramate treatment. There were significant differences in the cognitive impulsivity subscale and total score of the Barratt Impulsivity scale after one month and the motor impulsivity subscale after three months. Thus, topiramate may be an effective treatment for impulsivity in children and adolescents as well as in adults with some psychiatric disorders. More studies with larger samples and control groups are needed to confirm the efficacy of topiramate for the treatment of aggression and impulsivity in all age groups.

Levetiracetam

There is preliminary evidence that levetiracetam, FDA approved as an adjunctive treatment for partial-complex seizures, may be effective in some psychiatric disorders characterized by affective lability, impulsivity, and anxiety (180–183). In an open-label prospective study of 10 autistic boys aged 4 to 10 years, levetiracetam significantly reduced hyperactivity, impulsivity, mood instability, and disruptive outbursts (180). Aggressive behavior showed significant improvement only in subjects who were not recently weaned from medications that reduced aggression (e.g., risperidone, carbamazepine, desipramine). However, in a 10-week, double-blind, placebo-controlled trial of levetiracetam in 20 autistic children aged 5 to 17 years, no significant difference was found between drug and placebo groups in terms of change in CGI-I, Aberrant Behavior Checklist, Children's Y-BOCS, or Conners' scales (184). These findings suggest that levetiracetam may not improve the behavioral disturbances of autism, but are limited by the small sample size and lack of stratification of the autistic sample at baseline.

In some studies, levetiracetam has actually increased aggression as a side effect. Dinkelacker et al. (185) reported 33 patients with long-standing histories of epilepsy who experienced aggressive episodes during levetiracetam therapy (3.5% of levetiracetam-treated patients vs. <1% of patients not receiving levetiracetam). Among these cases, 24 showed only moderate, transient irritability, with 10 patients requiring reduction or discontinuation of levetiracetam; but nine patients had severe aggressive symptoms with physical violence, two of whom needed psychiatric emergency treatment. Weber et al. (186) gave levetiracetam to 10 generalized epilepsy patients, and one patient with Lennox-Gastaut syndrome discontinued the drug because of aggression. In an observational survey, 128 (44.9%) of 285 pediatric patients (mean age 9.9 years) with refractory generalized and focal epilepsy reported mild to moderate side effects after receiving levetiracetam as an add-on open-label treatment (187). Behavioral changes were the second most frequent side effect after somnolence, included aggressive behavior in 44 patients (15.4%) and prompted discontinuation of the drug in 23 cases (8.1%). The most common behavioral adverse event was aggression, which was seen in 30 patients (10.5%) and was often severe. Two patients violently attacked others, which they had never done before. In another study (188), 11 (13%) of 85 pediatric patients (mean age 10.5 years) with refractory generalized and focal epilepsy, who received levetiracetam as add-on treatment, reported mild to moderate side effects, consisting most frequently of general behavioral changes, aggression, and sleep disturbances, which ceased after decreasing the levetiracetam dosage.

In sum, levetiracetam may reduce impulsivity, mood instability, and aggression in some populations, but studies in other patient populations, including BPD, are warranted. Morever, because of reports of increased aggression, the behavioral tolerability of levetiracetam should be monitored carefully, especially in patients with histories of aggression.

Gabapentin

Gabapentin increases CNS GABA, a neurotransmitter important for the control of aggressive behavior and has been reported to have antiaggressive effects across several disorders (189). Thus, several studies have reported significant improvement with gabapentin of aggressive behavior in dementia patients (190,191). In a retrospective chart review, Hawkins et al. (192) examined the use of gabapentin for the treatment of aggressive and agitated behaviors in 24 nursing home patients with DSM-IV-diagnosed dementia. On the CGR-I, 17 of 22 patients were rated as much or greatly improved, four were minimally improved, and one remained unchanged. Two patients discontinued the medication because of excessive sedation. No other significant side effects were noted after treatment for up to two years. Alkhalil et al. (193) described three dementia nursing home residents whose sexual disinhibition was effectively treated with gabapentin.

McManaman and Tan (194) described a patient with Lesch-Nyhan syndrome (an X-linked disorder of purine metabolism) whose SIB was effectively treated with gabapentin. Gupta et al. (195) described a patient with aggression and violent behavior due to DSM-IV-diagnosed conduct disorder whose symptoms were controlled with gabapentin after he failed a trial of valproate. In another case (196), gabapentin treatment resulted in a decrease in the frequency and intensity of violent episodes in a young patient with IED, ADHD, organic mood disorder secondary to a TBI, and a simple partial seizure disorder. Cherek et al. (189) measured aggression in 20 adult parolees with a pattern of antisocial behavior ($N = 2$ females), using the Point Subtraction Aggression Paradigm, which provided subjects aggressive, escape, and monetary reinforced response options. Ten subjects had a history of conduct disorder (CD^+) and 10 had no history of conduct disorder (non-CD). Acute doses (200, 400, and 800 mg) of gabapentin had similar effects on aggressive responses among both CD^+ and non-CD control subjects. Aggressive responses of CD^+ and non-CD subjects increased at lower gabapentin doses and decreased at the highest dose (800 mg). Specifically, gabapentin increased escape responses for both groups at the lowest dose, but then produced dose-related decreases at the two higher doses in both groups. No changes in monetary reinforced responses were observed, suggesting an absence of CNS stimulation or sedation.

Phenytoin
Although phenytoin did not improve aggressive behavior in children with temper tantrums in one early study (197), it has been reported to reduce the frequency of impulsive-aggressive behavior in a variety of conditions (115,198), to alter mid-latency-evoked potentials (199), and to significantly reduce violent outbursts in psychiatric patients with episodic dyscontrol syndrome (200,201). Thus, incarcerated inmates with impulsive-aggressive behavior showed significant reductions in the frequency and intensity of aggressive acts, normalization of event-related potentials (ERPs) (i.e., increased P300 amplitude), and improved mood state measures during a six-week, double-blind, placebo-controlled trial of phenytoin (300 mg/day) (202,203). Further, inmates whose aggressive behavior was considered premeditated did not show improvement (203). Stanford et al. (199) corroborated and extended these findings in a double-blind, placebo-controlled, crossover study of a noninmate population. Individuals meeting previously established criteria for impulsive aggression were given phenytoin and placebo during separate six-week conditions. Compared with baseline and placebo, the frequency of impulsive-aggressive outbursts significantly decreased during phenytoin treatment. Phenytoin also affected sensory/attentional processing (measured by ERPs) as indicated by increased P1 amplitude, longer-evoked potential latencies, and the suggestion of reduced N1 amplitude. In a double-blind, placebo-controlled, parallel group design, impulsive-aggressive men were randomly assigned to one of four six-week treatments: phenytoin ($N = 7$), carbamazepine ($N = 7$), valproate ($N = 7$), or placebo ($N = 8$) (199). A significant reduction in impulsive aggression (as measured by the OAS global severity index) was found during all three AED conditions compared with placebo. Compared with phenytoin and valproate, there was a slightly delayed effect during carbamazepine treatment.

In sum, these findings suggest that phenytoin could have a significant impact in the control of impulsive aggression in mental health and criminal populations. Further, because the antiaggressive properties of phenytoin appear selective for impulsive aggression, it suggests that biological mechanisms may distinguish impulsive from premeditated aggression (204).

DISCUSSION

Effective treatment of impulsivity and aggression depends on determining the cause(s) of these behaviors and selecting treatments accordingly. Pharmacological treatments may reduce impulsivity or aggression and normalize arousal by reducing dopaminergic activity, enhancing serotonergic activity, shifting the balance of amino acid neurotransmitter from excitatory (glutamatergic) toward inhibitory (GABAergic) transmission, and/or reducing or stabilizing nonadrenergic effects. Pharmacological and nonpharmacological treatment, like behavioral strategies aimed at reducing aggressive or impulsive behavior, may be most effective for the long-term treatment of the underlying chronic or recurrent illness (114). In general, there is no treatment of choice for impulse control and cluster B personality disorders. Many drugs from different classes seem to offer some benefit to selected individuals depending on their symptom presentations. For example, BPD patients with prominent cognitive and/or perceptual distortion may respond to antipsychotics, while those with depressed mood may respond best to antidepressants. Biological and behavioral dimensions may underlie treatment response in personality disorder patients (4,21). There may be several developmental trajectories to impulsivity and aggression (e.g., ADHD, bipolar spectrum, and trait impulsivity) and various routes to altering motivational circuitry, like modulating of corticostriatal-limbic circuits. We suggest that core symptoms within disorders should be treated and appropriate outcome measures should be used to determine targeted treatment response.

On the basis of the evidence presented here, AEDs appear to be effective for treating the symptom domains of impulsivity and aggression across a wide range of psychiatric disorders and for impulse control and cluster B personality disorders in particular. It is suggested that interventions should be directed at the brain circuitry, which modulates core symptoms that may be shared across disorders rather than DSM diagnoses. In addition to core symptom domains like impulsivity, affective instability, and aggression, clinicians should identify comorbid conditions and associated symptoms related to brain systems as they can also influence overall treatment response. AEDs may be effective for the treatment of the brain circuitry related to impulsivity, aggression, comorbid affective instability, and traumatic arousal, by modulating GABA, glutamate, serotonin, and norepinephrine.

Since ICDs and cluster B personality disorders have been found to be highly comorbid with other psychiatric disorders, the most effective and best-tolerated medication may vary depending on the comorbidity (101). Thus, AEDs, traditionally used to treat bipolar disorder, can also be effective for ICDs and cluster B personality disorders when there are associated bipolar symptoms. When treating the core symptoms of impulsivity and aggression, the associated bipolar and mood lability symptoms may improve as well. Clinicians should treat target symptoms like impulsivity and aggression regardless of their overall diagnosis, while taking into account comorbid disorders (e.g., bipolar disorder, ADHD), associated symptoms, developmental trajectory, and family history. For example, while SSRIs may be effective in treating pathological gambling with a comorbid obsessive-compulsive spectrum disorder or obsessive-compulsive features, they may not be the optimal treatment of pathological gambling with comorbid ADHD or a bipolar spectrum disorder (205,206). Clinicians must be careful when treating patients at risk for bipolar disorder, as SSRI-induced manic behaviors could emerge in those with a history of, or at risk for, mania or hypomania (44). Thus, a mood-stabilizing

AED like valproate may be a better treatment option for ICD patients with a comorbid bipolar disorder.

Accordingly, BPD patients with comorbid bipolar II disorder or subclinical bipolar symptomology may benefit from mood-stabilizing AEDs, like carbamazepine, if irritability is pronounced (63). Preliminary data indicate personality disorders with aggressive behavior, and emotionally unstable character disorder with mood swings, respond to AEDs. A variety of personality factors and comorbid conditions overrepresented in BPD patients, like premenstrual syndrome, bulimia, agoraphobia, major affective disorder (e.g., bipolar II), and hypersomnia, often complicate the clinical picture. Depending on the mix of these factors, certain drugs may need to be avoided, nonstandard drug combinations may need to be used, and safer drugs may need to be used in place of more effective drugs (102).

The growing experience of psychiatrists in treating ICDs, cluster B personality disorders, and impulsivity and aggression across disorders should compliment the knowledge obtained from research. This will lead to a better understanding of the brain mechanisms underlying impulsive and aggressive symptom domains within DSM disorders and to more targeted treatments with improved outcomes.

REFERENCES

1. Asconape JJ. Some common issues in the use of antiepileptic drugs. Semin Neurol 2002; 22:27–39.
2. Evenden JL. Varieties of impulsivity. Psychopharmacology 1999; 146:348–361.
3. Moeller G, Barratt ES, Dougherty DM, et al. Psychiatric aspects of impulsivity. Am J Psychiatry 2001; 158:1783–1793.
4. Coccaro EF. Impulsive aggression: a behavior in search of clinical definition. Harv Res Psychiatry 1998; 5:336–339.
5. Virkkunen M. Reactive hypoglycemic tendency among habitually violent offenders. Nutr Rev 1975; 44:94–103.
6. Pattison E, Kahan J. The deliberate self-harm syndrome. Am J Psychiatry 1983; 140: 867–872.
7. Cold JW. Axis II disorders and motivation for serious criminal behavior. In: Skodal AE, ed. Psychopathology and Violent Crime. Washington, DC: American Psychiatric Press, 1998.
8. Hollander E, Berlin HA. Neuropsychiatric aspects of aggression and impulse control disorders. In: Yudofsky SC, Hales RE, eds. American Psychiatric Press Textbook of Neuropsychiatry and Clinical Neurosciences. Washington, DC: American Psychiatric Press, (in press).
9. Hollander E, Tracy KA, Swann AC, et al. Divalproex in the treatment of impulsive aggression: efficacy in cluster B personality disorders. Neuropsychopharmacology 2003; 28: 1186–97.
10. Critchfield KL, Levy KN, Clarkin JF. The relationship between impulsivity, aggression, and impulsive-aggression in borderline personality disorder: an empirical analysis of self-report measures. J Personal Disord 2004; 18:555–570.
11. Hollander E, Rosen J. Impulsivity. J Psychopharmacol 2000; 14:S39–S44.
12. Delville Y, Melloni RH Jr., Ferris CF. Behavioral and neurobiological consequences of social subjugation during puberty in golden hamsters. J Neurosci 1998; 18:2667–2672.
13. Davidson JR. Anxiety and affective style: role of prefrontal cortex and amygdala. Biol Psychiatry 2002; 51:68–80.
14. Davis M, Whalen PJ. The amygdala: vigilance and emotion. Mol Psychiatry 2001; 6:13–34.
15. Rolls ET, Hornak J, Wade D, et al. Emotion-related learning in patients with social and emotional changes associated with frontal lobe damage. J Neurol Neurosurg Psychiatry 1994; 57:1518–1524.

16. Hornak J, Bramham J, Rolls ET, et al. Changes in emotion after circumscribed surgical lesions of the orbitofrontal and cingulate cortices. Brain 2003; 126:1691–1712.

17. Hornak J, O'Doherty J, Bramham J, et al. Reward-related reversal learning after surgical excisions in orbitofrontal and dorsolateral prefrontal cortex in humans. J Cogn Neurosci 2004; 16:463–478.

18. Hornak J, Rolls ET, Wade D. Face and voice expression identification in patients with emotional and behavioural changes following ventral frontal lobe damage. Neuropsychologia 1996; 34:247–261.

19. Drevets WC. Functional neuroimaging studies of depression: the anatomy of melancholia. Annu Rev Med 1998; 49:341–361.

20. Van Reekum R. Acquired and developmental brain dysfunction in borderline personality disorder. Can J Psychiatry 1993; 38:S4–S10.

21. Berlin HA, Rolls ET, Iversen SD. Borderline personality disorder, impulsivity, and the orbitofrontal cortex. Am J Psychiatry 162:2360–2373.

22. Rolls ET. The Brain and Emotion. Oxford, UK: Oxford University Press, 1999.

23. Baxter MG, Parker A, Lindner CC, et al. Control of response selection by reinforcer value requires interaction of amygdala and orbital prefrontal cortex. J Neurosci 2000; 20:4311–4319.

24. Herpertz SC, Dietrich TM, Wenning B, et al. Evidence of abnormal amygdala functioning in borderline personality disorder: a functional MRI study. Biol Psychiatry 2001; 50: 292–298.

25. Tebartz van Elst L, Hesslinger B, Thiel T, et al. Frontolimbic brain abnormalities in patients with borderline personality disorder: a volumetric magnetic resonance imaging study. Biol Psychiatry 2003; 54:163–171.

26. Pietrini P, Guazzelli M, Basso G. Neural correlates of imaginal aggressive behavior assessed by positron emission tomography in healthy subjects. Am J Psychiatry 2000; 157:1772–1781.

27. Siever LJ, Buchsbaum MS, New AS, et al. d,l-fenfluramine response in impulsive personality disorder assessed with [18F]fluorodeoxyglucose positron emission tomography. Neuropsychopharmacology 1999; 20:413–423.

28. Drevets WC. Prefrontal cortical-amygdalar metabolism in major depression. Ann N Y Acad Sci 1999; 877:614–637.

29. Herpertz SC, Dietrich TM, Wenning B, et al. Evidence of abnormal amygdala functioning in borderline personality disorder: a functional MRI study. Biol Psychiatry 2001; 50: 292–298.

30. LeDoux JE. The Emotional Brain. New York: Simon and Schuster, 1996.

31. Whalen PJ, Rauch SL, Etcoff NL, et al. Masked presentations of emotional facial expressions modulate amygdala activity without explicit knowledge. J Neurosci 1998; 18: 411–418.

32. Morgan MA, Romanski LM, LeDoux JE. Extinction of emotional learning: contribution of medial prefrontal cortex. Neuroscience 1993; 163:109–113 (letter).

33. Rauch SL, Shin LM, Whalen PJ. Neuroimaging and the neuroanatomy of posttraumatic stress disorder. CNS Spectrums 1998; 3(suppl 2):30–41.

34. American Psychiatric Association (APA) . Diagnostic and Statistical Manual of Mental Disorders IV-TR. Washington, DC: APA, 2000.

35. Slutske WS, Eisen S, Xian H, et al. A twin study of the association between pathological gambling and antisocial personality disorder. J Abnorm Psychol 2001; 110:297–308.

36. Potenza MN, Steinberg MA, Skudlarski P, et al. Gambling urges in pathological gambling: a functional magnetic resonance imaging study. Arch Gen Psychiatry 2003; 60: 828–836.

37. Potenza MN, Leung HC, Blumberg HP, et al. An FMRI Stroop task study of ventromedial prefrontal cortical function in pathological gamblers. Am J Psychiatry 2003; 160: 1990–1994.

38. Bechara A, Damasio H, Damasio AR, et al. Different contributions of the human amygdala and ventromedial prefrontal cortex to decision-making. J Neurosci 1999; 19:5473–5481.

39. O'Doherty J, Kringelbach ML, Rolls ET, et al. Abstract reward and punishment representations in the human orbitofrontal cortex. Nat Neurosci 2001; 4:95–102.

40. Berlin HA, Rolls ET, Kischka U. Impulsivity, time perception, emotion, and reinforcement sensitivity in patients with orbitofrontal cortex lesions. Brain 2004; 127:1108–1126.

41. Hollander E, Pallanti S, Rossi NB, et al. Imaging monetary reward in pathological gamblers. World J Biol Psychiatry 2005; 6(2):113–120.

42. Hollander E, Buchalter AJ, DeCaria CM. Pathological gambling. Psychiatr Clin North Am 2000; 23:629–642.

43. Hollander E, Frenkel M, DeCaria C, et al. Treatment of pathological gambling with clomipramine. Am J Psychiatry 1992; 149:710–711 (letter).

44. Hollander E, DeCaria CM, Mari E, et al. Short-term single-blind fluvoxamine treatment of pathological gambling. Am J Psychiatry 1998; 155:1781–1783.

45. Hollander E, DeCaria CM, Finkell JN, et al. A randomized double-blind fluvoxamine/ placebo crossover trial in pathologic gambling. Biol Psychiatry 2000; 47:813–817.

46. Dannon PN, Lowengrub K, Gonopolski Y, et al. Topiramate versus fluvoxamine in the treatment of pathological gambling: a randomized, blind-rater comparison study. Clin Neuropharmacol 2005; 28:6–10.

47. Kim SW. Opioid antagonists in the treatment of impulse-control disorders. J Clin Psychiatry 1998; 59:159–164.

48. Moskowitz JA. Lithium and lady luck: use of lithium carbonate in compulsive gambling. N Y State J Med 1980; 80:785–788.

49. Pallanti S, Quercioli L, Sood E, et al. Lithium and valproate treatment of pathological gambling: a randomized single-blind study. J Clin Psychiatry 2002; 63:559–64.

50. Hollander E, Pallanti S, Allen A, et al. Does sustained-release lithium reduce impulsive gambling and affective instability versus placebo in pathological gamblers with bipolar spectrum disorders? Am J Psychiatry 2005; 162:137–145.

51. Haller R, Hinterhuber H. Treatment of pathological gambling with carbamazepine. Pharmacopsychiatry 1994; 27:129.

52. Dannon PN. Topiramate for the treatment of kleptomania: a case series and review of the literature. Clin Neuropharmacol 2003; 26:1–4.

53. Shapira NA, Lessig MC, Murphy TK, et al. Topiramate attenuates self-injurious behaviour in Prader–Willi Syndrome. Int J Neuropsychopharmacol 2002; 5:141–145.

54. Shapira NA, Lessig MC, Lewis MH, et al. Effects of topiramate in adults with Prader–Willi syndrome. Am J Ment Retard 2004; 109:301–309.

55. Lochner C, Seedat S, Niehaus DJ, et al. Topiramate in the treatment of trichotillomania: an open-label pilot study. Int Clin Psychopharmacol 2006; 21:255–259.

56. De Dios Perrino C, Santo-Domingo Carrasco J, Lozano Suarez M. Pharmacological treatment of the intermittent explosive disorder. Report of three cases and literature review. Actas Luso Esp Neurol Psiquiatr Cienc Afines 1995; 23:74–77.

57. Denicoff KD, Meglathery SB, Post RM, et al. Efficacy of carbamazepine compared with other agents: a clinical practice survey. J Clin Psychiatry 1994; 55:70–76.

58. Adu L, Lessig M, Shapira N. Topiramate in the treatment of trichotillomania. Presented at: The Southern Association for Research in Psychiatry 14th Annual Meeting, Gainesville, Florida, 2001.

59. Kaufman KR, Kugler SL, Sachdeo RC. Tiagabine in the management of postencephalitic epilepsy and impulse control disorder. Epilepsy Behav 2002; 3:190–194.

60. Nickel M, Nickel C, Leiberich P, et al. Psychosocial characteristics in people who often change their psychotherapists. Wien Med Wochenschr 2004; 154:163–169.

61. Skodol AE, Gunderson JG, Pfohl B, et al. The borderline diagnosis I: psychopathology, comorbidity, and personality structure. Biol Psychiatry 2002; 51:936–950.

62. Skodol AE, Siever LJ, Livesley WJ, et al. The borderline diagnosis II: biology, genetics, and clinical course. Biol Psychiatry 2002; 51:951–963.

63. Stone MH. The role of pharmacotherapy in the treatment of patients with borderline personality disorder. Psychopharmacol Bull 1989; 25:564–571.

64. Swartz M, Blazer D, George L, et al. Estimating the prevalence of borderline personality disorder in the community. J Personality Dis 1990; 4:257–272.

65. Maier W, Lichtermann D, Klinger T, et al. Prevalences of personality disorders (DSM-III-R) in the community. J Personality Dis 1992; 6:187–196.

66. Hollander E. Managing aggressive behavior in patients with obsessive-compulsive disorder and borderline personality disorder. J Clin Psychiatry 1999; 60:38–44.
67. Skodol AE, Bender DS. Why are women diagnosed borderline more than men? Psychiatr Q 2003; 74:349–360.
68. Kass F, Skodol A, Spitzer CE, et al. Scaled ratings of DSM-III personality disorders. Am J Psychiatry 1985; 142:627–630.
69. Piersma HL. The MCMI as a measure of DSM-III axis II diagnoses: an empirical comparison. J Clin Psychol 1987; 43:478–483.
70. Gunderson JG. Pharmacotherapy for patients with borderline personality disorder. Arch Gen Psychiatry 1986; 43:698–700.
71. Cowdry R, Gardner DL. Pharmacotherapy of borderline personality disorder. Alprazolam, carbamazepine, trifluoperazine, and tranylcypromine. Arch Gen Psychiatry 1988; 45: 111–9.
72. Gitlin MJ. Pharmacotherapy of personality disorders: conceptual framework and clinical strategies. J Clin Psychopharmacol 1993; 13:343–353.
73. New AS, Trestman RL, Siever LJ. The pharmacotherapy of borderline personality disorder. CNS Drugs 1994; 5:347–354.
74. Zanarini MC. Update on pharmacotherapy of borderline personality disorder, Curr Psychiatry Rep 2004; 6:66–70.
75. Coryell W. Rapid cycling bipolar disorder: clinical characteristics and treatment options. CNS Drugs 2005; 19:557–569.
76. Stein DJ, Simeon D, Frenkel M, et al. An open trial of valproate in borderline personality disorder. J Clin Psychiatry 1995; 56:506–510.
77. Wilcox JA. Divalproex sodium as a treatment for borderline personality disorder. Ann Clin Psychiatry 1995; 7:33–37.
78. Kavoussi RJ, Coccaro EF. Divalproex sodium for impulsive aggressive behavior in patients with personality disorder. J Clin Psychiatry 1998; 59:676–680.
79. Davis LL, Ryan W, Adinoff B, et al. Comprehensive review of the psychiatric uses of valproate. J Clin Psychopharmacol 2000; 20(suppl 1):S1–S17.
80. Hollander E, Allen A, Lopez RP, et al. A preliminary double-blind, placebo-controlled trial of divalproex sodium in borderline personality disorder. J Clin Psychiatry 2001; 62: 199–203.
81. Frankenburg FR, Zanarini MC. Divalproex sodium treatment of women with borderline personality disorder and bipolar II disorder: a double-blind placebo-controlled pilot study. J Clin Psychiatry 2002; 63:442–446.
82. Townsend MH, Cambre KM, Barbee JG. Treatment of borderline personality disorder with mood instability with divalproex sodium: series of ten cases. J Clin Psychopharmacol 2001; 21:249–251.
83. Hollander E, Swann AC, Coccaro EF, et al. Impact of trait impulsivity and state aggression on divalproex versus placebo response in borderline personality disorder. Am J Psychiatry 2005; 162:621–624.
84. Berlin HA, Rolls ET. Time perception, impulsivity, emotionality, and personality in self-harming borderline personality disorder patients. J Personal Disord 2004; 18:358–378.
85. Gardner DL, Cowdry RW. Positive effects of carbamazepine on behavioral dyscontrol in borderline personality disorder. Am J Psychiatry 1986; 143:519–522.
86. Cowdry RW, Gardner DL. Pharmacotherapy of borderline personality disorder. Alprazolam, carbamazepine, trifluoperazine, and tranylcypromine. Arch Gen Psychiatry 1988; 45:111–119.
87. De la Fuente JM, Lotstra F. A trial of carbamazepine in borderline personality disorder. Eur Neuropsychopharmacol 1994; 4:479–486.
88. Gardner DL, Cowdry RW. Development of melancholia during carbamazepine treatment in borderline personality disorder. J Clin Psychopharmacol 1986; 6:236–239.
89. Bellino S, Paradiso E, Bogetto F. Oxcarbazepine in the treatment of borderline personality disorder: a pilot study. J Clin Psychiatry 2005; 66:1111–1115.
90. Nickel MK, Nickel C, Mitterlehner FO, et al. Topiramate treatment of aggression in female borderline personality disorder patients: a double-blind, placebo-controlled study. J Clin Psychiatry 2004; 65:1515–1519.

91. Nickel MK, Nickel C, Kaplan P, et al. Treatment of aggression with topiramate in male borderline patients: a double-blind, placebo-controlled study. Biol Psychiatry 2005; 57:495–499.
92. Teter CJ, Early JJ, Gibbs CM. Treatment of affective disorder and obesity with topiramate, Ann Pharmacother 2000; 34:1262–1265.
93. Janowsky DS, Kraus JE, Barnhill J, et al. Effects of topiramate on aggressive, self-injurious, and disruptive/destructive behaviors in the intellectually disabled: an open-label retrospective study. J Clin Psychopharmacol 2003; 23:500–504.
94. Loew TH, Nickel MK, Muehlbacher M, et al. Topiramate treatment for women with borderline personality disorder: a double-blind, placebo-controlled study. J Clin Psychopharmacol 2006; 26:61–66.
95. Killaspy H. Topiramate improves psychopathological symptoms and quality of life in women with borderline personality disorder. Evid Based Ment Health 2006; 9:74.
96. do Prado-Lima PA, Kristensen CH, Bacaltchuk J. Can childhood trauma predict response to topiramate in borderline personality disorder? J Clin Pharm Ther 2006; 31: 193–196.
97. Pinto OC, Akiskal HS. Lamotrigine as a promising approach to borderline personality: an open case series without concurrent DSM-IV major mood disorder. J Affect Disord 1998; 51:333–343.
98. Preston GA, Marchant BK, Reimherr FW, et al. Borderline personality disorder in patients with bipolar disorder and response to lamotrigine. J Affect Disord 2004; 79: 297–303.
99. Tritt K, Nickel C, Lahmann C, et al. Lamotrigine treatment of aggression in female borderline-patients: a randomized, double-blind, placebo-controlled study. J Psychopharmacol 2005; 19:287–291.
100. Weinstein W, Jamison KL. Retrospective case review of lamotrigine use for affective instability of borderline personality disorder. CNS Spectr 2007; 12:207–210.
101. Stein G. Drug treatment of the personality disorders. Br J Psychiatry 1992; 161:167–184.
102. Hori A. Pharmacotherapy for personality disorders. Psychiatry Clin Neurosci 1998; 52: 13–19.
103. Coccaro EF, Kavoussi RJ. Biological and pharmacological aspects of borderline personality disorder. Hosp Community Psychiatry 1991; 42:1029–1033.
104. Pelissolo A, Lepine JP. Pharmacotherapy in personality disorders: methodological issues and results. Encephale 1999; 25:496–507.
105. Biancosino B, Facchi A, Marmai L, et al. Gabapentin treatment of impulsive-aggressive behaviour. Can J Psychiatry 2002; 47:483–484.
106. Morana HC, Olivi ML, Daltio CS. Use of gabapentin in group B – DSM-IV personality disorders. Rev Bras Psiquiatr 2004; 26:136–137.
107. Morana HC, Camara FP. International guidelines for the management of personality disorders. Curr Opin Psychia 2006; 19:539–543
108. Herranz JL. Gabapentin: its mechanisms of action in the year 2003. Rev Neurol 2003; 12: 1159–1165.
109. Soloff PH. Psychopharmacology of borderline personality disorder. Psychiatr Clin North Am 2000; 23:169–192.
110. Fava M. Psychopharmacologic treatment of pathologic aggression. Psychiatr Clin North Am 1997; 20:427–451.
111. Salpekar JA, Conry JA, Doss W, et al. Clinical experience with anticonvulsant medication in pediatric epilepsy and comorbid bipolar spectrum disorder. Epilepsy Behav 2006; 9:327–334.
112. Fleminger S, Greenwood RJ, Oliver DL. Pharmacological management for agitation and aggression in people with acquired brain injury. Cochrane Database Syst Rev 2006; 18(4): CD003299.
113. Golden AS, Haut SR, Moshe SL. Nonepileptic uses of antiepileptic drugs in children and adolescents. Pediatr Neurol 2006; 34:421–432.
114. Swann AC. Neuroreceptor mechanisms of aggression and its treatment. J Clin Psychiatry 2003; 64(suppl 4):26–35.

115. Barratt ES. The use of anticonvulsants in aggression and violence. Psychopharmacol Bull 1993; 29:75–81.
116. Tariot PN, Schneider LS, Mintzer JE, et al. Safety and tolerability of divalproex sodium in the treatment of signs and symptoms of mania in elderly patients with dementia: results of a double-blind, placebo-controlled trial. Curr Ther Res 2001; 62:51–67.
117. Wulsin L, Bachop M, Hoffman D. Group therapy in manic-depressive illness. Am J Psychother 1988; 42:263–271.
118. Donovan SJ, Susser ES, Nunes EV, et al. Divalproex treatment of disruptive adolescents: a report of 10 cases. J Clin Psychiatry 1997; 58:12–15.
119. Donovan SJ, Stewart JW, Nunes EV, et al. Divalproex treatment for youth with explosive temper and mood lability: a double-blind, placebo-controlled crossover design. Am J Psychiatry 2000; 157:818–820.
120. Fesler FA. Valproate in combat-related posttraumatic stress disorder. J Clin Psychiatry 1991; 52:361–364.
121. Szymanski HV, Olympia J. Divalproex in posttraumatic stress disorder. Am J Psychiatry 1991; 148:1086–1087.
122. Petty F, Davis LL, Nugent AL, et al. Valproate therapy for chronic combat-induced posttraumatic stress disorder. J Clin Psychopharmacol 2002; 22:100–101.
123. Giakas WJ, Seibyl JP, Mazure CM. Valproate in the treatment of temper outbursts. J Clin Psychiatry 1990; 51:525.
124. Horne M, Lindley SE. Divalproex sodium in the treatment of aggressive behavior and dysphoria in patients with organic brain syndromes. J Clin Psychiatry 1995; 56:430–431.
125. Wroblewski BA, Joseph AB, Kupfer J, et al. Effectiveness of valproic acid on destructive and aggressive behaviours in patients with acquired brain injury. Brain Inj 1997; 11:37–47.
126. Haas S, Vincent K, Holt J, et al. Divalproex: a possible treatment alternative for demented elderly aggressive patients. Ann Clin Psychiatry 1997; 9:145–147.
127. Buchalter EN, Lantz MS. Treatment of impulsivity and aggression in a patient with vascular dementia. Geriatrics 2001; 56:53–54.
128. Porsteinsson AP, Tariot PN, Erb R, et al. Placebo-controlled study of divalproex sodium for agitation in dementia. Am J Geriatr Psychiatry 2001; 9:58–66.
129. Porsteinsson AP, Tariot PN, Jakimovich LJ, et al. Valproate therapy for agitation in dementia: open-label extension of a double-blind trial. Am J Geriatr Psychiatry 2003; 11: 434–440.
130. Hollander E, Dolgoff-Kaspar R, Cartwright C, et al. An open trial of divalproex sodium in autism spectrum disorders. J Clin Psychiatry 2001; 62:530–534.
131. Lindenmayer JP, Kotsaftis A. Use of sodium valproate in violent and aggressive behaviors: a critical review. J Clin Psychiatry 2000; 61:123–128.
132. Vitiello B, Behar D, Hunt J, et al. Subtyping aggression in children and adolescents. J Neuropsychiatry Clin Neurosci 1990; 2:189–192.
133. Meinhold JM, Blake LM, Mini LJ, et al. Effect of divalproex sodium on behavioural and cognitive problems in elderly dementia. Drugs Aging 2005; 22:615–626.
134. Hellings JA, Nickel EJ, Weckbaugh M, et al. The overt aggression scale for rating aggression in outpatient youth with autistic disorder: preliminary findings. J Neuropsychiatry Clin Neurosci 2005; 17:29–35.
135. Lopez-Larson M, Frazier JA. Empirical evidence for the use of lithium and anticonvulsants in children with psychiatric disorders. Harv Rev Psychiatry 2006; 14:285–304.
136. Connor DF, Carlson GA, Chang KD, et al. Stanford/Howard/AACAP workgroup on juvenile impulsivity and aggression. Juvenile maladaptive aggression: a review of prevention, treatment, and service configuration and a proposed research agenda. J Clin Psychiatry 2006; 67:808–820.
137. Miyazaki M, Ito H, Saijo T, et al. Favorable response of ADHD with giant SEP to extended-release valproate. Brain Dev 2006; 28:470–472
138. Steiner H, Petersen ML, Saxena K, et al. Divalproex sodium for the treatment of conduct disorder a randomized controlled clinical trial. J Clin Psychiatry 2003; 64:936–942.
139. Barzman DH, DelBello MP, Adler CM, et al. efficacy and tolerability of quetiapine versus divalproex for the treatment of impulsivity and reactive aggression in adolescents with co-occurring bipolar disorder and disruptive behavior disorder(s). J Child Adolesc Psychopharmacol 2006; 16:665–670.

140. Gobbi G, Gaudreau PO, Leblanc N. Efficacy of topiramate, valproate, and their combination on aggression/agitation behavior in patients with psychosis. J Clin Psychopharmacol 2006; 26:467–473.
141. MacMillan CM, Korndorfer SR, Rao S, et al. A comparison of divalproex and oxcarbazepine in aggressive youth with bipolar disorder. J Psychiatr Pract 2006; 12:214–222.
142. State RC, Frye MA, Altshuler LL, et al. Chart review of the impact of attention-deficit/hyperactivity disorder comorbidity on response to lithium or divalproex sodium in adolescent mania. J Clin Psychiatry 2004; 65:1057–1063.
143. Barzman DH, McConville BJ, Masterson B, et al. Impulsive aggression with irritability and responsive to divalproex: a pediatric bipolar spectrum disorder phenotype? J Affect Disord 2005; 88:279–285.
144. Saxena K, Howe M, Simeonova D, et al. Divalproex sodium reduces overall aggression in youth at high risk for bipolar disorder. J Child Adolesc Psychopharmacol 2006; 16: 252–259.
145. Mattes JA. Psychopharmacology of temper outbursts: a review. J Nerv Ment Dis 1986; 174:464–470.
146. Cueva JE, Overall JE, Small AM, et al. Carbamazepine in aggressive children with conduct disorder: a double-blind and placebo-controlled study. J Am Acad Child Adolesc Psychiatry 1996; 35:480–90.
147. De Vogelaer J. Carbamazepine in the treatment of psychotic and behavioral disorders: a pilot study. ACTA Psychiatr Belg 1981; 81:532–541.
148. Thibaut F, Colonna L. Carbamazepine and aggressive behavior: a review. Encephale 1993; 19:651–656.
149. Young AL, Hillbrand M. Carbamazepine lowers aggression: a review. Bull Am Acad Psychiatry Law 1994; 22:52–61
150. Tariot PN, Erb R, Podgorski CA, et al. Efficacy and tolerability of carbamazepine for agitation and aggression in dementia. Am J Psychiatry 1998; 155:54–61.
151. Chatham-Showalter PE. Carbamazepine for combativeness in acute traumatic brain injury. J Neuropsychiatry Clin Neurosci 1996; 8:96–969.
152. Azouvi P, Jokic C, Attal N, et al. Carbamazepine in agitation and aggressive behaviour following severe closed-head injury: results of an open trial. Brain Inj 1999; 13:797–804.
153. Freymann N, Michael R, Dodel R, Jessen F. Successful treatment of sexual disinhibition in dementia with carbamazepine – a case report. Pharmacopsychiatry 2005; 38:144–145.
154. Kafantaris V, Campbell M, Padron-Gayol MV, et al. Carbamazepine in hospitalized aggressive conduct disorder children An open pilot study. Psychopharmacol Bull 1992; 28: 193–199.
155. Mattes JA. Comparative effectiveness of carbamazepine and propranolol for rage outbursts. J Neuropsychiatry Clin Neurosci 1990; 2:159–64.
156. Munoz P, Gonzalez Torres MA. Organic personality disorder: response to carbamazepine. Actas Luso Esp Neurol Psiquiatr Cienc Afines 1997; 25:197–200.
157. Morikawa M, Iida J, Tokuyama A, et al. Successful treatment using low-dose carbamazepine for a patient of personality change after mild diffuse brain injury. Nihon Shinkei Seishin Yakurigaku Zasshi 2000; 20:149–53.
158. Lewin J, Sumners D. Successful treatment of episodic dyscontrol with carbamazepine. Br J Psychiatry 1992; 161:261–2.
159. American Psychiatric Association. Practice guideline for the treatment of patients with bipolar disorder. Am J Psychiatry 2002; 159:4–5, 9–10, 24 (revision).
160. Mattes JA. Oxcarbazepine in patients with impulsive aggression: a double-blind, placebo-controlled trial. J Clin Psychopharmacol 2005; 25:575–9.
161. Gaudino MP, Smith MJ, Matthews DT. Use of oxcarbazepine for treatment-resistant aggression. Psychiatr Serv 2003; 54:1166–7.
162. Cordas TA, Tavares H, Calderoni DM, et al. Oxcarbazepine for self-mutilating bulimic patients. Int J Neuropsychopharmacol 2006; 9:769–71.
163. Nickel C, Lahmann C, Tritt K, et al. Topiramate in treatment of depressive and anger symptoms in female depressive patients: a randomized, double-blind, placebo-controlled study. J Affect Disord 2005; 87:243–52.
164. Smathers SA, Wilson JG, Nigro MA, Topiramate effectiveness in Prader-Willi Syndrome. Pediatr Neurol 2003; 28:130–133.

165. Shapira NA, Goldsmith TD, McElroy SL. Treatment of binge-eating disorder with topiramate: a clinical case series. J Clin Psychiatry 2000; 61:368–372.

166. McElroy SL, Arnold LM, Shapira NA, et al. Topiramate in the treatment of binge eating disorder associated with obesity: a randomized, placebo-controlled trial. Am J Psychiatry 2003; 160:255–261.

167. Pederson KJ, Roerig JL, Mitchell JE. Towards the pharmacotherapy of eating disorders. Expert Opin Pharmacother 2003; 4:1659–1678.

168. Appolinario JC, McElroy SL. Pharmacological approaches in the treatment of binge eating disorder. Curr Drug Targets 2004; 5:301–7.

169. Carter WP, Hudson JI, Lalonde JK, et al. Pharmacologic treatment of binge eating disorder. Int J Eat Disord 2003; 34:S74–S88.

170. Appolinario JC, Fontenelle LF, Papelbaum M, et al. Topiramate use in obese patients with binge eating disorder: an open study. Can J Psychiatry 2002; 47:271–273.

171. McElroy SL, Shapira NA, Arnold LM, et al. Topiramate in the long-term treatment of binge-eating disorder associated with obesity. J Clin Psychiatry 2004; 65:1463–1469.

172. Zilberstein B, Pajecki D, Garcia de Brito AC, et al. Topiramate after adjustable gastric banding in patients with binge eating and difficulty losing weight. Obes Surg 2004; 14:802–805.

173. Dolberg OT, Barkai G, Gross Y, et al. Differential effects of topiramate in patients with traumatic brain injury and obesity–a case series. Psychopharmacology (Berl) 2005; 179: 838–845.

174. Guerdjikova AI, Kotwal R, McElroy SL. Response of recurrent binge eating and weight gain to topiramate in patients with binge eating disorder after bariatric surgery. Obes Surg 2005; 15:273–277.

175. De Bernardi C, Ferraris S, D'Innella P, et al. Topiramate for binge eating disorder. Prog Neuropsychopharmacol Biol Psychiatry 2005; 29:339–41.

176. Nickel C, Lahmann C, Tritt K, et al. Topiramate in treatment of depressive and anger symptoms in female depressive patients: a randomized, double-blind, placebo-controlled study. J Affect Disord 2005; 87:243–252.

177. Chengappa KNR, Rathore D, Levine J, et al. Topiramate as add-on treatment for patients with bipolar mania. Bipolar Dis 1999; 1:42–53.

178. Cassano P, Lattanzi L, Pini S, et al. Topiramate for self-mutilation in a patient with borderline personality disorder. Bipolar Disord 2001; 3:161.

179. Dolengevich Segal H, Rodriguez Salgado B, Conejo Garcia A, et al. Efficacy of topiramate in children and adolescent with problems in impulse control: preliminary results. Actas Esp Psiquiatr 2006; 34:280–282.

180. Rugino TA, Samsock TC. Levetiracetam in autistic children: an open-label study. J Dev Behav Pediatr 2002; 23:225–30.

181. Grunze H, Langosch J, Born C, et al. Levetiracem in the treatment of acute mania: an open add-on study with an on-off-on design. J Clin Psychiatry 2003; 64:781–784.

182. Kaufman KR. Monotherapy treatment of bipolar disorder with levetiracetam. Epilepsy Behav 2004; 5:1017–1020.

183. Simon NM, Worthington JJ, Doyle AC, et al. An open-label study of levetiracetam for the treatment of social anxiety disorder. J Clin Psychiatry 2004; 65:1219–22.

184. Wasserman S, Iyengar R, Chaplin WF, et al. Levetiracetam versus placebo in childhood and adolescent autism: a double-blind placebo-controlled study. Int Clin Psychopharmacol 2006; 21:363–367.

185. Dinkelacker V, Dietl T, Widman G, et al. Aggressive behavior of epilepsy patients in the course of levetiracetam add-on therapy: report of 33 mild to severe cases. Epilepsy Behav 2003; 4:537–547.

186. Weber S, Beran RG. A pilot study of compassionate use of Levetiracetam in patients with generalised epilepsy. J Clin Neurosci 2004; 11:728–731.

187. Opp J, Tuxhorn I, May T, et al. Levetiracetam in children with refractory epilepsy: a multicenter open label study in Germany. Seizure 2005; 14:476–484.

188. Neuwirth M, Saracz J, Hegyi M, et al. Experience with levetiracetam in childhood epilepsy. Ideggyogy Sz 2006; 59:179–82.

189. Cherek DR, Tcheremissine OV, Lane SD, et al. Acute effects of gabapentin on laboratory measures of aggressive and escape responses of adult parolees with and without a history of conduct disorder. Psychopharmacology (Berl) 2004; 171:405–412.
190. Herrmann N, Lanctôt K, Myszak M. Effectiveness of gabapentin for the treatment of behavioral disorders in dementia. J Clin Psychopharmacol 2000; 20:90–93.
191. Miller LJ. Gabapentin for treatment of behavioral and psychological symptoms of dementia. Ann Pharmacother 2001; 35:427–431.
192. Hawkins JW, Tinklenberg JR, Sheikh JI, et al. A retrospective chart review of gabapentin for the treatment of aggressive and agitated behavior in patients with dementias. Am J Geriatr Psychiatry 2000; 8:221–5.
193. Alkhalil C, Tanvir F, Alkhalil B, et al. Treatment of sexual disinhibition in dementia: case reports and review of the literature. Am J Ther 2004; 11:231–235.
194. McManaman J, Tam DA. Gabapentin for self-injurious behavior in Lesch-Nyhan Syndrome. Pediatr Neurol 1999; 20:381–382.
195. Gupta S, Frank BL, Masand PS. Gabapentin in the treatment of aggression associated with conduct disorder, primary care companion. J Clin Psychiatry 2000; 2:60–61.
196. Ryback R, Ryback L. Gabapentin for behavioral dyscontrol. Am J Psychiatry 1995; 152: 1399 (letter).
197. Looker A, Conners CK. Diphenylhydantoin in children with severe temper tantrums. Arch Gen Psychiatry 1970; 23:80–9.
198. Stanford MS, Helfritz LE, Conklin SM, et al. A comparison of anticonvulsants in the treatment of impulsive aggression. Exp Clin Psychopharmacol 2005; 13:72–77.
199. Stanford MS, Houston RJ, Mathias CW, et al. A double-blind placebo-controlled crossover study of phenytoin in individuals with impulsive aggression. Psychiatry Res 2001; 103:193–203.
200. Maletzky BM. The episodic dyscontrol syndrome. Dis Nerv Syst 1973; 34:178–185.
201. Maletzky BM, Klotter J. Episodic dyscontrol: a controlled replication. Dis Nerv Syst 1974; 35:175–179.
202. Barratt ES, Kent TA, Bryant SG, et al. A controlled trial of phenytoin in impulsive aggression. J Clin Psychopharmacol 1991; 6:388–389.
203. Barratt ES, Stanford MS, Felthous AR, et al. The effects of phenytoin on impulsive and premeditated aggression: a controlled study. J Clin Psychopharmacol 1997; 17:341–9.
204. Keele NB. The role of serotonin in impulsive and aggressive behaviors associated with epilepsy-like neuronal hyperexcitability in the amygdala. Epilepsy Behav 2005; 7:325–35.
205. Hollander E, Begaz T, DeCaria CM. Pharmacological approaches in the treatment of pathological gambling. CNS Spectrums 1998; 3:72–80.
206. Hollander E, Sood E, Pallanti S, et al. Pharmacological treatments of pathological gambling. J Gambl Stud 2005; 21:99–108.

18 Antiepileptic Drugs and Borderline Personality Disorder

Mary C. Zanarini
Laboratory for the Study of Adult Development, McLean Hospital, Belmont and the Department of Psychiatry, Harvard Medical School, Boston, Massachusetts, U.S.A.

INTRODUCTION

Several cross-sectional studies have documented the high percentage of patients with borderline personality disorder (BPD) who have a lifetime history of taking anticonvulsant mood stabilizers (1,2). More recently, a study of the longitudinal course of BPD (3) documented high rates of the use of anticonvulsant mood stabilizers throughout six years of prospective follow-up. More specifically, about a quarter of the patients with BPD studied took such a mood stabilizer during the first two years after their index admission, 22% took such a mood stabilizer during the third and fourth years after their entry into the study, and 18% during their fifth and sixth years of study participation.

This high rate of use is probably due to two factors. The first is the overlap of some of the symptoms of BPD (particularly pronounced mood lability and impulsivity) and some of the symptoms of bipolar disorder. The second is the belief of some mental health professionals (4) that BPD is actually an attenuated form of bipolar disorder—a belief that is not consistent with the results of longitudinal studies that have found that most borderline patients do not develop a bipolar disorder over time (5,6).

Despite the high rate of use mentioned above, surprisingly few open-label or controlled medication trials of anticonvulsant mood stabilizers in particular or antiepileptic drugs (AEDs) in general in the treatment of patients with BPD have been conducted. Below is a careful review of first-generation and second-generation studies. Only published studies will be described, and only studies limited to patients with BPD have been included.

FIRST-GENERATION STUDIES

Gardner and Cowdry (7) conducted a six-week, placebo-controlled crossover study. They found that carbamazepine was superior to placebo in the treatment of behavior dyscontrol in a sample of 11 women with BPD and histories of severe impulsivity. The average daily dose of carbamazepine was 820 mg. Somewhat later, De la Fuente and Lotstra (8) conducted a double-blind, placebo-controlled trial of carbamazepine in a sample of inpatients with BPD ($N = 20$) and no co-occurring axis I disorders. They failed to find any significant differences in any sector of borderline psychopathology between those treated with carbamazepine and those treated with placebo.

This between-study difference in outcome may be due to the fact that Gardner and Cowdry were studying women with BPD plus a history of severe problems with behavior dyscontrol. However, the subjects in the study of De la Fuente and Lotstra were inpatients and thus were acutely ill.

SECOND-GENERATION STUDIES

Divalproex Sodium

Two open-label studies of *Diagnostic and Statistical Manual of Mental Disorders-Third Edition, Revised* (DSM-III-R) borderline patients treated with divalproex sodium have been conducted. Stein et al. (9) studied 11 outpatients in an eight-week trial. All subjects were in psychotherapy and none had a current major depression or a history of bipolarity or a psychotic disorder. Eight of the eleven subjects (73%) completed the trial and half of them were responders. However, when the scores of all 11 subjects were examined, significant decreases in psychopathology were found for only two of the study's five main outcomes: subjective irritability as measured by the Modified Overt Aggression Scale (also called the Overt Aggression Scale-Modified; OAS-M) (10) and general psychopathology as assessed by the Symptom Checklist-90 (SCL-90) (11).

Wilcox (12) also conducted an open-label trial of divalproex sodium. He studied 30 inpatients without comorbid disorders meeting DSM-III-R criteria for BPD. The trial lasted for six weeks, and seven of the subjects were on a concurrent medication. Wilcox found significant decreases in the study's outcome measures— general psychopathology as measured by the Brief Psychiatric Rating Scale (BPRS) (13)— and number of minutes in seclusion (which was viewed as a measure of agitation). The author concluded that the medication had its greatest effect on anxiety (as rated by the BPRS) and that reduced anxiety led to reduced agitation.

Hollander et al. (14) completed the first placebo-controlled, double-blind study of the efficacy of divalproex sodium in criteria-defined patients with BPD. They conducted a 10-week trial and studied 16 patients with DSM-IV BPD, 12 randomized to divalproex sodium and 4 to placebo. Fifty percent of the subjects on active medication dropped out of the study, and 100% of those taking placebo dropped out before completing the study. No significant between-group differences were found. However, 42% of subjects taking divalproex sodium were judged to be responders, while none of the subjects being treated with placebo were judged to be responders. In addition, substantial reductions in aggression and depression were found for subjects treated with divalproex sodium.

Hollander et al. (15) conducted a second double-blind, placebo-controlled trial of divalproex sodium versus placebo in a sample of 50 patients meeting DSM-IV criteria for BPD. Exclusion criteria included lifetime bipolar I disorder and bipolar II disorder within the past year. In this 12-week study, data were analyzed for 18 subjects assigned to the active group and 32 subjects assigned to the placebo group. The mean modal dose of divalproex sodium was 1325 mg/day. Borderline patients treated with divalproex had a significantly greater decrease in their impulsive aggression as measured by the OAS-M. In addition, those borderline patients taking divalproex who were high in state impulsivity and trait aggression at baseline had a significantly greater decrease in impulsive aggression than similar subjects taking placebo.

Frankenburg and Zanarini (16) also conducted a double-blind, placebo-controlled trial of divalproex sodium in the treatment of symptomatic volunteers meeting rigorous criteria for BPD. However, these investigators conducted a six-month long trial of 30 women meeting the revised Diagnostic Interview for Borderlines (DIB-R) (17) and DSM-IV criteria for BPD and DSM-IV criteria for comorbid bipolar II disorder. Twenty of these subjects were randomized to divalproex sodium and 10 were randomized to placebo; most had histories of outpatient treatment.

Those on active treatment were found to have experienced significantly greater reductions in three of the study's outcome measures: interpersonal sensitivity, anger, and hostility as measured by the SCL-90 and the total score of the OAS-M. However, depression as assessed by the SCL-90 did not show a significant between-group difference. The average dose of divalproex sodium was 850 mg (SD = 249). The groups gained, on average, a small but not significantly different amount of weight [2.6 pounds (SD = 5.6) vs. 0.3 pounds (SD = 4.0)]. Retention was quite good through the first eight weeks of the study (70% of those treated with active compound and 60% of those treated with placebo). However, only 35% of the subjects treated with divalproex sodium and 40% of the subjects treated with placebo remained in the study all 24 weeks. Given the design of the study, it is not clear whether the mild bipolarity of the subjects was treated or their borderline lability or a combination of the two.

More recently, Simeon et al. (18), in conjunction with Hollander, conducted an open-label trial of divalproex extended release (ER). This 12-week trial assessed the efficacy of this compound in 20 adults meeting DSM-IV criteria for BPD. None were in any kind of psychiatric treatment. The mean end dose of divalproex was 1350 mg/day. The attrition rate was high (50%). However, the following areas of borderline psychopathology saw significant improvement: overall symptoms, overall functioning, irritability, and aggression.

Lamotrigine

Pinto and Akiskal (19) studied eight DSM-IV borderline outpatients under their clinical care in an open-label trial of lamotrigine. None of the patients had a history of a major mood disorder of a unipolar or bipolar nature. Three of these severely ill patients were judged to be responders. The investigators reported in a series of case reports that the impulsive behaviors of these patients were completely eradicated and that they no longer met criteria for BPD.

Tritt et al. (20) have conducted the only double-blind, placebo-controlled trial of lamotrigine. They assessed 27 female outpatients meeting DSM-IV criteria for BPD, 18 women taking lamotrigine and 9 taking placebo. Over the course of this eight-week trial, the dose of lamotigine was titrated from 50 mg/day during the first two weeks of the trial to 200 mg/day during the final three weeks of the trial. In terms of dropouts, only 6% of those being treated with lamotrigine failed to complete the trial, while 22% of those in the placebo group dropped out prior to trial completion. Tritt et al. found that the active compound was superior to placebo on all five aspects of anger studied: state, trait, inward, outward, and control of anger.

TOPIRAMATE

Nickel et al. (21,22), who are part of the same research team as Tritt et al., conducted two placebo-controlled trials of topiramate. They studied the effects of topiramate versus placebo on the anger of female (N = 21 vs. 10) and male (N = 22 vs. 22) samples of patients meeting DSM-IV criteria for BPD. The female sample, who participated in an eight-week trial, consisted primarily of outpatients and the male sample, who participated in a 10-week trial, was a combination of outpatients and symptomatic volunteers. The titrated dose for those in both groups was 250 mg/day in the sixth week. Over 90% of those in both groups in both studies completed the trial. They found in both studies that treatment with top-iramate was superior to treatment with placebo on four of the five anger scales studied (i.e., all but anger directed inward). They also found that topiramate-treated subjects lost significantly more weight over the course of the trial than subjects treated with placebo (males = 5 kg and females = 2.3 kg).

The same group conducted a second study of topiramate treatment of females with BPD (23). A somewhat larger sample (28 vs. 28) was studied for 10 weeks with a dose of topiramate that was titrated to 200 mg/day in week 6. Attrition was low for both study groups (4% for active compound and 11% for placebo). It was found that topiramate was superior to placebo on six scales of the SCL-90: somatization, interpersonal sensitivity, anxiety, hostility, phobic anxiety, and global severity. Significant differences were also found on all eight scales of the SF-36 Health Survey (24). In addition, significant differences were found on four of the eight scales of the Inventory of Interpersonal Problems (25): overly autocratic, overly competitive, overly introverted, and overly expressive. They also found that topiramate-treated subjects lost significantly more weight over the course of the trial than subjects treated with placebo (4.3 kg).

Other AEDs

Bellino et al. (26) conducted an open-label trial of oxcarbazepine, a medication related to carbamazepine. They studied the effectiveness of this medication in treating 17 outpatients meeting DSM-IV criteria for BPD. None of these subjects had ever met criteria for bipolar I disorder or bipolar II disorder. They found that this medication was broadly effective, with the severity of anxiety symptoms, borderline (including affective instability and general impulsivity) symptoms, and overall symptoms declining significantly over the course of this 12-week trial. The retention rate in this trial was high (76%) and no serious adverse events were reported. The mean daily dose of oxcarbazepine, which was administered twice per day, was 1315 mg.

Limitations of Existing Studies and Directions for Future Research

In general, the methodology of the papers reviewed above is quite good. Firstly, it is particularly important for interpretability that studies either exclude borderline patients with histories of bipolarity or limit themselves to such patients. Secondly, studies involving larger samples would lessen the chances of type II errors. Thirdly, studies may often have included subjects who were not particularly symptomatic in the areas studied and, thus, substantial improvement in these symptoms would be unlikely. In fact, controlled studies of carbamazepine (7) and divalproex sodium (15) were only found to be effective in samples comprising subjects with serious emotional dysregulation and/or impulsive aggression.

CONCLUSIONS

Taken together, the results of these studies suggest several important findings. The first is that most of the AEDs studied in controlled trials were found to be efficacious. The second finding is that most of these medications were useful in treating symptoms of affective dysregulation and impulsive aggression, which have been suggested as the core dimensions of psychopathology underlying BPD (27). The third finding is that although each of these medications took the edge off of BPD symptomatology, none were curative for BPD. In fact, second-generation antidepressant and antipsychotic agents have also been found to be efficacious but not definitive in the treatment of BPD (28). However, helping borderline patients attain a moment to reflect without swinging into action is no small accomplishment and may set the stage for more adaptive behaviors. It may also allow borderline patients to better engage in psychotherapy. This is particularly important as there are now four forms of therapy that have been found to be efficacious in the treatment of BPD—dialectical behavior therapy (DBT) (29), mentalization-based treatment (MBT) (30), schema-focused therapy (SFT) (31), and transference-focused psychotherapy (TFP) (32).

REFERENCES

1. Bender DS, Dolan RT, Skodol AE, et al. Treatment utilization by patients with personality disorders. Am J Psychiatry 2001; 158(2):295–302.
2. Zanarini MC, Frankenburg FR, Khera GS, et al. Treatment histories of borderline inpatients. Compr Psychiatry 2001; 42(2):144–150.
3. Zanarini MC, Frankenburg FR, Hennen J, et al. Mental health service utilization of borderline patients and axis II comparison subjects followed prospectively for six years. J Clin Psychiatry 2004; 65(1):28–36.
4. Akiskal HS, Chen SE, Davis GC, et al. Borderline: an adjective in search of a noun. J Clin Psychiatry 1985; 46(2):41–48.
5. Gunderson JG, Weinberg I, Daversa MT, et al. Descriptive and longitudinal observations on the relationship of borderline personality disorder and bipolar disorder. Am J Psychiatry 2006; 163(7):1173–1178.
6. Zanarini MC, Frankenburg FR, Hennen J, et al. Axis I comorbidity in patients with borderline personality disorder: 6-year follow-up and prediction of time to remission. Am J Psychiatry 2004; 161(11):2108–2114.
7. Gardner DL, Cowdry RW. Positive effects of carbamazepine on behavioral dyscontrol in borderline personality disorder. Am J Psychiatry 1986; 143(4):519–522.
8. De la Fuente JM, Lotstra F. A trial of carbamazepine in borderline personality disorder. Eur Neuropsychopharmacol 1994; 4(4):479–486.
9. Stein DJ, Simeon D, Frenkel M, et al. An open trial of valproate in borderline personality disorder. J Clin Psychiatry 1995; 56(11):506–510.
10. Coccaro EF, Harvey PH, Kupshaw-Lawrence E, et al. Development of neuropharmacologically based assessments of impulsive aggressive behavior. J Neuropsychiatry 1991; 3(suppl):44–51.
11. Derogatis LR, Lipman RS, Covi L. SCL-90: an outpatient psychiatric rating scale–preliminary report. Psychopharmacol Bull 1973; 9(1):13–28.
12. Wilcox JA. Divalproex sodium as a treatment for borderline personality disorder. Ann Clin Psychiatry 1995; 7(1):33–37.
13. Overall JE, Gorham DR. The brief psychiatric rating scale. Psychol Rep 1962; 10:799–812.
14. Hollander E, Allen A, Lopez RP, et al. A preliminary double-blind, placebo-controlled trial of divalproex sodium in borderline personality disorder. J Clin Psychiatry 2001; 62(3): 199–203.
15. Hollander E, Swann AC, Coccaro EF, et al. Impact of trait impulsivity and state aggression on divalproex versus placebo response in borderline personality disorder. Am J Psychiatry 2005; 162(3):621–624.
16. Frankenburg FR, Zanarini MC. Divalproex sodium treatment of women with borderline personality disorder and bipolar II disorder: a double-blind placebo-controlled pilot study. J Clin Psychiatry 2002; 63(5):442–446.
17. Zanarini MC, Gunderson JG, Frankenburg FR, et al. The revised diagnostic interview for borderlines: discriminating BPD from other axis II disorders. J Personal Disord 1989; 3(1): 10–18.

18. Simeon D, Baker B, Chaplin W, et al. An open-label trial of divalproex extended-release in the treatment of borderline personality disorder. CNS Spectr 2007; 12(6):439–443.
19. Pinto OC, Akiskal HS. Lamotrigine as a promising approach to borderline personality: an open case series without concurrent DSM-IV major mood disorder. J Affect Disord 1998; 51(3): 333–343.
20. Tritt K, Nickel C, Lahmann C, et al. Lamotrigine treatment of aggression in female borderline-patients: a randomized, double-blind, placebo-controlled study. J Psychopharmacol 2005; 19(3):287–291.
21. Nickel MK, Nickel C, Mitterlehner FO, et al. Topiramate treatment of aggression in female borderline personality disorder patients: a double-blind, placebo-controlled study. J Clin Psychiatry 2004; 65(11):1515–1519.
22. Nickel MK, Nickel C, Kaplan P, et al. Treatment of aggression with topiramate in male borderline patients: a double-blind, placebo-controlled study. Biol Psychiatry 2005; 57(5): 495–499.
23. Loew TH, Nickel MK, Muehlbacher M, et al. Topiramate treatment for women with borderline personality disorder: a double-blind, placebo-controlled study. J Clin Psychopharmacol 2006; 26(1):61–66.
24. Bullinger M, Kirchberger I. SF-36 Health Survey. Goettingen, Germany: Hogrefe, 1998.
25. Horowitz LM, Rosenberg SE, Baer BA, et al. Inventory of interpersonal problems: psychometric properties and clinical applications. J Consult Clin Psychol 1988; 56(6):885–892.
26. Bellino S, Paradiso E, Bogetto F. Oxcarbazepine in the treatment of borderline personality disorder: a pilot study. J Clin Psychiatry 2005; 66(9):1111–1115.
27. Siever LJ, Davis KL. A psychobiological perspective on the personality disorders. Am J Psychiatry 1991; 148(12):1647–1658.
28. Zanarini MC. Update on pharmacotherapy of borderline personality disorder. Curr Psychiatry Rep 2004; 6(1):55–70.
29. Linehan MM, Armstrong HE, Suarez A, et al. Cognitive-behavioral treatment of chronically parasuicidal borderline patients. Arch Gen Psychiatry 1991; 48(12):1060–1064.
30. Bateman A, Fonagy P. Effectiveness of partial hospitalization in the treatment of borderline personality disorder: a randomized controlled trial. Am J Psychiatry 1999; 156(10): 1563–1569.
31. Giesen-Bloo J, van Dyck R, Spinhoven P, et al. Outpatient psychotherapy for borderline personality disorder. Arch Gen Psychiatry 2006; 63(6):649–658.
32. Clarkin JF, Levy KN, Lenzenweger MF, et al. Evaluating three treatments for borderline personality: a multiwave study. Am J Psychiatry 2007; 164(6):922–928.

19 Antiepileptics in the Treatment of Sleep Disorders

David T. Plante
Department of Psychiatry, Massachusetts General Hospital and McLean Hospital, Harvard Medical School, Boston, Massachusetts, U.S.A.

John W. Winkelman
Divisions of Sleep Medicine and Psychiatry, Brigham & Women's Hospital, Harvard Medical School, Boston, and the Sleep Health Center®, affiliated with Brigham & Women's Hospital, Brighton, Massachusetts, U.S.A.

INTRODUCTION

Sleep is a complex behavior generated by specific physiological changes in the central nervous system (CNS). Sleep is divided into non–rapid eye movement (NREM) and rapid eye movement (REM) sleep on the basis of specific neurophysiological characteristics. Since sleep, like any behavior, is generated in the brain, it is not surprising that many antiepileptic drugs (AEDs) not only affect sleep, but may also be of value in the management of sleep disorders. This chapter will briefly discuss the effects of AEDs on sleep, and then discuss in greater detail evidence for the use of AEDs in specific sleep disorders.

EFFECTS OF ANTIEPILEPTIC DRUGS ON SLEEP

It has long been appreciated that the relationship between sleep and epilepsy occurs on many levels: sleep deprivation may influence the frequency of seizures, certain epilepsy syndromes may arise during specific sleep stages, sleep induction may mitigate seizure activity, most AEDs affect sleep structure in some way, and many sedating medications have anticonvulsant properties (1). Since AEDs enact their effects through myriad systems, it is likely that some AEDs affect the same mechanistic systems related to sleep induction. In general, effects of AEDs on sleep may be measured subjectively (e.g., daytime alertness, perceived sleep latency) or objectively (e.g., changes in sleep architecture measured by polysomnography). Multiple reviews have been published regarding the effects of AEDs on sleep, and thus this chapter will seek to update work already published (Table 1) (1,2). There are, however, basic principles and caveats related to AEDs and sleep that deserve mention.

In general, studies that examine the effects of AEDs on sleep have been predominantly conducted in patients with epilepsy (2). Since seizures themselves can have profound effects on sleep architecture and patients may be on multiple AEDs when studied, interpretation of the literature is complicated. Further confounding the literature are methodological differences across studies, such as dose of AED tested, timing, and duration of treatment (3). Finally, since AEDs enact their effects through a diversity of interactions within the CNS, it can be difficult to generalize an AED's mechanism of action to sleep independent of other effects.

TABLE 1 Summary of the Effects of AEDs on Sleep Architecture

AED	Sleep latency	Sleep efficiency	Stage 1 sleep	SWS	REM sleep	Daytime drowsiness
Barbiturates	↓	–	–	–	↓	↑
Benzodiazepines	↓	–	–	↓	↓	↑
Carbamazepine	–	–	–	–	↓	↑
Phenytoin	↓	–	↑	–	↓	↑
Valproic acid	–	–	↑	–	–	↑
Felbamate	?	?	?	?	?	↓
Gabapentin	–	–	↓	↑	– or ↑	?
Lamotrigine	–	–	–	↓	– or ↑	?
Levetiracetam[a]	?	– or ↑	–	– or ↑	– or ↑	?
Oxcarbazepine	?	?	?	?	?	?
Tiagabine[a]	–	↑ or –	–	↑	– or ↓	?
Topiramate	?	?	?	?	?	?
Vigabatrin	?	?	?	?	?	↑
Zonisamide	?	?	?	?	?	?
Pregablin[a]	↓	↑	?	↑	?	– or ↑

Note: – indicates no effect; ↓ indicates decreases; ↑ indicates increases; and ? indicates effects unknown.
[a]See text for additional references.
Abbreviations: AEDs, antiepileptic drugs; SWS, slow wave sleep. REM, rapid eye movement.
Source: Modified from Ref. 1 with permission from Wolters Kluwer Health.

Ideally, AEDs would be systematically tested in normal control subjects using a placebo-controlled design to determine their effects on sleep; however, this is logistically difficult, particularly if the AED in question has a high side-effect burden. Since some of the newer AEDs are more amenable to such studies, the effects of these agents on sleep have been reported in the recent literature.

Both pregabalin and levetiracetam, for example, are newer AEDs that have been evaluated in healthy subjects in placebo-controlled trials. Pregabalin, when compared to placebo, seems to produce modest reductions in sleep onset latency (SOL), increased slow-wave sleep (SWS), decreased REM sleep, and a decreased number of awakenings. Subjectively, it improves the ease of falling asleep and quality of sleep, but produces impairment after awakening (4). Two recent studies have evaluated the effects of levetiracetam on healthy subjects, with conflicting results. Bazil et al. found no major differences in sleep architecture between drug and placebo except for an increased number of awakenings in the drug group (5). Cicolin et al. demonstrated that levetiracetam significantly increased total sleep time (TST), sleep efficiency (SE), SWS, and wake after sleep onset (WASO) but did not affect daytime sleepiness (6).

ANTIEPILEPTIC DRUGS IN SPECIFIC SLEEP DISORDERS

In the last few decades, sleep medicine as a field has grown exponentially, largely because of increased awareness on the importance of sleep for overall health, as well as the improved ability to accurately diagnose and treat primary sleep disorders (7). Not surprisingly, many AEDs have been utilized as treatments of primary sleep disorders, in either controlled trials or in clinical practice. In general, the potential utility of an AED in the management of sleep disorders depends on several factors including: mechanism of action, effects on sleep architecture, and pharmacokinetics. The half-life of a drug is vitally important in the treatment of sleep disorders since the majority of sleep disorders require treatment only during sleep or during a defined period prior to sleep onset. Thus, selection of a drug is often based, in part, on half-life so it is present in sufficient quantities during the sleep period, but is not present in significant quantities during wakefulness (e.g., gabapentin, $t_{1/2}$ 5–7 hours) (8). However, there are certain AEDs used in the treatment of sleep disorders whose half-life may be greater than 24 hours (e.g., topiramate, $t_{1/2}$ 20–30 hours), largely because they have shown efficacy in the treatment of specific disorders (8). In such instances when active drug remains during wakefulness, intolerable side effects are more apt to limit use.

The following sections will detail the evidence base for the use of AEDs in specific sleep disorders. Although benzodiazepines are technically AEDs and are used for both the prevention (e.g., clonazepam) and termination of seizures (e.g., lorazepam), for the purpose of this chapter, we will not focus on these medications in the same depth of detail as other anticonvulsants. However, since benzodiazepines are a widely used class of medications in the management of sleep disorders, their use in specific disorders will be acknowledged throughout the chapter.

Insomnia

Insomnia, broadly defined as difficulty falling asleep, maintaining sleep, inadequate sleep quality, or short sleep duration when given enough time for sleep, is a common complaint in the general population and occurs in higher frequencies in psychiatric populations (9). When accompanied by significant impairment or distress, often because of heightened frequency and/or chronicity of the insomnia, an insomnia disorder may be diagnosed. Although multiple diagnostic schemas are used to categorize insomnia syndromes, the most frequently used by psychiatrists is the Diagnostic and Statistical Manual (DSM). The DSM-IV-TR differentiates between primary insomnia and insomnia related to another disorder (e.g., major depressive disorder). However, since there is growing evidence that insomnia is independently associated with significant morbidity, functional impairment, and health care expenditures, many favor the more pragmatic approach of treating the insomnia complaint even when it occurs concurrently with another psychiatric condition (10,11).

There is evidence for the effective treatment of insomnia with both psychotherapy (e.g., cognitive behavioral therapy) and pharmacotherapy (12). Early in the 20th century, the major pharmacological agents used to manage insomnia were the barbiturates (e.g., phenobarbital). The barbiturates were also some of the first AEDs (13). Because of their risk of tolerance, dependence, and accidental overdose due to a low therapeutic index, these drugs were eventually supplanted by the benzodiazepines in the 1960s and 1970s and were rarely prescribed as sedative hypnotics by the end of the 1980s (14). Currently, when pharmacotherapy is pursued, the agents with the most evidence supporting their use (and the only agents with regulatory approval for treatment of insomnia) are benzodiazepine receptor agonists (e.g., triazolam, temazepam, zolpidem, eszopiclone, zaleplon) or melatonin receptor agonists (e.g., ramelteon). However, other agents are often prescribed off label for insomnia by clinicians (15). It should be noted that some of these, in particular benzodiazepines (e.g., lorazepam, clonazepam), are also effective as AEDs, thus reiterating the close connection between sleep induction and seizure management.

The AEDs with the most potential in the treatment of insomnia are those that affect GABAergic neurotransmission (16). This is not surprising given that many sedative-hypnotics approved (or used off label) for the treatment of primary insomnia are thought to work via gamma-aminobutyric acid (GABA) receptors. Tiagabine has recently been the subject of two double-blind, randomized, placebo-controlled studies in the treatment of primary insomnia (17,18). Walsh et al. found that tiagabine significantly increased SWS, decreased REM sleep, showed a trend toward decreased WASO [except at the highest dose tested (16 mg) which achieved significance], and TST, but failed to decrease latency to persistent sleep in subjects with primary insomnia (17). Similarly, in a study that examined lower doses of tiagabine in elderly patients with primary insomnia, it increased SWS, but did not significantly affect WASO, TST, or latency to persistent sleep when compared with placebo (18). In both of these trials, the incidence of adverse events was dose dependent, and the most common side effects were dizziness and nausea (17,18).

Gabapentin has been used clinically off label for the treatment of insomnia, but there are no controlled data to support its use for this indication. On the other hand, there are uncontrolled case studies/series and trials in the treatment of patients with co-occurring alcohol abuse/dependence and insomnia (19–21). The majority of work in this area has been performed by the group of Karam-Hage and Brower. In one uncontrolled case series, these authors found that gabapentin at a mean dose of 953 mg significantly improved subjective measures of insomnia at follow-up four to six weeks after initiation in patients with alcohol dependence (20). Similarly, in a larger, uncontrolled clinical trial comparing trazodone and gabapentin in alcohol dependent patients, both agents were found to subjectively improve insomnia complaints, with improvement being significantly greater (though not necessarily clinically significantly so) in gabapentin-treated patients (21).

It may be noted that most AEDs are associated with sedation, but insomnia can also be a side effect of certain AEDs. Felbamate has been associated with insomnia; similarly, patients taking lamotrigine may develop intolerable insomnia necessitating discontinuation (22–24). Thus, clinicians should be aware that patients may develop insomnia with certain AEDs, and that the risk of insomnia may be theoretically increased in patients with a history of sleep disturbance.

Restless Legs Syndrome/Periodic Leg Movements in Sleep

Restless legs syndrome (RLS) is a neurological disorder that is a common cause of disturbed sleep. RLS is characterized by the primary symptom of a distressing need to move the legs, often with uncomfortable or unpleasant sensations in the legs that are increased by inactivity and relieved by movement. A key feature that distinguishes RLS from other lower extremity paresthesias is that RLS symptoms typically worsen in the evening or night (Table 2) (25–27). RLS is considered a sleep disorder in part because its deleterious effects on sleep are typically what prompt patients to seek treatment. Although the precise pathophysiology responsible for RLS is unknown, it is thought to be a disorder of the central rather than the peripheral nervous system, with dopaminergic dysfunction in subcortical systems likely playing a key role, possibly mediated in part by disturbed iron homeostasis in the CNS (28). RLS is often associated with periodic leg movements of sleep (PLMS) that may further disturb sleep. However, not all patients with RLS have PLMS and vice versa (27). When PLMS result in a clinically significant sleep disturbance that cannot be accounted for by another disorder, including RLS, the

TABLE 2 Essential Diagnostic Criteria for RLS

1	An urge to move the legs, which is usually accompanied or caused by uncomfortable and unpleasant sensations in the legs (Sometimes the urge to move is present without the uncomfortable sensations and sometimes the arms or other body parts are involved in addition to the legs.)
2	The urge to move or unpleasant sensations begin or worsen during periods of rest or inactivity such as lying or sitting
3	The urge to move or unpleasant sensations are partially or totally relieved by movement, such as walking or stretching, at least as long as the activity continues
4	The urge to move or unpleasant sensations are worse in the evening or night than during the day or only occur in the evening or night (When symptoms are very severe, the worsening at night may not be noticeable but must have been previously present.)

Abbreviation: RLS, restless legs syndrome.
Source: From Ref. 27 reprinted with permission from Elsevier.

diagnosis of periodic leg movement disorder (PLMD) is ascribed. Because RLS and PLMS are interrelated but different disorders, they are often confused by clinicians in general practice (26).

Clinical studies that examined the use of AEDs in RLS began in the 1980s with carbamazepine. To date, three published studies have assessed the use of carbamazepine in RLS; one double-blind, placebo-controlled, randomized, parallel-group trial and two open-label studies (29–31). In the placebo-controlled study, which was also the largest ($N = 174$), both placebo and carbamazepine (mean dose 236 mg daily) significantly decreased symptoms of RLS, but the difference was significantly greater with carbamazepine (29). Sleep was not objectively evaluated in this study, nor were the specific types of adverse events reported (except that in the carbamazepine group, 34 patients experienced adverse events and 6 withdrew from the study versus 20 and 2 in the placebo group, respectively) (29). Follow-up analysis failed to show any variable characterizing response versus nonresponse of RLS to carbamazepine treatment (32). Responders, however, tended to have a shorter duration of ailment, lower blood pressure, and experienced initially higher degrees of suffering than nonresponders (32). In the first open-label study ($N = 6$), which utilized a crossover design with a placebo phase, carbamazepine (200–600 mg daily) subjectively improved symptoms of RLS (30). However, this study failed to employ a statistical analysis, and only three patients chose to continue carbamazepine at study conclusion (30). Two patients complained of side effects: one had gastritis during both placebo and carbamazepine treatment, the other had diaphoresis, dizziness, and vomiting during carbamazepine treatment (30). Finally, a small ($N = 9$) open-label trial of carbamazepine (3–7 mg/kg/day) in patients with RLS and PLMS found that carbamazepine significantly improved symptoms of RLS, including sleep efficiency and latency, decreased WASO and stage 1 sleep, but did not affect PLMS symptoms (31). Adverse events were not reported (31).

Although research regarding the use of AEDs to treat RLS or PLMS began with carbamazepine, recent studies have been performed using gabapentin, likely because of its more favorable side-effect profile and reduced frequency of drug-drug interactions. To date, five studies have examined the use of gabapentin in RLS: one randomized, double-blind, placebo-controlled, crossover study (33) and four open-label trials (34–37). The most convincing data that gabapentin is effica-cious in RLS and PLMS comes from the randomized placebo-controlled trial (33). Although this study was of moderate size ($N = 24$, 22 idiopathic, 2 secondary to iron deficiency), compared to placebo, gabapentin was associated with reduced symptoms of RLS on all rating scales, a decreased PLMS index, and improved sleep architecture (increased TST, SE, SWS, and decreased stage 1 sleep) (33). Mean dose at the end of the treatment period was 1855 mg daily (administered at noon and 6 pm), although therapeutic effects were observed at lower doses in many patients. Forty eight percent of patients taking gabapentin (vs. 20.8% taking placebo) reported adverse events. There was no significant difference between the types of adverse events reported between groups, and common complaints were malaise, abdominal pain, somnolence, headache, and dyspepsia (33). Patients with pain complaints seemed to do best with gabapentin treatment (33).

Open-label studies have tended to corroborate that gabapentin is useful in the treatment of RLS, with variable findings regarding objective sleep measurements. One small open-label trial ($N = 9$) found gabapentin (mean dose 733 mg) significantly decreased the subjective symptoms of RLS, and that at follow-up, patients continued to maintain improvement, often with a reduction in total daily dose (mean dose at follow-up 533 mg) (35). In this study, there was also a significant decrease in PLMS compared with baseline (35). There was no significant difference in sleep architecture between pre- and posttreatment polysomnography, but there was limited power to detect such a difference (35). Side effects were considered mild and included numbness, dizziness, sleepiness, and headache (35). An open-label trial comparing gabapentin with an active comparator, ropinirole (a dopamine agonist) ($N = 16$, eight in each group), found that gabapentin improved subjective RLS symptoms (mean dose 800 mg) similar to ropinirole, though these patients generally had mild RLS symptoms (36). As in the earlier study, PLMS (as well as arousals due to PLMS) decreased with gabapentin use, but other polysomnographic characteristics did not significantly change from baseline (36). Side effects were transient and included numbness, dizziness, sleepiness, and headache (36). Another open-label study found that 50% of patients (4 out of 8) with RLS showed improvement with gabapentin (mean dose 1163 mg daily), with dizziness (3), nausea (1), and drowsiness (1) being the most common side effects (37). Finally, a case series of gabapentin treated patients ($N = 16$) reported a robust improvement with at least 50% improvement in RLS symptoms among all subjects (34). Four patients reported adverse events including dizziness (2), drowsiness (1), and enhanced alcohol effect (1,34).

XP13512, an experimental gabapentin prodrug, has also shown promise in the treatment of idiopathic RLS (38). A recent exploratory (phase 2b), double blind, randomized, controlled study illustrated that XP13512 (600 mg–1200 mg) significantly improved RLS symptoms, decreased WASO, stage 1 sleep, PLMS, and increased SWS (38). The most common side effects of XP13512 were somnolence and dizziness (38).

Other AEDs have been studied in RLS/PLMS, but not as extensively as carbamazepine or gabapentin. In one randomized, double-blind, placebo-controlled, crossover study comparing slow-release valproic acid (valproate) to levodopa/benserazid ($N = 20$), valproate significantly improved subjective RLS complaints, but did not significantly affect PLMS frequency or other polysomnographic parameters (39). Side effects reported for each drug were similar, with drowsiness, initial insomnia, and headache the most common for valproate (39). In an open-label trial, valproate significantly improved sleep architecture (decreased stage 1 sleep, increased SWS, and improved SE) in six patients with PLMD (and without RLS), but showed only a trend toward decreased PLMS (40). More recently, case reports illustrating sustained effectiveness of levetiracetam in treatment of both

RLS and PLMS in patients in whom dopaminergic therapy had to be discontinued have been published (41). Also, a small ($N = 4$) pilot trial of lamotrigine in the treatment of RLS has shown that this agent (mean dose 360 mg daily) may be of some benefit in reducing RLS (42).

Secondary RLS is associated with a number of conditions including iron deficiency anemia, pregnancy, neurological conditions, and renal failure. It may also be precipitated or worsened by numerous drugs. Hemodialysis (HD) patients are at particularly elevated risk compared with the general population of developing RLS and PLMS, with an associated increased risk of morbidity and mortality as a result (43–45). One randomized, double-blind, placebo-controlled trial and one open-label trial have examined the use of gabapentin in patients with RLS on HD. The controlled trial, a small ($N = 16$), double-blind, crossover study found that 11 patients responded to gabapentin (200–300 mg after HD) but not to placebo, while one patient responded to both gabapentin and placebo and one to placebo alone (46). Two patients dropped out of the study because of complaints of lethargy (thought secondary to gabapentin), and one patient died from myocardial infarction (46). The small ($N = 15$) open-label trial, comparing gabapentin (200 mg after HD) with levodopa, found gabapentin to be significantly better at improving measures of sleep quality, sleep latency, and sleep disturbance (47).

When RLS is induced by medications, it is typically managed by discontinuing or switching agents. However, there are clinical situations in which adding a medication to treat the RLS may be indicated. One case study on the use of oxcarbazepine (total dose 300 mg daily) showed that this strategy may be useful in some patients with selective serotonin reuptake inhibitor (SSRI)-induced RLS. It should be noted, however, that there may be numerous other strategies, including the addition of gabapentin or carbamazepine, which have not yet been reported (48).

Despite growing evidence that AEDs are good therapeutic modalities in the treatment of RLS and PLMD, there is no consensus regarding their use. In 1999, the American Academy of Sleep Medicine (AASM) published both comprehensive reviews and practice parameters for the treatment of RLS and PLMD that, for AEDs, recommended carbamazepine ahead of gabapentin, largely because of the data available at that time (49,50). Since then, the AASM has published updated reviews and practice parameters on the use of dopaminergic agonists, considered to be the widely accepted first-line agents in the treatment of RLS, but has yet to update recommendations regarding other agents (51,52). More recently, published practice parameters from the European Federation of Neurological Societies (EFNS) have considered there to be level A evidence (established as useful) for the use of gabapentin (800–1800 mg daily) in idiopathic RLS, level B (established as probably useful) evidence for its use in RLS secondary to HD, and level B evidence for carbamazepine (100–300 mg daily) and slow release valproate (600 mg daily) in idiopathic RLS (53,54). Clinically, practitioners typically use gabapentin over carbamazepine and valproate likely because of its lower side-effect burden and greater tolerability. More recent treatment recommendations reflect the growing acceptance of gabapentin in the treatment of RLS, and it seems likely that the AASM may revise practice parameters accordingly in the future (55,56).

An important confounding issue in the studies of AEDs in RLS is the soporific effects of many of these agents, which may produce an apparent improvement in RLS severity, at least temporarily. As sleep complaints are considered by patients with RLS to be the most troublesome symptom of the disorder, some benefit may accrue from the sedative effect of a medication, without addressing its effects on the core RLS symptoms of restlessness and dysesthesia. This is also the case for benzodiazepines, which have also been examined in the treatment of RLS and PLMD. Although a detailed discussion of these reports is beyond the scope of this chapter, clonazepam is the most studied benzodiazepine in the treatment of both RLS and PLMD. As is the case for other AEDs, studies of benzodiazepines tend to be limited by small sample size, modest treatment effects, and difficulty in differentiating nonspecific/soporific effects from specific therapeutic effects on RLS and PLMD symptoms (50). A further discussion of benzodiazepines in RLS and PLMD can be found elsewhere (50,53).

Parasomnias

The parasomnias are a group of disorders that are broadly defined as undesirable physical or experiential events that occur during sleep. They are customarily categorized on the basis of whether they occur during REM or NREM sleep. NREM parasomnias include disorders of arousal such as confusional arousals, sleep-walking, and sleep terrors. REM parasomnias include such disorders as REM behavior disorder and nightmare disorder. In the following sections, the evidence for the use of AEDs in selected parasomnias will be reviewed.

NREM Parasomnias

In general, there is little evidence for the use of AEDs (except benzodiazepines) in the majority of NREM parasomnias. There are sporadic cases of success with carbamazepine, but it is possible that such instances reflect treatment of an underlying nocturnal frontal lobe epilepsy (NFLE) rather than a NREM para-somnia (57). Typically, if pharmacological agents are pursued in the management of NREM parasomnias, benzodiazepines (particularly clonazepam) are considered first-line agents. Since there are no controlled trials on the use of benzodiazepines in NREM parasomnias, this practice is largely based on clinical experience and open-label data. The largest study of long-term benzodiazepine use in a group of patients with sleepwalking/sleep terrors ($N = 69$) found that clonazepam allowed complete or substantial reduction of symptoms, though the average dose did increase by roughly 40% over the course of treatment (58).

Unlike the aforementioned classical NREM parasomnias, sleep-related eating disorder (SRED) is a recently described parasomnia for which AEDs may presently represent the treatment of choice. SRED may be conceptualized as a disorder in which the binge eating behavior of an eating disorder occurs within the context of the disordered arousal and confusional behavior that are typical of NREM para-somnias. Unlike other NREM parasomnias, patients with SRED may report being "half awake" or "half asleep" and the level of awareness of the binge eating is highly variable (59). SRED is similar in many ways to night eating syndrome (NES), a disorder of nighttime hyperphagia that occurs with full consciousness. Concep-tually, it is most useful to consider SRED and NES as occurring along a spectrum of nocturnal binge eating disorders (60). There is growing evidence that topiramate may be of clinical utility in the management of NES and SRED. A small open-label case series of patients with either NES or SRED ($N = 4$) found topiramate (mean dose 218 mg) was associated with moderate to marked improvement in self-reported nocturnal eating (61). A more recent, retrospective chart review of patients with SRED, prescribed topiramate ($N = 25$) showed that over two-thirds of patients responded to the drug (62). In addition, 28% of patients reported a decrease in body weight greater than 10% (62). Eighty four percent of patients reported adverse events, the most common of which were paresthesias (20%), excessive daytime sleepiness (16%), and sexual dysfunction (12%) (62). A recent study of 17 consecutive patients treated with topiramate for SRED found that 11 patients had substantial or full remission of night eating with weight loss (63). Six subjects discontinued topiramate because of inefficacy ($N = 4$) or side effects ($N = 2$) of pruritis and weight gain; paresthesias ($N = 2$) and vitreal floaters ($N = 1$) were the only reported adverse events in subjects who continued therapy (63).

REM Parasomnias

REM sleep behavior disorder (RBD) refers to a condition in which the atonia of REM sleep is partially absent, allowing patients to act out their dreams, often in a violent manner (64). As is the case for most NREM parasomnias, clonazepam is considered first-line treatment in RBD. However, there is a single case report of successful treatment of RBD using carbamazepine (65). Furthermore, in a cohort of overlap disorders of NREM and REM parasomnias (sleepwalking, sleep terrors, and RBD), a small proportion showed clinical improvement with alprazolam and/ or carbamazepine; however, it is unclear which individual agent was responsible for effectiveness on the basis of the reported results (66).

Nightmare disorder is a REM parasomnia in which recurrent dreams, often frightening, awaken the patient from sleep, often with heightened autonomic arousal and difficulty returning to sleep (59). It can be noted that the DSM-IV separates the parasomnia nightmare disorder and the nightmares that occur as part of posttraumatic stress disorder (PTSD) into two distinct entities, whereas the International Classification of Sleep Disorders, Second Edition (ICSD-2) considers PTSD a predisposing factor for nightmare disorder (10,67). Multiple AEDs may be of use in the management of nightmares associated with PTSD. Interpretation of studies assessing AEDs in PTSD nightmares, however, is complicated by the fact that nightmare data are typically presented in conjunction with the more inclusive re-experiencing/intrusive symptom cluster of PTSD. Nonetheless, a small case series and an open-label data review that suggested topiramate considerably diminished PTSD nightmares was later supported by a larger, prospective open-label trial that showed 17 out of 18 (94%) trial patients with premorbid nightmares experienced remission within four weeks of therapy (68–70). Similarly, carbamazepine was also found to significantly diminish both the frequency and severity of dreams about combat in an open-label trial (71,72). There are also case reports of successful diminution of PTSD nightmares with valproate and lamotrigine.

Larger case series tend to examine reduction of PTSD symptoms by cluster, thus making it difficult to interpret what effects these agents have on nightmares specifically (73–77). Valproate has been reported to decrease intrusive symptoms of PTSD in three open trials in male veterans (74,75,77). These effects, however, are difficult to interpret since nearly half of the subjects in these studies were allowed to continue previously prescribed psychotropic medications including sleep promoting agents (e.g., benzodiazepines, sedating antidepressants) (74,75,77). A more recent open-label study of valproate monotherapy (though subjects were allowed to use benzodiazepine receptor agonists for sleep complaints) failed to show that valproate improved any specific PTSD symptom clusters (78). In fact, valproate may have detrimental effects on nightmares, as a reported case of beneficial PTSD treatment with this agent had the side effect of more vivid nighttime dreaming with sleepwalking episodes (74).

Nocturnal Frontal Lobe Epilepsy

NFLE represents a spectrum seizure disorder that may present as many varied behavioral disturbances in sleep, broadly categorized as paroxysmal arousals, nocturnal paroxysmal dystonia, and episodic nocturnal wanderings (79). It is not uncommon for NFLE to be misdiagnosed, most commonly as a parasomnia, and thus it is important that clinicians include NFLE in the differential diagnosis of sleep-related behavioral problems, regardless of the specific nature of the behavior (80,81). There exists both an idiopathic as well as a more recently described autosomal dominant nocturnal frontal lobe epilepsy (ADNFLE) related to a mutation in the neuronal nicotinic acetylcholine receptor (82,83). NFLE is typically managed with carbamazepine, and there exists clinical and in vitro evidence that ADNFLE responds favorably to carbamazepine (79,80,84). A recent case series suggests topiramate may also be effective in patients with NFLE (85).

Other Sleep Disorders

Cataplexy, the sudden loss of muscle tone triggered by strong emotional or physical stimuli, is a cardinal symptom of narcolepsy and is thought to be related to the inappropriate intrusion of REM-related phenomenon (paralysis of the voluntary muscles) into wakefulness. Typically, cataplexy is managed with sodium oxybate, tricyclic antidepressants, or SSRIs (86). One case report of successful treatment of cataplexy with carbamazepine in a patient who either could not tolerate or had no response to typical agents has been reported (87). Despite this report, there have been no further follow-up studies systematically examining carbamazepine in cataplexy, possibly because of its unfavorable side-effect profile when compared to other agents.

Obstructive sleep apnea syndrome (OSAS) is a common sleep disorder in which sleep is disturbed by transient upper airway occlusion resulting in cessation of breathing (apnea), hypoxemia, and subsequent arousal from sleep, resulting in excessive daytime sleepiness (88). The greatest risk factor for OSAS is obesity (although obesity is not necessary for the development of the disease) and thus AEDs that cause weight gain may exacerbate or lead to OSAS (89). The gold standard of treatment is continuous positive airway pressure (CPAP), but lifestyle modifications, particularly weight loss, may profoundly affect the severity of OSAS. There is anecdotal evidence suggesting topiramate-induced weight loss may be an effective treatment for some patients with OSAS, although topiramate is not an approved pharmacotherapy for weight loss (90).

Bruxism, jaw clenching, or grinding of teeth that typically occurs during sleep, are common sleep complaint. The use of intraoral devices, discontinuation of causative medications (often psychotropic), and management of underlying sleep disorders may all be of benefit in the management of bruxism. Unfortunately, it is often difficult to discontinue medications that may cause bruxism in patients with significant psychiatric difficulties. Interestingly, there are reported cases of successful management of bruxism with gabapentin (300 mg nightly) and tiagabine (4–8 mg nightly) in patients for whom discontinuation of the causative agent was not possible (91,92). Unlike the majority of studies on bruxism that tend to be based on case report, a recent single-blind, nonrandomized, crossover study of 10 patients showed that clonazepam 1 mg significantly improved the bruxism index, as well as increased TST, SE, and SOL (93).

CONCLUSIONS

It is not surprising that AEDs can be of therapeutic value in the treatment of sleep disorders, as the mechanisms underlying sleep initiation and maintenance may involve some of the same CNS systems by which AEDs exert their anticonvulsant activity. Much of the evidence supporting the use of AEDs in sleep disorders is uncontrolled, except for the use of benzodiazepines in insomnia. There is growing evidence that specific AEDs may be of use in the treatment of multiple sleep disorders, but at this time, no AED is approved by the FDA for treatment of a specific sleep disorder (except benzodiazepines for insomnia). However, agents that alter GABAergic neurotransmission show promise in the treatment of insomnia. Gabapentin is widely used in the treatment of RLS, and topiramate is currently the treatment of choice in SRED. Hopefully, future studies into the use of AEDs in sleep disorders may lead to broadened treatment options for these conditions.

REFERENCES

1. Bazil CW. Effects of antiepileptic drugs on sleep structure: are all drugs equal? CNS Drugs 2003; 17(10):719–728.
2. Sammaritano M, Sherwin A. Effect of anticonvulsants on sleep. Neurology 2000; 54(5 suppl 1):S16–S24.
3. Foldvary-Schaefer N. Sleep complaints and epilepsy: the role of seizures, antiepileptic drugs and sleep disorders. J Clin Neurophysiol 2002; 19(6):514–521.
4. Hindmarch I, Dawson J, Stanley N. A double-blind study in healthy volunteers to assess the effects on sleep of pregabalin compared with alprazolam and placebo. Sleep 2005; 28(2):187–193.
5. Bazil CW, Battista J, Basner RC. Effects of levetiracetam on sleep in normal volunteers. Epilepsy Behav 2005; 7(3):539–542.
6. Cicolin A, Magliola U, Giordano A, et al. Effects of levetiracetam on nocturnal sleep and daytime vigilance in healthy volunteers. Epilepsia 2006; 47(1):82–85.
7. Shepard JW, Buysse DJ, Cheson AL, et al. History of the development of sleep medicine in the united states. J Clin Sleep Med 2005; 1(1):61–82.
8. Perucca E. The clinical pharmacokinetics of the new antiepileptic drugs. Epilepsia 1999; 40(suppl 9), S7–S13.
9. Ohayon MM. Epidemiology of insomnia: what we know and what we still need to learn. Sleep Med Rev 2002; 6(2):97–111.
10. American Psychiatric Association. Diagnostic and Statistical Manual of Mental Disorders. 4th ed. Text Revision. Washington, DC: American Psychiatric Association, 2000.
11. Buysse DJ, Germain A, Moul D, et al. Insomnia. In: Buysse DJ, ed. Sleep Disorders and Psychiatry. Vol 24. Washington, D.C.: American Psychiatric Publishing, Inc., 2005:29–75.
12. Smith MT, Perlis ML, Park A, et al. Comparative meta-analysis of pharmacotherapy and behavior therapy for persistent insomnia. Am J Psychiatry 2002; 159(1):5–11.
13. Doghramji PP. Trends in the pharmacologic management of insomnia. J Clin Psychiatry 2006; 67(suppl 13):5–8.
14. Wysowski DK, Baum C. Outpatient use of prescription sedative-hypnotic drugs in the United States, 1970 through 1989. Arch Intern Med 1991; 151(9):1779–1783.
15. Curry DT, Eisenstein RD, Walsh JK. Pharmacologic management of insomnia: past, present, and future. Psychiatr Clin North Am 2006; 29(4):871–893 (abstract vii–viii).
16. Bateson AN. Further potential of the GABA receptor in the treatment of insomnia. Sleep Med 2006; 7(suppl 1):S3–S9.
17. Walsh JK, Zammit G, Schweitzer PK, et al. Tiagabine enhances slow wave sleep and sleep maintenance in primary insomnia. Sleep Med 2006; 7(2):155–161.
18. Roth T, Wright KP Jr., Walsh J. Effect of tiagabine on sleep in elderly subjects with primary insomnia: a randomized, double-blind, placebo-controlled study. Sleep 2006; 29(3):335–341.

19. Rosenberg KP. Gabapentin for chronic insomnia. Am J Addict 2003; 12(3):273–274.
20. Karam-Hage M, Brower KJ. Gabapentin treatment for insomnia associated with alcohol dependence. Am J Psychiatry 2000; 157(1):151.
21. Karam-Hage M, Brower KJ. Open pilot study of gabapentin versus trazodone to treat insomnia in alcoholic outpatients. Psychiatry Clin Neurosci 2003; 57(5):542–544.
22. Leppik IE. Antiepileptic drugs in development: prospects for the near future. Epilepsia 1994; 35(suppl 4):S29–S40.
23. Sadler M. Lamotrigine associated with insomnia. Epilepsia 1999; 40(3):322–325.
24. Richens A. Safety of lamotrigine. Epilepsia 1994; 35(suppl 5):S37–S40.
25. Earley CJ. Clinical practice. restless legs syndrome. N Engl J Med 2003; 348(21):2103–2109.
26. Kushida CA. Clinical presentation, diagnosis, and quality of life issues in restless legs syndrome. Am J Med 2007; 120(suppl 1), S4–S12.
27. Allen RP, Picchietti D, Hening WA, et al. Restless legs syndrome: diagnostic criteria, special considerations, and epidemiology. A report from the restless legs syndrome diagnosis and epidemiology workshop at the National Institutes of Health. Sleep Med 2003; 4(2):101–119.
28. Winkelman JW. Considering the causes of RLS. Eur J Neurol 2006; 13(suppl 3):8–14.
29. Telstad W, Sorensen O, Larsen S, et al. Treatment of the restless legs syndrome with carbamazepine: a double blind study. Br Med J (Clin Res Ed) 1984; 288(6415):444–446.
30. Lundvall O, Abom PE, Holm R. Carbamazepine in restless legs. A controlled pilot study. Eur J Clin Pharmacol 1983; 25(3):323–324.
31. Zucconi M, Coccagna G, Petronelli R, et al. Nocturnal myoclonus in restless legs syndrome effect of carbamazepine treatment. Funct Neurol 1989; 4(3):263–271.
32. Larsen S, Telstad W, Sorensen O, et al. Carbamazepine therapy in restless legs. Discrimination between responders and non-responders. Acta Med Scand 1985; 218(2):223–227.
33. Garcia-Borreguero D, Larrosa O, de la Llave Y, et al. Treatment of restless legs syndrome with gabapentin: a double-blind, cross-over study. Neurology 2002; 59(10):1573–1579.
34. Mellick GA, Mellick LB. Management of restless legs syndrome with gabapentin (neurontin). Sleep 1996; 19(3):224–226.
35. Happe S, Klosch G, Saletu B, et al. Treatment of idiopathic restless legs syndrome (RLS) with gabapentin. Neurology 2001; 57(9):1717–1719.
36. Happe S, Sauter C, Klosch G, et al. Gabapentin versus ropinirole in the treatment of idiopathic restless legs syndrome. Neuropsychobiology 2003; 48(2):82–86.
37. Adler CH. Treatment of restless legs syndrome with gabapentin. Clin Neuropharmacol 1997; 20(2):148–151.
38. Kushida C, Becker PM, Ellenbogen AL, et al. XP13512 is well tolerated and effective in treating moderate to severe restless legs syndrome in a 2-week randomized, double-blind, placebo-controlled, exploratory trial. Presented at: The American Academy of Neurology; April 2, 2006: San Diego, CA.
39. Eisensehr I, Ehrenberg BL, Rogge Solti S, et al. Treatment of idiopathic restless legs syndrome (RLS) with slow-release valproic acid compared with slow-release levodopa/ benserazid. J Neurol 2004; 251(5):579–583.
40. Ehrenberg BL, Eisensehr I, Corbett KE, et al. Valproate for sleep consolidation in periodic limb movement disorder. J Clin Psychopharmacol 2000; 20(5):574–578.
41. Della Marca G, Vollono C, Mariotti P, et al. Levetiracetam can be effective in the treatment of restless legs syndrome with periodic limb movements in sleep: report of two cases. J Neurol Neurosurg Psychiatry 2006; 77(4):566–567.
42. Youssef EA, Wagner ML, Martinez JO, et al. Pilot trial of lamotrigine in the restless legs syndrome. Sleep Med 2005; 6(1):89.
43. Kavanagh D, Siddiqui S, Geddes CC. Restless legs syndrome in patients on dialysis. Am J Kidney Dis 2004; 43(5):763–771.
44. Winkelman JW, Chertow GM, Lazarus JM. Restless legs syndrome in end-stage renal disease. Am J Kidney Dis 1996; 28(3):372–378.
45. Pressman M, Benz RL, Paterson D. Periodic leg movements in sleep index predicts mortality in end stage renal disease patients. Sleep Res 1995; 24:416.
46. Thorp ML, Morris CD, Bagby SP. A crossover study of gabapentin in treatment of restless legs syndrome among hemodialysis patients. Am J Kidney Dis 2001; 38(1): 104–108.

47. Micozkadioglu H, Ozdemir FN, Kut A, et al. Gabapentin versus levodopa for the treatment of restless legs syndrome in hemodialysis patients: an open-label study. Ren Fail 2004; 26(4):393–397.
48. Ozturk O, Eraslan D, Kumral E. Oxcarbazepine treatment for paroxetine-induced restless leg syndrome. Gen Hosp Psychiatry 2006; 28(3):264–265.
49. Chesson AL Jr., Wise M, Davila D, et al. Practice parameters for the treatment of restless legs syndrome and periodic limb movement disorder. An American Academy of Sleep Medicine Report. Standards of Practice Committee of the American Academy of Sleep Medicine. Sleep 1999; 22(7):961–968.
50. Hening W, Allen R, Earley C, et al. The treatment of restless legs syndrome and periodic limb movement disorder. An American Academy of Sleep Medicine Review. Sleep 1999; 22(7):970–999.
51. Littner MR, Kushida C, Anderson WM, et al. Practice parameters for the dopaminergic treatment of restless legs syndrome and periodic limb movement disorder. Sleep 2004; 27(3):557–559.
52. Hening WA, Allen RP, Earley CJ, et al. An update on the dopaminergic treatment of restless legs syndrome and periodic limb movement disorder. Sleep 2004; 27(3):560–583.
53. Vignatelli L, Billiard M, Clarenbach P, et al. EFNS guidelines on management of restless legs syndrome and periodic limb movement disorder in sleep. Eur J Neurol 2006; 13(10): 1049–1065.
54. Brainin M, Barnes M, Baron JC, et al. Guidance for the preparation of neurological management guidelines by EFNS scientific task forces–revised recommendations 2004. Eur J Neurol 2004; 11(9):577–581.
55. Hening WA. Current guidelines and standards of practice for restless legs syndrome. Am J Med 2007; 120 (suppl 1):S22–S27.
56. Silber MH, Ehrenberg BL, Allen RP, et al. An algorithm for the management of restless legs syndrome. Mayo Clin Proc 2004; 79(7):916–922.
57. Kavey NB, Whyte J, Resor SR Jr., et al. Somnambulism in adults. Neurology 1990; 40(5): 749–752.
58. Schenck CH, Mahowald MW. Long-term, nightly benzodiazepine treatment of injurious parasomnias and other disorders of disrupted nocturnal sleep in 170 adults. Am J Med 1996; 100(3):333–337.
59. Plante DT, Winkelman JW. Parasomnias. Psychiatr Clin North Am 2006; 29(4):969–987.
60. Winkelman JW. Sleep-related eating disorder and night eating syndrome: sleep disorders, eating disorders, or both? Sleep 2006; 29(7):876–877.
61. Winkelman JW. Treatment of nocturnal eating syndrome and sleep-related eating disorder with topiramate. Sleep Med 2003; 4(3):243–246.
62. Winkelman JW. Efficacy and tolerability of open-label topiramate in the treatment of sleep-related eating disorder: a retrospective case series. J Clin Psychiatry 2006; 67(11): 1729–1734.
63. Schenck C, Mahowald M. Topiramate therapy of sleep related eating disorder (SRED). Sleep 2006; 29(suppl):A268.
64. Schenck CH, Mahowald MW. Rapid eye movement sleep parasomnias. Neurol Clin 2005; 23(4):1107–1126.
65. Bamford CR. Carbamazepine in REM sleep behavior disorder. Sleep 1993; 16(1):33–34.
66. Schenck CH, Boyd JL, Mahowald MW. A parasomnia overlap disorder involving sleepwalking, sleep terrors, and REM sleep behavior disorder in 33 polysomnographically confirmed cases. Sleep 1997; 20(11):972–981.
67. American Academy of Sleep Medicine. International classification of sleep disorders: diagnostic and coding manual. 2nd ed. Westchester, IL: American Academy of Sleep Medicine, 2005.
68. Berlant JL. Prospective open-label study of add-on and monotherapy topiramate in civilians with chronic nonhallucinatory posttraumatic stress disorder. BMC Psychiatry 2004; 4:24.
69. Berlant J, van Kammen DP. Open-label topiramate as primary or adjunctive therapy in chronic civilian posttraumatic stress disorder: a preliminary report. J Clin Psychiatry 2002; 63(1):15–20.

70. Berlant JL. Topiramate in posttraumatic stress disorder: preliminary clinical observations. J Clin Psychiatry 2001; 62(suppl 17):60–63.
71. Lipper S, Davidson JR, Grady TA, et al. Preliminary study of carbamazepine in posttraumatic stress disorder. Psychosomatics 1986; 27(12):849–854.
72. Wolf ME, Alavi A, Mosnaim AD. Posttraumatic stress disorder in Vietnam veterans clinical and EEG findings; possible therapeutic effects of carbamazepine. Biol Psychiatry 1988; 23(6):642–644.
73. Ford N. The use of anticonvulsants in posttraumatic stress disorder: case study and overview. J Trauma Stress 1996; 9(4):857–863.
74. Fesler FA. Valproate in combat-related posttraumatic stress disorder. J Clin Psychiatry 1991; 52(9):361–364.
75. Clark RD, Canive JM, Calais LA, et al. Divalproex in posttraumatic stress disorder: an open-label clinical trial. J Trauma Stress 1999; 12(2):395–401.
76. Hertzberg MA, Butterfield MI, Feldman ME, et al. A preliminary study of lamotrigine for the treatment of posttraumatic stress disorder. Biol Psychiatry 1999; 45(9):1226–1229.
77. Petty F, Davis LL, Nugent AL, et al. Valproate therapy for chronic, combat-induced posttraumatic stress disorder. J Clin Psychopharmacol 2002; 22(1):100–101.
78. Otte C, Wiedemann K, Yassouridis A, et al. Valproate monotherapy in the treatment of civilian patients with non-combat-related posttraumatic stress disorder: an open-label study. J Clin Psychopharmacol 2004; 24(1):106–108.
79. Provini F, Plazzi G, Montagna P, et al. The wide clinical spectrum of nocturnal frontal lobe epilepsy. Sleep Med Rev 2000; 4(4):375–386.
80. Scheffer IE, Bhatia KP, Lopes-Cendes I, et al. Autosomal dominant nocturnal frontal lobe epilepsy. A distinctive clinical disorder. Brain 1995; 118:61–73.
81. Zucconi M, Ferini-Strambi L. NREM parasomnias: arousal disorders and differentiation from nocturnal frontal lobe epilepsy. Clin Neurophysiol 2000; 111(suppl 2), S129–S135.
82. Steinlein OK, Mulley JC, Propping P, et al. A missense mutation in the neuronal nicotinic acetylcholine receptor alpha 4 subunit is associated with autosomal dominant nocturnal frontal lobe epilepsy. Nat Genet 1995; 11(2):201–203.
83. Combi R, Dalpra L, Tenchini ML, et al. Autosomal dominant nocturnal frontal lobe epilepsy: a critical overview. J Neurol 2004; 251(8):923–934.
84. Picard F, Bertrand S, Steinlein OK, et al. Mutated nicotinic receptors responsible for autosomal dominant nocturnal frontal lobe epilepsy are more sensitive to carbamazepine. Epilepsia 1999; 40(9):1198–1209.
85. Oldani A, Manconi M, Zucconi M, et al. Topiramate treatment for nocturnal frontal lobe epilepsy. Seizure 2006; 15(8):649–652.
86. Thorpy MJ. Cataplexy associated with narcolepsy: epidemiology, pathophysiology and management. CNS Drugs 2006; 20(1):43–50.
87. Vaughn BV, D'Cruz OF. Carbamazepine as a treatment for cataplexy. Sleep 1996; 19(2): 101–103.
88. Flemons WW. Clinical practice. Obstructive sleep apnea. N Engl J Med 2002; 347(7): 498–504.
89. Lambert MV, Bird JM. Obstructive sleep apnoea following rapid weight gain secondary to treatment with vigabatrin (sabril). Seizure 1997; 6(3):233–235.
90. Weber MV. Topiramate for obstructive sleep apnea and snoring. Am J Psychiatry 2002; 159(5):872–873.
91. Brown ES, Hong SC. Antidepressant-induced bruxism successfully treated with gabapentin. J Am Dent Assoc 1999; 130(10):1467–1469.
92. Kast RE. Tiagabine may reduce bruxism and associated temporomandibular joint pain. Anesth Prog 2005; 52(3):102–104.
93. Saletu A, Parapatics S, Saletu B, et al. On the pharmacotherapy of sleep bruxism: placebo-controlled polysomnographic and psychometric studies with clonazepam. Neuropsychobiology 2005; 51(4):214–225.

Use of Antiepileptics in Fibromyalgia

Sharon B. Stanford and Lesley M. Arnold
Department of Psychiatry, University of Cincinnati College of Medicine, Cincinnati, Ohio, U.S.A.

INTRODUCTION

In 1904, Gowers first coined the term "fibrositis" to describe a chronic painful condition of muscles thought to be due to inflammation. However, pathological inflammatory changes in the muscles were never discovered (1). In 1990, the multicenter criteria committee of the American College of Rheumatology (ACR) adopted the term "fibromyalgia," rather than "fibrositis," because of the lack of inflammatory changes in the muscles of affected individuals (2). Fibromyalgia is currently thought to be the prototype for a fundamentally different type of pain syndrome in which pain is not due to tissue damage or inflammation (inflammatory pain) and not due to known damage to or of a lesion of the nervous system (neuropathic pain). Fibromyalgia pain is likely due to an abnormal responsiveness or function of the nervous system (3).

DIAGNOSIS AND CLINICAL PRESENTATION OF FIBROMYALGIA

The criteria for the ACR classification of fibromyalgia include widespread pain of at least three months duration and tenderness at 11 or more of 18 specific tender point sites on the body (2). Although only widespread pain and tenderness are included in the ACR criteria, other symptoms commonly occur in patients with fibromyalgia, and the clinical presentation of fibromyalgia is heterogeneous. In the study that established the ACR criteria, 73% to 85% of patients with fibromyalgia reported fatigue, sleep disturbance (nonrestorative sleep or insomnia), and morning stiffness. "Pain all over," paresthesias, headache, history of depression, and anxiety were experienced by 45% to 69% of patients and co-occurring irritable bowel syndrome, sicca symptoms, and Raynaud's phenomenon were less common (<35%) (2). Many patients with fibromyalgia also report weakness, forgetfulness, concentration difficulties, urinary frequency, dysmenorrhea history, subjective swelling, and restless legs.

Alternative diagnostic criteria for fibromyalgia, developed by Pope and Hudson (4), may be helpful for mental health professionals who do not perform routine physical exams. These criteria include some of the characteristic symptoms of fibromyalgia in addition to pain and tender points (Table 1). Using the format of the Structured Clinical Interview for DSM-IV (SCID) (5), Pope and Hudson (4) incorporated their criteria for fibromyalgia into a structured interview, which has been used in family studies and clinical trials (6–8).

In studies of both community and clinic groups, fibromyalgia is strongly associated with anxiety and depressive symptoms, with about one-third of patients reporting major current problems with anxiety or depression. (9,10). In clinical studies of patients with ACR-defined fibromyalgia, any current anxiety disorder has been found in 27% to 60% of patients with fibromyalgia (11,12), and any lifetime anxiety disorder (both current and past) has been reported in 35% to 62% of patients (11,12). The rates of current major depressive disorder have ranged from

TABLE 1 Pope and Hudson Criteria for Fibromyalgia

A. Generalized pain affecting the axial, plus upper and lower segments, plus left and right sides of the body Either "B" or "C":
B. At least 11 of 18 reproducible tender points
C. At least 4 of the following symptoms:
    i.   Generalized fatigue
    ii. Generalized headache (of a type, severity, or pattern that is different from headaches the patient may have had in the premorbid state)
    iii. Sleep disturbance (hypersomnia or insomnia)
    iv. Neuropsychiatric complaints (1 or more of the following: forgetfulness, excessive irritability, confusion, difficulty thinking, inability to concentrate, depression)
    v.   Numbness, tingling sensations
    vi. Symptoms of irritable bowel syndrome (periodically altered bowel habits with lower abdominal pain or distension usually relieved or aggravated by bowel movements; no blood)
D. It cannot be established that the disturbance is due to another systemic condition.

14% to 23% (11,13,14), while lifetime diagnoses of major depressive disorder have varied between 58% and 86% (11,13–15). Arnold et al. (15) also reported that individuals with fibromyalgia were significantly more likely than those without fibromyalgia to have comorbid bipolar disorder.

EPIDEMIOLOGY

Fibromyalgia is common in the United States, with an estimated prevalence of 2% in the adult population. Fibromyalgia disproportionately affects women, with a prevalence of 3.4% in women compared with 0.5% in men (9). The community prevalence of fibromyalgia in Europe, South Africa, and Canada varies from 0.7% to 4.5%, with a greater prevalence in women compared with men (16–22). The prevalence of fibromyalgia in adults increases with age, rising sharply in middle age (ages 50–59 years) and then dropping off in the oldest age groups ($\geq$80 years) (9). The average age of onset is between 30 and 50 years. In the general population, fibromyalgia is most common in women aged 50 years and older (9).

ETIOLOGY OF FIBROMYALGIA

Genetic Factors

The etiology of fibromyalgia is unknown, although both genetic and environmental factors probably contribute to the liability to fibromyalgia.

Fibromyalgia aggregates strongly in families (6). Fibromyalgia also coaggregates in families with major mood disorders (6) as well as with mood disorders, anxiety disorders, eating disorders, irritable bowel disorder, and migraine, taken collectively (23). These results, and the findings that mood and anxiety disorders are frequently comorbid with fibromyalgia, suggest that fibromyalgia may share a common pathophysiological abnormality with some psychiatric and medical disorders (15).

Stress

Environmental stressors have been associated with the development of fibromyalgia, and patients with fibromyalgia often report the onset of their symptoms after a period of substantial stress. Patients with fibromyalgia report higher levels of stress as measured by daily hassles than patients with rheumatoid arthritis (24) and experience more stressful, negative lifetime events than healthy controls (25). Fibromyalgia patients have significantly higher prevalence rates of all forms of childhood and adult victimization than patients with rheumatoid arthritis (26).

Chronic stress might promote disturbances in the stress response system that could lead to the development of fibromyalgia. Patients with fibromyalgia have disturbances in the two major interacting stress response systems, the autonomic nervous system, and the hypothalamic-pituitary-adrenal (HPA) axis (27). Trauma or chronic stress may promote dysfunction of the stress systems that leads to the development of disorders like fibromyalgia (28). Genetic differences in the activity of the stress response system could also predispose individuals to fibromyalgia.

Central Nervous System Processing of Pain

There is emerging evidence that fibromyalgia is associated with aberrant central nervous system (CNS) processing of pain (27,29–31). Although the ACR criteria for fibromyalgia require tenderness in 11 out of 18 discrete regions, patients with fibromyalgia have increased sensitivity to pain throughout the body. Fibromyalgia patients often develop an increased response to painful stimuli (hyperalgesia) and experience pain from normally nonnoxious stimuli (allodynia) (30). Both hyperalgesia and allodynia reflect an enhanced CNS processing of painful stimuli that is characteristic of central sensitization (32).

Painful stimuli, such as one that occurs after an injury, may initiate the process in susceptible individuals that leads to central sensitization. Indeed, many patients with fibromyalgia report the onset of symptoms after physical trauma or repetitive injuries (33). Various injuries, including trauma and infections, can also induce a CNS-immune response that leads to subsequent production of proinflammatory cytokines, which have been implicated in the generation of chronic pain states (31,34).

Abnormalities in central monoaminergic neurotransmission may play a role in the development of central pain sensitization of fibromyalgia. There is evidence of a functional reduction in serotonergic activity in patients with fibromyalgia and reduced concentrations of the primary norepinephrine metabolite, 3-methoxy-4-hydroxyphenethylene (MHPG), in the cerebrospinal fluid (CSF) of fibromyalgia patients (35–38). Both norepinephrine and serotonin are involved in the descending inhibitory pain pathways in the brain and spinal cord that act to diminish pain (39,40). A reduction of serotonin and norepinephrine-mediated descending pain inhibitory pathways is a possible mechanism for the development of pain in fibromyalgia.

Substance P, an important nociceptive neurotransmitter, was found to be elevated in the CSF of individuals with fibromyalgia, compared with healthy controls (41,42). Substance P, along with pronociceptive excitatory amino acids acting at the N-methyl-D-aspartate (NMDA) receptor, and other neuropeptides may also play a role in the generation of central pain sensitization (43). Substance P levels might be influenced by serotonin activity as evidenced by a recent study that found a strong negative correlation between serum concentrations of the primary serotonin metabolite, 5-hydroxyindoleacetic acid (5-HIAA) and substance P, pain, and insomnia (38).

Neuroimaging studies of patients with fibromyalgia have provided evidence for central augmentation of pain sensitivity in fibromyalgia. In a study using functional magnetic resonance imaging, the pattern of cerebral activation during the application of painful pressure was assessed in fibromyalgia patients, compared with controls (44). The results showed an overlap between activations in patients and activations evoked by greater stimulus pressures in controls. In addition, application of mild pressure to both fibromyalgia patients and controls resulted in a greater number of activated regions in the patients. Both of these findings provide evidence that pain sensitivity is augmented in fibromyalgia (44).

Sleep

A common sleep problem described by fibromyalgia patients involves frequent awakenings during the night and nonrestorative sleep (feeling tired upon awakening). This sleep problem is sometime associated with an abnormality consisting of inappropriate intrusion of alpha waves (normally seen during wakefulness or REM sleep) into deep sleep (characterized by delta waves) (45). Alpha-delta sleep intrusion was thought to contribute to the musculoskeletal pain and fatigue of fibromyalgia (45); however, the sleep abnormality is not specific to fibromyalgia and is found in other disorders (46).

THE ROLE OF ANTIEPILEPTIC DRUGS IN TREATING FIBROMYALGIA

Pharmacological and nonpharmacological treatment options for patients with fibromyalgia have expanded substantially in recent years (47). Among the most promising pharmacological agents for fibromyalgia are some of the antiepileptic drugs (AEDs). AEDs are frequently used to treat chronic pain disorders, particularly neuropathic pain disorders and migraine (48–55). Although each AED's specific mechanism of action may differ, all of these agents generally reduce excitability, decrease ectopic discharge, and reduce neurotransmitter release, consequences that may contribute to their antiepileptic and antinociceptive effects (56).

Several possible mechanisms of action may account for the AED's efficacy in chronic pain disorders and include sodium channel blockade, calcium channel blockade, enhancement of GABAergic transmission, inhibition of glutamatergic transmission, free radical scavenging, inhibition of nitric oxide formation, and enhancement of monoamine transmission (51).

Two AEDs with a similar mechanism of action, pregabalin and gabapentin, have been studied in randomized, placebo-controlled trials of fibromyalgia. Both pregabalin and gabapentin bind to the α2-δ subunit of voltage-gated calcium cannels of neurons, reducing calcium influx at nerve terminals and thereby decreasing the synaptic release of several substances, including glutamate and substance P. This reduction in synaptic activity may account for pregabalin and gabapentin actions in vivo to reduce neuronal excitability and ultimately their analgesic activity (57–59).

Pregabalin

Pregabalin is the first medication to receive approval from the U.S. Food and Drug Administration (FDA) for treatment of fibromyalgia. In addition to fibromyalgia, pregabalin is approved in the United States in adults for the treatment of pain due to diabetic neuropathy or postherpetic neuralgia and as adjunctive therapy of partial seizures. In the European Union, it has been approved for treatment of peripheral and central neuropathic pain, for epilepsy as adjunctive therapy in adults with partial seizures with or without secondary generalization, and for the treatment of generalized anxiety disorder (60).

The first randomized, placebo-controlled, double-blind, multicenter, mono-therapy trial compared placebo with three doses of pregabalin, 150, 300, or 450 mg divided thrice daily (t.i.d.) in equal doses, for eight weeks (61). Men and women with primary fibromyalgia were eligible if they had a score of 40 mm or higher on the 100 mm visual analog scale (VAS) of the Short Form McGill Pain Questionnaire (SF-MPQ) at screening and randomization visits and a mean pain score of 4 or higher on a 0 to 10 pain rating scale (0 = no pain, 10 = worst possible pain) based on at least four daily pain diary entries in the week before randomization. Patients were excluded if they had previously failed to respond to gabapentin at dosages 1200 mg or higher daily for fibromyalgia pain, or if they had any other pain conditions that might interfere with fibromyalgia pain assessment. Patients were also excluded if they had a creatinine clearance less than or equal to 60 mL/min, were taking any other pain medications or CNS-active treatments (acetaminophen and aspirin up to 325 mg/day were allowed), or who were receiving or applying for disability. Those randomized to the 450-mg dose started at 300 mg daily with the dose increased to 450 mg after three days. Primary efficacy was measured using a daily paper diary in which patients were asked to rate the intensity of their pain (0–10) over the previous 24 hours. Secondary measures were included to obtain more information about the overall effect of pregabalin on other core symptoms of fibromyalgia. These included a daily diary which assessed sleep quality on a 0 to 10 scale (10 = worst possible sleep); the SF-MPQ, a self-reported rating scale with 15 descriptors, 11 sensory and 4 affective, related to pain; the Medical Outcomes Study (MOS) sleep measure, a 12-item self-reported sleep measure; the Multi-dimensional Assessment of Fatigue (MAF), a 16-item self-administered question-naire to measure fatigue; the Hospital Anxiety and Depression Scale (HADS), a self-report scale which assesses anxiety and depressive symptoms; the Short Form 36 (SF-36) health survey, a generic health-related quality of life measure with domains in physical functioning, role limitations due to physical health problems, bodily pain, social functioning, general mental health, role limitations due to emotional problems, vitality, energy or fatigue, and general health perceptions; the Manual Tender Point Survey, a measure of tenderness obtained during a stand-ardized tender point exam, in which the patient rates pain at each point on a 0 to 10 scale; the Patient Global Impression of Change (PGI-C), a self-assessment mea-sure allowing the patient to indicate change in overall status from 1 to 7 (1 = "very much improved," 7 = "very much worse"); and the Clinical Global Impression of Change (CGI-C), a clinician assessment of how ill the patient is on a 7-point scale from 1 to 7 (1 = "not at all ill," 7 = "among the most extremely ill patients").

Of the 529 patients who were randomized, 91% were female with a mean duration of fibromyalgia symptoms of nine years and a mean pain score of 7. Baseline mean depression and anxiety scores were in the mild range based on the HADS; 28% had moderate anxiety symptoms, 17% reported severe anxiety, 22% had moderate depressive symptoms, and 9% had severe depression.

The average pain score was significantly reduced in patients receiving pre-gabalin 450 mg/day when compared with placebo (-0.93 on the 0–10 scale, $p \leq 0.001$), and a significantly greater proportion of those randomized to the 450 mg/day dose (28.9%) reported 50% or greater reduction in pain scores than placebo group (13.2%). Patients in all pregabalin treatment groups compared with placebo reported improved sleep and had improved scores in the general health perception domain of the SF-36 (61). Most of the improvement in pain scores was found to be independent of the presence of anxiety or depressive symptoms at baseline and independent of improvements in HADS anxiety or depression scores (62).

The second monotherapy trial of pregabalin treatment of fibromyalgia enrolled 748 patients, of which 94% were female and 90% were white. Patients had a mean age of 49 years, a mean duration of symptoms of 9.3 years, and a mean pain score at baseline of 7.1. As in the first study, men and women with primary fibromyalgia were eligible if they did not have comorbid rheumatological disease or other severe pain disorders. Patients who had creatinine clearance less than or equal to 60 mL/min were taking CNS-active medications or pain medications other than acetaminophen or aspirin for cardiac prophylaxis or had been a previous participant in a pregabalin trial were excluded. Patients received pregabalin 300, 450, 600 mg, or placebo divided in twice daily (b.i.d.) dosing over 12 weeks, following a one-week baseline phase. Patients were asked to rate their pain at screening and during the baseline assessment and were required to have an average pain rating of at least 4 on the 0 to 10 rating scale and score at least 40 mm on the 100 mm VAS of the SF-MPQ at screening and randomization to be included in the study. All groups started with 150 mg daily dosing and were escalated to the fixed, goal dose over the first week of the treatment phase. Primary efficacy measures included mean pain scores as recorded in daily pain diaries using the 0 to 10 pain scale. Response was defined as at least 30% reduction in mean pain score from baseline to endpoint. If pain scores were improved, a second primary objective was to measure overall management of fibromyalgia, using scores on the PGI-C and Fibromyalgia Impact Questionnaire (FIQ). The FIQ contains 10 sub-scales, which are combined into a total score. Questions relate to physical functioning, pain, fatigue, stiffness, tiredness on awakening, difficulty working, days felt well, and symptoms of anxiety and depression. Secondary efficacy measures included sleep quality as rated in daily sleep diaries (using the 0–10 rating scale), the MOS sleep scale, the SF-36, the Sheehan Disability Scale (SDS), an assessment of impairment in occupational, social and family functioning, the Fibromyalgia Health Assessment Questionnaire (F-HAQ), an assessment of functional impairment in fibromyalgia, the SF-MPQ, the MAF, and the HADS.

Patients in all pregabalin treatment groups showed statistically significant improvement in mean pain scores at the end of the study when compared with the placebo group. Those in the 600-mg/day group showed the most improvement with a mean change of -0.66 ($p = 0.0070$) at endpoint. All three pregabalin groups significantly improved pain compared with the placebo group by the first week of therapy. Those in the 600-mg/day group were consistently improved at all visits throughout the study. However, those in the other two groups did not report pain scores significantly superior to placebo at four (out of 13) of the intermediate study assessments. The proportion of responders in the groups receiving pregabalin 300, 450, and 600 mg/day were 43%, 43%, and 44% compared with 35% for placebo. Although the percentage of responders was greater in the pregabalin groups, the difference compared with placebo did not achieve statistical significance. For the second primary objective, significant differences in the PGI-C response were observed in all the pregabalin groups when compared with placebo with $p = 0.0183$ for the 300-mg/day group, $p = 0.0467$ for the 450-mg/day group, and $p = 0.0127$ for the 600-mg/day group. The FIQ total score at endpoint did not show a statistically significant improvement for any of the pregabalin groups compared with placebo.

All three pregabalin dosages were associated with statistically significant improvement in sleep quality, improvement in the MOS sleep disturbance and Sleep Problem Index, and improvement on the MOS sleep quantity subscale. Other secondary measures did not show any statistical significance even though beneficial effects were seen on most measures in favor of pregabalin (63).

Another randomized, double-blind, placebo-controlled, monotherapy trial of pregabalin in fibromyalgia used a similar design but included a single-blind, placebo run-in phase (64). Inclusion criteria were similar to the previous studies, requiring patients to have a pain score of 40 mm or higher on the 100 mm VAS at screening and randomization. Exclusion criteria were also similar to the previous studies. However, this study allowed patients who had previously not responded to gabapentin. During the placebo run-in phase, patients must have completed at least four of seven daily entries in their pain diary, with a mean pain score of 4 or higher. Patients were also assessed at the end of the placebo run-in period and those who reported at least a 30% reduction on the pain VAS score were excluded from the trial as placebo responders. After this run-in, 750 patients were randomized to pregabalin 300, 450, 600 mg/day, or placebo administered b.i.d. for 14 weeks. Of those randomized, 94.5% were female and 91% were white, with a mean age of 50.1 years, a mean duration of symptoms of 10.0 years, and a mean pain score at baseline of 6.7. All pregabalin-treated patients were gradually escalated to goal dose over one to two weeks. The primary outcome was change in mean pain score derived from daily pain diaries as in the previous studies. Additional primary outcomes were the PGI-C and FIQ, to allow for an assessment of pregabalin's effect on the overall management of fibromyalgia. Secondary endpoints included sleep assessments as measured by the sleep quality diary and the MOS sleep scale, depressive and anxiety symptoms as measured by the HADS, fatigue measured by the MAF, and health-related quality of life as evaluated with the SF-36.

Patients in all pregabalin treatment groups showed statistically significant improvements in mean pain scores compared with the placebo-treated group. This difference occurred as early as week 1 and was sustained across all treatment groups throughout the trial with the exception of the 300-mg/day group at week 11. PGI-C and FIQ scores also showed significant improvement across all pregabalin groups compared with placebo with the exception of the FIQ score in the 300-mg/day group at endpoint (64). These results suggest that pregabalin improves pain, but also reduces the overall impact of fibromyalgia on patients.

Significant improvements were also noted in both sleep diary and MOS sleep scale scores in all of the pregabalin-treated groups compared with placebo. Several domains of the SF-36 showed significant improvement in scores in the 450- and 600-mg/day groups, including Social Functioning and Vitality for 450 mg/day and Mental Health, Vitality, and the Mental Component Summary for 600 mg/day. There was no difference noted in fatigue, depressive, or anxiety symptoms (except in the 600-mg/day group which showed a significantly improved HADS anxiety score compared with placebo) (64).

In addition to the studies showing efficacy of pregabalin for the acute treatment of fibromyalgia, a six-month double-blind, placebo-controlled study was conducted to evaluate the durability of pregabalin's efficacy on multiple symptom domains of fibromyalgia, including pain, fatigue, sleep, and global improvement in those who initially responded during a six-week, open-label phase (65). During initial open-label treatment, patients received pregabalin, which was gradually escalated to 300, 450, or 600 mg daily, depending on response and tolerability, with a reduction in dosage allowed during the first three weeks, followed by three weeks at a fixed dosage. Men and women with primary fibromyalgia were eligible if they had a VAS score of 40 mm or higher (0–100 mm scale) at open-label baseline. Patients were excluded for creatinine clearance less than or equal to 60 mL/min, use of prohibited medications (pain medications other than acetaminophen, sleep agents, and CNS-active agents), rheumatological disease, or unstable medical or psychiatric conditions. The primary outcome measure was time to loss of therapeutic response (measured in days). Loss of response was defined as either less than 30% reduction in VAS score relative to the open-label baseline value at two consecutive visits of the double-blind phase or worsening of fibromyalgia symptoms necessitating alternate treatment in the opinion of the investigator. Secondary measures included time to worsening of MOS sleep scale (8 point worsening), MAF (10 point worsening), and PGI-C (less improvement than "much improved"). Of those who enrolled in the study ($N = 1051$), 663 completed the open-label phase, 85% of which were classified as responders (at least 50% reduction in mean pain score and a PGI-C of "much" or "very much" improved over at least 2 visits). Patients who responded were randomized to continue on pregabalin (administered b.i.d.) ($N = 279$ subjects) or to placebo ($N = 287$ subjects) for 26 weeks. Of those randomized, 93% were female and 88% were white, with a mean age of 50 years and a mean duration of symptoms of 7.8 years. The mean VAS score at the open-label baseline was 78 (0–100 scale).

By the end of the double-blind phase of the study, nearly twice as many patients taking placebo had lost therapeutic response (61%) when compared with those taking pregabalin (32%). These results demonstrate a durable effect of pregabalin in pain relief for patients with fibromyalgia. Similar durability of effect was shown in measures of fatigue, sleep disturbance, and global improvement (65).

Dosing and Side Effects

Dosing for pregabalin is indicated at 300 to 450 mg/day divided b.i.d. for fibromyalgia, although the pregabalin studies reported efficacy up to 600 mg daily. However, there was a dose-related increase in adverse events, which contributed to the indicated maximum dose of 450 mg/day for fibromyalgia. The recommended starting dose is 150 mg administered in two divided doses per day (75 mg b.i.d.) and can be increased to 300 mg/day within one week, as tolerated. Further dosing up to the maximum indicated dose of 450 mg/day (225 mg b.i.d.) can occur by the end of the second week of therapy, as tolerated.

Pregabalin is generally well tolerated in the fibromyalgia population. The most common side effects include dizziness (>30% in all trials), somnolence (18–25%), weight gain (12–14%), peripheral edema (5–8%), and blurred vision (7.5–8.9%). Other side effects include euphoria, dry mouth, constipation, and poor concentration. Side effects are dose dependent, with smaller doses being better tolerated; however, in these studies, side effects lessened within days (61,63–65). If side effects are problematic, patients may tolerate once daily dosing near bedtime, initially with gradual increase to b.i.d. to t.i.d. dosing as side effects dissipate.

Metabolism

Pregabalin undergoes negligible metabolism in the body and is excreted largely unchanged in the urine. Its oral bioavailability is over 90%, with an elimination half-life of six hours. Pregabalin is absorbed more slowly when taken with food; however, there is no clinically relevant effect on total absorption with maximum plasma concentrations achieved within 1.5 hours on an empty stomach versus 3 hours with food.

Because pregabalin is excreted by the kidneys, care must be taken in individuals with renal insufficiency who may require a dose reduction on the basis of their creatinine clearance. Pregabalin is removed during dialysis, so dosing after hemodialysis is recommended (60).

Pregabalin does not affect levels of other AEDs or oral contraceptives and has minimal drug interactions, making it a good choice for patients on multiple medications. It should be noted, however, that alcohol and medications with sedating properties may augment the CNS effects of pregabalin, leading to more pronounced sedation and dizziness when taken together (60).

Gabapentin

Gabapentin was first approved by the FDA in 1993 for control of partial seizures and was later approved for use in controlling pain associated with postherpetic neuralgia (66). It was used widely off label for treating a variety of pain conditions, including fibromyalgia, although most evidence was anecdotal until recently.

The only placebo-controlled, double-blind study performed using gabapentin in the treatment of fibromyalgia was published in 2007 (67). This study was a 12-week, randomized, double-blind, placebo-controlled trial comparing gabapentin (1200–2400 flexible dosing) with placebo. Patients with primary fibromyalgia who scored 4 or higher on the average pain severity item of the Brief Pain Inventory (BPI) (in which patients rate their average pain severity over the last 24 hours) at screening and randomization were eligible for inclusion. Patients were excluded if they had unstable medical or psychiatric disorders, rheumatic disease, or were taking a prohibited medication (over-the-counter analgesics were allowed, including acetaminophen and nonsteroidal anti-inflammatory drugs; all other CNS-active treatments excluded). A total of 150 subjects were randomized (90% female, 97% white) with average pain scores of 5.7 in the gabapentin group and 6.0 in the placebo group. Gabapentin was administered beginning at 300 mg at bedtime for one week followed by 300 mg b.i.d. for one week, 300 mg b.i.d. and 600 mg q.h.s. for two weeks, 600 mg t.i.d. for two weeks, and then 600 mg b.i.d. and 1200 mg q.h.s. thereafter. If a patient was not able to tolerate 2400 mg/day, the dosing was reduced to a minimum of 1200 mg/day. The primary outcome measure was the BPI average pain severity score. Response to treatment was defined by a reduction in this score by at least 30%. Secondary outcomes included the BPI average pain interference score (which measures how much pain interferes in various aspects of the patient's life), the FIQ, the Mean Tender Point Pain Threshold (in which a Fischer dolorimeter is applied to the 18 tender point sites and pressure increased at a defined rate until the patient reports when first discomfort occurs), the C-GIS, the MOS sleep measure, and the Montgomery Asberg Depression Rating Scale (MADRS). Additional health outcomes were measured using the SF-36.

Over the course of the study, BPI average pain severity scores improved (-0.92; $p = 0.015$) in patients taking gabapentin versus patients on placebo. In addition, a significantly higher percentage of subjects in the gabapentin group achieved response (51%) versus placebo (31%). Compared with placebo, gabapentin was also found to be significantly effective at improving sleep, health-related quality of life, and global assessments but did not improve the mean tender point pain threshold or the MADRS (67) (Table 2).

TABLE 2 Summary of Anticonvulsant Trials of Fibromyalgia Treatment

Study (Ref.)	Drug (mg/day)	Study design (no. of patients)	Duration (wk)	Outcomes that significantly improved with treatment over placebo
Crofford et al. (61)	Pregabalin (150, 300 and 450)	Pregabalin vs. placebo, parallel (529)	8	Primary measure: Mean daily pain score (daily diaries) (450 mg only) Secondary measures: Sleep quality diary (300 mg, 450 mg), MAF global fatigue (300 mg, 450 mg), PGIC, CGIC (300 mg, 450 mg), SF-36 general health (150 mg, 300 mg, 450 mg), vitality (450 mg), bodily pain (450 mg), social functioning (450 mg)
Mease et al. (63)	Pregabalin (300, 450, 600)	Pregabalin vs. placebo, parallel (748)	13	Primary measure: Mean daily pain score (daily diaries) (300 mg, 450 mg, 600 mg) Secondary measures: PGIC (300 mg, 450 mg, 600 mg), sleep quality diary (300 mg, 450 mg, 600 mg), MOS sleep disturbance (300 mg, 450 mg, 600 mg), MOS sleep problem index (300 mg, 450 mg, 600 mg), MOS sleep quantity (300 mg, 450 mg, 600 mg)
Arnold et al. (64)	Pregabalin (300, 450, 600)	Pregabalin vs. placebo, parallel (750)	14	Primary measure: Mean daily pain score (daily diaries) (300 mg, 450 mg, 600 mg), PGIC (300 mg, 450 mg, 600 mg), FIQ score (450 mg, 600 mg) Secondary measures: Sleep quality diary (300 mg, 450 mg, 600 mg), MOS sleep quantity (300 mg, 450 mg, 600 mg), MOS sleep adequacy index (300 mg, 450 mg, 600 mg), MOS sleep problem index (300 mg, 450 mg, 600 mg), SF-36 mental health (600 mg), vitality (450 mg, 600 mg), mental component summary (600 mg), social functioning (450 mg)
Crofford et al. (65)	Pregabalin (300, 450, 600)	Pregabalin vs. placebo (1051)	26	Primary measure: Time to loss of therapeutic response Secondary measures: Time to worsening MOS sleep disturbance, adequacy, somnolence, sleep problem index, MAF, PGIC
Arnold et al. (67)	Gabapentin (1200–2400)	Gabapentin vs. placebo, parallel (150)	12	Primary measure: BPI average pain severity score Secondary measures: BPI pain interference score, FIQ score, MOS sleep problem index, CGI-S

Abbreviations: MAF, multidimensional assessment of fatigue; SF-36, Short form 36 health survey; MOS, medical outcomes study; FIQ, fibromyalgia impact; PGIC, patient global impression of change; CGI-C, clinician global impression of change; CGI-S, clinician global impression of severity.

Dosing and Side Effects

Side effects for gabapentin are similar to those for pregabalin, with the main effects during the study being dizziness (25%), sedation (24%), light-headedness (15%), edema (16%), and weight gain (8%), which is consistent with the general side-effect profile in other populations (66). In general, gabapentin was well tolerated in fibromyalgia patients with dosing of 1200 to 2400 mg daily divided t.i.d. (67). The maximum dose of gabapentin for other conditions is 3600 mg daily in divided doses (66). A slower titration may allow for better compliance and tolerability in patients with fibromyalgia.

Metabolism

The bioavailability of gabapentin decreases with increased doses and absorption is impaired when taken with certain antacids. Similar to pregabalin, gabapentin is not appreciably metabolized in the body and is excreted unchanged through the kidneys, so care must be taken when prescribing this medication to patients with renal insufficiency (66).

Summary of Studies

Across all trials involving pregabalin and in the single gabapentin trial, pain was improved in addition to improvement in patients' global assessment of change and the FIQ score, suggesting that pregabalin reduces the overall impact of fibromyalgia on patients.

Other symptom domains common in fibromyalgia, including mood disturbance, fatigue, subjective cognitive complaints, and sleep disturbance have a significant impact on patients with fibromyalgia. Indeed, sleep disturbance and fatigue are often more problematic than pain for many patients.

In addition to significant reduction in pain, pregabalin and gabapentin showed secondary improvements in several measures of sleep quality (Table 2). Pregabalin and gabapentin enhance slow-wave (delta wave) sleep in those with seizure disorders and healthy volunteers (68,69), and it may be this effect that contributes to improved sleep in fibromyalgia patients using the α2-δ ligands.

Differences Between Pregabalin and Gabapentin

Although pregabalin and gabapentin have similar mechanisms of action, there are several differences. Both act on the α2-δ protein subunit of voltage-gated calcium channels, but pregabalin has an increased binding affinity when compared with gabapentin. This may allow pregabalin to have more potent analgesic effects at smaller doses (70–72). The clinical significance of this effect is presently unknown, however, due to the lack of clinical studies directly comparing the two agents. Pregabalin also differs from gabapentin in its pharmacokinetics. Pregabalin exhibits a linear increase in plasma concentrations with increasing dose, whereas gabapentin is not as readily absorbed at higher doses (60,66). This feature allows pregabalin to be escalated to effective doses more rapidly than gabapentin (70–72). Pregabalin is a schedule V medication (73), whereas gabapentin is unscheduled. Cost and availability of gabapentin may provide a benefit for some patients, given its generic status in the United States.

Other Antiepileptic Drugs

Although studies are lacking, there may be a role for other AEDs in the treatment of fibromyalgia. Topiramate is indicated for the prophylaxis of migraine headaches and has evidence to support its use in neuropathic pain conditions (74). In the authors' clinical experience, topiramate can be especially useful in fibromyalgia patients with prominent comorbid migraines and in patients who experience weight gain with other medications. Other AEDs to consider in treating fibromyalgia include carbamazapine, valproic acid, lamotrigine, and oxcarbazapine. All have some evidence of efficacy in neuropathic pain (74) and may be useful in fibromyalgia patients with comorbid bipolar disorder. However, more study is needed to evaluate the safety and efficacy of these and other AEDs in the treatment of fibromyalgia.

SUMMARY

Since the publication of the ACR criteria, an expansion in research has increased our understanding of the possible genetic and environmental factors potentially involved in the etiology of fibromyalgia. Environmental stressors and genetic vulnerability could act alone or together to initiate a series of biological events in individuals that eventually leads to the development of fibromyalgia. These same CNS changes could also be involved in the development of symptoms of depression and other comorbid conditions.

AEDs, especially pregabalin and gabapentin, can play a significant role in the treatment of fibromyalgia, especially for those patients with prominent pain and sleep disturbance. More studies are needed to evaluate other AEDs with different mechanisms of action to determine how they may play a role in fibromyalgia treatment. Like major depressive disorder in which there are melancholic and atypical forms, fibromyalgia may be heterogeneous in its presentation and underlying pathophysiology, so care must be taken to evaluate the specific needs of each patient when deciding on a treatment regimen. All symptom domains that are present in fibromyalgia patients should be noted and medications adjusted for the specific needs of each patient.

REFERENCES

1. Reynolds MD. The development of the concept of fibrositis. J Hist Med Allied Sci 1983; 38:5–35.
2. Wolfe F, Smythe HA, Yunus MB, et al. The American college of rheumatology 1990 criteria for the classification of fibromyalgia. Arthritis Rheum 1990; 33:160–172.
3. Woolf CJ. Pain: moving from symptom control toward mechanism-specific pharmacologic management. Ann Intern Med 2004; 140(6):441–451.
4. Pope HG Jr., Hudson JI. A supplemental interview for forms of "affective spectrum disorder." Int J Psychiatry Med 1991; 21:205–232.
5. First MB, Spitzer RL, Gibbon M, et al. Structured Interview for the DSM-IV Axis I Disorders-Patient Edition (SCID-I/P), Version 2.0. New York, NY: Biometrics Research Department, New York State Psychiatric Institute, 1995.
6. Arnold LM, Hudson JI, Hess EV, et al. Family study of fibromyalgia. Arthritis Rheum 2004; 50(3):944–952.
7. Hudson JI, Mangweth B, Pope HG Jr., et al. Family study of affective spectrum disorder. Arch Gen Psychiatry 2003; 60:170–177.
8. Dwight MM, Arnold LM, O'Brien H, et al. An open clinical trial of venlafaxine treatment of fibromyalgia. Psychosomatics 1998; 39:14–17.
9. Wolfe F, Ross K, Anderson J, et al. The prevalence and characteristics of fibromyalgia in the general population. Arthritis Rheum 1995; 38:19–28.
10. White KP, Nielson WR, Harth M, et al. Chronic widespread musculoskeletal pain with or without fibromyalgia: psychological distress in a representative community adult sample. J Rheumatol 2002; 29:588–594.
11. Epstein SA, Kay G, Clauw D, et al. Psychiatric disorders in patients with fibromyalgia. Psychosomatics 1999; 40:57–63.
12. Malt EA, Berle JE, Olafsson S, et al. Fibromyalgia is associated with panic disorder and functional dyspepsia with mood disorders. A study of women with random sample population controls. J Psychosom Res 2000; 49:285–289.
13. Hudson JI, Goldenberg DL, Pope HG Jr., et al. Comorbidity of fibromyalgia with medical and psychiatric disorders. Am J Med 1992; 92:363–367.
14. Walker EA, Keegan D, Gardner G, et al. Psychosocial factors in fibromyalgia compared with rheumatoid arthritis: I. Psychiatric diagnoses and functional disability. Psychosom Med 1997; 59:565–571.

15. Arnold LM, Hudson JI, Keck PE, et al. Comorbidity of fibromyalgia and psychiatric disorders. J Clin Psychiatry 2006; 67:1219–1225.
16. Makela M, Heliovaara M. Prevalence of primary fibromyalgia in the Finnish population. BMJ 1991; 303:216–219.
17. Lyddell C, Meyers OL. The prevalence of fibromyalgia in a South African community. Scand J Rheumatol 1992; 21(suppl 94):8.
18. Raspe H, Baumgartner CH. The epidemiology of fibromyalgia syndrome (FMS) in a German town. Scand J Rheumatol 1992; 21(suppl 94):8.
19. Prescott E, Kjoller M, Jacobsen S, et al. Fibromyalgia in the adult Danish population: I. A prevalence study. Scand J Rheumatol 1993; 22:233–237.
20. Schochat T, Croft P, Raspe H. The epidemiology of fibromyalgia. Workshop of the standing committee on Epidemiology European League Against Rheumatism (EULAR), Bad Sackingen 19–21 November 1992. Br J Rheumatol 1994; 33:783–786.
21. White KP, Speechley M, Harth M, et al. The London fibromyalgia epidemiology study: the prevalence of fibromyalgia syndrome in London, Ontario. J Rheumatol 1999; 26:1570–1576.
22. Lindell L, Bergman S, Petersson IF, et al. Prevalence of fibromyalgia and chronic widespread pain. Scand J Prim Health Care 2000; 18:149–153.
23. Hudson JI, Arnold LM, Keck PE Jr., et al. Family study of fibromyalgia and affective spectrum disorder. Biol Psychiatry 2004; 56(11):884–891.
24. Dailey PA, Bishop GD, Russell IJ, et al. Psychological stress and the fibrositis/fibromyalgia syndrome. J Rheumatol 1990; 17:1380–1385.
25. Anderberg UM, Marteinsdottir I, Theorell T, et al. The impact of life events in female patients with fibromyalgia and in female healthy controls. Eur Psychiatry 2000; 15: 295–301.
26. Walker EA, Keegan D, Gardner G, et al. Psychosocial factors in fibromyalgia compared with rheumatoid arthritis: II. Sexual, physical and emotional abuse and neglect. Psychosom Med 1997; 59:572–577.
27. Pillemer SR, Bradley LA, Crofford LJ, et al. The neuroscience and endocrinology of fibromyalgia. Arthritis Rheum 1997; 40:1928–1939.
28. Heim C, Newport DJ, Heit S, et al. Pituitary-adrenal and autonomic responses to stress in women after sexual and physical abuse in childhood. JAMA 2000; 284:592–597.
29. Lautenbacher S, Rollman GB. Possible deficiencies of pain modulation in fibromyalgia. Clin J Pain 1997; 13:189–196.
30. Bennett RM. Emerging concepts in the neurobiology of chronic pain: evidence of abnormal sensory processing in fibromyalgia. Mayo Clin Proc 1999; 74:385–398.
31. Staud R. Evidence of involvement of central neural mechanisms in generating fibro-myalgia pain. Curr Rheumatol Rep 2002; 4:299–305.
32. Baranauskas G, Nistri A. Sensitization of pain pathways in the spinal cord: cellular mechanisms. Prog Neurobiol 1998; 54:349–365.
33. Buskila D, Neumann L. Musculoskeletal injury as a trigger for fibromyalgia/posttraumatic fibromyalgia. Curr Rheumatol Rep 2000; 2:104–108.
34. Wallace DJ, Linker-Israeli M, Hallegua D, et al. Cytokines play an aetiopathogenetic role in fibromyalgia: a hypothesis and pilot study. Rheumatology 2001; 40:743–749.
35. Russell IJ, Vaeroy H, Javors M, et al. Cerebrospinal fluid biogenic amine metabolites in fibromyalgia/fibrositis syndrome and rheumatoid arthritis. Arthritis Rheum 1992; 35: 550–556.
36. Russell IJ, Michalek JE, Vipraio GA, et al. Platelet 3H-imipramine uptake receptor density and serum serotonin levels in patients with fibromyalgia/fibrositis syndrome. J Rheumatol 1992; 19:104–109.
37. Yunus MB, Dailey JW, Aldag JC, et al. Plasma tryptophan and other amino acids in primary fibromyalgia: a controlled study. J Rheumatol 1992; 19:90–94.
38. Schwarz MJ, Spath M, Muller-Bardorff H, et al. Relationship of substance P, 5-hydroxyindole acetic acid and tryptophan in serum of fibromyalgia patients. Neurosci Lett 1999; 259:196–198.
39. Basbaum AI, Fields HL. Endogenous pain control systems: brainstem pathways and endorphin circuitry. Ann Rev Neurosci 1984; 7:309–338.

40. Clark FM, Proudfit HK. The projections of noradrenergic neurons in the A5 catechol-amine cell groups to the spinal cord in the rat: anatomical evidence that A5 neurons modulate nociception. Brain Res 1993; 616:200–213.

41. Vaeroy H, Helle R, Fokrre O, et al. Elevated CSF levels of substance P and high incidence of Raynaud phenomenon in patients with fibromyalgia: new features for diagnosis. Pain 1988; 32:21–26.

42. Russell IJ, Orr MD, Littman B, et al. Elevated cerebrospinal fluid levels of substance P in patients with fibromyalgia syndrome. Arthritis Rheum 1994; 37:1593–1601.

43. Watkins LR, Wiertelak EP, Furness LE, et al. Illness-induced hyperalgesia is mediated by spinal neuropeptides and excitatory amino acids. Brain Res 1994; 664:17–24.

44. Gracely RH, Petzke F, Wolf JM, et al. Functional magnetic resonance imaging evidence of augmented pain processing in fibromyalgia. Arthritis Rheum 2002; 46:1333–1343.

45. Moldofsky H, Scarisbrick P, England R, et al. Musculoskeletal symptoms and non-REM sleep disturbance in patients with "fibrositis syndrome" and healthy subjects. Psychosom Med 1975; 37:341–351.

46. Schneider-Helmert D, Whitehouse I, Kumar A, et al. Insomnia and alpha sleep in chronic non-organic pain as compared to primary insomnia. Neuropsychobiology 2001; 43:54–58.

47. Arnold LM. Biology and therapy of fibromyalgia. New therapies in fibromyalgia. Arthritis Res Ther 2006; 8:212.

48. Campbell FG, Graham JG, Zilkha KJ. Clinical trial of carbazepine (Tegretol) in trigeminal neuralgia. J Neurol Neurosurg Psychiatry 1966; 29:265–267.

49. Nicol CF. A four year double-blind study of Tegretol in facial pain. Headache 1969; 9:54–57.

50. Klapper JA. Divalproex sodium in migraine prophylaxis: a dose-controlled study. Cephalalgia 1997; 17:103–108.

51. Pappagallo M. Newer antiepileptic drugs: possible uses in the treatment of neuropathic pain and migraine. Clin Ther 2003; 25:2506–2538.

52. Rowbotham M, Harden N, Stacey B, et al. Gabapentin for the treatment of postherpetic neuralgia. JAMA 1998; 280:1837–1842.

53. Rice AS, Maton S. Gabapentin in postherpetic neuralgia: a randomized, double-blind, placebo controlled study. Pain 2001; 94:215–224.

54. Backonja M, Beydoun A, Edwards KR, et al. Gabapentin for the symptomatic treatment of painful neuropathy in patients with diabetes mellitus: a randomized controlled trial. JAMA 1998; 280:1831–1836.

55. Mathew NT, Rapoport A, Saper J, et al. Efficacy of gabapentin in migraine prophylaxis. Headache 2001; 41:119–128.

56. Rao SG. The neuropharmacology of centrally-acting analgesic medications in fibromyalgia. Rheum Dis Clin North Am 2002; 28:235–259.

57. Taylor CP, Angelotti T, Fauman E. Pharmacology and mechanism of action of pregabalin: the calcium channel $\alpha2-\delta$ (alpha2-delta) subunit as a target for antiepileptic drug discovery. Epilepsy Res 2007; 73(2):137–150.

58. Field MJ, Cox PJ, Stott E. Identification of the $\alpha2-\delta$ -1 subunit of voltage-dependent calcium channels as a molecular target for pain mediating the analgesic actions of pregabalin. PNAS 2006; 103:17537–17542.

59. Dooley DJ, Taylor CP, Donevan S, et al. Ca2+ channel $\alpha2\delta$ ligands: novel modulators of neurotransmission. Trends Pharmacol Sci 2007; 28:75–82.

60. Lyrica® [Package Insert] New York, NY: Pfizer; 2004.

61. Crofford LJ, Rowbotham MC, Mease PJ, et al. Pregabalin for the treatment of fibromyalgia syndrome: results of a randomized, double-blind, placebo-controlled trial. Arthritis Rheum 2005; 52:1264–1273.

62. Arnold LM, Crofford L, Martin SA, et al. The effect of anxiety and depression on improvements in pain in a randomized, controlled trial of pregabalin for treatment of fibromyalgia. Pain Med 2007; 8(8):633–638.

63. Mease PJ, Russell IJ, Arnold LM, et al. A randomized, double- blind, placebo-controlled, phase III trial of pregabalin in the treatment of patients with fibromyalgia. J Rheumatol 2008; 35(3):502–514.

64. Arnold LM, Russell IJ, Duan WR, et al. Pregabalin for management of fibromyalgia: A 14-week, randomized, double-blind, placebo-controlled, monotherapy trial. Presented at: The American Psychiatric Association Annual Meeting; May 2007; San Diego, CA.

65. Crofford LJ, Simpson S, Young JP, et al. A six-month, double-blind, placebo-controlled, durability of effect study of pregabalin for pain associated with fibromyalgia. Presented at: The American College of Rheumatology Annual Meeting; November 2006; Washington, DC.

66. Neurontin [package insert]. NewYork, NY: Pfizer, Inc.; 2004.

67. Arnold LM, Goldenberg DL, Stanford SB, et al. Gabapentin in the treatment of fibromyalgia. Arthritis Rheum 2007; 56:1336–1344.

68. Hindmarch I, Dawson J, Stanley N. A double-blind study in healthy volunteers to assess the effects on sleep of pregabalin compared with alprazolam and placebo. Sleep 2005; 28:187–193.

69. Legros B, Basil CW. Effects of antiepileptic drugs on sleep architecture: a pilot study. Sleep Med 2003; 4(1):51–55.

70. Frampton JE, Foster RH. Pregabalin in the treatment of postherpetic neuralgia. Drugs 2005; 65:111–118.

71. Frampton JE, Scott LJ. Pregabalin in the treatment of painful diabetic neuropathy. Drugs 2004; 64:2813–2820.

72. Sabatowski R, Galvez R, Cherry DA, et al. Pregabalin reduces pain and improves sleep and mood disturbances in patients with post-herpetic neuralgia: results of a randomised, placebo-controlled clinical trial. Pain 2004; 109:26–35.

73. Drug Enforcement Administration. Schedules of controlled substances: placement of pregabalin into schedule V. Final rule. Fed Regist 2005; 70:43633–43635.

74. Dworkin RH, O'Conner AB, Backonja M, et al. Pharmacologic management of neuropathic pain: evidence-based recommendations. Pain 2007; 132:237–251.

21 Psychotrophic Mechanisms of Action of Antiepileptic Drugs in Mood Disorder

Robert M. Post
Head, Bipolar Collaborative Network, Bethesda, Maryland, U.S.A.

INTRODUCTION

A number of conundrums complicate the interpretation of which biochemical effects of the antiepileptic drugs (AEDs) may be related to their mood-stabilizing and other psychotropic properties. We outline several of these issues prior to consideration of actions of specific drugs because these are crucial to the interpretation of the data. The first issue to consider is whether the mechanism of action of these agents in the seizure disorders mirrors those in the psychiatric illnesses. There are diverse mechanisms of the AEDs and these may be pertinent to efficacy in different epilepsy syndromes. Some of the AEDs are thought to act by enhancing gamma-aminobutyric acid (GABA)-benzodiazepine receptor inhibition, while others are thought to decrease overexcitation, inhibiting glutamate release, or its postsynaptic receptor effects (Fig. 1).

In either instance, these drugs tend to act against seizures either immediately or as quickly as therapeutic blood levels can be achieved (Fig. 2). In contrast, full anti-manic and antidepressant effects are slower to achieve, often requiring days to weeks for mania and two to four weeks for depression, even in those who are eventually highly responsive to carbamazepine, for example (Fig. 3). Thus, the time course of onset of either initial or maximum degree of therapeutic efficacy appears to dissociate the psychotropic from anticonvulsant effects of these agents. Therefore, it would appear that actions of AEDs that require longer time periods or chronic administration in order to be achieved will likely be related to the psychotropic effects, while acute effects are more likely relevant to efficacy in seizure disorders and pain syndromes. However, exceptions are beginning to emerge with very rapid onset of antidepressant effects seen with thyrotropin-releasing hormone (TRH) (1,2), the N-methyl-D-aspartate (NMDA) receptor antagonist ketamine (3), and a specific NR2B subunit antagonist (4).

Another important and perhaps clarifying factor is that all of the AEDs do not appear to possess a similar range of psychotropic effects. Specifically, a number of AEDs do not have acute antimanic efficacy (Table 1). In particular, many of those that increase brain GABA levels (topiramate, gabapentin, tiagabine) are not effective in mania, further dissociating these anticonvulsant and psychotropic effects (Table 2).

There are also a variety of psychiatric illness–related variables that are pertinent to the interpretation of which drug actions are important to their psychotropic profile. That is, a general strategy has been to search for common mechanisms among the mood-stabilizing drugs that appear to exert both antimanic and antide-pressant properties and assume that these should be in common with lithium carbonate (5,6). However, while this proposition has some theoretical merit, the issue of subtypes of responsive patients makes it suspect.

Lithium, carbamazepine, and valproate do share the very general psycho-tropic profile of better antimanic than antidepressant effects, both acutely and, perhaps to a lesser extent, in prophylaxis (7–9). However, considerable evidence suggests that individual patients are differentially responsive to one but not to

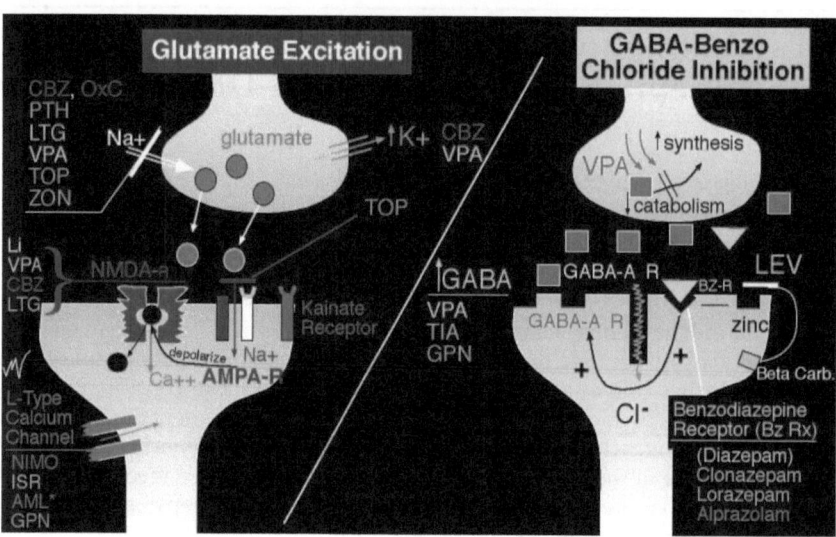

FIGURE 1 Mechanisms of anticonvulsant action. *Abbreviations*: CBZ, carbamazepine; OXC, oxcarbazepine; LTG, lamotrigine; VPA, valproic acid; NMDA, *N*-methyl-D-aspartate; AMPA, α-amino-3-hydroxy-5-methyl-4-isoxazole proprionic acid; GABA, gamma-aminobutyric acid; PTH, phenytoin; TOP, topiramate; ZON, zonisamide; GPN, gabapentin; TIA, tiagabine; LEV, levetiracetam; NIMO, nimodipine; ISR, isradipine; AML, amlodipine.

another of these drugs (10). For example, lithium-responsive patients are more likely to have classic euphoric manic episodes with discrete well intervals and a lack of anxiety and substance abuse comorbidity, as well as a positive family history for bipolar illness in first-degree relatives (11–13). In contrast, carbamazepine responders appear more likely to be bipolar II, atypical patients with substance abuse comorbidity, schizoaffective presentations, and rapid cycling patterns in the context of a negative family history of bipolar illness in first-degree relatives (13). Valproate responders are characterized by either euphoric or dysphoric mania in contrast to lithium's much greater degree of effectiveness in those with the euphoric compared with dysphoric subtype (14). These differential patient response characteristics suggest that in spite of some common mechanisms, each of these drugs may have biophysical effects that are sufficiently different (Table 2) to account for the differences in profiles of the subtypes of responsive patients.

This caveat is all the more important with respect to lamotrigine, which appears to have effects in the prevention of depressive episodes, and to a lesser extent, manic or mixed episodes. In addition, while several studies have suggested acute antidepressant efficacy (9,15–18), lamotrigine does not possess acute antimanic efficacy. Together, this differential profile of lamotrigine compared with that of lithium, carbamazepine, and valproate further implicates differential mechanisms of action. This conclusion is further supported by the preliminary clinical profiles of patients likely to respond to lamotrigine monotherapy (19–21). Lamotrigine-responsive patients appear more likely to have a positive family history of anxiety disorders in first-degree relatives as well as a personal history of anxiety comorbidity. They are also more likely to have more continuous cyclic courses of illness, as opposed to discrete episodes for lithium.

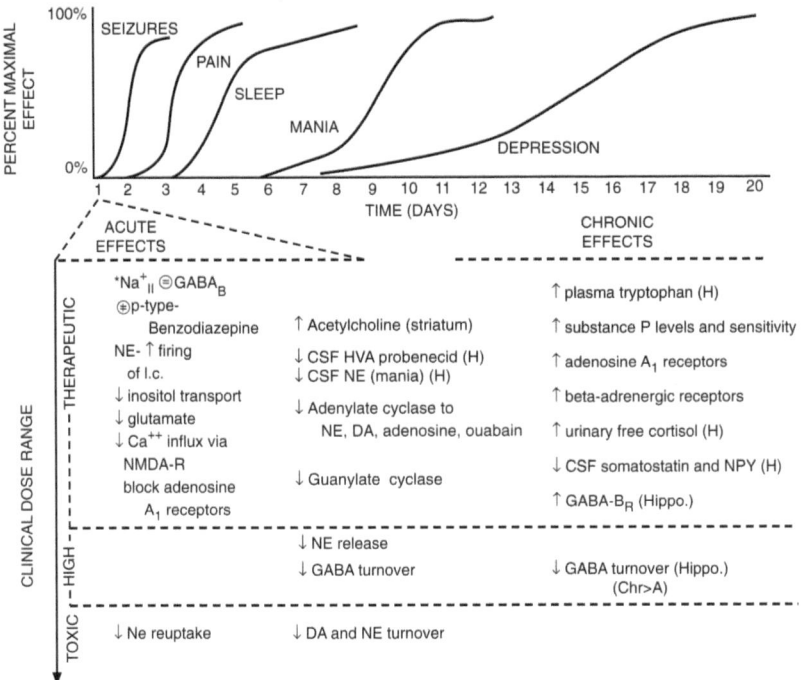

FIGURE 2 Schematic of comparative time course of clinical and biochemical effects of carbamazepine. *Abbreviations*: GABA, gamma-aminobutyric acid; NMDA, *N*-methyl-D-aspartate; HVA, homovanillic acid; NE, norepinephrine (noradrenaline); DA, dopamine; NPY, neuropeptide Y.

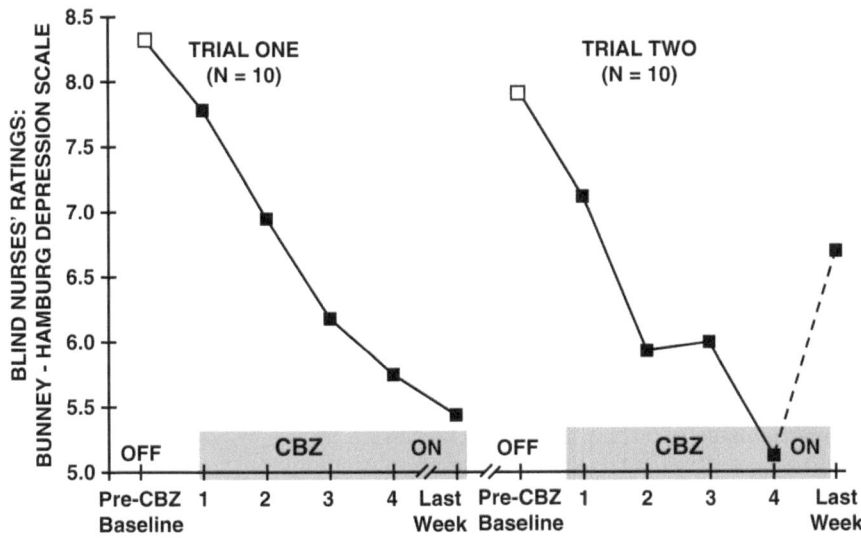

FIGURE 3 Confirmation of antidepressant response to CBZ in off-on-off-on design. *Abbreviation*: CBZ, carbamazepine.

TABLE 1   Spectrum of Psychotropic Action of Anticonvulsants

	Acute Efficacy			Prophylaxis		
	Mania	Depression	Anxiety	Mania	Depression	Other Effects
VPA	+++	++	+++	+++	+++	Migraine, panic, alcohol abstinence (PTSD)
CBZ	+++	++	++	++	+++	Paroxysmal pain syndrome, alcohol withdrawal, (PTSD)
OXC	(+++)	?	?	(++)	(++)	
LTG	0	+++	++	+	+++	(PTSD)
ZNS	(++)	(++)	?	?	?	Bulimia, overweight
PHT	(+++)	(++)	?	?	?	(Pain)
TPM	0	(+)	(+)	?	?	PTSD, bulimia, alcohol and cocaine abstinence, overweight, migraine
GPN	0,−	(+)	+++	(+)	(+)	Panic, social phobia, pain syndromes, alcohol withdrawal
PGN	(0)	(+)	+++	?	?	Panic, social phobia, pain syndromes
TIA	0	(±)	(+)	?	?	[a]May cause new onset seizures
LEV	(+)	(±)	(+)	?	?	
PB	(±)	(±)	+	0	0	(I.V.) anticatatonic effects
BZ	+	+	+	+	+	
FBM	?	?	?	?	?	Refractory seizures, overweight

[a]Adverse effect caution.

Abbreviations: PTSD, posttraumatic stress disorder; VPA, valproic acid; CBZ, carbamazepine; LTG, lamotrigine; OXC, oxcarbazepine; ZNS, zonisamide; PHT, phenytoin; TPM, topiramate; GPN, gabapentin; PGN, pregabalin; TIA, tiagabine; LEV, levetiracetam; PB, phenobarbital; BZ, benzodiazepine; FBM, felbamate.

+++, highly effective, placebo controlled data; ++, effective, substantial literature; +, likely effective; ±, possibly effective; (), ambiguous result; 0, no effect; −, worse.

Such distinctions are likely to be mechanistically relevant. For example, Du et al. (22) found that lamotrigine and riluzole, which are predominately antidepressant, enhanced surface expression of α-amino-3-hydroxy-5-methylisoxazole-4-propionic acid (AMPA) GluR1 and GluR2 receptors in cultured hippocampal neurons. Conversely, the predominately antimanic drug, valproate, significantly reduced expression of GluR1 and GluR2 subunits. Such divergent actions may ultimately be useful in the targeting and development of novel drugs with phase-selective effects.

Perhaps the most serious complicating factor is the lack of suitable animal models of manic-depressive illness in particular and only very cumbersome models for examining antidepressant actions. This contrasts with the situation in the epilepsies where a wide range of readily available animal models have been delineated for different seizure subtypes, further implying differences in mechanisms of action. Until this deficiency is ameliorated, it is highly likely that we will have to remain satisfied with only rough inferences about potential mechanisms of action related to psychotropic effects.

Lastly, a caveat about lithium's potential mechanisms of action would appear appropriate in this regard. It had been widely assumed that understanding lithium's mechanisms of action in manic-depressive illness would rapidly be converted to a better understanding of the pathophysiology of the disorder. This has not happened and, instead, lithium has been found to have a panoply of biochemical effects, none of which has been definitely linked to its psychotropic properties. It is of historical interest that lithium's actions in manic-depressive illness were first assumed to reside at the level of ion channels; then on neurotransmitter release and reuptake mechanisms presynaptically; later at postsynaptic

TABLE 2 Mechanism of Action of Anticonvulsants

	GABA levels	GABA_AR (indirect)	↓Na+	Voltage-gated Ca²⁺				NMDA Ca²⁺	Other mechanisms
				T	N	P	L		
VPA	↑		+	T			✓	→	↑ Inositol monophosphase; ↑ GABA synthesis and ↓ catabolism; ↑ K efflux; ↓ folate; ↑ GABA_B R(hippo); ↑Bcl-2; ↓ histone deacetylase; ↓ aspartate; ↑ Homocysteine
CBZ			++				✓?	(↓)	↑ Striatal choline; ↑5HT_hippo; ↓NE release; ↑AVP; ↑Sub P; ↓ SRIF; ↓ DA T.O.; ↓α4 subunit muscarinic Ach-R; ↑ K efflux; ↑ GABA_B R(hippo); ↓ Adenosine A₁R; GABA_AR α₁; ↓ Histone deacetylase; ↑ BDNF; ↓AA T.O.
OXC	(↑)26%	(↓)	+++		N,	P	✓		↑ K efflux
LTG		↑	+++		N,	(P/Q)	✓	(↓)	Amygdala slice,↓ glutamate and ↓ GABA; ↑ K efflux (weak ↓ folate)
ZNS			++	T			L		↓↓ CA (carbonic anhydrase inhibition), ↑,↓ DA and 5HT T.O., free radical scavenger; ↑glutamate, and ↓ GABA transporters
PHT		↑	+++	(T)			✓		↓ SRIF
TPM		↑	+++				✓ ↓R		↓↓ CA; ↓ AMPA/Kainate R; binds GluR₅ subunit K_R
GPN[a]		↑	+				✓ (L)		↓ Strychnine insensitive glycine receptors; ↓ glutamate; L-amino acid transporter; α₂ δ subunit of L-type Ca²⁺ channel
PGN[b]		↑			N,	(P/Q)	✓ (L)		↓α₂ δ subunit of L-type Ca²⁺ calcium channel
TIA		↑							GABA reuptake inhibitor
LEV		↑			N,	(P/Q)	✓		↓ Zn²⁺ and βcarboline negative modulation of GABA_AR; own CNS binding site (SV2-A); ↓ Delayed K+ rectifier
PB		↑ duration open time		+					
BZ		↑ frequency open time		+					
FBM		↑		++			✓	↓↓	Glycine; ↓ NR-1A and NR-2B subunits of NMDAR

Note: ✓ indicates VACC high voltage activated calcium channel.
a and b Act at α2 δ subunit of L-type calcium channel.

Abbreviations: GABA, gamma-aminobutyric acid; AMPA, α-amino-3-hydroxy-5-methylisoxazole-4-propionic acid; BDNF, brain-derived neurotrophic factor; T.O., turnover; VPA, valproic acid; CBZ, carbamazepine; LTG, lamotrigine; OXC, oxcarbazepine; ZNS, zonisamide; PHT, phenytoin; TPM, topiramate; GPN, gabapentin; PGN, pregabalin; TIA, tiagabine; LEV, levetiracetam; PB, phenobarbital; BZ, benzodiazepine; FBM, felbamate; DA, dopamine; AA, arachidonic acid; NR, NMDA receptor.
[Types of calcium channels: T, transient; N, neither nor; P, purkinje cell; L, long lasting]

receptors, second messengers, protein kinases, transcription factors; and ultimately at a variety of effects on gene expression, with most recent interest in its potential neurotrophic and neuroprotective effects.

Thus, candidate mechanisms for lithium's psychotropic actions have generally followed our increasingly detailed understanding of synaptic and intracellular transduction mechanisms and those of gene expression, but even this sequence has not necessarily propelled us to a more definitive relationship of a specific mechanism to a specific psychotropic effect. It therefore would appear prudent to be similarly cautious in our assumptions about what precise mechanisms underlie the psychotropic actions of the AEDs. We should continue to examine potential candidate mechanisms as important for clinical hypothesis testing (5), but should remain skeptical that we have as yet definitely identified the critical actions of any single drug.

PRESUMPTIVE ANTICONVULSANT MECHANISMS

As outlined in Table 2, among the AEDs there are a series of actions that appear to be pertinent for many members of a given subclass. Thus, many AEDs are blockers of type II bratrachotoxin-sensitive sodium channels. This property is thought to be related to their effects on complex partial and major motor seizures. Mishory and colleagues (23) have postulated that it is this set of actions of the AEDs that most likely underlies their antimanic efficacy. However, weighing against this proposition are the findings that lamotrigine and topiramate are sodium channel blockers but have no efficacy in mania.

A series of AEDs enhance chloride influx directly or indirectly via their effects on $GABA_A$ or benzodiazepine receptors. The high potency benzodiazepines such as clonazepam, lorazepam, and alprazolam are clearly anticonvulsant moieties, but the antimanic effects of the first two compounds remain somewhat ambiguous, and alprazolam can induce mania in isolated cases as opposed to treating or preventing it (24).

Drugs that exert major actions on GABA metabolism, brain GABA levels, or $GABA_A$ receptors directly are not necessarily antimanic. It had been hoped that since valproate increases brain GABA levels in animals and humans, enhances GABA synthesis, and decreases GABA breakdown, other GABA-active drugs might share its excellent profile in acute mania. This has not proven to be the case. Gabapentin does not have acute antimanic efficacy over placebo when used as an adjunct to lithium and/or valproate (25) or when used in high-dose monotherapy in treatment-refractory (predominantly bipolar) affectively ill patients (16,17).

Tiagabine is a relatively selective reuptake inhibitor of GABA that enhances intrasynaptic levels of GABA, and also increases brain GABA levels in animals and humans. Not only does it not appear to have acute antimanic efficacy, but, paradoxically, several psychiatric patients without a history of seizure disorders experienced seizures on this drug (26,27).

Convergent with this theme are the ambiguous antimanic effects of levetiracetam, which is thought to enhance the GABA/benzodiazepine receptor chloride ionophore indirectly (28). At this site, it blocks the actions of zinc and β carboline, which are endogenous negative modulators, thus indirectly potentiating actions at this ionophore. However, levetiracetam also has its own binding site in brain, which has recently been identified as the synaptic vesicle protein 2A component of the calcium-sensitive release mechanisms closely linked to synaptophysin or synaptotagmin. This mechanism could account for the drug's somewhat mysterious anticonvulsant properties where it fails to exert efficacy in standard models for grand mal and petit mal seizures, such as maximal electroshock and pentylenetrazol seizures, respectively (29–31).

Interestingly, levetiracetam, in concert with valproate and the high potency benzodiazepines, blocks both the development and fully expressed phases of amygdala-kindled seizures (Fig. 4). In contrast, carbamazepine, lamotrigine, and

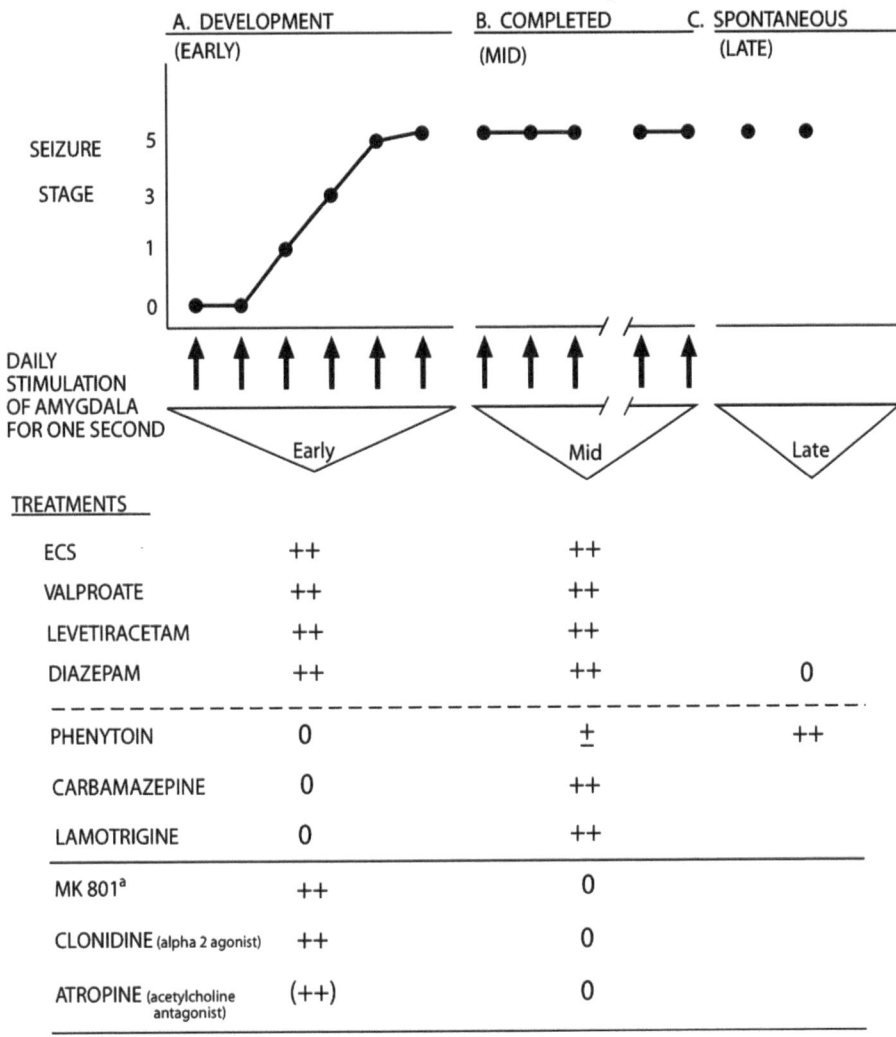

FIGURE 4 Dissociation of pharmacological responsivity as a function of phase of amygdala kindling evolution. [a]indicates glutamate NMDA R antagonist. *Abbreviations*: NMDA, N-methyl-D-aspartate; ++, highly effective, ±, ambiguous; 0, not effective; (), inconsistent data.

phenytoin do not block the early development phase and are only effective on completed or full-blown kindled seizures (32). Given its so far ambiguous psychotropic profile and the indirect enhancement of benzodiazepine GABA receptors, it would appear that further exploration of levetiracetam's potential antianxiety effects would be warranted even in the absence of a clear-cut demonstration of its antimanic efficacy.

Zonisamide has not been adequately tested for its acute antimanic efficacy in controlled clinical trials, but open studies suggest its promising effects in acute mania and a potentially useful side-effect profile regarding weight loss (33,34). Not only does it share this latter property with topiramate, but both drugs are also carbonic anhydrase inhibitors, which is thought to relate to their approximately 1% incidence of renal calculi, and dysaesthesias in a larger percentage of patients.

CONVERGENT MECHANISMS OF LITHIUM AND THE ANTICONVULSANT MOOD STABILIZERS, CARBAMAZEPINE AND VALPROATE

If one examines common mechanisms attributable to all three drugs (lithium, carbamazepine, and valproate) that are more effective in acute mania than in depression, one recognizes a series of potential candidates for their psychotropic effects (Table 3). These include: the ability to reduce dopamine turnover (35); to increase $GABA_B$ receptors in the hippocampus upon chronic, but not acute, administration (36); to acutely block the inositol transporter (37); and to moderately inhibit calcium influx through the NMDA receptor (38). It is of interest that this last mechanism is also shared by lamotrigine.

TABLE 3A Common Actions of Mood Stabilizers

	Li	VPA	CBZ	LTG
Common to Li and ACs				
↓ Inositol transport	+	+	+	?
↑ $GABA_B R_{hippo}$	+	+	+	?
↓ DA turnover	+	+	+	?
↓ Phospholipase A_2 and AA cascade	+	+	+	?
↓ Ca^{2+} influx via NMDA R	+	+	+	?
↑ BDNF	+	+	+	?
stroke neuroprotection	+	+	+	+
↓ GSK-3β	+	+	+	?
Common to two				
↓ PKC	+	+		
↑Bcl-2	+	+		
↓ β catenin	+	+		
↓ ras-erk-pathway	+	+		
↑ Akt	+	+		
↑ AP-1	+	+		
Block C-Amp	+		+	
↑ Substance P (striatum)	+		+	

Abbreviations: NMDA, *N*-methyl-ᴅ-aspartate, BDNF, brain-derived neurotrophic factor; GABA, gamma-aminobutyric acid; AMPA; valproic acid; CBZ, carbamazepine; LTG, lamotrigine; DA dopamine; AA, arachidonic acid; PKC, protein kinase C; +, positive effect; −, no effect; ↑, increase; ↓, decrease; ( ), ambiguous data.

TABLE 3B Common Actions of Anticonvulsant Mood Stabilizers

	Li	VPA	CBZ	LTG
Block Na$^+$ influx		(+)	+	+
↑ K$^+$ efflux		+	+	+
↓ Histone deacetylase		+	+	

Abbreviations: Li, lithium, VPA, valproic acid; CBZ, carbamazepine; LTG, lamotrigine.

TABLE 3C Divergent Actions of Mood Stabilizers

	Li	VPA	CBZ	LTG
Inositol monophosphotase	↓	↑	−	?
Absence seizures	−	↓	↑	↓
GABA levels	( )	↑	−	(↑)26%
AMPA receptor subunits Glu R1 and R2[a]		↓		↑

[a]From Ref. 22
Abbreviations: GABA, gamma-aminobutyric acid; Li, lithium, VPA, valproic acid; CBZ, carbamazepine; LTG, lamotrigine.

TABLE 3D Unique Effects of Mood Stabilizers

Lithium	CBZ	VPA	LTG
↑ NAA[a]	↓ SRIF[a]	↑ ER stress protein	↓ GABA release
↑ Grey Matter[a]	↓ choline (striatum)	GRP 78 & 94	
↓ BAX, P53	↓ Adenosine		
pilocarpine	A$_1$ receptors		
seizures and	↓ p-type Bz R		
↓sprouting	↓ Ne β R		
↓ CAMK-IV	↑ 5HT$_{hippo.}$		
↓ CAMK-II	α4subunit Ach R		
	(↑ GRP78) ±		

[a] in patients.
Abbreviations: NAA, *N*-acetylaspartate; GABA, gamma-aminobutyric acid; VPA, valproic acid; CBZ, carbamazepine; LTG, lamotrigine; ER, estrogen receptor.

The examination of the comparative effects of lithium and valproate are particularly intriguing from the perspective of potential neurotrophic and neuroprotective effects (Table 4, Fig. 5). Both of these agents increase brain-derived neurotrophic factor (BDNF) and Bcl-2 (39); lithium also decreases cell death factors Bax and p53 (40). Both seem to activate many elements of the mitogen-activated protein (MAP) kinase pathway (41), but valproate has the additional effects of being a histone deacetylase inhibitor (42). It is of interest that recently carbamazepine has been shown to exert this same activity (43), and this action could account for more readily available changes in gene expression based on altered DNA conformation.

Lithium and carbamazepine also have interesting shared mechanisms, including the ability to inhibit noradrenergic-stimulated adenylate cyclase and to increase substance P levels and substance P receptor sensitivity in the striatum and nucleus accumbens (NAcc).

Carbamazepine has unique effects in decreasing somatostatin levels in cerebrospinal fluid (CSF) and in acting as an indirect potentiator of vasopressin receptors. Additionally, it inhibits the release of corticotropin-releasing hormone (CRH)

TABLE 4 Neurotropic and Protective Effects of Psychotropic Drugs

	Lithium	Valproate	Antidepressants	Electro convulsive therapy	Atypical antipsychotic
In vitro					
Sprouting	↑	↑		↑	
Neurogenesis	↑		↑	↑	
BDNF	↑	↑	↑	↑	
Prevention of ↓ BDNF with stress			+ [a]	+	+
↑ Bcl-2	↑	↑		↑	
Gliogenesis	↑	↑		↑	↓
In vivo NAA (neuronal integrity)					
Pfc (H)	↑	–			
Temporal lobe (H)	↑	↑			
Gray matter (MRI) Pfc and B25 (H)	↑				
Stroke neuroprotection	↑b/a	↑b/a		(↑)	
Hippocampal volume protection (in depressed patients) (H)			↑		

[a]Pramipexole.

Abbreviations: H, humans; b/a, before and after insult; BDNF, brain-derived neurotrophic factor; NAA, *N*-acetylaspartate.

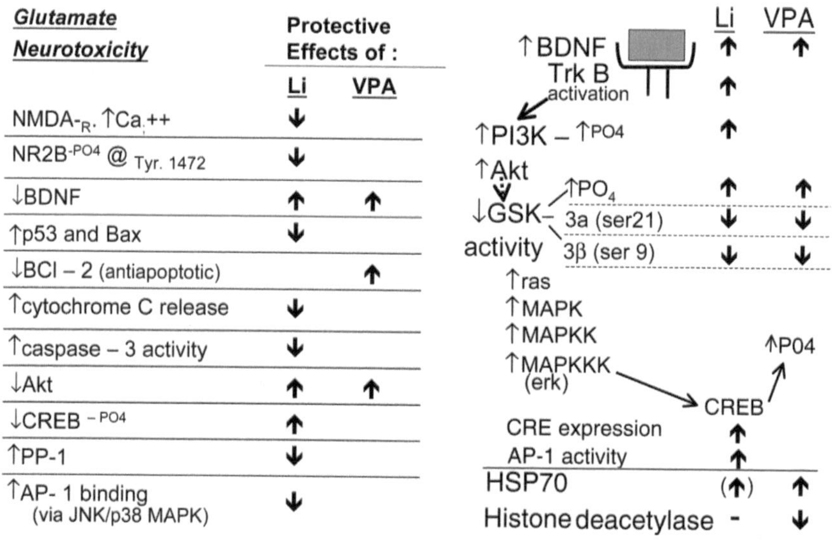

FIGURE 5 Lithium and valproate block glutamate toxicity and enhance growth factors. *Abbreviations*: VPA, valproic acid; NMDA, *N*-methyl-D-aspartate; BDNF, brain-derived neurotrophic factor. *Source*: From refs. 39–41.

from the hypothalamus and is uniquely able to increase 24-hour urinary free cortisol levels and produce false-positive escape from dexamethasone suppression.

Carbamazepine and valproate share the ability to enhance potassium channel–mediated efflux, and as noted previously, block batrachotoxin type II sodium channels.

Lithium is an inositol 1-monophosphate inhibitor and is capable of decreasing membrane inositol and inhibiting phosphoinositol turnover. Valproate is without effect on this system, and carbamazepine may have opposing effects (44,45), again highlighting potentially very different mechanisms of these drugs which could, in part, account for their differential profiles of clinical efficacy within individual patients.

Clinical Implications of the Mechanistic Differences Among the Antiepileptics

Since lamotrigine and carbamazepine share the ability to potently inhibit sodium influx through the type II channel, it is apparent that some other mechanism of action of lamotrigine must underlie its profile of being a better antidepressant than antimanic agent. In addition to blocking glutamate release (via the sodium channel blockade similar to that of carbamazepine), lamotrigine has the ability to inhibit GABA release. It also has effects on N- and P-type calcium channels that do not appear to be shared by carbamazepine.

However, if one is considering augmenting lamotrigine with another mood stabilizer, using lithium or valproate with their very different mechanistic profiles would be more worthy of consideration than adding carbamazepine, given the considerable mechanistic overlap between lamotrigine and carbamazepine. If valproate is used with lamotrigine, however, lamotrigine doses should be reduced by one half because valproate can double lamotrigine levels and increase the risk of rash. Nonetheless, when the two are used in combination in refractory seizure disorders, they appear to be particularly well tolerated.

Lithium and valproate are widely used together, but this combination poses increased risk from potentially additive side effects such as gastrointestinal distress, tremor, and weight gain. These are not particularly prominent side effects of carbamazepine or lamotrigine, and avoidance of side effects may provide an alternate rationale to therapeutic mechanistic considerations in the choice of agents.

Since the U.S. Food and Drug Administration (FDA) approval of new drugs is almost exclusively based on placebo-controlled, parallel group study designs which cannot distinguish individually responsive patients from nonresponders (46), there is great underappreciation in the literature that patients respond differentially to the mood stabilizers in general and the AEDs in particular. Each of the AEDs carries an approximately 50% response rate in uncomplicated patients, but unless one examines individual patients on a series of drugs or in an on-off-on fashion, one is not able to ascertain individual patient responsiveness or unique responsiveness to one compound and not another. Using more clinician-friendly longitudinal clinical designs, we have consistently seen that some patients respond to valproate and not to carbamazepine, while others showed good responses to carbamazepine but not to valproate (10).

In the past decade, valproate has surpassed lithium for a larger market share for first treatment of manic patients, but with the recent approval of a long-acting carbamazepine preparation, the clinician may also want to consider carbamazepine as a reasonable option for the patient inadequately responsive or intolerant to other agents. The extended-release capsule is suitable for single h.s. dosing, at least in bipolar illness, although not in those with epilepsy. There are only a few preliminary clinical hints of which patient may respond to which agent, as noted above, so one looks forward to the use of currently available single nucleotide polymorphism (SNP) profiling techniques to more formally and quantitatively help predict individual patient's likelihood of clinical response or severe side effects.

Oxcarbazepine is structurally similar to carbamazepine, differing only by a keto oxygen molecule in the middle ring instead of a double bond between carbon atoms in carbamazepine. It is thought to have a generally similar clinical profile and mechanism of action to carbamazepine, but has been much less well studied. Ambiguities about its range of efficacy are further supported by the negative study of Wagner et al. (47) in child and adolescent mania. The ability of oxcarbazepine to substitute for carbamazepine in psychiatric illness therefore requires further evaluation. It is a less potent inducer of hepatic enzymes, but more likely to cause hyponatremia. It does not have a black box warning for hematological side effects and may be an appropriate drug to explore clinically in those who do not wish to risk these very rare, but serious side effects.

POTENTIAL NEUROTROPHIC AND NEUROPROTECTIVE EFFECTS OF LITHIUM, VALPROATE, AND THE UNIMODAL ANTIDEPRESSANTS

Recent data indicate that all of the antidepressant modalities, as well as the mood stabilizers lithium, carbamazepine, and valproate, are capable of increasing both BDNF and neurogenesis (48,49) (Table 4). For example, Sheline and colleagues (50) found that depressed patients treated with antidepressants more of the time had no evidence of hippocampal atrophy compared with those with less antidepressant treatment. Taken together with preclinical data, these findings suggest that antidepressants may be pertinent to sustaining hippocampal volume in unipolar depressed humans, possibly by enhancing neural production and survival via increasing BDNF (49).

Preliminary evidence also suggests that lithium not only increases N-acetyl aspartate (NAA), a marker of neuronal integrity, but also increases gray matter volume in patients with bipolar disorder (but not in normal controls) (51,52). These findings raise the possibility that enhancing neurogenesis and gliogenesis and changing the ratio of cell survival factors (BDNF and Bcl-2) to cell death factors (Bax and p53) in favor of survival factors could be important to the therapeutic action of these drugs (40).

There is considerable evidence, as summarized in Figure 6, for deficits in prefrontal cortical neuronal and glial elements, biochemistry, and physiology in recurrent mood disorder. The extent to which some of our therapeutic agents could either help reverse these deficits or prevent their progression raises an entirely new perspective about long-term prophylaxis of bipolar illness. It is not only possible that these treatments could help decrease recurrence of both manic and depressive episodes, but they might also reverse or prevent progression of some of the biochemical and physiological alterations associated with the recurrent mood episodes as well as the underlying affective illness.

A number of the pathological findings in both unipolar and bipolar mood disorders have been shown to vary either as a function of illness duration or prior number of episodes (53,54). While it is unclear as to whether greater degrees of abnormalities are causally linked to a more adverse course of illness or whether a more adverse course of illness is etiologically involved in more severe biochemical abnormalities, the findings at least raise the question of whether episode

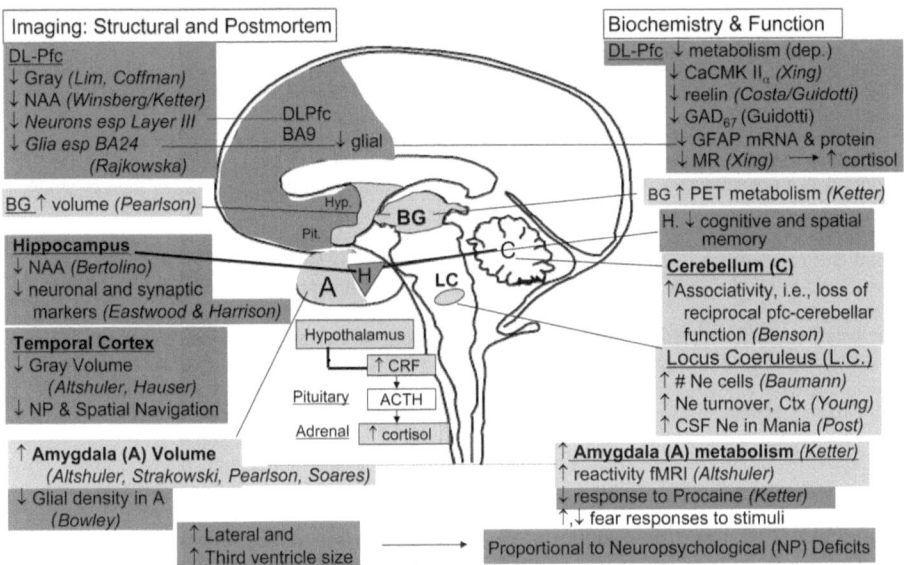

FIGURE 6 Convergence of structural, biochemical, and functional abnormalities in bipolar illness. *Source*: From Ref. 84.

prophylaxis with these agents may also alter the underlying neurobiology of the illness.

The bulk of the literature supports the clinical validity of the sensitization and kindling hypothesis which postulates that having recurrent mood episodes increases the vulnerability to subsequent episodes and to their occurring more autonomously from psychosocial stressors (54–56). This evidence, along with findings that patients with greater numbers of prior episodes and more rapid-cycling forms of the illness are, in general, more refractory to most treatments for bipolar disorder, further raises the urgency of attempting to initiate effective prophylaxis earlier in the course of illness.

At the least, the benefit of acting on this proposition would be a reduction in number of episodes. On the basis of the sensitization and kindling hypothesis and the data alluded to here, the maximal benefit would be to also alter some of the biochemical consequences of illness recurrence, decrease sensitization phenomenon, reduce vulnerability to recurrences, and potentially change the course of illness. This might be associated with not only fewer neurobiological alterations but a less treatment-refractory type of illness. Even if the sensitization and kindling notions of progressive changes associated with recurrent episodes are not entirely validated, the patient and clinician have little to lose and much to gain from earlier and concerted attempts at episode prophylaxis (Table 5).

However, early and sustained prophylactic intervention in bipolar illness is neither readily achieved nor high in the public health consciousness of many physicians and patients in the United States. The lag from illness onset to first treatment averaged 10 years in our large outpatient series (57,58) and was inversely associated with age of onset (59). Moreover, those with the earliest ages of onset

TABLE 5 Testable Clinical Predictions About Therapeutic Approaches to Tolerance Development to be Explored Based on the Preclinical Model

Preclinical study findings in amygdala-kindled seizures	Future studies: Are there parallel findings for clinical tolerance in affective illness?
A. Tolerance to anticonvulsant effects slowed by: higher doses (except with LTG)	A. Would tolerance be slowed by: maximum tolerated doses rather than minimally effective doses
not escalating doses	stable dosing
more efficacious drugs (VPA > CBZ)	valproate compared with carbamazepine
treatments initiated early in course of kindled seizures	early treatment more effective (as observed with lithium)[a]
combination treatment (CBZ + VPA)	combination treatment rather than monotherapy
reducing illness drive (stimulation intensity)	treatment or prevention of comorbidities and concomitant stressors
B. Treatment response in tolerant animals restored by: period of drug discontinuation, then re-exposure	B. Would treatment response be restored by: period of time off-CBZ in tolerant patients (randomized study of discontinuation and re-treatment needed)
agents with different mechanisms of action, i.e., no cross tolerance	anticonvulsant cross tolerances (as summarized in Table 6A) may or may not be predictive of cross tolerances in affective illness

[a]Supported by clinical studies.
Abbreviations: VPA, valproic acid; CBZ, carbamazepine; LTG, lamotrigine.

were at highest risk for an adverse course of bipolar illness, as assessed both retrospectively in the Systematic Treatment Enhancement Program for Bipolar Disorder (STEP-BD) network (60) and prospectively in our collaborative network (53,54). These are the very patients who have the longest time between first symptoms with dysfunction and first treatment for manic or depressive illness.

Indeed, in our subgroup of patients with illness onset prior to age 13 years, the lag to first treatment averaged about 15 years (59). This inverse relationship between age of onset and lag time to first treatment was also found in the epidemiological studies of Kessler and colleagues (61). Together, these data speak to the importance of earlier recognition of the illness and institution of more effective treatment in the hope of altering what can otherwise be a very difficult illness course, including one associated with a relatively high rate of lethality. These data and implications contrast somewhat with those of Baldessarini et al. (62) who found that delay to initiating prophylaxis (with lithium) was not associated with differential outcome. However, their sample was from Italy and Germany where universal health care is available, prophylaxis (rather than acute treatment) was examined, lithium was used in more than 90% of patients, and shorter time to institute prophylaxis was confounded by increased severity of baseline psychopathology. Thus, their (62) findings may not generalize to other populations.

Fortunately, there appears to be increased recognition of early-onset bipolar illness in children and adolescents. Lange and McInnis (63) analyzed the literature on this issue and concluded that there is substantial evidence for both cohort (year of birth) and anticipation (generational) effects. Together, the cohort and anticipation effects convey a greater incidence and earlier age of onset of both unipolar and bipolar illness in each generation since World War I. Given this increasing recognition of childhood-onset bipolar illness, one needs to raise a further caveat about the mechanism of action of AEDs. It is not at all clear whether the same degree of clinical responsivity occurs in children as it does in adults. This could be partially attributable to differences in maturity of various aspects of the developing central nervous system (CNS). Pertinent to this point are the observations that the GABA$_B$ antagonist baclofen is effective as an anticonvulsant in very young animals, but not in older animals, and the considerable evidence for altered GABAergic function across different stages of development (64). In the youngest animals, for example, GABA receptor activity is paradoxically associated with excitation, and only later in development do alterations in GABAergic tone convey their inhibitory properties.

Thus, how the mechanisms of action of GABAergic and other mechanistically acting drugs play out in relationship to efficacy in children remains a further conundrum, and one that requires new reassessment of the efficacy of each drug in children and adolescents to see whether or not it parallels that observed in adults.

Finally, as one moves toward notions of identifying those at highest risk and beginning to intervene very early in the course of illness (secondary prevention), and even prior to illness onset (i.e., primary prevention), one also needs to consider the possibility, on the basis of the striking data evident in the kindling model, that different agents may be effective in different phases of illness evolution and that what works against fully developed episodes may not prevent their initial developmental stages. Carbamazepine, lamotrigine, and phenytoin are potent against fully developed seizures, but ineffective against their development (Fig. 4). By contrast, valproate, diazepam, and levetiracetam are effective in the developmental stage of kindling. Perhaps in the most remarkable dissociation, the high potency benzodiazepines are effective in the early (or developmental) and mid (or completed) stages of kindling, but are not effective in the late, spontaneous seizures associated with kindling (65). Conversely, phenytoin is ineffective in preventing the development of kindling, has mixed effects on fully kindled seizures, but is highly effective in preventing the spontaneous variety. Thus, the psychotropic drugs and their associated mechanistic properties that are associated with prevention of the development of syndromal unipolar and bipolar illness may be different from those that are effective in the mid phases of the illnesses or even, again, in the very latest (or spontaneous) phases, where there appears to be the greatest amount of automaticity and rapid cycling independent of specific psychosocial stressors.

Lastly, one must caution patients and family members that effectiveness of a treatment regimen in the short or intermediate term (e.g., two years) may not guarantee long-term freedom from illness burden, even with excellent compliance. A subset of patients (perhaps from 25% to 35% of those with initially highly treatment-responsive presentations) may begin to show a progression of minor intermittent to more frequent and major breakthrough episodes in a fashion that suggests the development of pharmacodynamic tolerance. This should not be used as a "negative" with patients, but as a "positive" in helping them maintain long-term full or steady-dose prophylaxis, since lowering doses appears to enhance the onset and likelihood of tolerance development (Table 5).

In addition, from a mechanistic perspective, the development of inefficacy through drug tolerance may show cross tolerance to some, but not to other AEDs (32,66) (Table 6). Moreover, it is unknown whether one can directly extrapolate via drug classes and/or mechanisms from AED tolerance to psychotropic tolerance (Table 5,6), but using drugs clinically which do not show cross tolerance in the

TABLE 6A Cross-Tolerance Patterns in Contingent Anticonvulsant Effects on Amygdala-Kindled Seizures

Drug; tolerance from	Cross tolerance to	No cross tolerance to
CBZ	PK11195 CBZ-10,11-epoxide Valproate[a]	Clonazepam Diazepam Phenytoin LEV[b]
LTG	CBZ	Valproate MK801a Gabapentin[c]
LEV	CBZ[a]	

[a]Cross tolerance from CBZ to valproate may occur because of the observed failure to upregulate the $\alpha 4$ subunit of the $GABA_A$ receptor during CBZ tolerance.
[b]Unidirection cross tolerance from LEV to CBZ, not CBZ to LEV.
[c]These drugs slow the development of tolerance to LTG.
Abbreviations: GABA, gamma-aminobutyric acid; CBZ, carbamazepine; LTG, lamotrigine; LEV, levetiracetam.

TABLE 6B Differential Effects of CBZ and LTG on Anticonvulsant Tolerance Development

	CBZ (15 mg/kg)	LTG (15 mg/kg)
Rapid tolerance to anticonvulsant effects (amygdala kindling)	+++	+++
Cross tolerance	+++	+++
Duration of "time-off" effect (seizures enhance efficacy)	4–5 days	4–5 days
Seizure threshold change with tolerance	Decrease	Increase (possible residual drug effect)
Using high doses	Slows tolerance	Speeds tolerance and are proconvulsant
Alternating high and low doses	?	Slows tolerance
Chronic noncontingent drug dosing	Slows tolerance	?
MK801 on tolerance development	No effect	Slows (NMDA implicated)
Cross tolerance to valproate	Yes	No
Valproate combination	Slows tolerance	?
Gabapentin augmentation (2 hr pretreatment)	?	Slows tolerance
(½ hr pretreatment)	No effect	↓ Stage VI seizures
(Tolerance reversal)	?	+++

Abbreviations: LTG, lamotrigine; CBZ, carbamazepine; NMDA, *N*-methyl-D-aspartate.

kindled seizure model may be a more appropriate first approximation for a given individual than crossing over to a drug with known AED cross tolerance. If this proposition is proven empirically in the clinic, it may be one other reason to consider presumptive mechanisms of action in choice of a therapeutic agent.

Electroconvulsive therapy (ECT) is not only acutely effective in depression and mania, it is also a potent anticonvulsant (67). Recent data, however, indicate that depressive relapses/remissions occur rapidly after the last ECT treatment, at a rate of 4% per day over the first 10 days (68,69). These data suggest that mechanisms induced even by ECT only convey therapeutic effects in the short-term.

TABLE 7 Topiramate: Not Antimanic but Potentially Useful in Comorbidities

Comorbidities	Study (Refs.)
Alcohol use	Johnson et al., 2007; Johnson 2004 (78,79)
Cocaine use	Johnson, 2005 (80)
PTSD	Berlant, 2002; Berlant, 2001; (74,75) Tucker et al., 2007 (85)
Bulimia	McElroy et al., 2007; McElroy et al., 2004 (73,81)
Weight Loss	McElroy et al., 2007 (73)
Depression	McIntyre et al., 2002 (82)
Migraine	Dahlof et al., 2007 (83)
Side effects	
Renal calculi and parasthesia related to carbonic anhydrase inhibition	
Decreased word retrieval/memory probably related to blockage of AMPA receptors	

By contrast, vagal nerve stimulation (VNS) is an adjunctive anticonvulsant modality for refractory epilepsy and appears unique in both seizure disorders and affective illness in that effectiveness increases progressively over the first year of treatment (70,71). Thus, changes occurring over the long-term may be most pertinent to its therapeutic effectiveness. How these (72) interact with the diverse pharmacotherapies with which it is typically administered require further study. While there are ambiguities about the magnitude of VNS effects in both seizure disorders and affective illness, the trend for increasing effectiveness over time, in contrast to ECT and most other long-term treatments in bipolar illness, suggest active effects that are likely not placebo effects.

Bipolar illness is also associated with a multiplicity of comorbid conditions, and some AEDs that lack antimanic or mood-stabilizing effects may nonetheless be helpful in treating a co-occurring syndrome. In this fashion, topiramate shows substantial evidence for decreasing alcohol and cocaine use in those with these primary substance use disorders (Table 7). It is also effective in binge eating disorder and bulimia nervosa (73) and may be helpful in posttraumatic stress disorder (PTSD) (74,75). These actions of the drug may thus be dissociated from those that are required for effective mood stabilization.

Similarly, gabapentin and pregabalin have a range of effects in anxiety syndromes, such as panic disorder and social phobia and are particularly effective in pain syndromes (76,77). Whether these effects are based on their ability to increase brain GABA levels or to inhibit the α_2-δ subunit of the L-type calcium channel requires further investigation.

The therapeutics of bipolar illness have progressed over the past 50 years from just one or two effective agents to an entire range of agents from multiple classes with multiple drugs within each class. We have some preliminary understanding of the mechanisms of action of the AEDs, but much work remains in identifying those crucially related to a given syndrome and to individual clinical responsivity. We look forward to this phase of individualized medicine rapidly becoming realized so that bipolar patients can be more readily treated with the most appropriate therapeutic regimens right from the outset, thus sparing many individuals from the very considerable morbidity and dysfunction associated with the recurrent affective disorders in general, and bipolar illness in particular.

REFERENCES

1. Marangell LB, George MS, Callahan AM, et al. Effects of intrathecal thyrotropin-releasing hormone (protirelin) in refractory depressed patients. Arch Gen Psychiatry 1997; 54:214–222.
2. Szuba MP, Amsterdam JD, Fernando AT III, et al. Rapid antidepressant response after nocturnal TRH administration in patients with bipolar type I and bipolar type II major depression. J Clin Psychopharmacol 2005; 25:325–330.
3. Maeng S, Zarate CA Jr., Du J, et al. Cellular mechanisms underlying the antidepressant effects of ketamine: role of alpha-amino-3-hydroxy-5-methylsoxazole-4-propionic acid receptors. Biol Psychiatry 2008; 63(4):349–352.
4. Preskorn SD, Baker B, Omo K, et al. A placebo- controlled trial of the NR2B specific NMDA antagonist CP-101, 606 plus paroxetine for treatment resistant depression. 160th Annual Meeting of the American Psychiatric Association, San Diego, CA, 2007 (New Research Abstracts No.362).
5. Manji HK, Duman RS. Impairments of neuroplasticity and cellular resilience in severe mood disorders: implications for the development of novel therapeutics. Psychopharmacol Bull 2001; 35:5–49.
6. Zarate CA Jr., Singh JB, Carlson PJ, et al Efficacy of a protein kinase C inhibitor (tamoxifen) in the treatment of acute mania: a pilot study. Bipolar Disord 2007; 9:561–570.
7. Post RM, Speer AM, Obrocea, GV, et al Acute and prophylactic effects of anticonvulsants in bipolar depression. Clin Neurosci Res 2002; 2:228–251.
8. Geddes JR, Burgess H, Hawton K, et al. Long-term lithium treatment therapy for bipolar disorder: systemic review and meta-analysis of randomized controlled trials. Am J Psychiatry 2004; 161(2): 217–22.
9. Cipriani A, Smith K, Burgess S, et al. Lithium versus antidepressants in the long-term treatment of unipolar affective disorder. Cochrane Database Syst Rev 2006; 168(4):CD003492.
10. Post RM, Berrettini W, Uhde TW, et al. Selective response to the anticonvulsant carbamazepine in manic–depressive illness: a case study. J Clin Psychopharmacol 1984; 4: 178–185.
11. Greil W, Kleindienst N. Lithium versus carbamazepine in the maintenance treatment of bipolar II disorder and bipolar disorder not otherwise specified. Int Clin Psychopharmacol 1999; 14(5):283–285.
12. Greil W, Kleindienst N. The comparative prophylactic efficacy of lithium and carbamazepine in patients with bipolar I disorder. Int Clin Psychopharmacol 1999; 14(5):277–281.
13. Greil W, Kleindienst N, Erazo N, et al. Differential response to lithium and carbamazepine in the prophylaxis of bipolar disorder. J Clin Psychopharmacol 1998; 18:455–460.
14. Bowden CL. Predictors of response to divalproex and lithium. J Clin Psychiatry 1995; 56(suppl 3):25–30.
15. Calabrese JR, Fatemi SH, Woyshville MJ. Antidepressant effects of lamotrigine in rapid cycling bipolar disorder. Am J Psychiatry 1996; 153:236.
16. Frye MA, Ketter TA, Kimbrell TA, et al. A placebo-controlled study of lamotrigine and gabapentin monotherapy in refractory mood disorders. J Clin Psychopharmacol 2000; 20:607–614.
17. Obrocea GV, Dunn RM, Frye MA, et al. Clinical predictors of response to lamotrigine and gabapentin monotherapy in refractory affective disorders. Biol Psychiatry 2002; 51: 253–260.
18. van der Loos ML, Kolling P, Knoppert-van der Klein EA et al. Lamotrigine as add-on to lithium in bipolar depression, 160th Annual Meeting American Psychiatric Association, San Diego, CA, New Research Abstract No.286, p.20.
19. Passmore MJ, Garnham J, Duffy A, et al. Phenotypic spectra of bipolar disorder in responders to lithium versus lamotrigine. Bipolar Disord 2003; 5:110–114.
20. Alda M. The phenotypic spectra of bipolar disorder. Eur Neuropsychopharmacol 2004; 14(suppl 2): S94–S99.
21. Grof P. Selecting effective long-term treatment for bipolar patients: monotherapy and combinations. J Clin Psychiatry 2003; 64(suppl 5):53–61.
22. Du J, Suzuki K, Wei Y, et al. The anticonvulsants lamotrigine, riluzole, and valproate differentially regulate AMPA receptor membrane localization: relationship to clinical effects in mood disorders. Neuropsychopharmacology 2007; 32:793–802.

23. Mishory A, Yaroslavsky Y, Bersudsky Y, et al. Phenytoin as an antimanic anticonvulsant: a controlled study. Am J Psychiatry 2000; 157:463–465.
24. Post RM, Speer AM. A brief history of anticonvulsant use in affective disorders. In: Trimble MR, Schmitz B, eds. Seizures, Affective Disorders and Anticonvulsant Drugs. Surrey, UK: Clarius Press, 2002:53–81.
25. Pande AC, Crockatt JG, Janney CA, et al. Gabapentin in bipolar disorder: a placebo-controlled trial of adjunctive therapy. Gabapentin Bipolar Disorder Study Group. Bipolar Disord 2000; 2(3 pt 2):249–255.
26. Grunze H, Erfurth A, Marcuse A, et al. Tiagabine appears not to be efficacious in the treatment of acute mania. J Clin Psychiatry 1999; 60:759–762.
27. Suppes T, Chisholm KA, Dhavale D, et al. Tiagabine in treatment-refractory bipolar disorder: a clinical case series. Bipolar Disord 2002; 4:283–289.
28. Post RM, Altshuler LL, Frye MA, et al. Preliminary observations on the effectiveness of levetiracetam in the open adjunctive treatment of refractory bipolar disorder. J Clin Psychiatry 2005; 66:370–374.
29. Rigo JM, Hans G, Nguyen L, et al. The anti-epileptic drug levetiracetam reverses the inhibition by negative allosteric modulators of neuronal GABA- and glycine-gated currents. Br J Pharmacol 2002; 136:659–672.
30. Klitgaard H. Levetiracetam: the preclinical profile of a new class of antiepileptic drugs? Epilepsia 2001; 4:13–18.
31. Klitgaard H, Matagne A, Gobert J, et al. Evidence for a unique profile of levetiracetam in rodent models of seizures and epilepsy. Eur J Pharmacol 1998; 353(2–3):191–206.
32. Post RM. Animal models of mood disorders: kindling as a model of affective illness progression. In: Schachter S, Holmes G, Kasteleijn-Nolst Trenité D, eds. Behavioral Aspects of Epilepsy: Principles and Practice. New York, NY: Demos Medical Publishing, 2008.
33. McElroy SL, Suppes T, Keck PE Jr., et al. Open-label adjunctive zonisamide in the treatment of bipolar disorders: a prospective trial. J Clin Psychiatry 2005; 66(5):617–624.
34. McElroy SL, Kotwal R, Guerdjikova AI, et al. Zonisamide in the treatment of binge eating disorder with obesity: a randomized controlled trial. J Clin Psychiatry 2006; 67(12):1897–1906.
35. Maitre M, Mandel P. [Properties allowing the attribution to gamma-hydroxybutyrate the quality of neurotransmitter in the central nervous system] C R Acad Sci III 1984; 298(12):341–345.
36. Motohashi N, Ikawa K, Kariya T. GABA$_B$ receptors are up-regulated by chronic treatment with lithium or carbamazepine: GABA hypothesis of affective disorders. Eur J Pharmacol 1989; 166:95–99.
37. van Calker D, Belmaker RH. The high affinity inositol transport system–implications for the pathophysiology and treatment of bipolar disorder. Bipolar Disord 2000; 2(2):102–107.
38. Hough CJ, Irwin RP, Gao XM, et al. Carbamazepine inhibition of N-methyl-D-aspartate-evoked calcium influx in rat cerebellar granule cells. J Pharmacol Exp Ther 1996; 276(1):143–149.
39. Manji HK, Moore GJ, Rajkowska G, et al. Neuroplasticity and cellular resilience in mood disorders. Mol Psychiatry 2000; 5(6):578–593.
40. Chuang DM, Chen RW, Chalecka-Franaszek E, et al. Neuroprotective effects of lithium in cultured cells and animal models of diseases. Bipolar Disord 2007; 4(2):129–136.
41. Einat H, Yuan P, Gould TD, et al. The role of the extracellular signal-regulated kinase signaling pathway in mood modulation. J Neurosci 2003; 13; 23(19):7311–7316.
42. Chen PS, Wang CC, Bortner CD, et al. Valproic acid and other histone deacetylase inhibitors induce microglial apoptosis and attenuate lipopolysaccharide-induced dopaminergic neurotoxicity. Neuroscience 2007; 149(1):203–212.
43. Beutler AS, Li S, Nicol R, et al. Carbamazepine is an inhibitor of histone deacetylases. Life Sci 2005; 76(26):3107–3115.
44. Sherman WR, Leavitt AL, Honchar MP, et al. Evidence that lithium alters phosphoinositide metabolism: chronic administration elevates primarily D-myo-inositol-1-phosphate in cerebral cortex of the rat. J Neurochem 1981; 36:1947–1951.

45. Post RM, Weiss SRB, Clark M, et al. Lithium, carbamazepine and valproate in affective illness. In Manji HK, Bowden CL, Belmaker RH, eds. Bipolar Medications: Mechanisms of Action. Washington, DC: Am Psychiatric Press, Inc., 2000:219–248.

46. Post RM, Luckenbaugh DA. Unique design issues in clinical trials of patients with bipolar affective disorder. J Psychiatr Res 2003; 37(1):61–73 (review).

47. Wagner KD, Kowatch RA, Emslie GJ, et al. A double-blind, randomized, placebo-controlled trial of oxcarbazepine in the treatment of bipolar disorder in children and adolescents. Am J Psychiatry 2006; 163(7):1179–1186.

48. Duman RS, Monteggia LM. A neurotrophic model for stress-related mood disorders. Biol Psychiatry 2006; 59(12):1116–1127.

49. Post RM. Role of BDNF in bipolar and unipolar disorder: clinical and theoretical implications. J Psychiatr Res 2007; 41(12):979–990.

50. Sheline YI, Wang PW, Gado MH, et al. Hippocampal atrophy in recurrent major depression. Proc Natl Acad Sci U S A 1996; 93(9):3908–3913.

51. Moore GJ, Bebchuk JM, Wilds IB, et al. Lithium-induced increase in human brain grey matter. Lancet 2000; 356:1241–1242.

52. Bearden CE, Thompson PM, Dalwani M, et al. Reply: lithium and Increased Cortical Gray Matter-More Tissue or More Water? Biol Psychiatry 2008; 63(3):E19.

53. Post RM, Denicoff KD, Leverich GS, et al. Morbidity in 258 bipolar outpatients followed for one year with daily prospective ratings on the NIMH-Life Chart Method. J Clin Psychiatry 2003; 64:680–690.

54. Post RM. Kindling and sensitization as models for affective episode recurrence, cyclicity, and tolerance phenomena. Neurosci Biobehav Rev 2007; 31(6):858–873.

55. Post RM. Transduction of psychosocial stress into the neurobiology of recurrent affective disorder. Am J Psychiatry 1992; 149: 999–1010.

56. Post RM, Leverich GS. The role of psychosocial stress in the onset and progression of bipolar disorder and its comorbidities: the need for earlier and alternative modes of therapeutic intervention. Dev Psychopathol 2006; 18:1181–1211.

57. Leverich GS, McElroy SL, Suppes T, et al. Early physical and sexual abuse associated with an adverse course of bipolar illness. Biol Psychiatry 2002; 51(4):288–297.

58. Leverich GS, Altshuler LL, Frye MA, et al. Factors associated with suicide attempts in 648 patients with bipolar disorder in the Stanley Foundation Bipolar Network. J Clin Psychiatry 2003; 64(5):506–515.

59. Leverich GS, Post RM, Keck PE Jr., et al. The poor prognosis of childhood-onset bipolar disorder. J Pediatr 2007; 150: 485–490.

60. Perlis RH, Miyahara S, Marangell LB, et al. Long-Term implications of early onset in bipolar disorder: data from the first 1000 participants in the systematic treatment enhancement program for bipolar disorder (STEP-BD). Biol Psychiatry 2004; 55(9):875–881.

61. Kessler RC, Berglund P, Demler O, et al. Lifetime prevalence and age-of-onset distributions of DSM-IV disorders in the National Comorbidity Survey Replication. Arch Gen Psychiatry 2005; 62(6):593–602.

62. Baldessarini RJ, Tondo L, Baethge CJ, et al. Effects of treatment latency on response to maintenance treatment in manic-depressive disorders. Bipolar Disord 2007; 9(4): 386–393.

63. Lange KJ, McInnis MG. Studies of anticipation in bipolar affective disorder. CNS Spectr 2002; 7(3):196–202.

64. Velísek L, Velíshková J, Ptachewich Y, et al. Age-dependent effects of gamma-aminobutyric acid agents on flurothyl seizures. Epilepsia 1995; 36(7): 636–643.

65. Pinel JP. Kindling-induced experimental epilepsy in rats: cortical stimulation. Exp Neurol 1981; 72(3):559–569.

66. Weiss SR, Clark M, Rosen JB, et al. Contingent tolerance to the anticonvulsant effects of carbamazepine: relationship to loss of endogenous adaptive mechanisms. Brain Res Rev 1995; 20:305–325.

67. Post R, Uhde T, Kramlinger K, et al. Carbamazepine treatment of mania: clinical and biochemical aspects. Clin Neuropharmacol 1986; 4:547–549.

68. Prudic J, Olfson M, Marcus SC, et al. Effectiveness of electroconvulsive therapy in community settings. Biol Psychiatry 2004; 55(3):301–312.

69. Sackeim HA, Prudic J, Olfson M. Response to Drs Abrams and Kellner: the cognitive effects of ECT in community settings. J ECT 2007; 23(2):65–67.
70. Rush AJ, Sackeim HA, Marangell LB, et al. Effects of 12 months of vagus nerve stimulation in treatment-resistant depression: a naturalistic study. Biol Psychiatry 2005; 58(5): 355–363.
71. Rush AJ, Marangell LB, Sackeim HA, et al. Vagus nerve stimulation for treatment-resistant depression: a randomized, controlled acute phase trial. Biol Psychiatry 2005; 58(5):347–354.
72. Nemeroff CB, Mayberg HS, Krahl SE, et al. VNS therapy in treatment-resistant depression: clinical evidence and putative neurobiological mechanisms. Neuropsychopharmacology 2006; 31(7):1345–1355.
73. McElroy SL, Hudson JI, Capece JA, et al. Topiramate for the treatment of binge eating disorder associated with obesity: a placebo-controlled study. Biol Psychiatry 2007; 61(9): 1039–1048.
74. Berlant JL. Topiramate in posttraumatic stress disorder: preliminary clinical observations. J Clin Psychiatry 2001; 62(suppl 17):60–63.
75. Berlant J, van Kammen DP. Open-label topiramate as primary or adjunctive therapy in chronic civilian posttraumatic stress disorder: a preliminary report. J Clin Psychiatry 2002; 63(1):15–20.
76. Pande AC, Davidson JR, Jefferson JW, et al. Treatment of social phobia with gabapentin: a placebo-controlled study. J Clin Psychopharmacol 1999; 19(4):341–348.
77. Pande AC, Pollack MH, Crockatt J, et al. Placebo-controlled study of gabapentin treatment of panic disorder. J Clin Psychopharmacol 2000; 20:467–471.
78. Johnson BA. Uses of topiramate in the treatment of alcohol dependence. Expert Rev Neurother 2004; 4(5):751–758.
79. Johnson BA, Rosenthal N, Capece JA, et al. Topiramate for treating alcohol dependence: a randomized controlled trial. JAMA 2007; 298(14):1641–1651.
80. Johnson BA. Recent advances in the development of treatments for alcohol and cocaine dependence: focus on topiramate and other modulators of GABA or glutamate function. CNS Drugs 2005; 19(10):873–896.
81. McElroy SL, Shapira NA, Arnold LM, et al. Topiramate in the long-term treatment of binge-eating disorder associated with obesity. J Clin Psychiatry 2004; 65(11):1463–1469.
82. McIntyre RS, Mancini DA, McCann S, et al. Topiramate versus bupropion SR when added to mood stabilizer therapy for the depressive phase of bipolar disorder: a preliminary single-blind study. Bipolar Disord 2002; 4(3):207–213.
83. Dahlof C, Loder E, Diamond M, et al. The impact of migraine prevention on daily activities: a longitudinal and responder analysis from three topiramate placebo-controlled clinical trials. Health Qual Life Outcomes 2007; 5(1):56.
84. Post RM, Speer AM, Hough CJ, et al. Neurobiology of bipolar illness: implications for future study and therapeutics. Ann Clin Psychiatry 2003; 15:85–94.
85. Tucker P, Trautman RP, Wyatt DB, et al. Efficacy and safety of topiramate monotherapy in civilian posttraumatic stress disorder: a randomized, double-blind, placebo-controlled study. J Clin Psychiatry 2007; 68(2):201–206.

Abbreviations

AASM: American Academy of Sleep Medicine

ABC: Aberrant Behavior Checklist

ACR: American College of Rheumatology

ACTH: adrenocorticotropic hormone

ADH: antidiuretic hormone

ADHD: attention deficit hyperactivity disorder

ADI-R: Autism Diagnostic Interview—Revised

ADNFLE: autosomal dominant nocturnal frontal lobe epilepsy

ADOS: Autism Diagnostic Observation Schedule

AED: antiepileptic drug

AMP: adenosine monophosphate

AMPA: alpha-amino-3-hydroxy-5-methyl-4-isoxazole proprionic acid

AN: anorexia nervosa

ANOVA: analysis or variance

API: Acute Panic Inventory

ASD: austism spectrum disorder

BAI: Beck Anxiety Inventory

Bcl-2: cytoprotective protein B-cell lymphoma/leukemia–2 gene

BDI: Beck Depression Inventory

BDNF: brain-derived neurotrophic factor

BED: binge eating disorder

BMI: body mass index

BN: bulimia nervosa

BPD: borderline personality disorder

BPI: Brief Pain Inventory

BPRS: Brief Psychiatric Rating Scale

BSPS: Brief Social Phobia Scale

CA: carbonic anhydrase

CAPS: Clinician Administered PTSD Scale

CCK-4:   cholecystokinin-tetrapeptide

CDC: Center for Disease Control

CGI-C: Clinical Global Impression of Change Scale

CGI-I: Clinical Global Impressions of Improvement Scale

CGI-S: Clinical Global Impressions of Severity Scale

CI: confidence interval

CIWA-Ar: Clinical Institute Withdrawal Assessment for Alcohol-Revised

CNS: central nervous system

CO: carbon monoxide

CPAP: continuous positive airway pressure

CrCl: creatinine clearance

CRH: corticotropin releasing hormone

CSD: cortical spreading depression

CSF: cerebrospinal fluid

C-YBOCS: Children's Yale–Brown Obsessive Compulsive Scale

DC: direct current

DC-MEG: direct current-magnetoencephalography

DGRP: Duke Global Rating for PTSD

DHD: 10,11-dihydro-10,11-trans-hydroxy carbamazepine

DSM: Diagnostic and Statistical Manual

DTS: Davidson Trauma Scale

ECT: electroconvulsive therapy

EFNS: European Federation of Neurological Societies

ER: extended release

ERK: extracellular signal–regulated kinase

ERP: event-related potential

FDA: Food and Drug Administration

F-HAQ: Fibromyalgia Health Assessment Questionnaire

FHM: familial hemiplegic migraine

FIQ: Fibromyalgia Impact Questionnaire

FMRI: functional magnetic resonance imaging

FMRI-BOLD: FMRI-blood oxygen–level dependent

GABA: gamma-aminobutyric acid

GAD: generalized anxiety disorder

GAF: Global Assessment of Functioning Scale

GAT: gamma-aminobutyric acid transaminase inhibitor

GSK-3: glycogen synthase kinase 3

GTN: glyceryltrinitrate

GVG: gamma-vinyl GABA

HADS: Hospital Anxiety and Depression Scale

HAM-A: Hamilton Rating Scale for Anxiety

HAM-D: Hamilton Rating Scale for Depression

HbAlc: glycosylated hemoglobin

HD: hemodialysis

HPA: hypothalamic-pituitary-adrenal

5-HIAA: 5-hydroxyindoleacetic acid

5-HT: serotonin

ICD: impulse control disorder

ICSD-2: International Classification of Sleep Disorders, Second Edition

IED: intermittent explosive disorder

ITT: intent-to-treat

LOCF: last observation carried forward

LSAS: Liebowitz Social Anxiety Scale

MADRS: Montgomery-Åsberg Depression Rating Scale

MAF: Multidimensional Assessment of Fatigue

MAOI: monoamine oxidase inhibitor

MAP: mitogen-activated protein

MBT: mentalization-based treatment

MEG: magnetoencephalography

MELAS: mitochondrial encephalopathy, lactic acidosis, and stroke-like episodes

mGluII: Group II metabotropic glutamate

MHD: 10,11-dihydro-10-hydroxy-5H-dibenzo (b,f) azepine-5-carboxamide

MHPG: 3-methoxy-4-hydroxyphenylglycol

MMRM: mixed models repeated-measures

MOS: Medical Outcomes Study

MRS: Mania Rating Scale

MWA: migraine with aura

MwoA: migraine without aura

NAA: *N*-acetylaspartate

NAcc: nucleus accumbens

nAChR: nicotinic acetylcholine receptor

NES: night eating syndrome

NFLE: nocturnal frontal lobe epilepsy

NMDA: *N*-methyl-D-aspartate

NNH: number needed to harm

NNT: number needed to treat

NOS: not otherwise specified

NREM: non-REM

NSAID: nonsteroidal anti-inflammatory drug

NYSOMH: New York State Office of Mental Health

OAS: Overt Aggression Scale

OAS-M: Overt Aggression Scale-Modified

OCD: obsessive-compulsive disorder

OFC: orbitofrontal cortex

OR: odds ratio

OSAS: obstructive sleep apnea syndrome

PAG: periaqueductal grey

PANSS: Positive and Negative Symptom Scale

PAS: Panic and Agoraphobia Scale

PCL-C: PTSD Checklist-Civilian Version

PCOS: Polycystic Ovarian Syndrome

PFC: prefrontal cortex

PGI-C: Patient Global Impression of Change Scale

PKC: protein kinase C

PLMD: periodic leg movement disorder

PLMS: periodic leg movements of sleep

POMS: Profile of Mood States

PSG: polysomnography

PSS: panic symptom scale

PTSD: posttraumatic stress disorder

PWS: Prader-Willi syndrome

RBC: red blood cell

RBD: REM-sleep behavior disorder

RCBF: regional cerebral blood flow

RCT: randomized controlled trial

REM: rapid eye movement

RIMA: reversible inhibitor of monoamine oxidase-A

RLS: restless leg syndrome

SANS: Schedule for Assessment of Negative Symptoms

SCID: Structured Clinical Interview for DSM-IV

SCL-90: Symptom Checklist 90

SD: spreading depression

SDS: Sheehan Disability Scale

SE: sleep efficiency

SF-36: Short Form 36 Health Survey

SF-MPQ: Short Form McGill Pain Questionnaire

SFT: schema-focused therapy

SGA: second generation (atypical) antipsychotic

SGRI: selective gaba reuptake inhibitor

SIADH: syndrome of inappropriate ADH secretion

SIB: self-injurious behavior

SMAP: stromal membrane associated protein

SNP: single nucleotide polymorphism

SNRI: serotonin-norepinephrine reuptake inhibitor

SOL: sleep onset latency

SPIN: Social Phobia Inventory

SR: slow release

SRED: sleep related eating disorder

SRI: serotonin reuptake inhibitor

SSRI: selective serotonin reuptake inhibitor

STAXI: State Trait Anger Expression Inventory

STEP-BD: Systematic Treatment Enhancement Program for Bipolar Disorder

SWS: slow wave sleep

TBI: traumatic brain injury

TFEQ: Three Factor Eating Questionnaire

TMS: transcranial magnetic stimulation

TOP-8:   Treatment Outcome PTSD scale

TRH: thyrotropin-releasing hormone

TST: total sleep time

UDP: uridine-5′-diphosphate

UGT: UDP-glucuronyl transferase

VAMS: Visual Analogue Mood Scale

VAS: visual analogue scale

VNS: vagal nerve stimulation

VTA: ventral tegmental area

WASO: wake after sleep onset

WHR: waist-to-hip ratio

XR: extended release

YBOCS-BE: Yale-Brown Obsessive Compulsive Scale Modified for Binge Eating

YBOCS-PG: Yale-Brown Obsessive Compulsive Scale Modified for Pathological Gambling

YMRS: Young Mania Rating Scale

Index